English-Chinese Collegiate Textbooks in Traditional
Chinese Medicine for Institutions of Traditional
Chinese Medicine of Higher Learning
Edited by Beijing University of Traditional
Chinese Medicine

普通高等中医药院校英汉对照中医本科系列教材
北京中医药大学　主编

Acupuncture and Moxibustion

针　灸　学

Academy Press [Xue Yuan]
学苑出版社

图书在版编目(CIP)数据

针灸学/唐玉秀、党毅、耿恩广主编.-北京:学苑出版社,1999
普通高等中医药院校英汉对照中医本科系列教材
ISBN 7—5077—1269—9

Ⅰ.针… Ⅱ.①唐…②党…③耿… Ⅲ.针灸学-医学院校-教材-英、汉 Ⅳ.R241

中国版本图书馆 CIP 数据核字(97)第 13610 号

责任编辑:东青 陈辉

学苑出版社出版 发行
社址:北京万寿路西街 11 号 邮政编码:100036
北京市广内印刷厂印刷 新华书店经销
787×1092 1/16 46.875 印张 1018 千字
1999 年 10 月北京第 1 版 1999 年 10 月北京第 1 次印刷
印数:0001—3000 册
定价:68 元($)

English-Chinese Collegiate Textbooks in Traditional
Chinese Medicine for Institutions of Traditional
Chinese Medicine of Higher Learning
Edited by Beijing University of Traditional
Chinese Medicine

普通高等中医药院校
英汉对照中医本科系列教材
北京中医药大学 主编

General Chief Editor: Long Zhixian
Associate Chief Editors: Zheng Shouzeng
He Min
He Xingdong
Suo Runtang
Liu Jinsheng
Gao Baozhong
Chen Jing
Chief Reviewers of Chinese: Wang Yuchuan
Yan Zhenghua

总 主 编：龙致贤
副总主编：郑守曾 何 珉
贺兴东 索润堂
刘金生 高宝忠
陈 静
中文主审：王玉川 颜正华

Acupuncture and Moxibustion

针 灸 学

Chief Editor of Chinese: Tang Yuxiu   Geng Enguang
Chief Editor of English: Dang Yi
Associate Editor of English: Sun Yilian
Translators: Dang Yi   Sun Yilian
Corey S. C. Wong
Lin Huanying   Lu Xiaozhen
Du Wei

中文主编：唐玉秀　耿恩广
英文主编：党　毅
英文副主编：孙一莲
译　　者：党　毅　孙一莲　黄顺昌
　　　　　林焕英　陆小珍　杜　巍

Specially Invited International Editors

Chief Reviewer: Fang Nengyu
Associate Reviewer: Concetta Maria Pirrone
Advisor: George Francis Mclean

特邀外籍审校人员

英文主审校：方能御
协　　　校：康西特·玛丽亚·皮罗尼
顾　　　问：乔治·弗郎西斯·麦克林

Preface

Beijing University of Chinese Medicine and Pharmacology under the auspices of the Department of Science and Education for the State Administration of Traditional Chinese Medicine has compiled the English-Chinese textbook series in traditional Chinese medicine (TCM) for undergraduate of college. These textbooks include Basic Theories of Traditional Chinese Medicine, Diagnostics of Traditional Chinese Medicine, Chinese Materia Medica, Formulas of Traditional Chinese Medicine, Traditional Chinese Internal Medicine, Acupuncture & Moxibustion and an English-Chinese Dictionary of Traditional chinese Medicine. This project is very scholastic and now is coming into publication for the first time domestically and abroad.

Traditional Chinese medicine possesses a unique theoretical system, rich clinical experience and excellent clinical effects. It has made great contributions to the health of mankind. Either now or future, based on its own potential, TCM will play an increasingly important role in promoting the development of a world medicine, and more attention of people in the world. More and more international friends are interested in TCM and they are studying and practicing TCM throughout the world. In order to overcome the language barrier and to understand TCM correctly they are eager for a set of TCM textbooks. They want these textbooks to be suitable for use in colleges of higher learning and with accurate in English translation.

Beijing University of Chinese Medicine and Pharmacology is a key university among the TCM teaching institutions of higher learning in China. The university began to enroll foreign students in 1957. Since then about one thousand foreign students coming form more than 70 countries and regions in the world graduated form it. At present, there are nearly 300 foreign students form 41 countries and regions studying at the university. Our university has accumulated rich experience in teaching foreign students and understands their special needs in the study of TCM. These years of practice in teaching has greatly helped the compilation of the TCM textbooks.

The authorities at our university highly evaluate the task of compiling and translating the TCM textbook series and organized a special working group of experienced professors and other professionals to compile the series. Based on the fifth edition of relevant all-China TCM textbooks of higher learning, the TCM textbooks absorb the latest achievements of scientific research in TCM lay more stress on logicality, scientificality and practicality, make every effort to contain more information and to build a rational framework of the content in an understandable and readable manner. This TCM textbook series in suitable for both foreign and Chinese students and all those who are interested in TCM, both at home and abroad.

In order to ensure academic standards and an accurate English translation of this textbook series, we invited well-known TCM experts Prof. Wang Yuchuan and Prof. Yan Zhenghua to examine and review the Chinese language experts Fang Nengyu, Concetta Maria Pirrone and George Francis Mclean to review the English translation.

The Acupuncture and Moxibustion has been published; it is devided into three parts, The Part I includes the anatomy of the meridians system, physiology of the the system, clinical application of the theory of the meridians, the course of the twelve regular meridians and the eight extra meridians and their principal indications, and the external anatomical location, regional anatomy, indications and needling and moxibustion method of the fourteen meridians points and the extraordinary points, etc. Part II, Acupuncture and moxibustion techniques, includes the filiform needling, moxibustion, other acupuncture therapies and so on. Part III, Acupuncture and moxibustion treatment includes the etiology and pathology, differentiation and prescription of more than 70 kinds of diseases.

Finally, any correction to errors and suggestions concerning its contents and format will be appreciated. We will take them into careful consideration in the next edition and we believe that with such help, these TCM textbooks will be much improved in the next edition.

During the compilation of the TCM textbook series, we have been greatly helped by the relevant official departments and experts and we would like to express our profound thanks to them.

The compiler and translator

前　言

北京中医药大学受国家中医药管理局科技教育司的委托,编译高等中医药院校英汉对照中医本科系列教材,包括《中医基础理论》、《中医诊断学》、《中药学》、《方剂学》、《中医内科学》、《针灸学》及《英汉中医药学词典》7种。这是中医高等教材汉译英方面空前盛大的工程,是一项大型科研活动。

中国医药学以其独特的理论体系、丰富的医疗实践、卓越的临床疗效,为人类的健康事业作出了巨大贡献。当今和未来,中医药学将发挥出更大的潜力,推动世界医学向前发展,引起世界人民更多更大的重视与关注。近年来,外国朋友中学习、研究、应用中医中药的人越来越多,但由于语言文字的差异,给学习带来一定的困难,他们迫切需要一套专业层次高、翻译准确的英汉对照教材,以便更好学习中医中药。

北京中医药大学是唯一的中国重点中医药大学,自1957年接受外国留学生以来,已为世界70多个国家和地区培养了近千名留学生。目前在校外国留学生近3百人,分别来自41个国家和地区,多年来,北京中医药大学积累了丰富的培养外国留学生的教学经验,了解他们学习的规律和特点,这为编写这套教材打下了良好的基础。

北京中医药大学领导十分重视这套教材,专门组织了教学经验丰富的专家、教授和专业骨干从事编写工作。全套教材在全国高等中医院校五版教材的基础上,扬长避短,吸收了中医药的最新科研成果,强调逻辑性、科学性、实用性,努力做到内容充实,重点突出,通俗易懂。

本套教材适用于留学生、国内学生及国内外研究中医药的学者。

为保证这套教材的学术与翻译水平,中文内容特请全国著名中医学专家王玉川教授、颜正华教授审定,英文译文特邀美籍专家Fang Nengyu（方能御）,Concetta Maria Pirrone,George Francis Mclean审校。

此次出版的《针灸学》共分为上、中、下三篇。上篇包括经络系统的组成、经络的生理功能及经络学说在临床上的应用、十二经脉和奇经八脉的循行病候以及十四经穴和经外奇穴的体表定位、层次解剖、主治病症、针灸方法等内容。中篇刺灸方法包括毫针刺法、灸法、其它针法以及耳针疗法。下篇针灸治疗包括70多种常见病的病因病机、辨证及处方。

由于时间紧迫,水平有限,不妥之处在所难免,真诚地欢迎国内外同道提出批评意见,以便再版时进行修改补充,使这套教材更加完善。

编译工作过程中,得到有关部门和专家的大力支持与协助,在此深表谢意。

编译者

CONTENTS

Introduction ··· (1)

Part I Meridians and Points

Chapter 1 A General Introduction to the Meridians ·················· (7)
  Section 1 Development of the Theory of the Meridians ············ (8)
  Section 2 The Composition of the Meridians System ··················· (8)
    1. The Twelve Regular Meridians ··· (9)
    2. The Eight Extra Meridians ·· (13)
    3. The Fifteen Collaterals ·· (14)
    4. The Twelve Divergent Meridians ·· (15)
    5. The Twelve Muscle Regions ·· (17)
    6. The Twelve Cutaneous Regions ·· (17)
  Section 3 The Gen, Jie, Biao, Ben, Qijie and the Four Seas of
          the Meridians ·· (18)
  Section 4 Physiological Functions of the Meridians System and
          Clinical Application of the Theory of the Meridians ········ (21)
    1. Physiological Function of the Meridians ····························· (21)
    2. Clinical Application of the Theory of the Meridians ········· (22)
  Section 5 The Courses of the Twelve Regular Meridians and Their
          Principal Symptoms ·· (23)
    1. Lung Meridian ··· (23)
    2. Large Intestine Meridian ··· (23)
    3. Stomach Meridian ·· (25)
    4. Spleen Meridian ··· (26)
    5. Heart Meridian ·· (27)
    6. Small Intestine Meridian ·· (28)
    7. Bladder Meridian ·· (29)
    8. Kidney Meridian ··· (30)

    9. Pericardium Meridian ……………………………………………… (31)
    10. Triple Energizer Meridian ……………………………………… (32)
    11. Gallbladder Meridian …………………………………………… (33)
    12. Liver Meridian …………………………………………………… (35)
  Section 6 The Course, Principal Symptoms and Crossing Acupoints
             of the Eight Extra Meridians ……………………………… (36)
    1. Governor Vessel …………………………………………………… (36)
    2. Conception Vessel ………………………………………………… (36)
    3. Thoroughfare Vessel ……………………………………………… (37)
    4. Belt Vessel ………………………………………………………… (38)
    5. Yin Link Vessel …………………………………………………… (38)
    6. Yang Link Vessel ………………………………………………… (39)
    7. Yin Heel Vessel …………………………………………………… (40)
    8. Yang Heel Vessel ………………………………………………… (40)
  Section 7 Acupoints, Courses, Principal Indications and Treatment
             of Fifteen Collaterals ……………………………………… (41)

Chapter 2 An Introduction to Acupoints ………………………………… (46)
  Section 1 The Essential Concept of Acupoints ……………………… (46)
  Section 2 The Development and Classification of Acupoints ……… (46)
  Section 3 The Nomenclature of Acupoints …………………………… (47)
  Section 4 The Properties of Acupoints ………………………………… (48)
  Section 5 The Concept and Classification of Specific Points ……… (49)
    1. Five Shu Points …………………………………………………… (49)
    2. Yuan-(Primary)Points and Luo-(Connecting)Points ………… (52)
      (1) Yuan-(Primary)Points ……………………………………… (53)
      (2) Luo-(Connecting)Points …………………………………… (54)
    3. Back-(Shu)Points and Front-(Mu)Points ……………………… (55)
      (1) Back-(Shu)Points …………………………………………… (55)
      (2) Front-(Mu)Points …………………………………………… (56)
    4. Eight Converging Points ………………………………………… (57)
    5. Xi-(Cleft)Points …………………………………………………… (58)
    6. Lower He-(Sea)Points …………………………………………… (59)
    7. Eight Confluent Points and Crossing Points ………………… (59)
  Section 6 Methods of Locating Acupoints …………………………… (65)

Chapter 3 The Fourteen Meridians' Acupuncture Points and the Extraordinary Points (70)

Section 1 The Acupuncture Points of Lung Meridian (70)
1. LU 1 Zhongfu (70)
2. LU 2 Yunmen (71)
3. LU 3 Tianfu (72)
4. LU 4 Xiabai (72)
5. LU 5 Chize (73)
6. LU 6 Kongzui (73)
7. LU 7 Lieque (73)
8. LU 8 Jingqu (74)
9. LU 9 Taiyuan (74)
10. LU 10 Yuji (74)
11. LU 11 Shaoshang (75)

Section 2 The Acupuncture Points of Large Intestine Meridian (75)
1. LI 1 Shangyang (76)
2. LI 2 Erjian (76)
3. LI 3 Sanjian (76)
4. LI 4 Hegu (76)
5. LI 5 Yangxi (77)
6. LI 6 Pianli (78)
7. LI 7 Wenliu (78)
8. LI 8 Xialian (78)
9. LI 9 Shanglian (78)
10. LI 10 Shousanli (79)
11. LI 11 Quchi (79)
12. LI 12 Zhouliao (79)
13. LI 13 Shouwuli (80)
14. LI 14 Binao (80)
15. LI 15 Jianyu (81)
16. LI 16 Jugu (81)
17. LI 17 Tianding (82)
18. LI 18 Futu (82)
19. LI 19 Kouheliao (82)
20. LI 20 Yingxiang (83)

Section 3 The Acupuncture Points of Stomach Meridian .... (83)
  1. ST 1 Chengqi .... (84)
  2. ST 2 Sibai .... (84)
  3. ST 3 Juliao .... (84)
  4. ST 4 Dicang .... (85)
  5. ST 5 Daying .... (85)
  6. ST 6 Jiache .... (85)
  7. ST 7 Xiaguan .... (86)
  8. ST 8 Touwei .... (86)
  9. ST 9 Renying .... (87)
  10. ST 10 Shuitu .... (87)
  11. ST 11 Qishe .... (88)
  12. ST 12 Quepen .... (88)
  13. ST 13 Qihu .... (88)
  14. ST 14 Kufang .... (88)
  15. ST 15 Wuyi .... (89)
  16. ST 16 Yingchuang .... (89)
  17. ST 17 Ruzhong .... (89)
  18. ST 18 Rugen .... (89)
  19. ST 19 Burong .... (90)
  20. ST 20 Chengman .... (90)
  21. ST 21 Liangmen .... (90)
  22. ST 22 Guanmen .... (90)
  23. ST 23 Taiyi .... (91)
  24. ST 24 Huaroumen .... (91)
  25. ST 25 Tianshu .... (92)
  26. ST 26 Wailing .... (92)
  27. ST 27 Daju .... (92)
  28. ST 28 Shuidao .... (92)
  29. ST 29 Guilai .... (93)
  30. ST 30 Qichong .... (93)
  31. ST 31 Biguan .... (93)
  32. ST 32 Futu .... (93)
  33. ST 33 Yinshi .... (94)
  34. ST 34 Liangqiu .... (94)

35. ST 35 Dubi ………………………………………………………… (94)
36. ST 36 Zusanli ……………………………………………………… (94)
37. ST 37 Shangjuxu …………………………………………………… (95)
38. ST 38 Tiaokou ……………………………………………………… (95)
39. ST 39 Xiajuxu ……………………………………………………… (96)
40. ST 40 Fenglong …………………………………………………… (96)
41. ST 41 Jiexi ………………………………………………………… (97)
42. ST 42 Chongyang …………………………………………………… (97)
43. ST 43 Xiangu ……………………………………………………… (97)
44. ST 44 Neiting ……………………………………………………… (98)
45. ST 45 Lidui ………………………………………………………… (98)

Section 4 The Acupuncture Points of Spleen Meridian …………… (98)
1. SP 1 Yinbai ………………………………………………………… (98)
2. SP 2 Dadu …………………………………………………………… (99)
3. SP 3 Taibai ………………………………………………………… (99)
4. SP 4 Gongsun ……………………………………………………… (100)
5. SP 5 Shangqiu ……………………………………………………… (100)
6. SP 6 Sanyinjiao …………………………………………………… (100)
7. SP 7 Lougu ………………………………………………………… (101)
8. SP 8 Diji …………………………………………………………… (101)
9. SP 9 Yinlingquan ………………………………………………… (102)
10. SP 10 Xuehai ……………………………………………………… (102)
11. SP 11 Jimen ……………………………………………………… (102)
12. SP 12 Chongmen ………………………………………………… (103)
13. SP 13 Fushe ……………………………………………………… (103)
14. SP 14 Fujie ……………………………………………………… (103)
15. SP 15 Daheng …………………………………………………… (104)
16. SP 16 Fuai ……………………………………………………… (104)
17. SP 17 Shidou …………………………………………………… (104)
18. SP 18 Tianxi …………………………………………………… (105)
19. SP 19 Xiongxiang ……………………………………………… (105)
20. SP 20 Zhourong ………………………………………………… (105)
21. SP 21 Dabao …………………………………………………… (106)

Section 5 The Acupuncture Points of Heart Meridian ……………… (106)
1. HT 1 Jiquan ……………………………………………………… (107)

2. HT 2 Qingling .... (107)
3. HT 3 Shaohai .... (107)
4. HT 4 Lingdao .... (108)
5. HT 5 Tongli .... (108)
6. HT 6 Yinxi .... (109)
7. HT 7 Shenmen .... (109)
8. HT 8 Shaofu .... (109)
9. HT 9 Shaochong .... (110)

Section 6 The Acupuncture Points of Small Intestine Meridian ...... (110)
1. SI 1 Shaoze .... (111)
2. SI 2 Qiangu .... (111)
3. SI 3 Houxi .... (111)
4. SI 4 Wangu .... (112)
5. SI 5 Yanggu .... (112)
6. SI 6 Yanglao .... (112)
7. SI 7 Zhizheng .... (113)
8. SI 8 Xiaohai .... (113)
9. SI 9 Jianzhen .... (113)
10. SI 10 Naoshu .... (113)
11. SI 11 Tianzong .... (114)
12. SI 12 Bingfeng .... (114)
13. SI 13 Quyuan .... (114)
14. SI 14 Jianwaishu .... (115)
15. SI 15 Jianzhongshu .... (115)
16. SI 16 Tianchuang .... (115)
17. SI 17 Tianrong .... (115)
18. SI 18 Quanliao .... (116)
19. SI 19 Tinggong .... (116)

Section 7 The Acupuncture Points of Bladder Meridian .... (118)
1. BL 1 Jingming .... (118)
2. BL 2 Cuanzhu .... (118)
3. BL 3 Meichong .... (119)
4. BL 4 Qucha .... (119)
5. BL 5 Wuchu .... (119)
6. BL 6 Chengguang .... (119)

7. BL 7 Tongtian ……………………………………………… (120)
8. BL 8 Luoque ………………………………………………… (120)
9. BL 9 Yuzhen ………………………………………………… (120)
10. BL 10 Tianzhu ……………………………………………… (121)
11. BL 11 Dazhu ………………………………………………… (121)
12. BL 12 Fengmen ……………………………………………… (121)
13. BL 13 Feishu ………………………………………………… (122)
14. BL 14 Jueyinshu …………………………………………… (122)
15. BL 15 Xinshu ………………………………………………… (122)
16. BL 16 Dushu ………………………………………………… (123)
17. BL 17 Geshu ………………………………………………… (123)
18. BL 18 Ganshu ……………………………………………… (124)
19. BL 19 Danshu ……………………………………………… (124)
20. BL 20 Pishu ………………………………………………… (124)
21. BL 21 Weishu ……………………………………………… (125)
22. BL 22 Sanjiaoshu ………………………………………… (125)
23. BL 23 Shenshu ……………………………………………… (125)
24. BL 24 Qihaishu …………………………………………… (126)
25. BL 25 Dachangshu ………………………………………… (126)
26. BL 26 Guanyuanshu ……………………………………… (126)
27. BL 27 Xiaochangshu ……………………………………… (126)
28. BL 28 Pangguangshu ……………………………………… (127)
29. BL 29 Zhonglushu ………………………………………… (127)
30. BL 30 Baihuanshu ………………………………………… (127)
31. BL 31 Shangliao …………………………………………… (128)
32. BL 32 Ciliao ………………………………………………… (128)
33. BL 33 Zhongliao …………………………………………… (128)
34. BL 34 Xialiao ……………………………………………… (128)
35. BL 35 Huiyang ……………………………………………… (129)
36. BL 36 Chengfu ……………………………………………… (129)
37. BL 37 Yinmen ……………………………………………… (129)
38. BL 38 Fuxi …………………………………………………… (129)
39. BL 39 Weiyang ……………………………………………… (130)
40. BL 40 Weizhong …………………………………………… (130)
41. BL 41 Fufen ………………………………………………… (130)

42. BL 42 Pohu ······ (131)
43. BL 43 Gaohuang ······ (132)
44. BL 44 Shentang ······ (132)
45. BL 45 Yixi ······ (132)
46. BL 46 Geguan ······ (132)
47. BL 47 Hunmen ······ (133)
48. BL 48 Yanggang ······ (133)
49. BL 49 Yishe ······ (133)
50. BL 50 Weicang ······ (133)
51. BL 51 Huangmen ······ (134)
52. BL 52 Zhishi ······ (134)
53. BL 53 Baohuang ······ (134)
54. BL 54 Zhibian ······ (134)
55. BL 55 Heyang ······ (135)
56. BL 56 Chengjin ······ (135)
57. BL 57 Chengshan ······ (135)
58. BL 58 Feiyang ······ (136)
59. BL 59 Fuyang ······ (136)
60. BL 60 Kunlun ······ (137)
61. BL 61 Pucan ······ (137)
62. BL 62 Shenmai ······ (137)
63. BL 63 Jinmen ······ (137)
64. BL 64 Jinggu ······ (138)
65. BL 65 Shugu ······ (138)
66. BL 66 Zutonggu ······ (138)
67. BL 67 Zhiyin ······ (139)

Section 8   The Acupuncture Points of Kidney Meridian ······ (139)
1. KI 1 Yongquan ······ (139)
2. KI 2 Rangu ······ (140)
3. KI 3 Taixi ······ (141)
4. KI 4 Dazhong ······ (141)
5. KI 5 Shuiquan ······ (142)
6. KI 6 Zhaohai ······ (142)
7. KI 7 Fuliu ······ (142)
8. KI 8 Jiaoxin ······ (143)

9. KI 9 Zhubin ………………………………………………………… (143)
10. KI 10 Yingu ………………………………………………………… (143)
11. KI 11 Henggu ……………………………………………………… (144)
12. KI 12 Dahe ………………………………………………………… (144)
13. KI 13 Qixue ………………………………………………………… (145)
14. KI 14 Siman ………………………………………………………… (145)
15. KI 15 Zhongzhu …………………………………………………… (145)
16. KI 16 Huangshu …………………………………………………… (146)
17. KI 17 Shangqu …………………………………………………… (146)
18. KI 18 Shiguan ……………………………………………………… (146)
19. KI 19 Yindu ………………………………………………………… (146)
20. KI 20 Futonggu …………………………………………………… (147)
21. KI 21 Youmen ……………………………………………………… (147)
22. KI 22 Bulang ……………………………………………………… (147)
23. KI 23 Shenfeng …………………………………………………… (148)
24. KI 24 Lingxu ……………………………………………………… (148)
25. KI 25 Shencang …………………………………………………… (148)
26. KI 26 Yuzhong …………………………………………………… (149)
27. KI 27 Shufu ………………………………………………………… (149)
Section 9   The Acupuncture Points of Pericardium Meridian ………… (149)
1. PC 1 Tianchi ……………………………………………………… (149)
2. PC 2 Tianquan …………………………………………………… (150)
3. PC 3 Quze ………………………………………………………… (150)
4. PC 4 Ximen ……………………………………………………… (151)
5. PC 5 Jianshi ……………………………………………………… (151)
6. PC 6 Neiguan ……………………………………………………… (152)
7. PC 7 Daling ……………………………………………………… (152)
8. PC 8 Laogong …………………………………………………… (152)
9. PC 9 Zhongchong ………………………………………………… (153)
Section 10   The Acupuncture Points of Triple Energizer Meridian … (153)
1. TE 1 Guanchong ………………………………………………… (154)
2. TE 2 Yemen ……………………………………………………… (154)
3. TE 3 Zhongzhu …………………………………………………… (155)
4. TE 4 Yangchi ……………………………………………………… (155)
5. TE 5 Waiguan …………………………………………………… (156)

6. TE 6 Zhigou ………………………………………………………… (156)
7. TE 7 Huizong ………………………………………………………… (156)
8. TE 8 Sanyangluo ……………………………………………………… (157)
9. TE 9 Sidu ……………………………………………………………… (157)
10. TE 10 Tianjing ……………………………………………………… (158)
11. TE 11 Qinglengyuan ………………………………………………… (158)
12. TE 12 Xiaoluo ……………………………………………………… (158)
13. TE 13 Naohui ………………………………………………………… (158)
14. TE 14 Jianliao ……………………………………………………… (159)
15. TE 15 Tianliao ……………………………………………………… (159)
16. TE 16 Tianyou ……………………………………………………… (159)
17. TE 17 Yifeng ………………………………………………………… (160)
18. TE 18 Chimai ………………………………………………………… (160)
19. TE 19 Luxi …………………………………………………………… (161)
20. TE 20 Jiaosun ……………………………………………………… (161)
21. TE 21 Ermen ………………………………………………………… (161)
22. TE 22 Erheliao ……………………………………………………… (162)
23. TE 23 Sizhukong …………………………………………………… (162)
Section 11   The Acupuncture Points of Gallbladder Meridian ……… (162)
1. GB 1 Tongziliao ……………………………………………………… (162)
2. GB 2 Tinghui ………………………………………………………… (163)
3. GB 3 Shangguan ……………………………………………………… (164)
4. GB 4 Hanyan ………………………………………………………… (164)
5. GB 5 Xuanlu ………………………………………………………… (164)
6. GB 6 Xuanli ………………………………………………………… (165)
7. GB 7 Qubin …………………………………………………………… (165)
8. GB 8 Shuaigu ………………………………………………………… (165)
9. GB 9 Tianchong ……………………………………………………… (166)
10. GB 10 Fubai ………………………………………………………… (166)
11. GB 11 Touqiaoyin …………………………………………………… (166)
12. GB 12 Wangu ………………………………………………………… (166)
13. GB 13 Benshen ……………………………………………………… (167)
14. GB 14 Yangbai ……………………………………………………… (167)
15. GB 15 Toulinqi ……………………………………………………… (167)
16. GB 16 Muchuang …………………………………………………… (168)

17. GB 17 Zhengying ·· (168)
18. GB 18 Chengling ·· (168)
19. GB 19 Naokong ·· (169)
20. GB 20 Fengchi ··· (169)
21. GB 21 Jianjing ··· (170)
22. GB 22 Yuanye ·· (170)
23. GB 23 Zhejin ··· (171)
24. GB 24 Riyue ·· (171)
25. GB 25 Jingmen ·· (171)
26. GB 26 Daimai ·· (172)
27. GB 27 Wushu ·· (172)
28. GB 28 Weidao ·· (172)
29. GB 29 Juliao ··· (173)
30. GB 30 Huantiao ·· (173)
31. GB 31 Fengshi ·· (173)
32. GB 32 Zhongdu ··· (174)
33. GB 33 Xiyangguan ····································· (174)
34. GB 34 Yanglingquan ·································· (174)
35. GB 35 Yangjiao ··· (175)
36. GB 36 Waiqiu ·· (175)
37. GB 37 Guangming ····································· (175)
38. GB 38 Yangfu ·· (176)
39. GB 39 Xuanzhong ····································· (176)
40. GB 40 Qiuxu ··· (177)
41. GB 41 Zulinqi ··· (177)
42. GB 42 Diwuhui ··· (177)
43. GB 43 Xiaxi ··· (178)
44. GB 44 Zuqiaoyin ······································· (178)

Section 12   The Acupuncture Points of Liver Meridian ········· (179)
1. LR 1 Dadun ··· (179)
2. LR 2 Xingjian ·· (180)
3. LR 3 Taichong ··· (180)
4. LR 4 Zhongfeng ······································· (180)
5. LR 5 Ligou ·· (181)
6. LR 6 Zhongdu ··· (181)

7. LR 7 Xiguan ……………………………………………………… (181)
8. LR 8 Ququan ……………………………………………………… (182)
9. LR 9 Yinbao ……………………………………………………… (182)
10. LR 10 Zuwuli …………………………………………………… (183)
11. LR 11 Yinlian …………………………………………………… (183)
12. LR 12 Jimai ……………………………………………………… (183)
13. LR 13 Zhangmen ………………………………………………… (183)
14. LR 14 Qimen …………………………………………………… (184)
Section 13　The Acupuncture Points of Governor Vessel …………… (184)
1. GV 1 Changqiang ………………………………………………… (185)
2. GV 2 Yaoshu …………………………………………………… (186)
3. GV 3 Yaoyangguan ……………………………………………… (186)
4. GV 4 Mingmen …………………………………………………… (187)
5. GV 5 Xuanshu …………………………………………………… (187)
6. GV 6 Jizhong …………………………………………………… (187)
7. GV 7 Zhongshu ………………………………………………… (187)
8. GV 8 Jinsuo …………………………………………………… (188)
9. GV 9 Zhiyang …………………………………………………… (188)
10. GV 10 Lingtai …………………………………………………… (188)
11. GV 11 Shendao ………………………………………………… (188)
12. GV 12 Shenzhu ………………………………………………… (189)
13. GV 13 Taodao ………………………………………………… (189)
14. GV 14 Dazhui ………………………………………………… (189)
15. GV 15 Yamen ………………………………………………… (189)
16. GV 16 Fengfu ………………………………………………… (190)
17. GV 17 Naohu ………………………………………………… (190)
18. GV 18 Qiangjian ……………………………………………… (191)
19. GV 19 Houding ……………………………………………… (191)
20. GV 20 Baihui ………………………………………………… (191)
21. GV 21 Qianding ……………………………………………… (192)
22. GV 22 Xinhui ………………………………………………… (192)
23. GV 23 Shangxing …………………………………………… (192)
24. GV 24 Shenting ……………………………………………… (192)
25. GV 25 Suliao ………………………………………………… (193)
26. GV 26 Shuigou ……………………………………………… (193)

27. GV 27 Duiduan ……………………………………………… (193)
28. GV 28 Yinjiao ……………………………………………… (193)
Section 14　The Acupuncture Points of Conception Vessel ………… (194)
　1. CV 1 Huiyin ………………………………………………… (194)
　2. CV 2 Qugu ………………………………………………… (195)
　3. CV 3 Zhongji ……………………………………………… (196)
　4. CV 4 Guanyuan …………………………………………… (196)
　5. CV 5 Shimen ……………………………………………… (196)
　6. CV 6 Qihai ………………………………………………… (197)
　7. CV 7 Yinjiao ……………………………………………… (197)
　8. CV 8 Shenque …………………………………………… (197)
　9. CV 9 Shuifen ……………………………………………… (198)
　10. CV 10 Xiawan …………………………………………… (198)
　11. CV 11 Jianli ……………………………………………… (198)
　12. CV 12 Zhongwan ………………………………………… (198)
　13. CV 13 Shangwan ………………………………………… (199)
　14. CV 14 Juque ……………………………………………… (199)
　15. CV 15 Jiuwei …………………………………………… (199)
　16. CV 16 Zhongting ………………………………………… (200)
　17. CV 17 Tanzhong ………………………………………… (200)
　18. CV 18 Yutang …………………………………………… (200)
　19. CV 19 Zigong …………………………………………… (200)
　20. CV 20 Huagai …………………………………………… (201)
　21. CV 21 Xuanji …………………………………………… (201)
　22. CV 22 Tiantu …………………………………………… (201)
　23. CV 23 Lianquan ………………………………………… (202)
　24. CV 24 Chengjiang ……………………………………… (202)

Chapter 4　Extraordinary Points …………………………………… (203)
　Section 1　Region of the Head and Neck ………………………… (203)
　　1. EX-HN 1 Sishencong …………………………………… (203)
　　2. EX-HN 3 Yintang ……………………………………… (203)
　　3. EX-HN 5 Taiyang ……………………………………… (203)
　　4. EX-HN 6 Erjian ………………………………………… (204)
　　5. EX-HN 7 Qiuhou ……………………………………… (205)

  6. EX-HN 8 Shangyingxiang ·················· (205)
  7. EX-HN 9 Neiyingxiang ···················· (205)
  8. EX-HN 10 Juquan ························ (205)
  9. EX-HN 12 Jinjin ·························· (206)
  10. EX-HN 13 Yuye ·························· (206)
  11. EX-HN 14 Yiming ························ (206)
  12. EX-HN 15 Jingbailao ···················· (207)
  13. EX-HN Shanglianquan ·················· (207)
  14. EX-HN Jingbi ···························· (207)
Section 2 The Points in the Region of the Chest and Abdomen ······ (208)
  1. EX-CA Weishang ·························· (208)
  2. EX-CA Sanjiaojiu ·························· (209)
  3. EX-CA Liniaoxue ·························· (209)
  4. EX-CA Qimenxue ·························· (210)
  5. EX-CA Tituo ······························ (210)
  6. EX-CA Zigongxue ·························· (210)
Section 3 The Points in the Region of the Back and Lumbar ········· (211)
  1. EX-B 1 Dingchuan ························ (211)
  2. EX-B 2 Jiaji ······························ (211)
  3. EX-B 3 Weiwanxiashu ···················· (212)
  4. EX-B 4 Pigen ···························· (212)
  5. EX-B 5 Xiajishu ·························· (212)
  6. EX-B 7 Yaoyan ·························· (212)
  7. EX-B 8 Shiqizhui ·························· (213)
  8. EX-B Xueyadian ·························· (213)
  9. EX-B Juqueshu ···························· (213)
  10. EX-B Jieji ································ (214)
Section 4 The Point in the Region of the Upper and Lower
  Extremities ·································· (214)
  1. EX-UE 1 Zhoujian ························ (214)
  2. EX-UE 2 Erbai ···························· (214)
  3. EX-UE 3 Zhongquan ······················ (214)
  4. EX-UE 4 Zhongkui ························ (215)
  5. EX-UE 5 Dagukong ······················ (215)
  6. EX-UE 6 Xiaogukong ···················· (216)

7. EX-UE 7 Yaotongdian .... (216)
8. EX-UE 8 Wailaogong .... (216)
9. EX-UE 9 Baxie .... (216)
10. EX-UE 10 Sifeng .... (217)
11. EX-UE 11 Shixuan .... (217)
12. EX-UE Wuhu .... (217)
13. EX-UE Shounizhu .... (218)
14. EX-UE Jianqian .... (218)
15. EX-LE 2 Heding .... (218)
16. EX-LE Baichongwo .... (219)
17. EX-LE 4 Neixiyan .... (219)
18. EX-LE 6 Dannang .... (220)
19. EX-LE 7 Lanwei .... (220)
20. EX-LE 10 Bafeng .... (220)
21. EX-LE 11 Duyin .... (220)
22. EX-LE 12 Qiduan .... (221)

Part II Acupuncture and Moxibustion Techniques

Chapter 1 Filiform Needle .... (222)
Section 1 The Structure and Specification .... (222)
Section 2 Needle Practice .... (223)
  1. Practice on Sheets of Paper .... (223)
  2. Practice on a Cotton Cushion .... (223)
  3. Practice on Your Own Body .... (224)
Section 3 Preparations Prior to Acupuncture Treatment .... (224)
  1. Inspection of the Instruments .... (224)
  2. Posture of the Patient .... (224)
  3. Sterilization .... (225)
Section 4 Manipulation .... (226)
  1. Insertion .... (226)
  2. Angle and Depth of Insertion .... (228)
  3. Manipulations and Arrival of Qi(needling sensation) ... (229)
  4. Reinforcing and Reducing Methods .... (232)
  5. Retaining and Withdrawing the Needle .... (235)
Section 5 Management of Possible Accidents .... (235)

1. Fainting ……………………………………………………………… (236)
2. Stuck Needle ………………………………………………………… (236)
3. Bent Needle ………………………………………………………… (237)
4. Broken Needle ……………………………………………………… (238)
5. Hematoma …………………………………………………………… (238)
Section 6 Precautions in Acupuncture Treatment ………………… (239)

Chapter 2 Moxibustion ………………………………………………… (240)
Section 1 Classification of Moxibustion ……………………………… (240)
1. Moxibustion with Moxa Cone …………………………………… (240)
2. Moxibustion with Moxa Roll …………………………………… (243)
3. Warming Needle Moxibustion …………………………………… (245)
4. Moxibustion with Mild Moxibustioner ………………………… (245)
Section 2 Moxibustion with Other Materials ………………………… (246)
1. Burning Rush Moxibustion ……………………………………… (246)
2. White Mustard Seed (Semen Sinapis Albae) Moxibustion ……… (246)
Section 3 Precautions ………………………………………………… (246)
1. Order of Moxibustion …………………………………………… (246)
2. Reinforcement and Reduction with Moxibustion ……………… (246)
Section 4 Contraindications of Moxibustion ………………………… (247)
Section 5 Management After Moxibustion ………………………… (247)
(Appendix: Cupping) ………………………………………………… (247)

Chapter 3 Other Acupuncture Therapies …………………………… (251)
Section 1 The Three-Edged Needle …………………………………… (251)
1. Manipulations ……………………………………………………… (251)
2. Indications ………………………………………………………… (252)
3. Precautions ………………………………………………………… (252)
Section 2 The Cutaneous Needle ……………………………………… (253)
1. Manipulation ……………………………………………………… (253)
2. Indications ………………………………………………………… (253)
3. Precautions ………………………………………………………… (254)
Section 3 The Intradermal Needle …………………………………… (254)
1. Manipulations ……………………………………………………… (254)
2. Indications ………………………………………………………… (254)

16

  3. Precautions ·· (255)

Section 4 Electro-Acupuncture ·· (255)

  1. Manipulation ·· (255)

  2. The Actions of the Electro-Pulsation and the Indications of
    Electro-Acupuncture ··· (256)

  3. Precautions ·· (257)

Section 5 Hydro-Acupuncture ··· (258)

  1. Commonly Used Drugs ··· (258)

  2. Administration ·· (259)

  3. Precautions ·· (260)

Chapter 4 Nine Needles in the Ancient Times and the Methods Listed in Internal Classic ··· (261)

Section 1 Nine Needles ··· (261)

Section 2 The Nine Needling Methods ···································· (263)

Section 3 The Twelve Needlings ·· (264)

Section 4 The Five Needling Techniques ································· (265)

Chapter 5 Scalp Acupuncture ··· (267)

Section 1 Locations and Indications of the Stimulating Areas ········ (267)

Section 2 Operations ·· (270)

Section 3 Indications ··· (271)

Section 4 Precautions ··· (272)

Chapter 6 Ear Acupuncture ·· (273)

Section 1 Relations between the Auricle and Zang-fu Organs and
     Meridians ··· (273)

Section 2 Anatomical Names of the Auricles Surface ··················· (274)

Section 3 Auricular Points ··· (276)

Section 4 Application of Ear Acupuncture ································ (291)

  1. Diagnosis by Auricular Points ·· (291)

  2. Selection of Points and Manipulation of Ear Acupuncture— ······ (291)

Section 5 Precautions ··· (293)

Section 6 Examples of Points Prescriptions for Some Common
     Diseases ·· (293)

Part III Acupuncture and Moxibustion Treatment

Chapter 1 Introduction .... (295)
  Section 1 Differentiation according to the Principles of Acupuncture
             and Moxibustion Therapy .... (295)
  Section 2 Principles of Acupuncture and Moxibustion .... (296)
  Section 3 Acupuncture and Moxibustion Prescription .... (297)
    1. Selection of Nearby Points .... (298)
    2. Selection of Distant Points .... (298)
    3. Selection of Symptomatic Points .... (299)
    4. Selection of Points by Reinforcing the Mother and Reducing the
       Son .... (300)
    5. Selecting Points by Earth Meridian Ebb-Flowing Rule .... (301)

Chapter 2 Acupuncture Therapy .... (304)
  Section 1 Internal Diseases .... (304)
    1. Stroke .... (304)
    2. Sunstroke .... (309)
    3. Syncope .... (310)
    4. Common Cold .... (312)
    5. Malaria .... (314)
    6. Cough .... (317)
    7. Asthma .... (320)
    8. Epigastric Pain .... (325)
    9. Vomiting .... (327)
    10. Hiccup .... (330)
    11. Diarrhea .... (332)
    12. Constipation .... (335)
    13. Abdominal Distention .... (338)
    14. Dysentery .... (339)
    15. Prolapse Ani .... (342)
    16. Jaundice .... (344)
    17. Edema .... (346)
    18. Enuresis .... (348)
    19. Hesitancy and Obstruction .... (350)

18

20. Urination Disturbance (352)
21. Impotence (355)
22. Spermatorrhea (357)
23. Insomnia (Appendix: Poor Memory) (359)
24. Palpitation and Severe Palpitation (363)
25. Depressive Madness (365)
26. Epilepsy (368)
27. Dizziness (370)
28. Melancholia (373)
29. Obesity (376)
30. Headache (378)
31. Facial Pain (380)
32. Pain in Hypochondriac Region (382)
33. Lumbago (384)
34. Blockage-Syndromes (Bi Syndromes) (387)
35. Wry Face (389)
36. Atrophy-Syndrome (Wei Syndromes) (391)

Section 2 Gynecological and Pediatric Diseases (394)
1. Irregular Menstruation (394)
2. Dysmenorrhea (397)
3. Amenorrhea (399)
4. Uterine Bleeding (402)
5. Morbid Leukorrhea (404)
6. Prolapse of Uterus (407)
7. Morning Sickness (409)
8. Malposition of Fetus (411)
9. Protracted Labour (412)
10. Insufficient Lactation (Appendix: Delactation) (414)
11. Acute Infantile Convulsion (416)
12. Chronic Infantile Convulsion (417)
13. Infantile Diarrhea (419)
14. Children's Malnutrition (420)
15. Infantile Paralysis (422)
16. Mumps (424)

Section 3 External Diseases (425)

1. Urticaria ······ (425)
2. Acne ······ (427)
3. Erysipelas ······ (429)
4. Herpes Zoster ······ (430)
5. Boils ······ (432)
6. Breast Abscess ······ (434)
7. Intestinal Abscess ······ (435)
8. Goiter ······ (437)
9. Sprain and Contusion (Appendix: Torticollis) ······ (439)

Section 4   Diseases and Syndromes of the Eye, Ear, Nose, Throat and Mouth ······ (442)
1. Tinnitus and Deafness ······ (442)
2. Congestion, Swelling and Pain of the Eye ······ (444)
3. Rhinorrhea with Turbid Discharge ······ (446)
4. Epistaxis ······ (447)
5. Toothache ······ (448)
6. Sore Throat with Swelling ······ (450)
7. Blindness with Insidious Onset ······ (451)
8. Myopia ······ (453)

目 录

绪 言 ·· (459)

上篇 经络腧穴

第一章 经络总论 ··· (462)
 第一节 经络学说的形成 ·· (462)
 第二节 经络系统的组成 ·· (462)
  1. 十二经脉 ··· (463)
  2. 奇经八脉 ··· (464)
  3. 十五络脉 ··· (465)
  4. 十二经别 ··· (466)
  5. 十二经筋 ··· (466)
  6. 十二皮部 ··· (466)
 第三节 经络的根结、标本与气街、四海 ··· (467)
 第四节 经络的生理功能及经络学说在临床上的应用 ························· (468)
  1. 经络的生理功能 ·· (468)
  2. 经络学说在临床上的应用 ·· (468)
 第五节 十二经脉的循行与病候 ·· (469)
  1. 手太阴肺经 ·· (469)
  2. 手阳明大肠经 ··· (470)
  3. 足阳明胃经 ·· (471)
  4. 足太阴脾经 ·· (472)
  5. 手少阴心经 ·· (473)
  6. 手太阳小肠经 ··· (474)
  7. 足太阳膀胱经 ··· (475)
  8. 足少阴肾经 ·· (476)
  9. 手厥阴心包经 ··· (477)
  10. 手少阳三焦经 ··· (478)
  11. 足少阳胆经 ··· (479)
  12. 足厥阴肝经 ··· (480)
 第六节 奇经八脉的循行、病候及交会腧穴 ····································· (481)

1. 督脉 ……………………………………………………………………………… (481)
2. 任脉 ……………………………………………………………………………… (482)
3. 冲脉 ……………………………………………………………………………… (483)
4. 带脉 ……………………………………………………………………………… (483)
5. 阴维脉 …………………………………………………………………………… (484)
6. 阳维脉 …………………………………………………………………………… (484)
7. 阴跷脉 …………………………………………………………………………… (485)
8. 阳跷脉 …………………………………………………………………………… (485)
第七节 十五络脉的穴名、循行、病候及治疗 ……………………………………… (486)

第二章 腧穴总论 …………………………………………………………………………… (488)
第一节 腧穴的基本概念 …………………………………………………………… (488)
第二节 腧穴的发展与分类 ………………………………………………………… (488)
第三节 腧穴的命名 ………………………………………………………………… (488)
第四节 腧穴的作用 ………………………………………………………………… (489)
第五节 特定穴的概念和分类 ……………………………………………………… (489)
1. 五腧穴 …………………………………………………………………………… (489)
2. 原穴、络穴 ……………………………………………………………………… (490)
   2.1. 原穴 ………………………………………………………………………… (490)
   2.2. 络穴 ………………………………………………………………………… (491)
3. 背俞穴、募穴 …………………………………………………………………… (491)
   3.1. 背俞穴 ……………………………………………………………………… (491)
   3.2. 募穴 ………………………………………………………………………… (492)
4. 八会穴 …………………………………………………………………………… (492)
5. 郄穴 ……………………………………………………………………………… (492)
6. 下合穴 …………………………………………………………………………… (493)
7. 八脉交会穴、交会穴 …………………………………………………………… (493)
第六节 腧穴的定位方法 …………………………………………………………… (495)

第三章 十四经穴和经外奇穴 ……………………………………………………………… (498)
第一节 手太阴肺经穴 ……………………………………………………………… (498)
1. 中府 ……………………………………………………………………………… (498)
2. 云门 ……………………………………………………………………………… (499)
3. 天府 ……………………………………………………………………………… (499)
4. 侠白 ……………………………………………………………………………… (499)
5. 尺泽 ……………………………………………………………………………… (499)
6. 孔最 ……………………………………………………………………………… (499)
7. 列缺 ……………………………………………………………………………… (500)
8. 经渠 ……………………………………………………………………………… (500)

9. 太渊 ……………………………………………………………………… (500)
　10. 鱼际 ……………………………………………………………………… (500)
　11. 少商 ……………………………………………………………………… (501)
第二节　手阳明大肠经穴 ……………………………………………………… (501)
　1. 商阳 ……………………………………………………………………… (501)
　2. 二间 ……………………………………………………………………… (502)
　3. 三间 ……………………………………………………………………… (502)
　4. 合谷 ……………………………………………………………………… (502)
　5. 阳溪 ……………………………………………………………………… (502)
　6. 偏历 ……………………………………………………………………… (503)
　7. 温溜 ……………………………………………………………………… (503)
　8. 下廉 ……………………………………………………………………… (503)
　9. 上廉 ……………………………………………………………………… (503)
　10. 手三里 …………………………………………………………………… (503)
　11. 曲池 ……………………………………………………………………… (503)
　12. 肘髎 ……………………………………………………………………… (504)
　13. 手五里 …………………………………………………………………… (504)
　14. 臂臑 ……………………………………………………………………… (504)
　15. 肩髃 ……………………………………………………………………… (505)
　16. 巨骨 ……………………………………………………………………… (505)
　17. 天鼎 ……………………………………………………………………… (505)
　18. 扶突 ……………………………………………………………………… (505)
　19. 口禾髎 …………………………………………………………………… (506)
　20. 迎香 ……………………………………………………………………… (506)
第三节　足阳明胃经 …………………………………………………………… (506)
　1. 承泣 ……………………………………………………………………… (506)
　2. 四白 ……………………………………………………………………… (507)
　3. 巨髎 ……………………………………………………………………… (507)
　4. 地仓 ……………………………………………………………………… (507)
　5. 大迎 ……………………………………………………………………… (508)
　6. 颊车 ……………………………………………………………………… (508)
　7. 下关 ……………………………………………………………………… (508)
　8. 头维 ……………………………………………………………………… (509)
　9. 人迎 ……………………………………………………………………… (509)
　10. 水突 ……………………………………………………………………… (509)
　11. 气舍 ……………………………………………………………………… (509)
　12. 缺盆 ……………………………………………………………………… (509)
　13. 气户 ……………………………………………………………………… (509)
　14. 库房 ……………………………………………………………………… (510)

15. 屋翳	(510)
16. 膺窗	(510)
17. 乳中	(510)
18. 乳根	(510)
19. 不容	(511)
20. 承满	(511)
21. 梁门	(511)
22. 关门	(511)
23. 太乙	(511)
24. 滑肉门	(511)
25. 天枢	(511)
26. 外陵	(512)
27. 大巨	(512)
28. 水道	(512)
29. 归来	(512)
30. 气冲	(512)
31. 髀关	(512)
32. 伏兔	(513)
33. 阴市	(513)
34. 梁丘	(513)
35. 犊鼻	(513)
36. 足三里	(513)
37. 上巨虚	(514)
38. 条口	(514)
39. 下巨虚	(514)
40. 丰隆	(514)
41. 解溪	(514)
42. 冲阳	(515)
43. 陷谷	(515)
44. 内庭	(515)
45. 厉兑	(515)

第四节　足太阴脾经穴 ……………………………………………………… (515)

1. 隐白	(515)
2. 大都	(516)
3. 太白	(516)
4. 公孙	(517)
5. 商丘	(517)
6. 三阴交	(517)
7. 漏谷	(517)

8. 地机 ……………………………………………………………… (517)
9. 阴陵泉 …………………………………………………………… (518)
10. 血海 …………………………………………………………… (518)
11. 箕门 …………………………………………………………… (518)
12. 冲门 …………………………………………………………… (518)
13. 府舍 …………………………………………………………… (518)
14. 腹结 …………………………………………………………… (519)
15. 大横 …………………………………………………………… (519)
16. 腹哀 …………………………………………………………… (519)
17. 食窦 …………………………………………………………… (519)
18. 天溪 …………………………………………………………… (519)
19. 胸乡 …………………………………………………………… (519)
20. 周荣 …………………………………………………………… (520)
21. 大包 …………………………………………………………… (520)

第五节 手少阴心经穴 ……………………………………………… (520)

1. 极泉 ……………………………………………………………… (521)
2. 青灵 ……………………………………………………………… (521)
3. 少海 ……………………………………………………………… (521)
4. 灵道 ……………………………………………………………… (521)
5. 通里 ……………………………………………………………… (521)
6. 阴郄 ……………………………………………………………… (522)
7. 神门 ……………………………………………………………… (522)
8. 少府 ……………………………………………………………… (522)
9. 少冲 ……………………………………………………………… (522)

第六节 手太阳小肠经 ……………………………………………… (522)

1. 少泽 ……………………………………………………………… (522)
2. 前谷 ……………………………………………………………… (523)
3. 后溪 ……………………………………………………………… (523)
4. 腕骨 ……………………………………………………………… (524)
5. 阳谷 ……………………………………………………………… (524)
6. 养老 ……………………………………………………………… (524)
7. 支正 ……………………………………………………………… (524)
8. 小海 ……………………………………………………………… (524)
9. 肩贞 ……………………………………………………………… (525)
10. 臑俞 …………………………………………………………… (525)
11. 天宗 …………………………………………………………… (525)
12. 秉风 …………………………………………………………… (525)
13. 曲垣 …………………………………………………………… (525)
14. 肩外俞 ………………………………………………………… (525)

15. 肩中俞 …………………………………………………………………… (526)
16. 天窗 ……………………………………………………………………… (526)
17. 天容 ……………………………………………………………………… (526)
18. 颧髎 ……………………………………………………………………… (526)
19. 听宫 ……………………………………………………………………… (527)

第七节　足太阳膀胱经穴 ……………………………………………………… (527)
1. 睛明 ……………………………………………………………………… (527)
2. 攒竹 ……………………………………………………………………… (527)
3. 眉冲 ……………………………………………………………………… (527)
4. 曲差 ……………………………………………………………………… (527)
5. 五处 ……………………………………………………………………… (529)
6. 承光 ……………………………………………………………………… (529)
7. 通天 ……………………………………………………………………… (529)
8. 络却 ……………………………………………………………………… (529)
9. 玉枕 ……………………………………………………………………… (529)
10. 天柱 …………………………………………………………………… (530)
11. 大杼 …………………………………………………………………… (530)
12. 风门 …………………………………………………………………… (531)
13. 肺俞 …………………………………………………………………… (531)
14. 厥阴俞 ………………………………………………………………… (531)
15. 心俞 …………………………………………………………………… (531)
16. 督俞 …………………………………………………………………… (531)
17. 膈俞 …………………………………………………………………… (531)
18. 肝俞 …………………………………………………………………… (532)
19. 胆俞 …………………………………………………………………… (532)
20. 脾俞 …………………………………………………………………… (532)
21. 胃俞 …………………………………………………………………… (532)
22. 三焦俞 ………………………………………………………………… (532)
23. 肾俞 …………………………………………………………………… (533)
24. 气海俞 ………………………………………………………………… (533)
25. 大肠俞 ………………………………………………………………… (533)
26. 关元俞 ………………………………………………………………… (533)
27. 小肠俞 ………………………………………………………………… (533)
28. 膀胱俞 ………………………………………………………………… (533)
29. 中膂俞 ………………………………………………………………… (534)
30. 白环俞 ………………………………………………………………… (534)
31. 上髎 …………………………………………………………………… (534)
32. 次髎 …………………………………………………………………… (534)
33. 中髎 …………………………………………………………………… (534)

34. 下髎 ··· (534)
　　35. 会阳 ··· (535)
　　36. 承扶 ··· (535)
　　37. 殷门 ··· (535)
　　38. 浮郄 ··· (535)
　　39. 委阳 ··· (535)
　　40. 委中 ··· (535)
　　41. 附分 ··· (536)
　　42. 魄户 ··· (536)
　　43. 膏肓 ··· (537)
　　44. 神堂 ··· (537)
　　45. 譩譆 ··· (537)
　　46. 膈关 ··· (537)
　　47. 魂门 ··· (537)
　　48. 阳纲 ··· (537)
　　49. 意舍 ··· (538)
　　50. 胃仓 ··· (538)
　　51. 肓门 ··· (538)
　　52. 志室 ··· (538)
　　53. 胞肓 ··· (538)
　　54. 秩边 ··· (538)
　　55. 合阳 ··· (538)
　　56. 承筋 ··· (539)
　　57. 承山 ··· (539)
　　58. 飞扬 ··· (539)
　　59. 跗阳 ··· (539)
　　60. 昆仑 ··· (539)
　　61. 仆参 ··· (540)
　　62. 申脉 ··· (540)
　　63. 金门 ··· (540)
　　64. 京骨 ··· (540)
　　65. 束骨 ··· (540)
　　66. 足通谷 ·· (541)
　　67. 至阴 ··· (541)
　第八节　足少阴肾经 ··· (541)
　　1. 涌泉 ··· (541)
　　2. 然谷 ··· (541)
　　3. 太溪 ··· (542)
　　4. 大钟 ··· (543)

- 5. 水泉 ………………………………………………………………………… (543)
- 6. 照海 ………………………………………………………………………… (543)
- 7. 复溜 ………………………………………………………………………… (543)
- 8. 交信 ………………………………………………………………………… (543)
- 9. 筑宾 ………………………………………………………………………… (544)
- 10. 阴谷 ………………………………………………………………………… (544)
- 11. 横骨 ………………………………………………………………………… (544)
- 12. 大赫 ………………………………………………………………………… (544)
- 13. 气穴 ………………………………………………………………………… (544)
- 14. 四满 ………………………………………………………………………… (545)
- 15. 中注 ………………………………………………………………………… (545)
- 16. 肓俞 ………………………………………………………………………… (545)
- 17. 商曲 ………………………………………………………………………… (545)
- 18. 石关 ………………………………………………………………………… (545)
- 19. 阴都 ………………………………………………………………………… (546)
- 20. 腹通谷 ……………………………………………………………………… (546)
- 21. 幽门 ………………………………………………………………………… (546)
- 22. 步廊 ………………………………………………………………………… (546)
- 23. 神封 ………………………………………………………………………… (546)
- 24. 灵墟 ………………………………………………………………………… (546)
- 25. 神藏 ………………………………………………………………………… (547)
- 26. 彧中 ………………………………………………………………………… (547)
- 27. 俞府 ………………………………………………………………………… (547)

第九节 手厥阴心包经穴 …………………………………………………… (547)

- 1. 天池 ………………………………………………………………………… (547)
- 2. 天泉 ………………………………………………………………………… (548)
- 3. 曲泽 ………………………………………………………………………… (548)
- 4. 郄门 ………………………………………………………………………… (548)
- 5. 间使 ………………………………………………………………………… (548)
- 6. 内关 ………………………………………………………………………… (549)
- 7. 大陵 ………………………………………………………………………… (549)
- 8. 劳宫 ………………………………………………………………………… (549)
- 9. 中冲 ………………………………………………………………………… (549)

第十节 手少阳三焦经 ……………………………………………………… (550)

- 1. 关冲 ………………………………………………………………………… (550)
- 2. 液门 ………………………………………………………………………… (550)
- 3. 中渚 ………………………………………………………………………… (550)
- 4. 阳池 ………………………………………………………………………… (550)
- 5. 外关 ………………………………………………………………………… (551)

6. 支沟 …………………………………………………………………………… (551)
  7. 会宗 …………………………………………………………………………… (551)
  8. 三阳络 ………………………………………………………………………… (551)
  9. 四渎 …………………………………………………………………………… (551)
  10. 天井 ………………………………………………………………………… (552)
  11. 清冷渊 ……………………………………………………………………… (552)
  12. 消泺 ………………………………………………………………………… (552)
  13. 臑会 ………………………………………………………………………… (552)
  14. 肩髎 ………………………………………………………………………… (552)
  15. 天髎 ………………………………………………………………………… (552)
  16. 天牖 ………………………………………………………………………… (553)
  17. 翳风 ………………………………………………………………………… (553)
  18. 瘈脉 ………………………………………………………………………… (553)
  19. 颅息 ………………………………………………………………………… (553)
  20. 角孙 ………………………………………………………………………… (554)
  21. 耳门 ………………………………………………………………………… (554)
  22. 耳和髎 ……………………………………………………………………… (554)
  23. 丝竹空 ……………………………………………………………………… (554)
第十一节　足少阳胆经穴 …………………………………………………… (554)
  1. 瞳子髎 ………………………………………………………………………… (554)
  2. 听会 …………………………………………………………………………… (555)
  3. 上关 …………………………………………………………………………… (555)
  4. 颔厌 …………………………………………………………………………… (556)
  5. 悬颅 …………………………………………………………………………… (556)
  6. 悬厘 …………………………………………………………………………… (556)
  7. 曲鬓 …………………………………………………………………………… (556)
  8. 率谷 …………………………………………………………………………… (556)
  9. 天冲 …………………………………………………………………………… (556)
  10. 浮白 ………………………………………………………………………… (557)
  11. 头窍阴 ……………………………………………………………………… (557)
  12. 完骨 ………………………………………………………………………… (557)
  13. 本神 ………………………………………………………………………… (557)
  14. 阳白 ………………………………………………………………………… (557)
  15. 头临泣 ……………………………………………………………………… (558)
  16. 目窗 ………………………………………………………………………… (558)
  17. 正营 ………………………………………………………………………… (558)
  18. 承灵 ………………………………………………………………………… (558)
  19. 脑空 ………………………………………………………………………… (558)
  20. 风池 ………………………………………………………………………… (559)

21. 肩井 ………………………………………………………………………………… (559)
22. 渊腋 ………………………………………………………………………………… (559)
23. 辄筋 ………………………………………………………………………………… (560)
24. 日月 ………………………………………………………………………………… (560)
25. 京门 ………………………………………………………………………………… (560)
26. 带脉 ………………………………………………………………………………… (560)
27. 五枢 ………………………………………………………………………………… (560)
28. 维道 ………………………………………………………………………………… (561)
29. 居髎 ………………………………………………………………………………… (561)
30. 环跳 ………………………………………………………………………………… (561)
31. 风市 ………………………………………………………………………………… (561)
32. 中渎 ………………………………………………………………………………… (561)
33. 膝阳关 ……………………………………………………………………………… (562)
34. 阳陵泉 ……………………………………………………………………………… (562)
35. 阳交 ………………………………………………………………………………… (562)
36. 外丘 ………………………………………………………………………………… (562)
37. 光明 ………………………………………………………………………………… (562)
38. 阳辅 ………………………………………………………………………………… (562)
39. 悬钟 ………………………………………………………………………………… (563)
40. 丘墟 ………………………………………………………………………………… (563)
41. 足临泣 ……………………………………………………………………………… (563)
42. 地五会 ……………………………………………………………………………… (563)
43. 侠溪 ………………………………………………………………………………… (563)
44. 足窍阴 ……………………………………………………………………………… (564)

第十二节 足厥阴肝经穴 …………………………………………………………… (564)

1. 大敦 ………………………………………………………………………………… (564)
2. 行间 ………………………………………………………………………………… (565)
3. 太冲 ………………………………………………………………………………… (565)
4. 中封 ………………………………………………………………………………… (565)
5. 蠡沟 ………………………………………………………………………………… (565)
6. 中都 ………………………………………………………………………………… (565)
7. 膝关 ………………………………………………………………………………… (566)
8. 曲泉 ………………………………………………………………………………… (566)
9. 阴包 ………………………………………………………………………………… (566)
10. 足五里 ……………………………………………………………………………… (566)
11. 阴廉 ………………………………………………………………………………… (566)
12. 急脉 ………………………………………………………………………………… (567)
13. 章门 ………………………………………………………………………………… (567)
14. 期门 ………………………………………………………………………………… (567)

第十三节　督脉穴 ……………………………………………………………………(567)
    1. 长强 ………………………………………………………………………………(567)
    2. 腰俞 ………………………………………………………………………………(568)
    3. 腰阳关 ……………………………………………………………………………(568)
    4. 命门 ………………………………………………………………………………(568)
    5. 悬枢 ………………………………………………………………………………(569)
    6. 脊中 ………………………………………………………………………………(569)
    7. 中枢 ………………………………………………………………………………(569)
    8. 筋缩 ………………………………………………………………………………(570)
    9. 至阳 ………………………………………………………………………………(570)
    10. 灵台 ……………………………………………………………………………(570)
    11. 神道 ……………………………………………………………………………(570)
    12. 身柱 ……………………………………………………………………………(570)
    13. 陶道 ……………………………………………………………………………(570)
    14. 大椎 ……………………………………………………………………………(571)
    15. 哑门 ……………………………………………………………………………(571)
    16. 风府 ……………………………………………………………………………(571)
    17. 脑户 ……………………………………………………………………………(571)
    18. 强间 ……………………………………………………………………………(571)
    19. 后顶 ……………………………………………………………………………(572)
    20. 百会 ……………………………………………………………………………(572)
    21. 前顶 ……………………………………………………………………………(572)
    22. 囟会 ……………………………………………………………………………(572)
    23. 上星 ……………………………………………………………………………(572)
    24. 神庭 ……………………………………………………………………………(572)
    25. 素髎 ……………………………………………………………………………(573)
    26. 水沟 ……………………………………………………………………………(573)
    27. 兑端 ……………………………………………………………………………(573)
    28. 龈交 ……………………………………………………………………………(573)
第十四节　任脉穴 ……………………………………………………………………(573)
    1. 会阴 ………………………………………………………………………………(573)
    2. 曲骨 ………………………………………………………………………………(574)
    3. 中极 ………………………………………………………………………………(574)
    4. 关元 ………………………………………………………………………………(574)
    5. 石门 ………………………………………………………………………………(575)
    6. 气海 ………………………………………………………………………………(575)
    7. 阴交 ………………………………………………………………………………(575)
    8. 神阙 ………………………………………………………………………………(575)
    9. 水分 ………………………………………………………………………………(575)

10. 下脘 (575)
11. 建里 (576)
12. 中脘 (576)
13. 上脘 (576)
14. 巨阙 (576)
15. 鸠尾 (576)
16. 中庭 (576)
17. 膻中 (577)
18. 玉堂 (577)
19. 紫宫 (577)
20. 华盖 (577)
21. 璇玑 (577)
22. 天突 (577)
23. 廉泉 (578)
24. 承浆 (578)

第四章 经外奇穴 (579)
第一节 头颈部 (579)
1. 四神聪 (579)
2. 印堂 (579)
3. 太阳 (579)
4. 耳尖 (580)
5. 球后 (580)
6. 上迎香 (580)
7. 内迎香 (580)
8. 聚泉 (580)
9. 金津 (580)
10. 玉液 (581)
11. 翳明 (581)
12. 颈百劳 (581)
13. 上廉泉 (581)
14. 颈臂 (582)

第二节 胸腹部 (582)
1. 胃上 (582)
2. 三角灸 (582)
3. 利尿穴 (582)
4. 气门 (583)
5. 提托 (583)
6. 子宫穴 (583)

第三节 背腰部 ……………………………………………………………………… (583)
1. 定喘 ……………………………………………………………………………… (583)
2. 夹脊 ……………………………………………………………………………… (584)
3. 胃脘下俞 ………………………………………………………………………… (584)
4. 痞根 ……………………………………………………………………………… (585)
5. 下极俞 …………………………………………………………………………… (585)
6. 腰眼 ……………………………………………………………………………… (585)
7. 十七椎 …………………………………………………………………………… (585)
8. 血压点 …………………………………………………………………………… (585)
9. 巨阙俞 …………………………………………………………………………… (585)
10. 接脊 …………………………………………………………………………… (585)

第四节 四肢部 ……………………………………………………………………… (586)
1. 肘尖 ……………………………………………………………………………… (586)
2. 二白 ……………………………………………………………………………… (586)
3. 中泉 ……………………………………………………………………………… (586)
4. 中魁 ……………………………………………………………………………… (586)
5. 大骨空 …………………………………………………………………………… (586)
6. 小骨空 …………………………………………………………………………… (587)
7. 腰痛点 …………………………………………………………………………… (587)
8. 外劳宫 …………………………………………………………………………… (587)
9. 八邪 ……………………………………………………………………………… (587)
10. 四缝 …………………………………………………………………………… (588)
11. 十宣 …………………………………………………………………………… (588)
12. 五虎 …………………………………………………………………………… (588)
13. 手逆注 ………………………………………………………………………… (588)
14. 肩前 …………………………………………………………………………… (589)
15. 鹤顶 …………………………………………………………………………… (589)
16. 百虫窝 ………………………………………………………………………… (589)
17. 内膝眼 ………………………………………………………………………… (589)
18. 胆囊 …………………………………………………………………………… (589)
19. 阑尾 …………………………………………………………………………… (589)
20. 八风 …………………………………………………………………………… (590)
21. 独阴 …………………………………………………………………………… (590)
22. 气端 …………………………………………………………………………… (590)

中篇 刺灸方法

第一章 毫针刺法 ………………………………………………………………………… (591)

第一节 毫针的构造、规格 …………………………………………………………… (591)
第二节 针刺练习 …………………………………………………………………… (591)
　1. 纸垫练针法 …………………………………………………………………… (592)
　2. 棉球练习法 …………………………………………………………………… (592)
　3. 自身试针 ……………………………………………………………………… (592)
第三节 针刺前的准备 ……………………………………………………………… (592)
　1. 检查用具 ……………………………………………………………………… (592)
　2. 选择体位 ……………………………………………………………………… (592)
　3. 消毒 …………………………………………………………………………… (594)
第四节 操作 ………………………………………………………………………… (594)
　1. 进针法 ………………………………………………………………………… (594)
　2. 针刺的角度和深度 …………………………………………………………… (595)
　3. 行针与得气 …………………………………………………………………… (596)
　4. 针刺补泻 ……………………………………………………………………… (598)
　5. 留针与出针 …………………………………………………………………… (599)
第五节 异常情况处理及预防 ……………………………………………………… (599)
　1. 晕针 …………………………………………………………………………… (599)
　2. 滞针 …………………………………………………………………………… (600)
　3. 弯针 …………………………………………………………………………… (600)
　4. 断针 …………………………………………………………………………… (600)
　5. 血肿 …………………………………………………………………………… (601)
第六节 针刺注意事项 ……………………………………………………………… (601)

第二章 灸法 ………………………………………………………………………… (602)
第一节 常用灸法 …………………………………………………………………… (602)
　1. 艾炷灸 ………………………………………………………………………… (602)
　2. 艾卷灸 ………………………………………………………………………… (604)
　3. 温针灸 ………………………………………………………………………… (605)
　4. 温灸器灸 ……………………………………………………………………… (605)
第二节 其它灸法 …………………………………………………………………… (605)
　1. 灯草灸 ………………………………………………………………………… (605)
　2. 白芥子灸 ……………………………………………………………………… (605)
第三节 注意事项 …………………………………………………………………… (606)
第四节 施灸的禁忌 ………………………………………………………………… (606)
第五节 灸后处理 …………………………………………………………………… (606)
　〔附〕拔罐法 …………………………………………………………………… (606)

第三章 其它针法 …………………………………………………………………… (610)
第一节 三棱针 ……………………………………………………………………… (610)

1. 操作方法 ……………………………………………………………… (610)
　　2. 适用范围 ……………………………………………………………… (610)
　　3. 注意事项 ……………………………………………………………… (610)
　第二节　皮肤针 …………………………………………………………… (611)
　　1. 操作方法 ……………………………………………………………… (611)
　　2. 适应范围 ……………………………………………………………… (612)
　　3. 注意事项 ……………………………………………………………… (612)
　第三节　皮内针 …………………………………………………………… (612)
　　1. 操作方法 ……………………………………………………………… (612)
　　2. 适应范围 ……………………………………………………………… (612)
　　3. 注意事项 ……………………………………………………………… (612)
　第四节　电针 ……………………………………………………………… (613)
　　1. 操作方法 ……………………………………………………………… (613)
　　2. 脉冲电流作用和电针的适应症 ……………………………………… (613)
　　3. 注意事项 ……………………………………………………………… (614)
　第五节　水针 ……………………………………………………………… (614)
　　1. 常用药物 ……………………………………………………………… (614)
　　2. 治疗方法 ……………………………………………………………… (615)
　　3. 注意事项 ……………………………………………………………… (615)

第四章　古代九针和《内经》刺法 ………………………………………… (616)
　第一节　九针 ……………………………………………………………… (616)
　第二节　九刺 ……………………………………………………………… (617)
　第三节　十二刺 …………………………………………………………… (618)
　第四节　五刺 ……………………………………………………………… (619)

第五章　头针疗法 …………………………………………………………… (620)
　第一节　刺激区线的定位及主治 ………………………………………… (620)
　第二节　操作方法 ………………………………………………………… (622)
　第三节　适应范围 ………………………………………………………… (623)
　第四节　注意事项 ………………………………………………………… (623)

第六章　耳针疗法 …………………………………………………………… (624)
　第一节　耳与脏腑经络的关系 …………………………………………… (624)
　第二节　耳廓表面的解剖名称 …………………………………………… (624)
　第三节　耳针穴位 ………………………………………………………… (625)
　第四节　耳穴的应用 ……………………………………………………… (631)
　　1. 探查耳穴诊病 ………………………………………………………… (631)
　　2. 耳穴的选穴与操作 …………………………………………………… (631)

第五节　注意事项 ………………………………………………………………… (632)
　第六节　常见病症处方举例 ……………………………………………………… (632)

下篇　针灸治疗

第一章　治疗总论 …………………………………………………………………… (633)
　第一节　针灸辨证 ………………………………………………………………… (633)
　第二节　针灸立法 ………………………………………………………………… (633)
　第三节　针灸处方 ………………………………………………………………… (634)
　　1. 近部取穴 ……………………………………………………………………… (634)
　　2. 远部取穴 ……………………………………………………………………… (634)
　　3. 对症选穴 ……………………………………………………………………… (635)
　　4. 补母泻子法 …………………………………………………………………… (635)
　　5. 子午流注纳子法取穴 ………………………………………………………… (636)

第二章　治疗各论 …………………………………………………………………… (637)
　第一节　内科病症 ………………………………………………………………… (637)
　　1. 中风 …………………………………………………………………………… (637)
　　2. 中暑 …………………………………………………………………………… (639)
　　3. 昏厥 …………………………………………………………………………… (639)
　　4. 感冒 …………………………………………………………………………… (640)
　　5. 疟疾 …………………………………………………………………………… (641)
　　6. 咳嗽 …………………………………………………………………………… (642)
　　7. 哮喘 …………………………………………………………………………… (643)
　　8. 胃痛 …………………………………………………………………………… (645)
　　9. 呕吐 …………………………………………………………………………… (646)
　　10. 呃逆 ………………………………………………………………………… (647)
　　11. 泄泻 ………………………………………………………………………… (648)
　　12. 便秘 ………………………………………………………………………… (649)
　　13. 腹胀 ………………………………………………………………………… (650)
　　14. 痢疾 ………………………………………………………………………… (651)
　　15. 脱肛 ………………………………………………………………………… (652)
　　16. 黄疸 ………………………………………………………………………… (653)
　　17. 水肿 ………………………………………………………………………… (654)
　　18. 遗尿 ………………………………………………………………………… (655)
　　19. 癃闭 ………………………………………………………………………… (655)
　　20. 淋证 ………………………………………………………………………… (657)
　　21. 阳痿 ………………………………………………………………………… (658)

22. 遗精 ……………………………………………………………… (658)
23. 失眠(附:健忘) ………………………………………………… (659)
24. 惊悸、怔忡 ……………………………………………………… (661)
25. 癫狂 ……………………………………………………………… (662)
26. 痫症 ……………………………………………………………… (663)
27. 眩晕 ……………………………………………………………… (664)
28. 郁症 ……………………………………………………………… (665)
29. 肥胖症 …………………………………………………………… (667)
30. 头痛 ……………………………………………………………… (667)
31. 面痛 ……………………………………………………………… (669)
32. 胁痛 ……………………………………………………………… (670)
33. 腰痛 ……………………………………………………………… (671)
34. 痹证 ……………………………………………………………… (672)
35. 面瘫 ……………………………………………………………… (673)
36. 痿证 ……………………………………………………………… (674)

第二节 妇儿科病症 ………………………………………………… (675)
1. 月经不调 ………………………………………………………… (675)
2. 痛经 ……………………………………………………………… (676)
3. 经闭 ……………………………………………………………… (677)
4. 崩漏 ……………………………………………………………… (678)
5. 带下 ……………………………………………………………… (679)
6. 阴挺 ……………………………………………………………… (680)
7. 妊娠恶阻 ………………………………………………………… (681)
8. 胎位不正 ………………………………………………………… (682)
9. 滞产 ……………………………………………………………… (682)
10. 乳少(附:回乳) ………………………………………………… (683)
11. 急惊风 …………………………………………………………… (684)
12. 慢惊风 …………………………………………………………… (685)
13. 小儿腹泻 ………………………………………………………… (685)
14. 小儿疳积 ………………………………………………………… (686)
15. 小儿瘫痪 ………………………………………………………… (687)
16. 痄腮 ……………………………………………………………… (687)

第三节 外科病症 …………………………………………………… (688)
1. 风疹 ……………………………………………………………… (688)
2. 痤疮 ……………………………………………………………… (689)
3. 丹毒 ……………………………………………………………… (689)
4. 蛇丹 ……………………………………………………………… (690)
5. 疔疮 ……………………………………………………………… (691)
6. 乳痈 ……………………………………………………………… (692)

7. 肠痈 …………………………………………………………… (692)
　　8. 瘿病 …………………………………………………………… (693)
　　9. 扭伤（附：落枕） …………………………………………… (694)
　第四节　五官科病症 ……………………………………………… (695)
　　1. 耳鸣、耳聋 …………………………………………………… (695)
　　2. 目赤肿痛 ……………………………………………………… (696)
　　3. 鼻渊 …………………………………………………………… (697)
　　4. 鼻衄 …………………………………………………………… (697)
　　5. 牙痛 …………………………………………………………… (698)
　　6. 咽喉肿病 ……………………………………………………… (699)
　　7. 青盲 …………………………………………………………… (699)
　　8. 近视 …………………………………………………………… (700)

INTRODUCTION

The science of acupuncture and moxibustion, which includes four aspects, i.e, the meridians and collaterals, acupoints, manipulating methods, and clinical treatment, is an important component of Traditional Chinese Medicine (TCM). It is a practical science of preventing and treating diseases with acupuncture and moxibustion under the guidance of the TCM theory.

With such advantages as wide range of indications, distinct curative effect, simple application, low cost, safety, etc., acupuncture and moxibustion has been very popular in the broad masses of the people, and it has made a great contribution to the prosperity of the Chinese nation for thousands of years.

The science of acupuncture and moxibustion was developed by Chinese people and doctors through the ages during their struggle against diseases. Acupuncture and moxibustion developed before the creation of Chinese characters.

At that time, the primitive people lived in the wild and open field and got food through fighting against fierce beasts. When they fell ill, they often pressed certain location on their body instinctively with their fingers or pieces of stone, and sometimes the pain was relieved unexpectedly, and so the treatment of diseases with Bianshi (stone needles) gradually developed in that way through a long-term accumulation of experience. In 1963, a roundstone needle, which is determined as the primitive tool for acupuncture therapy, was unearthed in the relics of the Neolithic Age at Toudaowa, Dolun Banner, Inner Mongolia. Therefore, the origin of Bianshi can be traced back to the Neolithic Age which was four to ten thousand years ago.

With the invention of metal casting techniques, needle tools were improved from stone, bone, bamboo needles to metal ones made from bronze, iron, gold, silver or other materials.

Nowadays stainless steel needles are widely used. In 1978, a bronze needle was found for the first time in the archaeological finds at Shulinzhao Commune, Dalata Banner, Inner Mongolia. In 1968, nine needles, made of gold or silver, were found in the excavation of Liusheng tomb of the West Han Dynasty at

Mancheng, Hebei Province, which proved the continuous development of metal needles.

Moxibustion was brought into being after discovery and use of fire. People found the pain in certain parts of the body alleviated or relieved when warmed by fire. And this resulted in moxibustion therapy through a long-term of practice using materials from tree branches to moxa, and it has branched to many kinds of moxibustion with the development of medicine in later ages. This is referred by the book *Plain Question*: "For the fullness and oppression due to cold in Zang-organs, moxibustion is indicated to be applied."

With the improvement of the instruments for acupuncture and moxibustion, the curative effect was increased, and this greatly promoted the study of acupuncture and moxibustion

So acupuncture and moxibustion as a science has undergone a long course of development. In 1973, the two ancient books, *Moxibustion Classic with Eleven Foot-Hand Meridians* and *Moxibustion Classic with Yin-Yang Meridians*, which record meridians and collaterals, were unearthed in the medical silk scrolls of the No. 3 Han Tomb at Mawangdui, Changsha City, Hunan Province. They described the courses and distributions of the eleven meridians, signs and symptoms of diseases and moxibustion treatment. The results of preliminary identification showed that the books were written before *Canon of Medicine* and the primitive theory about meridians and collaterals can be seen a little here.

The book *Canon of Medicine* discussed meridians and collaterals, acupoints, manipulation, indications and contraindications of acupuncture and moxibustion in detail, especially in one part of the book called *Miraculous Pivot*. It recorded the theory of acupuncture and moxibustion more abundantly and systematically. So, another name for *Miraculous Pivot* is *Canon of Acupuncture*. Thus, acupuncture and moxibustion theories were shown relatively matured at that time, which built up the theoretical basis for the development of acupuncture and moxibustion.

A—B Classic of Acupuncture and Moxibustion, the early classic on acupuncture and moxibustion in addition to *Canon of Acupuncture* was compiled by Huang Fumi in the Jin Dynasty, on the basis of *Canon of Medicine* and *An Outline of Points for Acupuncture and Moxibustion* (Lost). Not only does it discuss the theories of viscera and bowels, meridians and collaterals, but also based on *Canon of Medicine* tells the locations and indications of 349 acupoints according to the part of the body such as head, face, chest, belly and back, etc., and it also describes the manipulations of acupuncture, contraindications and treatment of common diseases. This book, which was another summary of acupuncture and moxibustion after *Canon of Medicine*, is a link between the past and following time. Ge Hong in the East Jin Dynasty wrote the book *A Handbook of Prescriptions for Emergencies* which recorded 109 prescriptions, 99 of which are about moxibustion, which brought more attention to moxibustion and promoted the further development of moxibustion along with acupuncture. In the Tang Dynasty, Sun Simiao compiled the book entitled *Prescriptions with the Worth of Thousand Gold Pieces* which introduces the location and application of Ashi points. He also made the multicolored *Charts of Three Views* in which he drew the twelve regular meridians and the eight extra meridians on the front, back and side of the human body with different colors. What is worth great esteem is that he proposed methods of preventing diseases by moxibustion which made contribution to the preventive medicine.

After that, in his book entitled The *Medical Secrets of An Official*, Wang Tao in the Tang Dynasty elaborated the moxibustion therapy, which promoted the popularization of moxibustion. In the Sui and Tang Dynasty, the Imperial Medical Bureau was set up to take charge of the medical education. In the Bureau, acupuncture and moxibustion was a special subject which had professional staff for acupuncture and moxibustion such as professors, assistants, instructors, etc. to do the educational work. In the North Song Dynasty, Wang Weiyi compiled the book *Illustrated Manual of Acupoints of the Bronze Figure* which included meridians, collaterals, acupoints and so on, and did textual research on 354 acupoints. The whole book was carved on a stone tablet in Bianjin (Now Kaifeng in Henan Province) for people who want to learn acupuncture and moxibustion to make rubbings. The next year, he designed and cast two bronze figures which are the earliest models of acupuncture and moxibustion in China and very helpful for recognizing the acupoints and teaching. In the Yuan Dynasty, Hua Boren had the opinion that although the Conception and Governor Vessel belong to the extra meridians, they have special acupoints and therefore should also be considered in the same breath with the regular meridians to make up the fourteen meridians. His book *Exposition of the Fourteen Meridians*, in which he elaborated systematically the courses of meridians and collaterals and their relative acupoints were quite profitable later on to study acupoints.

Acupuncture and moxibustion had a prosperous time of development in the Ming Dynasty. Yang Jizhou wrote the book *Compendium of Acupuncture and Moxibustion* on the basis of his ancestor's book *Mysterious Secrets of Acupuncture and Moxibustion* combined with his own clinical experience. The book, collecting acupuncture and moxibustion works through the ages is very rich in content, and is another compendium of acupuncture and moxibustion after *Canon of Medicine* and *A—B Classic of Acupuncture and Moxibustion*. Today it is still the main reference book to study acupuncture and moxibustion. In that period, many famous doctors were emerged with exclusive works on acupuncture and moxibustion, for instance, *Canon of Shenying* written by Chen Hui, *A Complete Collection of Acupuncture and Moxibustion* by Xu Feng, *An Exemplary Collection of Acupuncture and Moxibustion* by Gao Wu, *Questions and Answers to Acupuncture and Moxibustion* by Gao Wu, *Questions and Answers to Acupuncture and Moxibustion* by Wang Ji, and *A Study on the Eight—Extra Meridians* by Li Shizhen. They formed different schools of thought with their own advantages, contending with each other and promoted the development of acupuncture and moxibustion.

In the Qing Dynasty, there were the books *Golden Mirror of Medicine*, *Essentials of Acupuncture and Moxibustion in Verse* by Wu Qian and his collaborators, and *A Collection of Acupuncture and Moxibustion* by . Liao Runhong, and so on, but only few development was made. In the late of the Qin Dynasty, acupuncture and moxibustion went on the wane. In 1822, the acupuncture and moxibustion department was abolished and the acupuncture and moxibustion treatment was not allowed to practise or teach in the Imperial Medicine College anymore, under the absurd pretext that needle inserting and firing moxa were not suitable to be applied to the Emperor. So the Confucian doctors paid more attention to decoctions while ignoring acupuncture and moxibustion. After China was defeated in Opium War, the imperialists invaded China and set up some missionary hospitals and medical colleges excluding TCM. Thus, TCM, including acupuncture and moxibustion, went on further decline.

After the foundation of the P. R. China, TCM as well as acupuncture and moxibustion was reestablished and developed prosperously due to the implementation of the policies for TCM. Colleges, hospitals of TCM, specialities and departments for acupuncture and moxibustion, and special research institutes were set up throughout China, so that great achievements have been made in many aspects of acupuncture and moxibustion such as in teaching, clinical treatment, scientific research and others.

In the past 30 years, lots of books on acupuncture and moxibustion have been compiled and published. Unified textbooks of acupuncture and moxibustion are used in TCM colleges. Revision and annotation works have been made about *Canon of Medicine*, *Classic on Medical Problems*, *A—B Classic of Acupuncture and Moxibustion*, and *Compendium of Acupuncture and Moxibustion*. Over 10,000 treatises on acupuncture and moxibustion have been published in medical journals in the whole country. All of these have offered a good condition for studying and also enriched the acupuncture and moxibustion.

Great progress of acupuncture and moxibustion has been made in the clinical medicine and more and more diseases can be treated by acupuncture. It is proved by clinical experience that acupuncture and moxibustion are effective to treat more than 300 kinds of diseases in internal medicine, surgery, gynecology, pediatrics and other fields, about 100 of which with a good or very good effect. Acupuncture and moxibustion are effective to treat cardiovascular and cerebral vascular diseases, cholelithes, bacillary dysentery, etc, which is not only proved scientifically, also the mechanism have been disclosed by means of modern physiology, biochemistry, microbiology, immunology and so on. Many materials have been collected. In 1960s, Chinese doctors succeeded in performing surgical operations by using acupuncture anaesthesia. This new development caused world-wide attention and greatly promoted the development of acupuncture and moxibustion.

In recent decades, intensive cross and inter-disciplinary researches on the mechanism of acupuncture have been made by broad co-operation. It is proved that acupuncture has effects on regulating the functions of physiological systems and can increase body ability of defending diseases. The studies on the mechanism of acupuncture analgesia have deepened to the level of molecular biochemistry such as researches about nerve cells, eletrophysiology and neurotransmitters, e.g. enkephalin and others.

Researches on meridians with plenty of general survey have affirmed the objective existence of propagation of acupuncture sensation. Much has been done on the rules, objective indices and determination method of the phenomena of propagated sensation, and this has provided important clues for further studies about the nature of meridians. Meanwhile, researches on the manipulation of acupuncture in many areas have got preliminary achievements.

The acupuncture has contributed to the health care not only for the Chinese people but also for people in other countries for thousands of years. Acupuncture and moxibustion was introduced abroad long ago. In the sixth century A. D., acupuncture and moxibustion spread to Korea with *A-B Classic of Acupuncture and Moxibustion* and other books as textbooks. An ancient Chinese called Zhi Cong came to Japan with *Charts of Three Views* and *A-B Classic of Acupuncture and Moxibustion* in 562 A.D. In 701 A.D., the acupuncture was set up in the medical education system in Japan, and today there are still some colleges of acupuncture and moxibustion which are very popular in Japan. In the later period of 17th century acupuncture and moxibustion came to Europe. Besides, special clinic of acupuncture, special institutes were also established for the study of acupuncture, and many international symposiums on acupuncture and moxibustion were held. International acupuncture training centres have been set up in some provinces and cities of China and have trained a lot of acupuncturists from many countries. So far, acupuncture is used and studied in more than 100 countries all over the world. The unique acupuncture in China has been an important part of world medicine and will have an active and wide influence on it.

In order to inherit and promote TCM, it is an important task for those who want to research on the TCM, the nature of meridians and the mechanism of acupuncture by means of modern science in addition to teach TCM and use the theory of TCM in medical practice. As long as we try to use dialectical materialistic point of view in our work, it is sure that the medicine of acupuncture and moxibustion will get rich harvest and contribute more to the health care of mankind.

Part I Meridians and Points

Chapter 1
A General Introduction to the Meridians

The Meridians is a comprehensive term of "Jingluo" in Traditional Chinese Medicine. They are the passages through which the Qi can be conducted. The meridians mainly refer to the paths of main trunks which run up and down, interiorly and exteriorly within the body. The branches of meridians are called collaterals which imply the networks, thinner and smaller than meridians, run crisscrossly over the body. The chapter, *Discussion on the Measurement of Meridians* (Chapter 17) in *Miraculous Pivot* says: "The meridians are internal trunks, its transversing branches are collaterals, the subdivisions of collaterals are minute collaterals."

The meridians and its collaterals belong to the Zang-Fu organs interiorly and extend to the extremities and joints exteriorly integrating the Zang, the Fu, tissues and organs into an organic whole, by which they transport Qi of blood and regulate Yin and Yang, keeping the functions and activities of all parts of the body in harmony and balance relatively. In the practice of acupuncture, the signs-symptoms differentiation, the corresponding meridian point selection, and the needling for reinforcing and reducing are all based on the theory of the meridians. The chapter "Discussion on the Divergent Meridian" (Chapter 7) in *Miraculous Pivot* says: "The so-called twelve meridians are what life is based on, what diseases are caused by, what patients are cured by, what disorders originated from, what the medical sciences are developed from and what the skills are perfected with." which illustrated the significance of meridians for physiology, pathology, diagnosis and treatment.

The theory of the meridians deals with the courses and distributions, physiological functions, pathological changes of the meridians of the human body, and their relations to the Zang-Fu organs. It guides the diagnosis and treatment for clinic of Traditional Chinese Medicine and it links tightly with the theory of acupuncture.

Section 1   Development of the Theory of the Meridians

The theory of the meridians is formed through long-time practice and observation of Chinese people. Based on the analysis of records, the formation is as follows:

1. Observation of Needling Sensation: Acupuncture produces sensation of soreness, numbness, distension or heaviness. This sensation usually goes to the distal region along a definite pathway.

2. The Summary of the Therapeutic Effects of Acupoint: The acupoints which have similar clinical effects are regularly lined on the same course.

3. Reference of the Pathological Phenomenon on the Body Surface: When there appears the disorder in a certain organ, then on the corresponding areas of the body surface appear tenderness, tubercles, skin rash and changes of the skin color, this is also another way of discovering the system of meridians.

4. Suggestions from knowledge of Anatomy and Physiology: With the help of anatomy, Chinese doctors in ancient times got to know the position, the appearance and some physiological functions of internal organs, and observed the tunnel-like and the cord-like structures are distributed over the body and connected with four limbs as well. The phenomenon of the circulation of blood can be seen in same blood vessels.

Above-mentioned statements indicate that there are various ways of discovering meridians, different understandings can be inter-supplemented, inter-proved and inter-suggestive, thus we may know more and more about the meridians. According to documents remained today, the theory of the meridians had been formed over 2000 years ago.

Section 2   The Composition of the Meridians System

The system of meridians consists of main meridians and their collaterals. The meridians include the Twelve Regular Meridians, the Eight Extra Meridians and those subordinate to the Twelve Regular Meridians, the Twelve Divergent

Meridians, the Twelve Muscle Regions and the Twelve Cutaneous Regions. The collaterals consist of the Fifteen Collaterals, the Superficial Collaterals, and the Minute Collaterals. The composition of the system of the meridians and collaterals is shown in the following in table:

Table 1-1 The Composition of the System of the Meridians and their Collaterals

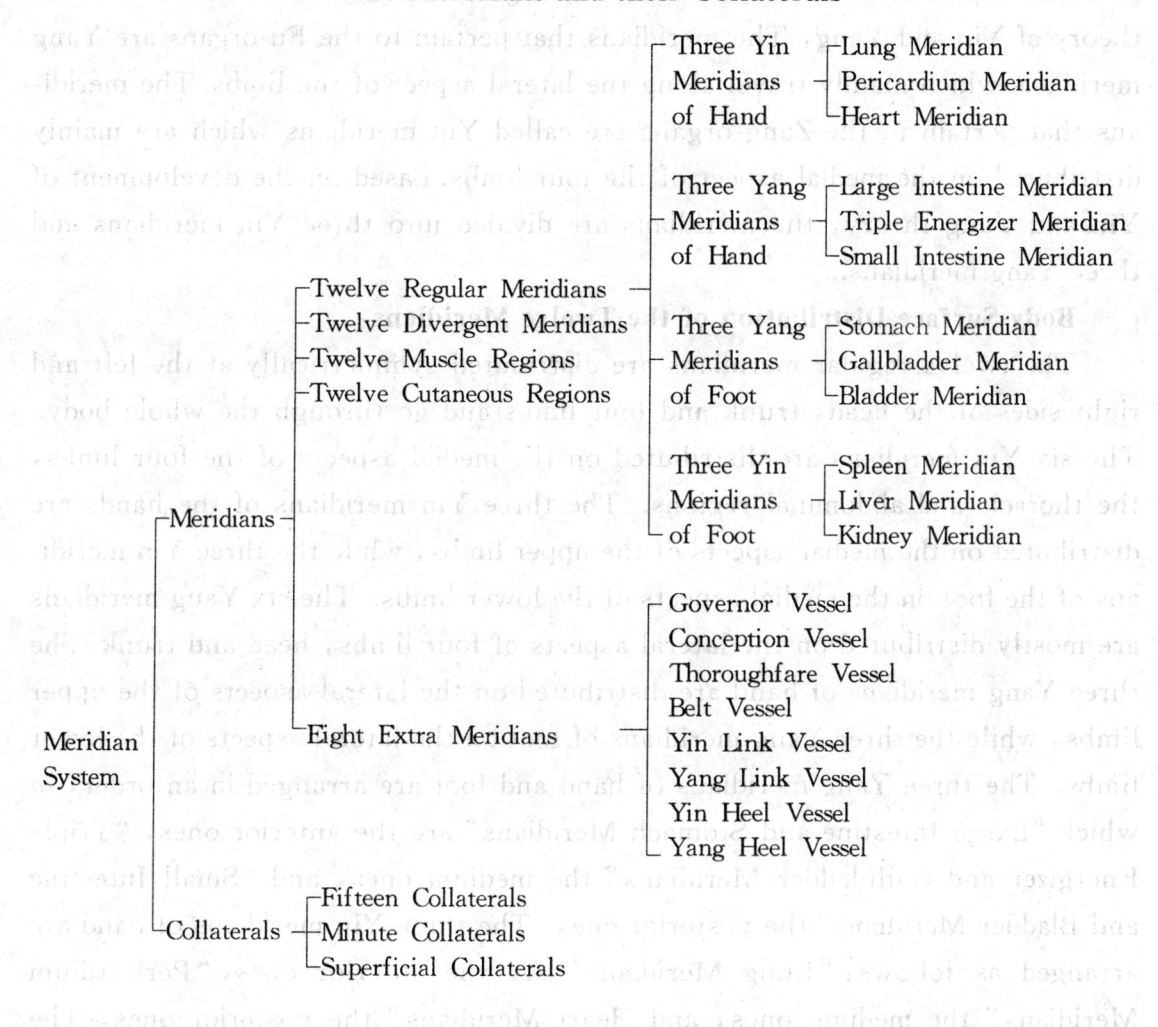

```
                    ┌─ Twelve Regular Meridians ─┬─ Three Yin Meridians of Hand ─┬─ Lung Meridian
                    │                            │                               ├─ Pericardium Meridian
                    │                            │                               └─ Heart Meridian
                    │                            │
                    │                            ├─ Three Yang Meridians of Hand ─┬─ Large Intestine Meridian
                    │                            │                                ├─ Triple Energizer Meridian
                    │                            │                                └─ Small Intestine Meridian
                    │                            │
                    │                            ├─ Three Yang Meridians of Foot ─┬─ Stomach Meridian
         ┌─ Meridians ─┤                         │                                ├─ Gallbladder Meridian
         │          │  ├─ Twelve Divergent Meridians                              └─ Bladder Meridian
         │          │  ├─ Twelve Muscle Regions  │
         │          │  └─ Twelve Cutaneous Regions
         │          │                            └─ Three Yin Meridians of Foot ─┬─ Spleen Meridian
Meridian ┤                                                                       ├─ Liver Meridian
System   │                                                                       └─ Kidney Meridian
         │          ┌─ Eight Extra Meridians ─┬─ Governor Vessel
         │                                    ├─ Conception Vessel
         │                                    ├─ Thoroughfare Vessel
         │                                    ├─ Belt Vessel
         │                                    ├─ Yin Link Vessel
         │                                    ├─ Yang Link Vessel
         │                                    ├─ Yin Heel Vessel
         │                                    └─ Yang Heel Vessel
         │
         └─ Collaterals ─┬─ Fifteen Collaterals
                         ├─ Minute Collaterals
                         └─ Superficial Collaterals
```

1. Twelve Regular Meridians

The Twelve Regular Meridians include Three Yin Meridians of Hand(Lung, Pericardium and Heart), Three Yang Meridians of Hand(Large Intestine, Triple Energizer and Small Intestine), Three Yang Meridians of Foot(Stomach, Gallbladder and Bladder), Three Yin Meridians of Foot (Spleen, Liver and Kidney). They are the major trunks of the system of the meridians, so they are called the

Twelve Regular Meridians.

The nomenclature of the Twelve Regular Meridians is based on the three factors: a) hand or foot, b) Yin or Yang, and c) Zang or Fu organ. The Twelve Regular Meridians pertain to the twelve Zang and Fu organs correspondingly, each regular meridian is named after the organ to which it pertains. In consideration of the factors, such as hand or foot, interior or exterior, anterior, middle or posterior aspect of the meridian travels through, and also in accordance with the theory of Yin and Yang, The meridians that pertain to the Fu-organs are Yang meridians which mainly travel along the lateral aspect of the limbs. The meridians that pertain to the Zang-organs are called Yin meridians which are mainly distributed on the medial aspect of the four limbs. Based on the development of Yin and Yang theory, the meridians are divided into three Yin meridians and three Yang meridians.

Body-Surface Distribution of the Twelve Meridians:

The twelve regular meridians are distributed symmetrically at the left and right sides of the head, trunk and four limbs and go through the whole body. The six Yin meridians are distributed on the medial aspects of the four limbs, the thoracic and abdominal regions. The three Yin meridians of the hands are distributed on the medial aspects of the upper limbs, while the three Yin meridians of the foot on the medial aspects of the lower limbs. The six Yang meridians are mostly distributed on the lateral aspects of four limbs, head and trunk. The three Yang meridians of hand are distributed on the lateral aspects of the upper limbs, while the three Yang meridians of foot on the lateral aspects of the lower limbs. The three Yang meridians of hand and foot are arranged in an order, in which "Large Intestine and Stomach Meridians" are the anterior ones, "Triple Energizer and Gallbladder Meridians" the medium ones, and "Small Intestine and Bladder Meridians" the posterior ones. The three Yin meridians of hand are arranged as follows: "Lung Meridians" are the anterior ones, "Pericardium Meridians" the medium ones, and Heart Meridians" the posterior ones, The three Yin meridians of foot are to the aspects of the lower limbs and instep. They are arranged in an order in which Liver Meridians are the anterior ones, Spleen Meridians are the medium ones, Kidney Meridians are the posterior ones, under the lever 8 cun above the medial malleolus, Liver Meridians and Spleen Meridians are crossed, then, Spleen Meridian is in the anterior aspect, Liver Meridian in the medium aspect, Kidney Meridian in the posterior aspect.

The Exterior-Interior and Pertaining Relation of the Twelve Regular Meridians:

The Twelve Regular Meridians pertain to Zang-Fu organs interiorly, there is an exterior-interior and corresponding relation between Zang and Fu organs, an exterior-interior and pertaining relation between Yin meridians and Yang meridians. That is, the Lung Meridian has an exterior and interior relations with the Large Intestine Meridian, the Stomach Meridian with the Spleen Meridian, the Heart Meridian with the Small Intestine Meridian, the Bladder Meridian with the Kidney Meridian, the Pericardium Meridian with the Triple Energizer Meridian, and the Gallbladder Meridian with the Liver Meridian. There is a pertaining and communicative relation between the Yin meridians and Yang meridians connected interiorly-exteriorly in the body. The Yin meridians pertain to the Zang-organs, and communicate with the Fu-organs, while the Yang meridians pertain to the Fu-organs, and communicate with the Zang-organs. For example, the Lung Meridian pertains to the lung and communicates with the large intestine, the Large Intestine Meridian pertains to the large intestine and communicates with the lung. The relation of interior and exterior meridians is reinforced by linking the collaterals in the four limbs. Thus six pairs of the interior-exterior, pertaining and communicative relations are formed among Zang and Fu, Yin and Yang and meridians. There is a close relation physiologically among the interior-exterior meridians. They are inter-affected during the pathological changes and inter-action during treatment.

Courses and Links of the Twelve Meridians:

The Courses of The Twelve Meridians: Three Yin meridians of hand start from the chest to the hands.

Three Yang meridians of hand run from hands to the head. Three Yang meridians of foot run from the head to the feet. Three Yin meridians of foot run from the feet to abdomen and chest.

Links of the Twelve Regular Meridians:

(1) The Yin Meridians link with the Yang meridians mainly in the limbs. For instance, the Lung Meridian links with the Large Intestine Meridian on the tip of the index finger. The Stomach Meridian connects with the Spleen Meridian on the tip of the great toe, the Bladder Meridian reaches the lateral side of the tip of the little toe where it links with the Kidney Meridian. The Gallbladder Meridian runs to the distal portion of the great toe and terminates at its hairy re-

gion where it links with the Liver Meridian.

(2) The Yang meridians and Yang meridians (with the same nomenclature) are met on the head. For instance, both the Large Intestine meridian and the Stomach Meridian go to both sides of the nose. Both the Small Intestine Meridian and the Bladder Meridian reach the inner canthus, and both the Triple Energizer Meridian and the Gallbladder Meridian reach the outer canthus.

(3) The Yin meridians and Yin meridians are met in the chest region. For instance, the Spleen Meridian links with the Heart Meridian in the heart, the Kidney Meridian links with the Pericardium Meridian in the chest, and the Liver Meridian links with the Lung Meridian in the lung.

The Twelve Meridians are connected with each other through the hand-foot, Yin-Yang, and interior-exterior relations, so they form the system of a cyclic flow, and the Qi and blood can travel all over the body to the Zang-Fu organs interiorly and to the muscles and superficies exteriorly, nourish the whole body. See the table as follows:

Table 1-2 The Twelve Meridian's distribution on the body surface, their circulation, and their relations with Zang-Fu organs.

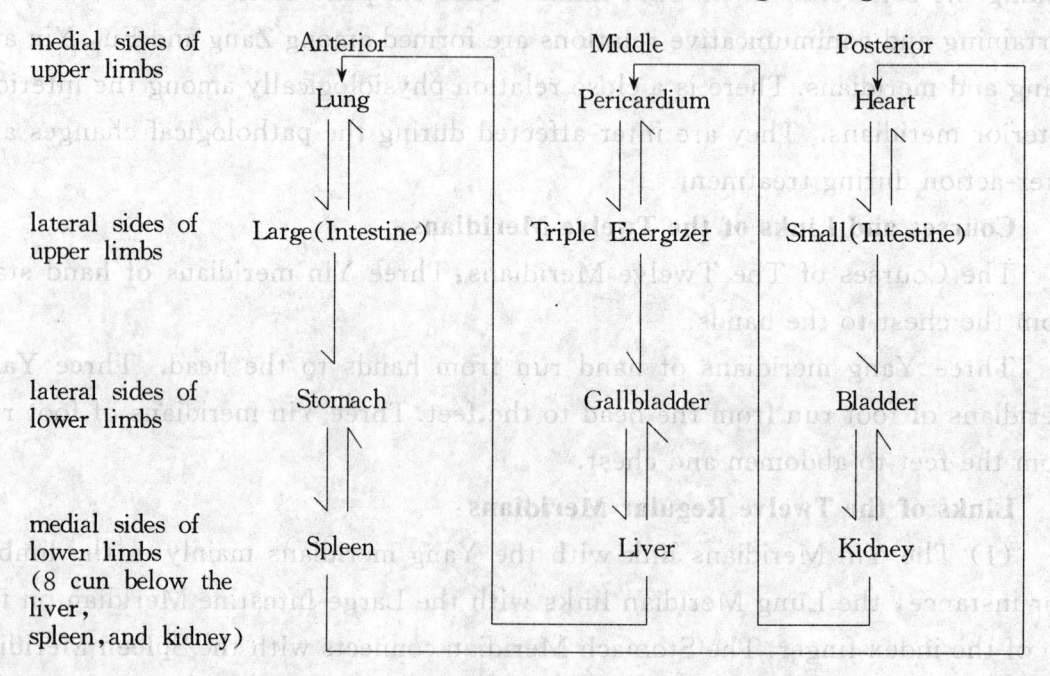

	Anterior	Middle	Posterior
medial sides of upper limbs	Lung ⇅	Pericardium ⇅	Heart ⇅
lateral sides of upper limbs	Large (Intestine) ↓	Triple Energizer ↓	Small (Intestine) ↓
lateral sides of lower limbs	Stomach ⇅	Gallbladder ⇅	Bladder ⇅
medial sides of lower limbs (8 cun below the liver, spleen, and kidney)	Spleen	Liver	Kidney

12

2. Eight Extra Meridians

The Eight Extra Meridians are the Governor Vessel, Conception Vessel, Thoroughfare Vessel, Belt Vessel, Yin Link Vessel, Yang Link Vessel, Yin Heel Vessel, Yang Heel Vessel. Unlike the Twelve Regular Meridians, none of them pertain to the Zang-Fu organs. And they are not exteriorly-interiorly related. Their courses are unique, and hence, they are called extra meridians.

The Governor, Conception and Thoroughfare Vessels arise from the lower abdomen and emerge from the perineum, so they are called three streams of one source. The Governor Vessel runs posteriorly along the interior of the spinal column and reaches the head. The Conception Vessel goes along the interior of the abdomen, passes through the cheek and enters the infraorbital region. The Thoroughfare Vessel runs parallel to the Kidney Meridian and curves around the lips. The Belt Vessel originates below the hypochondriac region and runs transversely around the waist like a belt. The Yin Link Vessel starts from the medial aspect of the leg and ascends along the medial aspect of the thigh to the abdomen, reaches the throat and communicates with the Conception Vessel. The Yang Link Vessel emerges from the external malleolus, ascending along the external side of the leg, then reaches the back of the neck where it communicates with the Governor Vessel. The Yin Heel Vessel starts from the medial side of the heel, and ascends along the Kidney Meridian, it reaches the inner canthus and communicates with the Yang Heel Vessel. The Yang Heel Vessel starts from the lateral side of the heel and ascends along the Bladder Meridians, then it enters inner canthus to communicate with the Yin Heel Vessel, it runs upward along the Bladder Meridian to the forehead and reaches the back of the neck where it meets the Gallbladder Meridians.

The Eight Extra Meridians are distributed among the Twelve Regular Meridians. They contain two main functions.

(1) They can strengthen the relationships among the Twelve Regular Meridians. The Eight Extra Meridians communicate with the other meridians which have the related aspects and the similar functions. They assume the responsibility to control, store the Qi and blood of each meridian and regulate Yin and Yang. The Governor Vessel meets all the Yang meridians, thus it is called "The sea of the Yang Meridians", its function is to govern the Qi of all the Yang meridians of the body. The Conception Vessel meets all the Yin meridians, thus it is called "the sea of the Yin Meridians", its function is to receive and bear the

Qi of the Yin meridians. The Thoroughfare Vessel meets the Conception Vessel, the Governor Vessel, the Stomach Meridians, the Kidney Meridians, so it is termed "the sea of the Twelve Regular Meridians" or "the sea of blood". Its function is to reserve the Qi and blood of the Twelve Regular Meridians. The Belt Vessel performs a function of binding up all the meridians of foot on trunk. The Yang Link Vessel is connected with all Yang meridians and dominates the exterior of the whole body, the Yin Link Vessel is connected with all the Yin meridians and dominates the interior of the whole body. The Yin and Yang Heel Vessel dominate the Yang activity and the Yin calmness, and control the movement of lower limbs and sleep.

(2) The Eight Extra meridians can regulate the Qi and blood of the regular meridians, when the Qi and blood of Zang-Fu organs are vigorous, the Eight Extra Meridian can store them; while the body needs them for its activity, they can be supplied by The Eight Extra Meridians. Acupoints of the Thoroughfare, Belt, Heel and Link Vessels pertain to the Twelve Regular Meridians and the Conception and Governor Vessels. The Conception and the Governor Vessels which have their own acupoints together with the Twelve Regular Meridians are called "the Fourteen Meridians". The Fourteen Meridians contain the regular courses, symptoms and their own acupoints, they are main parts of the system of the meridians. They are basic factors for acupuncture treatment and classification of medicinals according to the meridians on which their therapeutic action is manifested. The distribution of the Fourteen Meridians is as follows: (Fig. 1-1)

3. Fifteen Collaterals

The Fifteen Collaterals include the twelve collaterals which branch out from the Twelve Regular Meridians, the collaterals of the Conception, the Governor and the Major Collateral of the Spleen. They are named respectively after the names of the points from where they start. The collaterals of the Twelve Meridians branch out from the regular meridians below the elbow and knee, go toward their interiorly-exteriorly related meridians. The collateral of the Conception Vessel comes out from Jiuwei (CV 15) and spreads over the abdomen. The Collateral of the Governor Vessel arises from Changqiang (GV 1) and spreads over the top of the head. It goes along the Bladder Meridians on the right and left sides. The Major Collateral of the Spleen Meridian begins from Dabao (SP 21) and spreads through the chest and hypochondriac region. Among the collaterals of the whole body, the Fifteen Collaterals are larger, "Superficial Collaterals"

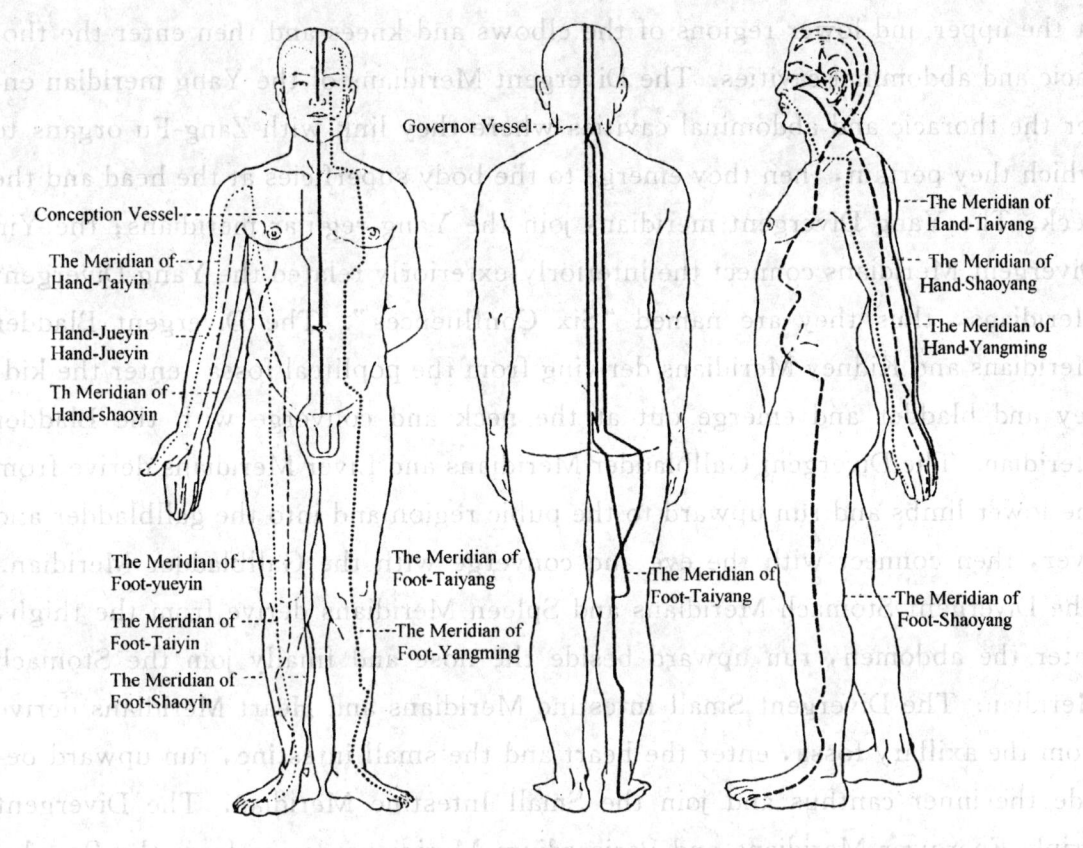

Fig. 1-1　Distributions of the Fourteen Meridians

are those which are distributed on the superficies of the body, and the smallest branches of the collaterals are called "Minute Collaterals". They are innumerable and are distributed all over the body.

　　The collaterals of the twelve meridians strengthen the relations of the Yin-Yang and the Exterior-interior meridians. The collaterals of the Conception Vessel communicate with the Qi of meridian in the abdominal region. The collaterals of the Governor Vessel communicate with the Qi of meridian in the back region. The Major Collateral of the Spleen Meridian communicates with the Qi of meridian in the lateral side of the chest. Minute Collaterals are very thin and distributed densely, their functions are to transport Qi and blood and nourish the tissues.

4. Twelve Divergent Meridians

　　The Twelve Divergent Meridians are the branches which derive from, enter, leave and join the Twelve Regular Meridians which, in turn, reach the deeper parts of the body through these branches.

　　Most of the Twelve Divergent Meridians derive from the Regular Meridians

15

at the upper and lower regions of the elbows and knees and then enter the thoracic and abdominal cavities. The Divergent Meridians of the Yang meridian enter the thoracic and abdominal cavities where they link with Zang-Fu organs to which they pertain, then they emerge to the body superficies at the head and the neck. The Yang Divergent meridians join the Yang regular meridians; the Yin Divergent Meridians connect the interiorly-exteriorly related the Yang Divergent Meridians, thus they are named "Six Confluences". The Divergent Bladder Meridians and Kidney Meridians deriving from the popliteal fossa, enter the kidney and bladder and emerge out at the neck and converge with the Bladder Meridian. The Divergent Gallbladder Meridians and Liver Meridians derive from the lower limbs and run upward to the pubic region and into the gallbladder and liver, then connect with the eye and converge with the Gallbladder Meridian. The Divergent Stomach Meridians and Spleen Meridians derive from the thigh, enter the abdomen, run upward beside the nose and finally join the Stomach Meridian. The Divergent Small Intestine Meridians and Heart Meridians derive from the axillary fossa, enter the heart and the small intestine, run upward beside the inner canthus and join the Small Intestine Meridian. The Divergent Triple Energizer Meridians and Pericardium Meridians derive from the Regular Meridians, enter the chest, cross Triple Energizer, emerge out behind the ear, then converge with the Triple Energizer Meridian. The Divergent Large Intestine Meridians and Lung Meridians derive from the Regular Meridians, connect with the lung and disperse in the large intestine, emerge out upward from Quepen(ST 12) and converge with the Large Intestine Meridian. Thus, the Twelve Divergent Meridians strengthen the connections between the Zang and Fu organs by the distribution of branching out from the Twelve Regular Meridians. They bring the Twelve Regular Meridians and all parts of the body closer, and extend the scope of indications of the acupoints (the Liver Meridian not included), For example, the Yin meridians don't run in the head region, but the Yin Divergent Meridians join the exterior-interior Yang meridians on the head, this strengthens the relations between the Yin meridians and the head. The diseases of the head and sense organs can be cured by needling the acupoints of the three Yin meridians of Hand-Foot because of the relations of the divergent meridians. Select Lieque (LU 7), Taiyuan(LU 9) for headache and migraine, Taixi(KI 3)and Zhaohai(KI 6) for toothache and throat conditions.

5. Twelve Muscle Regions

The Twelve Muscle Regions are the conduits which distribute the Qi of the Twelve Regular Meridians to the muscles, tendons and joints, They are external connecting regions of the Twelve Regular Meridians.

The distribution of the muscle regions is parallel to the body superficies course of the Regular Meridians. All the muscle regions start from the terminals of the limbs and run on to the head and trunk. Instead of entering Zang-Fu organs, they travel along the body surface and connect with the joints and bones. Three Yang Muscle Regions of Foot start from toes and ascend along the lateral aspect of the leg and end at the face. Three Yin Muscle Regions of Foot originate from the toes, and ascend along the medial aspect of the leg and to the genital region. Three Yang Muscle Regions of Hand start from the fingers and proceed up along the lateral side of arm and end at the angle of forehead. Three Yin Muscle Regions of Hand start from the finger, run along the medial side of the arm and end in the thoracic cavity. In their circulations, the Twelve Muscle Regions connect with ankle, popliteal fossa, knee, thigh, wrist, elbow, axilla, shoulder and neck. Especially the Liver Muscle Region knots with the genital region and connects with all the other muscle regions.

The main functions of the muscle regions are to connect with all the bones and control them to ease flexing and extending of the joints and normal motion of the body. This refers to in the Chapter "Discussion on Flaccidity-Syndrome" (Chapter 44) in *Plain Questions* "The tendons control and connect with bone to ensure proper joint."

6. Twelve Cutaneous Regions

The Twelve Cutaneous Regions refer to the body superficies on which the functions of the Twelve Regular Meridians are reflected, and the sites where the Qi of the collaterals spreads. In the Chapter "Discussion on the Cutaneous Regions" (Chapter 56) in *Plain Questions* Says: "The Twelve Meridians and Collaterals are also demonstrated over the Twelve Cutaneous Regions." The Cutaneous Regions are within the domains of the Twelve Regular Meridians. In the Chapter "Discussion on the Cutaneous Regions" (Chapter 56) in *Plain Questions*, it points out "The Cutaneous Regions are marked by the regular meridians." Since the Cutaneous Regions are the most superficial part of the body tissues, they render protection to the organism.

The system of the meridians consist of the collaterals, the Twelve Regular Meridians, the Eight Extra Meridians above-mentioned, the Twelve Divergent Meridians, the Twelve Muscle Regions and the Twelve Cutaneous Regions. They frame up to a close-related integrated system.

Section 3 The Gen, Jie, Biao, Ben, Qijie, and the Four Seas of the Meridians

The theory of the meridians includes the concept of the Gen, Jie, Biao, Ben, Qijie and four seas. From another angle, it explains the relations between the meridians system and the various organs of the body.

The Chapter "Discussion on the Gen and Jie" (Chapter 5) in *Miraculous Pivot* points out the Gen of the six meridians of foot locate at Jing(well)point of the terminals of the limbs, the Jie are in the fixed regions of the head, chest and abdomen regions. (See Table 1-3)

Table 1-3 Gen and Jie of Six Meridians of Foot

Meridian	Gen	jie
Bladder Meridian	Zhiyin(BL 67)	Jingming(BL 1)
Stomach Meridian	Lidui(ST 45)	Touwei(ST 8)
Gallbladder Meridian	Zuqiaoyin(GB 44)	Tinggong(SI 19)
Spleen Meridian	Yinbai(SP 1)	Zhongwan(CV 12)
Kidney Meridian	Yongquan(KI 1)	Lianquan(CV 23)
Liver Meridian	Dadun(LR 1)	Yutang(CV 18) Tanzhong(CV 17)

In the essay *Biao Chu Fu* Dou Hanqing further explained the four Gen and the three Jie of the Twelve Regular Meridians, that the limbs were regarded as the Gen and the head, chest, and abdomen as the Jie.

The Chapter"Discussion on the Defence-Qi"(Chapter 52)in *Miraculous Pivot* stated Biao and Ben of the twelve meridians. Generally, Ben remains in the limbs, and Biao in the head and trunk. Their distributions are wider than those of the Gen and Jie. (See Table 1-4)

Table 1-4 Locations of Biao and Ben of the Twelve Meridians

	Meridians	Locations of Ben	Locations of Biao
Three Foot Yang	Bladder Meridian	between heel and 5 cun above heel	Eyes
	Gallbladder Meridian	Zuqiaoyin(GB 44)	Anterior ear
	Stomach Meridian	Lidui(ST 45)	Neck, cheek, Hangsang
Three Foot Yin	Kidney Meridian	Jiaoxin(KI 8)	Beishu and two meridians below the tongue
	Liver Meridian	the dorsum of foot	Beishu
	Spleen Meridian	between medial ankle and 4 cun above ankle	Beishu and the root of tongue
Three Hand Yang	Small Intestine Meridian	the dorsum of wrist	1 cun above the eyes
	Triple Energizer Meridian	Zhongzhu(TE 3)	In the depression at the lateral end of eyebrow
	Large Intestine Meridian	Elbow	lateral to the nose
Three Hand Yin	Lung Meridian	in the depression on the radial side of the radial artery(Cunkou)	in the axillary artery
	Heart Meridian	at the ulna end of the transverse crease of the wrist	Beishu
	Pericardium Meridian	2 cun above the transverse crease of the wrist, between the tendons of medial palmaris longus and medial flexor radials	3 cun below the axilla

The positions of Gen and Ben and Jie and Biao are quite close or same, and their significances are very similar. Gen and Ben locate in the lower parts of the body, they are the source of the meridian Qi. Jie and Biao locate in the upper parts of the body, they are the terminals of the meridian Qi.

The theory of Biao, Ben, Gen and Jie explains the cyclical flow of the meridian Qi. The Chapter "Discussion on the Meridian" (Chapter 10) in *Miraculous Pivot*, the Chapter "Discussion on the going against, conform to, fat and thin"

(Chapter 38) in *Miraculous Pivot*, and the Chapter "Discussion on the Nutrient-Qi" (Chapter 16) in *Miraculous Pivot* state the system of the cyclical flow of the twelve meridians, which promotes the flow of Qi and blood endlessly and nourishes the whole body. This theory not only explains the close relationship between the four limbs, the head and the trunk. but also emphasizes that the limbs are the Gen and the Ben of the meridian Qi. In clinical practice, doctors puncture the acupoints in the limbs region, which easily stimulates the meridian Qi and regulates the function of the meridian and collaterals of Zang-Fu organs, so the acupoints in the lower regions of the elbow and knees contain a wide scope of indications. These acupoints can be applied not only for the local treatment, but also for the distal treatment, such as the diseases of the Zang-Fu organs, head and sense organs.

Qijie refers to the common passages through which the meridian Qi circulates. The Chapter "Discussion on the Defence-Qi" (Chapter 52) in *Miraculous Pivot* says: "There are passages for the chest Qi, abdomen Qi, head Qi and the leg Qi."

The Qijie locates mainly in the regions of the Jie and the Biao. Based on this theory, the diseases of the local region and internal organs can be cured by stimulating acupoints distributed on the head and the trunk, some acupoints can be applied for the disease of the limbs.

The Chapter "Discussion on the Sea" (Chapter 33) in *Miraculous Pivot* points out that there are four seas in the body, brain referring to the sea of medulla, Tanzhong referring to the sea of Qi, stomach referring to the sea of grain and water, Thoroughfare Vessel referring to the sea of the Twelve Meridians and also called the sea of blood.

There is a similarity in the locations of the four seas and the Qijie. The sea of medulla is in the head, the sea of Qi in the chest, the sea of grain and water in the upper abdomen. the sea of blood in the lower abdomen. They are connected one another and dominate the Qi, blood and body fluid of the whole body.

The region of brain is regarded as the sea of medulla, which is the origin of the vital energy. It dominates the activities of the meridians of Zang-Fu organs. The thoracic region is the sea of Qi, where the pectoral energy is stored. It promotes the movement of lung and the circulation of heart blood. The region of stomach is the sea of grain and water. It is the source of nutrient Qi and defensive Qi. The Thoroughfare Vessel starts from the womb, named blood chamber concerning with menstruation. So Thoroughfare Vessel is called the sea of blood. Classic on Medical Problems says: "The lower part of the navel where Qi is moving in between the kidneys." The basis of the twelve meridians is the Yuan Qi (primary Qi), spreading over five Zang and six Fu organs through Triple Energizer Meridian. It is the energy resource of the vital activity of the body. The vital energy consists of pectoral Qi, defensive Qi, nutrient Qi and primary Qi. The vital energy going through the meridians is called the meridian Qi, thus the theory of the four seas further indicates the formation and the origin of the meridian Qi.

Section 4 Physiological Functions of the Meridian System and Clinical Application of the Theory of the Meridian

1. The Physiological Functions of the Meridians

The meridians have the function of connecting: the human body contains the five Zang-organs, the six Fu-organs, four limbs, all the bones of the body, five sense organs, nine body orifices, skin, muscle, tendon and bone. Each of them has its own physiological function, but contributes the organism an organic integral activity. The Twelve Regular Meridians run vertically and horizontally, communicate with all parts, upper and lower, interior or exterior of the body and ensure the proper coordination and unification of the various functions of the body. These connections and coordinations are fulfilled by the function of the meridian system. The Chapter "Discussion on the Sea" (Chapter 33) in *Miraculous Pivot* says: "These Twelve Regular Meridians pertain to the Zang-Fu organs interiorly and communicate with the limbs and joints exteriorly."

The function of nourishing: The Chapter "Discussion on the Important Basis of Zang Organs" (Chapter 47) in *Miraculous Pivot* says: "the circulation of Qi and blood, nourish the Yin and Yang, soften the tendon and bones, lubricate the joints." That implies the meridian system can circulate Qi and blood, regulate Yin and Yang, and nourish the entire body. All the Zang-Fu organs need to be nourished by Qi and blood, then maintain their normal physiological functions. The Qi and blood provide a material base for the vital activities of the body. It is through the meridians that the Qi and blood are transported to all the parts of the body.

The function of resisting exopathogens: Because the meridians can transport the Qi and blood, nourish Yin and Yang, the nutrient Qi circulates the meridians interiorly, the defensive Qi runs along the meridians exteriorly. This makes the nutrient Qi and the defensive Qi spread over the whole body and strengthen the body resistance against the disease. They work to resist exopathogens and defend the organism. The Chapter "Discussion on the Important Basis of Zang-Organs" (Chapter 47) in *Miraculous Pivot* says "The softness of the skin and the tightness of interspace are resulted from proper muscular structure and the harmony of defensive Qi."

2. Clinical Application of the Theory of the Meridians

Guiding the clinical diagnosis: As each meridian or collateral has its own specific course and specific Zang or Fu organ to which it pertains, so that disorder of the Zang or Fu organs will reflect symptoms and sign along the course of the meridian. Taking this into account can be the basis for clinical diagnosis. For instance, headache, pain in the forehead is diagnosed as pathogenic changes of the Yangming Meridians, pain in both sides of the head is diagnosed as pathogenic changes of the Shaoyang Meridians, pain in the neck is connecting with pathogenic changes of Taiyang Meridians, pain in the top of head is linking with pathogenic changes of the Jueyin Meridians. Besides, doctors can diagnose diseases according to reactive changes along the courses of meridians such as sensitive tenderness, tubercles and cord-like things, for instance, if one has got appendicitis, sensitive tenderness can be found at Shangjuxu (ST 37) of the Stomach Meridian. Tenderness appears at Yanglingquan (GB 34) of the Gallbladder Meridian when one gets cholecystitis. Doctors can make clinical diagnosis by pressing along the courses of the meridians or testing electric resistance of the skin.

Guiding the treatment: The acupuncture is a therapy by needling or fuming certain acupoint with moxa smoke to transport Qi and blood, and regulate the function of the Zang-Fu organs. Based on the principle "the diseases can be cured when the affected meridians or the affected Zang-Fu organs are cleared." The selection of points along the course of meridians is the basic principle. It refers to selection of points from the affected meridian or from the meridian pertaining to the affected Zang or Fu organs, just as mentioned in *the Song of Four Major Acupoints*: "To needle Zusanli (ST 36) for stomach and abdomen disorder, to needle Weizhong (BL 40) for lumbar and back disorder, to puncture Lieque (LU 7) for head and neck disorder and to puncture Hegu (LI 4) for facial and mouth disorder."

Besides, in view of the close relation of the cutaneous region to the meridians and collaterals and Zang-Fu organs, diseases of the meridians and collaterals and Zang-Fu organs can be treated by using plum-flower needle to tap the skin or embedding an intradermal needle and needling the collaterals to let blood out.

Section 5   Courses of the Twelve Regular Meridians and Their Principal Symptoms

1. Lung Meridian

The Chapter "Discussion on the Meridians" (Chapter 10) in *Miraculous Pivot*: the Lung Meridian originates from the middle energizer, running downward to connect with the large intestine. Winding back, it goes along the upper orifice of the stomach, passes upward through the diaphragm, and enters the lung, its pertaining organ. From the lung, it comes out transversely from the axilla, running downward along the medial aspect of the upper arm, it reaches the cubital fossa, then it goes continuously downward along the anterior border of the radial side in the medial aspect of the forearm and enters Cunkou. Passing the thenar eminence, and going along its radial border, it ends at the medial side of the tip of the thumb. The branch emerges from the posterior wrist and runs along the dorsum of the hand onto the radial side of the tip of the index finger. (Fig. 1-2)

Principal Symptoms: The main symptoms from disorder of Lung Meridian are lung congestion, dyspnea, cough, and pain in the supraclavicular fossa. The pain may be so sharp that the patient clasps his hands across the chest with blurred vision, which is named "Bijue" in TCM. A disorder of the meridian, affected by lung disease, is symptomatized by cough, asthma, thirst, impatience, chest congestion, pain and a cold feeling along the anterior border of the medial aspect of the arm, and a burning sensation in the palms. One whose Qi of the meridian is excessive has a pain in the shoulder and the back, or coryza caused by wind and cold, or sweat due to catching pathogenic wind, or frequency of micturition and oliguria. One whose Qi of the meridian is deficient has pain and cold feeling in the shoulder and the back, or has difficulty in breathing or the colour change of his urine.

2. Large Intestine Meridian

The Chapter "Discussion on the Meridians" (Chapter 10) in *Miraculous Pivot* says: the Large Intestine Meridian starts from the tip of the index finger, running

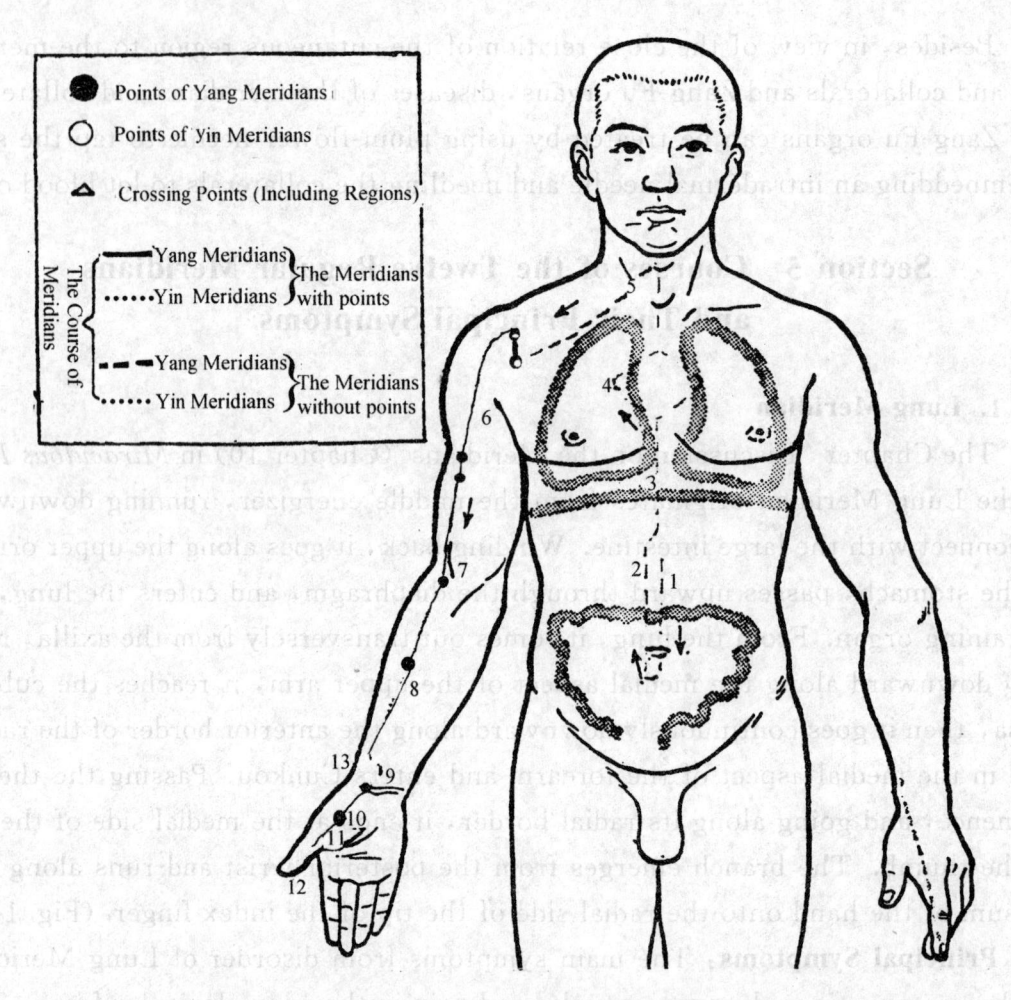

- ● Points of Yang Meridians
- ○ Points of Yin Meridians
- △ Crossing Points (Including Regions)

The Course of Meridians:
- ——— Yang Meridians / ······ Yin Meridians } The Meridians with points
- - - - Yang Meridians / ······ Yin Meridians } The Meridians without points

Fig. 1-2 The Lung Meridian of Hand-Taiyin

upward along the radial side of the index finger and passing through the interspace of the 1st and 2nd metacarpal bones, it enters the depression between the tendons of m. extensor pollcis longus and brevis. Then, running on along the anterior aspect of the forearm, it reaches the lateral side of the elbow. Then it ascends along the lateral anterior aspect of the upper arm to the highest point of the shoulder, then along the anterior border of the acromion, it goes up to the cervical vertebra and descends to Quepen (ST 12) and connects with lung. Then it passes through the diaphragm and enters the large intestine, its pertaining organ.

The branch from Quepen (ST 12) runs upward to the neck, passes through the cheek and enters the lower gums. Then it turns back to the upper lip and crosses the opposite meridian at Renzhong(the philtrum). The left meridian goes to the right and the right meridian to the left, to the contralateral sides of the nose. (Fig. 1-3)

Principal Symptoms: Disorder of the meridian causes toothache and swelling of the neck. Disease of the large intestine and the disorder of the body fluid the disease affects, gives rise to icteric sclera, dry mouth, epistaxis, pharyngitis, pain along the anterior border of the shoulder and the upper arm, and limitation of the index finger. Those whose Qi of the meridian is excessive probably suffer from heat and swelling of the regions where the meridian passes, while those whose Qi of the meridian is deficient often suffer from severe shivering.

3. Stomach Meridian

The Stomach Meridian starts from the lateral side of ala nosi. It ascends to the bridge of the nose, where it meets the Bladder Meridian, turning downward along the lateral side of the nose, it enters the upper gum. Reemerging, it

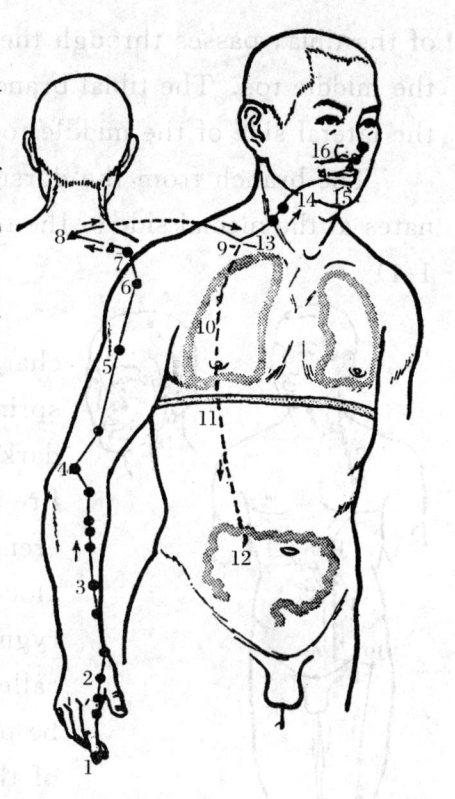

Fig. 1-3 The Large Intestine Meridian of Hand-Yangming

curves round the lips, descends to meet Chengjiang (CV 24), then it runs posterior laterally across the lower position of the cheek at Daying (ST 5). Winding along the angle of the mandible-Jiache, it ascends in front of the ear and traverses Shangguan (GB 3) then it follows the anterior hairline, and reaches the forehead.

The branch emerging in front of Daying (ST 5) runs downwards to Renying (ST 9), it goes along the throat and enters the supraclavicular fossa. Descending, it passes through the diaphragm, enters the stomach, the pertaining organ, and meets the spleen.

The branch emerging from the supraclavicular fossa runs downward passing through the nipple. It descends by the umbilicus and enters Qichong (ST 30) on the lateral side of the lower abdomen.

The branch from the lower orifice of the stomach descends inside the abdomen and joins the previous portion of the meridian at Qichong (ST 30), running downward, traversing Biguan (ST 31), and reaching Futu (ST 32) and then the knee. It continues downward along the anterior border of the lateral aspect of the tibia, passes through the dorsum of the foot and enters the medial side of the middle toe. The tibial branch emerges from 3 cun below the knee and enters the lateral side of the middle toe.

The branch from the dorsum of the foot rises from the dorsum and terminates at the medial side of the tip of the great toe and comes out at the tip. (Fig. 1-4)

Principal Symptoms: Disease of the meridian is characterized by shivering with a feeling of cold water sprinkling over the body, groaning and yawning, and dark complexion. In fulminat stage, it shows fear to fire and people, frightened by woody sound and preference of staying alone. Serious case shows singing aloud on height or running around nakedly. Borborygmus and abdominal distension may exist and is called "Ganjue" in TCM. Some symptoms that may be present due to blood trouble caused by a disorder of the stomach meridian are: mania, malaria, febrile disease, sweating, epistaxis, wry mouth, lip boil, swelling of the neck, sorethroat, ascites, swelling and pain of the patella, pain along the course of the meridian in the chest, breast, Qichong(ST 30), thigh, Futu (ST 32), the anterior-lateral aspect of the tibia and the dorsum of the foot, and limitation of the middle toe. A patient whose of the meridian is excessive may feel hot in the anterior part of the body. Hyperfunction of the stomach will lead to rapid digestion, hunger, and yellowish urine. The patient whose Qi of the meridian is deficient may have frequent shiver in the anterior part of the body. If his stomach trouble is caused by pathogenic cold, he will have abdominal distension.

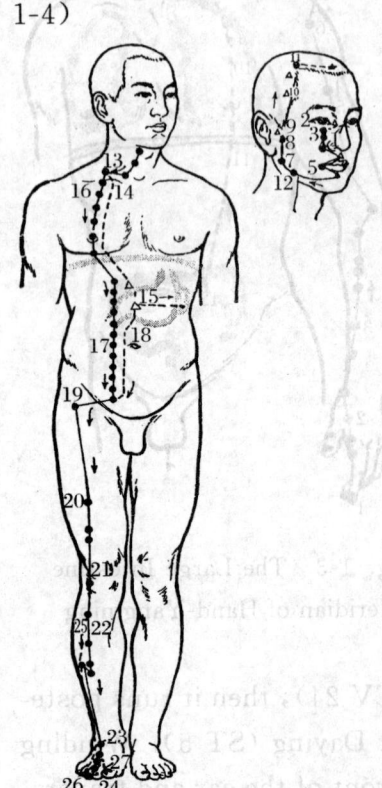

Fig. 1-4 The Stomach Meridian of Foot-Yangming

4. Spleen Meridian

The Chapter "Discussion on the Meridians" (Chapter 10) in *Miraculous Pivot* says: the Spleen Meridian starts from the tip of the big toe. It runs along the medial aspect of the big toe between the red and white skin and ascends to the front of the medial malleolus and further up to the medial aspect of the leg. It follows the posterior aspect of the tibia and passes through the front of the Liver Meridian. Going on along the anterior medial aspect of the knee and then the thigh, it enters the abdomen, reaches the spleen, its pertaining organ, and connects with the stomach. Passing through the disphragm and running alongside the esophagus, it reaches the root of the tongue, and spreads over under the tongue.

A branch goes upwards through the stomach and the diaphragm, then flows into the heart. (Fig. 1-5)

Principal Symptoms: The most obvious symptoms of the meridian disorder are as follows: stiff tongue, vomiting after meals, stomachache, flatulence and frequent eructation which may be alleviated after bowels movement or passing flatus, and heaviness sensation of the whole body. As for symptoms due to a disorder of the spleen, they are mainly in the form of pains in the root of the tongue, askinesia, inappetence, vexation, acute pain in the upper abdomen, loose stool or dysentery, dysuria, jaundice, being unable to lie flat and difficulty in standing, swelling of the medial aspect of the thigh and knee, cold extremities, and disability of the great toe.

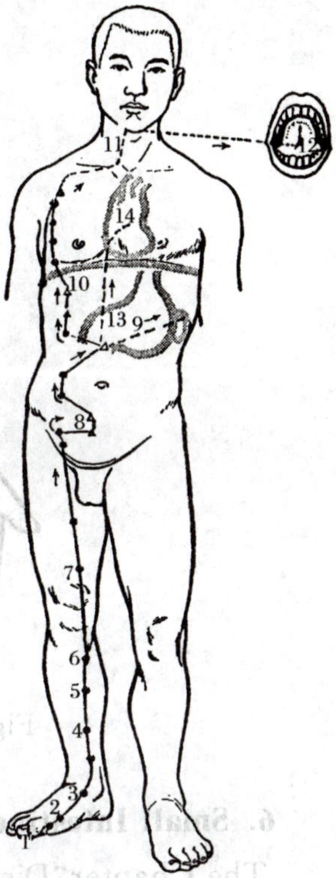

5. Heart Meridian

The Chapter ""Discussion on the Meridian"(Chapter 10) in *Miraculous Pivot* says: the Heart Meridian originates from the heart, spreads over the heart system. It goes down through the diaphragm to connect with the small intestine. The ascending portion of the meridian from the heart system runs alongside the esophagus to connect with the eye system. The straight portion of the meridian from the heart system goes upward to the lung, then it runs out from the axilla, it goes along the posterior border of the medial aspect of the upper arm behind the Lung Meridian and Pericardium Meridian, it runs downward the medial aspect of the elbow and descends along the posterior border of the medial aspect of the forearm to the pisiform region proximal to the palm and enters the palm, it follows the medial aspect of the little finger to its tip. (Fig. 1-6)

Fig. 1-5 The Spleen Meridian of Foot-Taiyin

Principal Symptoms: Dry throat, precordial pain and thirst are the most common symptoms of heart meridian disorder which is called "Bijue"in TCM. A disorder of heart gives rise to icteric sclera, painful hypochondrium and posterior the medial aspect of the upper extremities, cold hands and feet, and hot palms.

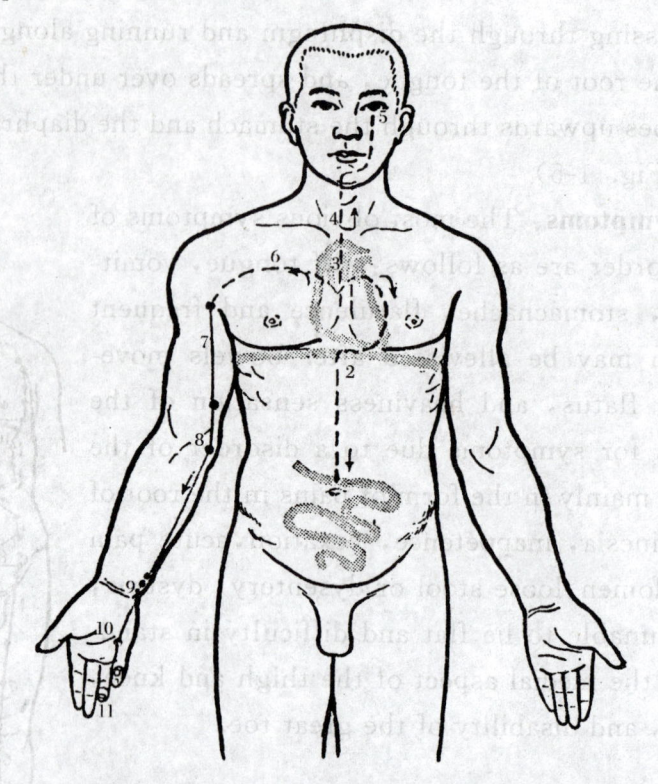

Fig. 1-6   The Heart Meridian of Hand-Shaoyin

6. Small Intestine Meridian

The Chapter "Discussion on the Meridians" (Chapter 10) in *Miraculous Pivot* says: The Small Intestine Meridian starts from the ulnar side of the tip of the little finger. Following the ulnar side of the dorsum of the hand, it reaches the wrist. Then it goes out from the styloid process of the ulna, ascends along the posterior border of the lateral aspect of the forearm, passes between the olecranon of the ulna and the medial epicondyle of the humerus and runs along the posterior border of the lateral aspect of the upper arm to the shoulder joint. Circling around the scapular region, it meets the superior aspect of the shoulder, then turns downward to the supraclavicular fossa. It connects with the heart. From there, then it descends along the esophagus, passes through the diaphragm, reaches the stomach and enters the small intestine, its pertaining organ.

The branch from the supraclavicular fossa ascends along the neck to the cheek, reaches the outer canthus and enters the ear.

The branch from the cheek runs upward to the infraobital region and further to the lateral side of the nose, then it reaches the inner canthus. (Fig. 1-7)

Principal Symptoms: The main symptoms of meridian disorder are as follows: sore throat, swelling of the chin, stiff neck, unbearable pain in the shoulder as if extracted, and severe pain of the upper arm as if fractured. The main symptoms due to fluid trouble that is caused by small intestine disease are deafness, icteric sclera, swelling of the cheek, and pains along the posterior border of the lateral aspect of the neck, the chin, the shoulder, the upper arm, the elbow and the forearm.

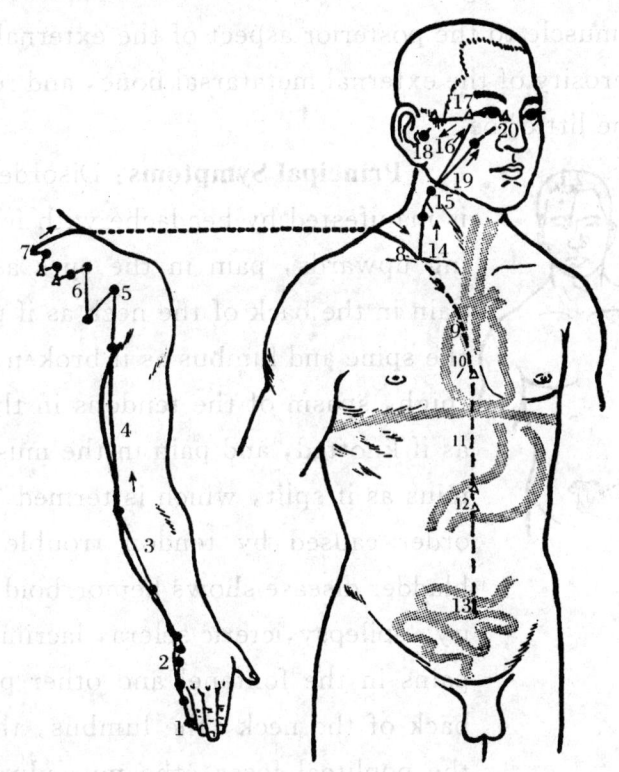

Fig. 1-7 The Small Intestine Meridian of Hand-Taiyang

7. Bladder Meridian

The Chapter "Discussion on the Meridian" (Chapter 10) in *Miraculous Pivot* says: The Bladder Meridian starts from the inner canthus and then ascends to the forehead, and joins the vertex.

A branch arises from the vertex, runs to the temple.

The straight portion of the meridian enters and communicates with the brain from the vertex. It comes out and bifurcates to descend along the posterior aspect of the neck. and then downward along the medial aspect of the scapula region and paralleled to the vertebral column. It reaches the lumber region where it enters the body cavity via the paravertebral muscle to connect with the kidney and join its pertaining organ, the urinary bladder.

The branch of the lumbar region descends through the gluteal region and ends in the popliteal fossa.

The branch from the posterior aspect of the neck runs straight downward along the medial border of the scapula, passes through the gluteal region and downward along the lateral aspect of the thigh, to meet the preceding branch descending from the lumbar region in the popliteal fossa, then descends through the gastrocnemius muscle to the posterior aspect of the external malleolus, then runs along the tuberosity of the external metatarsal bone, and reaches the lateral side of the tip of the little toe.

Principal Symptoms: Disorder of the meridian is manifested by headache with feeling of Qi rushing upwards, pain in the eyes as if gouged out, pain in the back of the neck as if pulled up, pain in the spine and lumbus as if broken, acampsia of the thigh, spasm of the tendons in the popliteal fossa as if knotted, and pain in the musculus gastrocnemius as if split, which is termed "Huai Jue". Disorder caused by tendon trouble due to urinary bladder disease shows hemorrhoid, malaria, insanity, epilepsy, icteric sclera, lacrimation, epistaxis, pains in the fontanel and other parts such as the back of the neck, the lumbus, the sacral region, the popliteal fossa, the musculus gastrocnemius, and the foot, and dysfunction of the small toes. (Fig. 1-8)

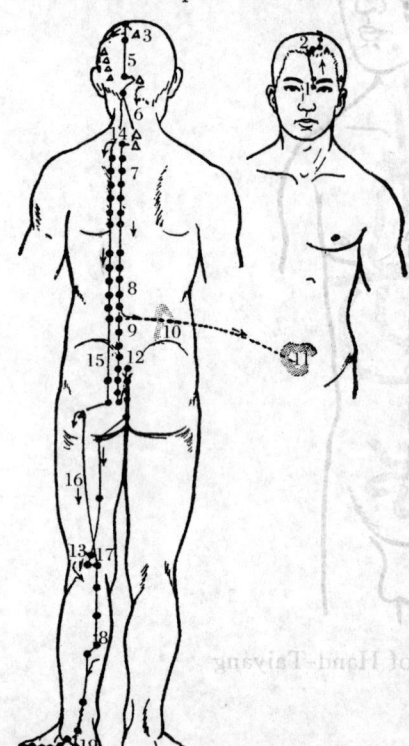

Fig. 1-8   The Bladder Meridian of Foot-Taiyang

8. Kidney Meridian

The Chapter "Discussion on the Meridian" (Chapter 10) in *Miraculous Pivot* says: The Kidney Meridian starts from the inferior aspect of the small toe and runs obliquely towards the sole. It comes out from Rangu(KI 2), runs behind the medial malleolus and enters the heel. Then it ascends along the medial side of the leg to the medial side of the popliteal fossa and goes further upward along the posterior medial aspect of the thigh towards the vertebral column, where it enters the kidney, its pertaining organ, and connects with the bladder.

The straight portion of meridian re-emerges from the kidney. Ascending and passing through the liver and diaphragm, it enters the lung, runs along the throat and terminates at the root of the tongue.

A branch springs from the lung, joins the heart, and runs into the chest. (Fig. 1-9)

Principal Symptoms: Disorder of the meridian is characterized by feeling hungry but no taste for food, dark complexion, hemoptysis, branchial wheezing, and blurred vision and uncomfortable when sitting. the patient feels so hungry that he feels heart hung in the air. Qi deficiency in the meridian shows nervousness, palpitation with fear of being caught, which is termed "Bone Jue". Meridian disorder with kidney disease is symptomized by burning sensation of mouth, dry tongue, swollen throat, inspiratory dyspnea, dry sore pharynx, vexation, precordial pain, jaundice, dysentery, pains in the spine and the posterior border of the medial aspect of thigh, syncope, flaccidity, somnolence, and painful soles with burning sensation.

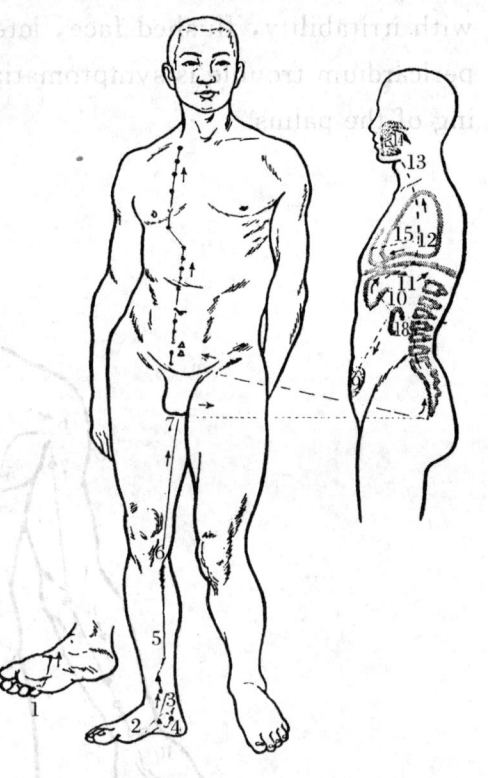

Fig. 1-9 The Kidney Meridian of Foot-Shaoyin

9. Pericardium Meridian

The Chapter "Discussion on the Meridian" (Chapter 10) in *Miraculous Pivot* says: The Pericardium Meridian starts from the chest, and enters its pertaining organ, the pericardium. It descends through the diaphragm to connect successively with the upper, middle and lower energizer.

A branch arising from the chest runs inside the chest, comes out from the costal region below the axilla and ascends to the axilla. Following the medial aspect of the upper arm, it runs between the Lung Meridian and Heart Meridian to the cublital fossa, further downward to the forearm between the tendons of m. palmaris longus and m. flexor carpi radiadis, enters the palm, then passes along the middle finger right down to its tip.

Another branch arising from the palm runs along the ring finger to its tip.

31

(Fig. 1-10)

Principal Symptoms: Disorder of the meridian is symptomatized by feverish sensation in the palm center, spasm and contracture of the arm and elbow, swelling of the axilla, chest and hypochondria congestion, violent palpitation with irritability, flushed face, icteric sclera and mania. Meridian disorder with pericardium trouble is symptomatized by vexation, precordial pain, and hot feeling of the palms.

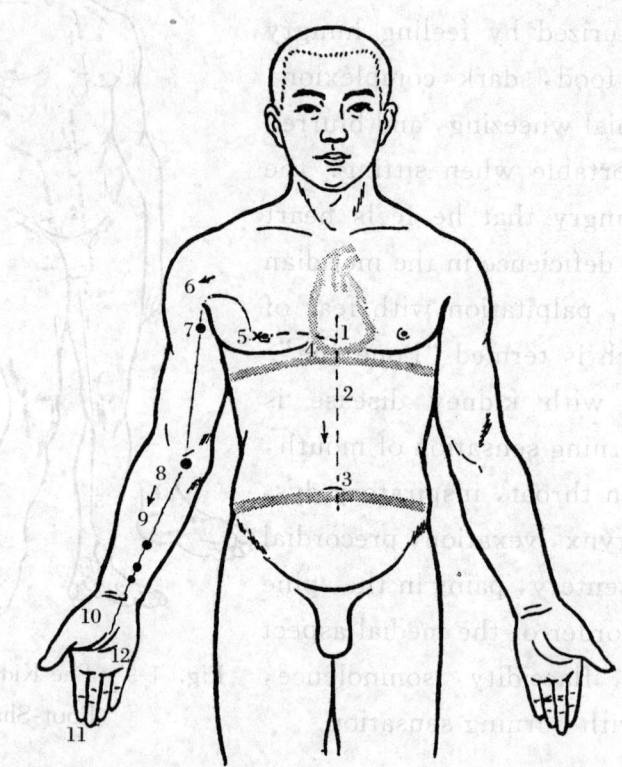

Fig. 1-10 The Pericardium Meridian of Hand-Jueyin

10. Triple Energizer Meridian

The Chapter "Discussion on the Meridians" (Chapter 10) in *Miraculous Pivot* says: The Triple Energizer Meridian originates from the tip of the ring finger, runs upward between the 4th and 5th metacarpal bones along the dorsal aspect of the wrist to the lateral aspect of the forearm between the radius and ulna then ascends through the olecranon and goes along the lateral aspect of the upper arm, reaches the shoulder region, across and passes behind the Gallbladder Meridian winding over to supraclavicular fossa, and spreads in the chest to connect with the pericardium. It then descends through diaphragm and joins its pertaining organ, the upper, middle and lower energizer.

A branch starts from the chest (Tanzhong)(CV 17) runs upward and comes out from the supraclavicular fossa, then ascends to the neck, runs along the posterior border of the ear and further to the corner of the anterior hairline. Then it runs downward to the neck and terminates in the infraorbital region.

The branch arises from the retroauricular region and enters the ear, comes out at the front of ear, crosses the previous branch at the cheek and reaches the outer canthus. (Fig. 1-11)

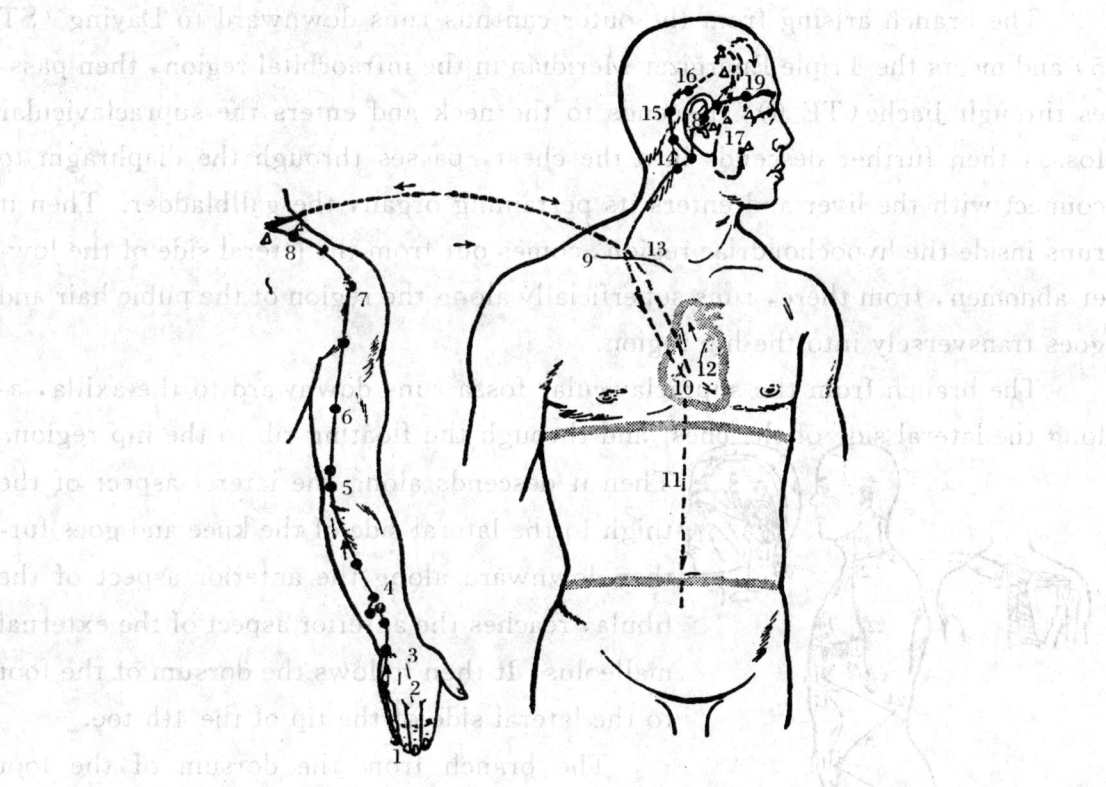

Fig. 1-11 The Triple Energizer Meridian of Hand-Shaoyang

Principal Symptoms: Symptoms of disorder of the meridian include: deafness, tinnitus, swelling of the pharynx and sore throat. When its Qi is troubled, or when its relevant organ is diseased, it has the followig manifestations: hidrosis, pain in the outer canthus of the eye, pain in the cheek, pains in the posterior border of the ear and along the lateral aspect of the shoulder, upper arm, elbow and forearm, and dysfunction of the ring finger.

11. Gallbladder Meridian

The Chapter "Discussion on the Meridians"(Chapter 10) in *Miraculous Pivot* says: The Gallbladder Meridian starts from the outer canthus, ascends to the corner of the forehead, then curves downward to the retroauricual region and rounds along the side of the neck in front of the Triple Energizer Meridian to the shoulder, then turns back, transverses and passes behind the Triple Energizer Meridian, down to the supraclavicular fossa.

The branch arises from the rectroauricular region and enters into the ear. It comes out and passes the preauricular region to the posterior aspect of the outer canthus.

The branch arising from the outer canthus runs downward to Daying (ST 5) and meets the Triple Energizer Meridian in the infraorbital region, then passes through Jiache (TE 6), descends to the neck and enters the supraclavicular fossa, then further descends into the chest, passes through the diaphragm to connect with the liver and enters its pertaining organ, the gallbladder. Then it runs inside the hypochondriac region, comes out from the lateral side of the lower abdomen, from there, runs superficially along the region of the pubic hair and goes transversely into the hip region.

The branch from the supraclavicular fossa runs downward to the axilla, along the lateral side of the chest and through the floating rib to the hip region. Then it descends along the lateral aspect of the thigh to the lateral side of the knee and goes further downward along the anterior aspect of the fibula, reaches the anterior aspect of the external malleolus, It then follows the dorsum of the foot to the lateral side of the tip of the 4th toe.

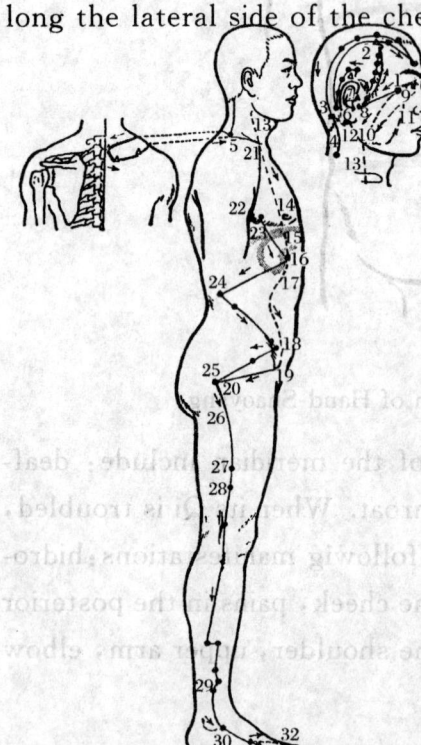

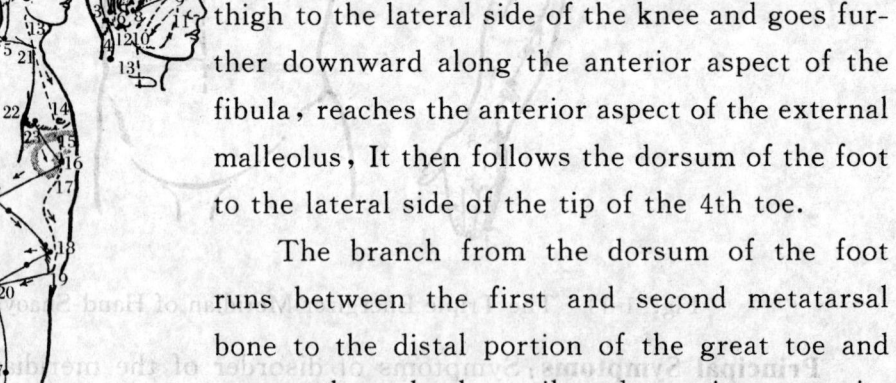

The branch from the dorsum of the foot runs between the first and second metatarsal bone to the distal portion of the great toe and passes through the nail and terminates at its hairy region. (Fig. 1-12)

Principal Symptoms: Disorder of the meridian is symptomized by bitter taste, frequent sighing, precordial and hypochondriac pains, unable to turn round, sallow complexion (in serious cases), dry skin, and hot feeling of the lateral aspect of the dorsum of the foot, which is called "Yang Jue" in TCM. Bone disorder caused by

Fig. 1-12 The Gallbladder Meridian of Foot-Shaoyang

gallbladder trouble may have headache, pains in the chin, in the outer canthus of the eye, and in the supraclavicular fossa, edema of the axilla, tuberculosis of the lymph nodes, sweating, shivering, malaria, and pains along the course of this meridian such as the chest, hypochondrium, rib, thigh, lateral aspect of the part from knee to fibula and its lower part, external malleolus and joints, and dysfunction of the 4th toe.

12. Liver Meridian

The Chapter "Discussion on the Meridians" (Chapter 10) in *Miraculous Pivot* says: The Liver Meridian starts from the dorsal hair of the great toe, runs upward along the dorsum of the foot through the point, 1 cun in front of the medial malleolus, ascends to the area 8 cun above the medial malleolus when it runs across and behind the Spleen Meridian. Then it runs further upward to the medial side of the knee, and along the medial side of the thigh to the pubic hair region where it curves around the external genitalia and goes up to the lower abdomen. It then runs upward and curves around the stomach to enter the liver, its pertaining organ, and connects with the gallbladder. It ascends, passing through the diaphragm and branching out in the costal and hypochondriac regions. Then it ascends along the posterior aspect of the throat to the nasopharynx and connects with the eye. Running upward, it comes out from the forehead and meets the Governor Vessel at the vertex.

The branch arising from the eye runs downward into the cheek and curves around the inner surface of the lips.

The branch arising from the liver passes through the diaphragm, runs upward into the lung. (Fig. 1-13)

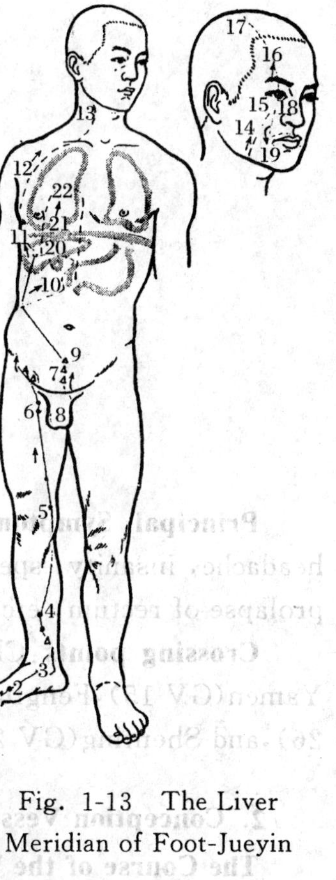

Principal Symptoms: Disorder of the meridian is symptomized by lumbago which prevents the patient from bending, swollen painful testis, edema of the lower abdomen in females, dry throat in heavy cases and sallow complexion. Meridian disorder from liver disease is manifested by chest congestion, vomiting, watery diarrhea containing undigested food, inguinal hernia, bed-wetting and dysuria.

Fig. 1-13 The Liver Meridian of Foot-Jueyin

Section 6 Courses, Principal Symptoms and Crossing Acupoints of the Eight Extra Meridians.

1. Governor Vessel

The Course of the Vessel: It arises from the lower abdomen and comes out from the perineum. It runs posteriorly along the interior side of the spinal column to Fengfu(GV 16) at the nape where it enters the brain. It further ascends to the vertex and goes down along the forehead to the nasal column. (Fig. 1-14)

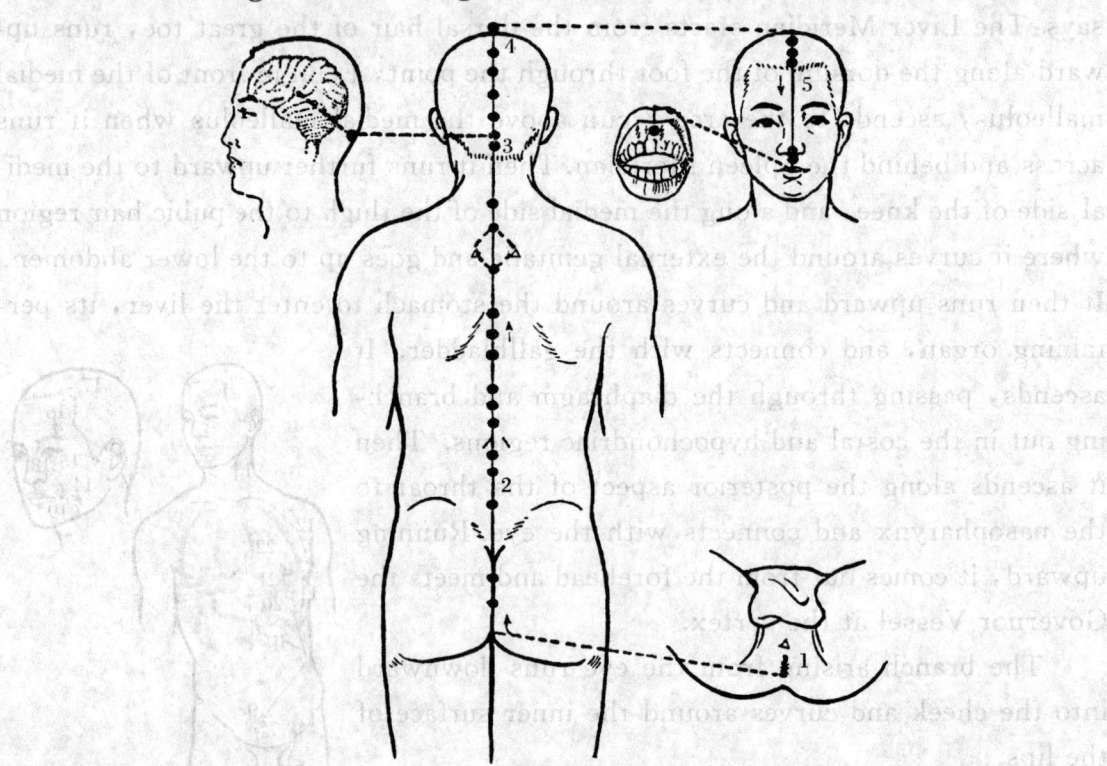

Fig. 1-14 The Governor Vessel

Principal Symptoms: Rigid spine, opisthotonus, rachialgia, dorsalgia, headache, insanity, spermatorrhea, impotence, premature ejaculation, infertility prolapse of rectum, etc.

Crossing points: Changqiang(GV 1), Taodao (GV 13), Dazhui (GV 14), Yamen(GV 15), Fengfu (GV 16), Naoshu(GV 17), Baihui(GV 20), Shuigou(GV 26), and Shenting(GV 24).

2. Conception Vessel

The Course of the Vessel: It starts from the inside of the lower abdomen and comes out from the perineum. It goes anteriorly to the pubic region and ascends along the interior side of the abdomen, passes through Guanyuan (CV 4) and reaches the throat. Ascending further, it curves around the lips, passes through the cheek and enters the infraorbital region Chengqi (ST 1). (Fig. 1-15)

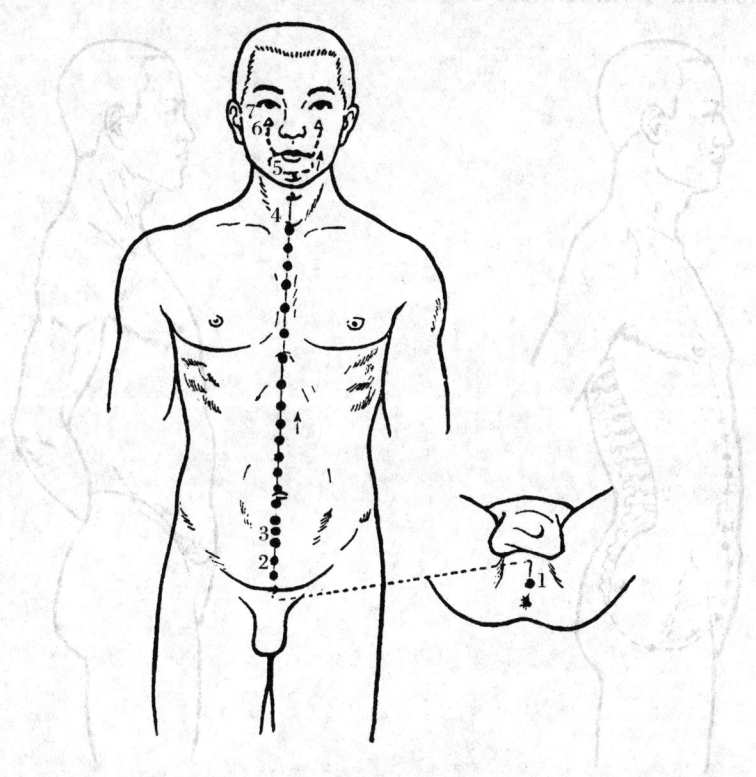

Fig. 1-15 The Conception Vessel

Principal Symptoms: Menoxenia, infertility, abortion, profuse leukorrhea, hernia, mass in the abdomen, sore throat, etc.

Crossing points: Huiyin (CV 1), Qugu (CV 2), Zhongji (CV 3), Guanyuan (CV 4), Yinjiao (CV 7), Xiawan (CV 10), Zhongwan (CV 12), Shangwan (CV 13), Tiantu (CV 22), Lianquan (CV 23) and Chengjiang (CV 24).

3. Thoroughfare Vessel

The Course of the Vessel: It starts from the inside of the lower abdomen and comes out at the perineum. Ascending, it runs the inside of the spinal column where its superficial branch passes through the region of Qichong (ST 30) and communicates with the Kidney Meridian, running along both sides of the abdomen. It goes up to the throat and curves around the lips. (Fig. 1-16)

Principal Symptoms: Cramps due to rebellious abdominal Qi.

Crossing Points: Huiyin(CV 1), Yinjiao(CV 7), Qichong(ST 30), Henggu (KI 11), Dahe(KI 12), Qixue(KI 13), Siman(KI 14), Zhongzhu(KI 15), Huangshu(KI 16), Shangqu (KI 17), Shiguan (KI 18), Yindu (KI 19), Tonggu (abdomen)(KI 20) and Youmen(KI 21).

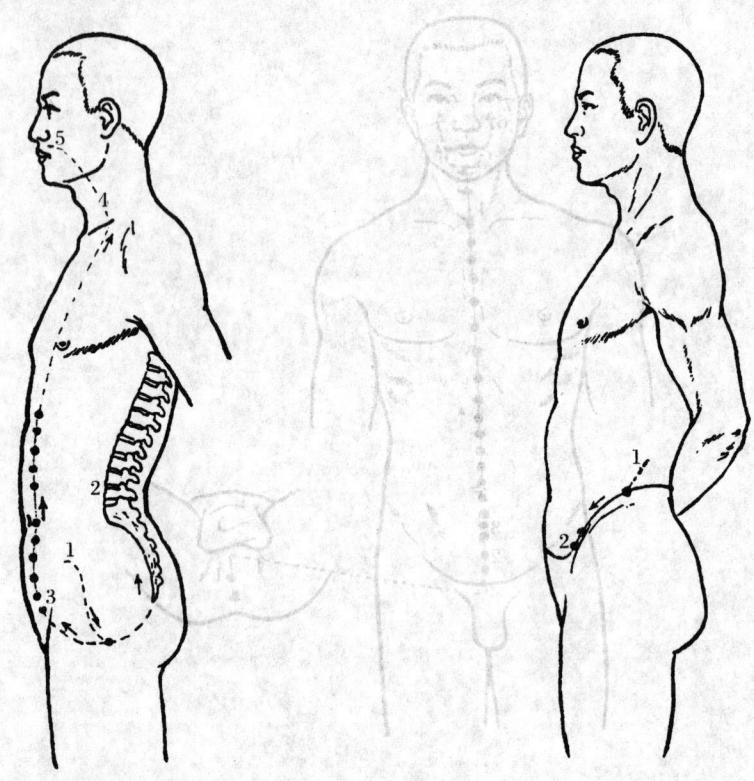

Fig. 1-16

The Thoroughfare Vessel

Fig. 1-17

The Belt Vessel

4. Belt Vessel

The Course of the Vessel: It starts below the hypochondriac region and runs obliquely downward through Daimai (GB 26), Wushu (GB 27) and Weidao (GB 28) then runs transversely around the waist like a belt. (Fig. 1-17)

Principal Symptoms: Abdominal distention, cold sensation in the lumbar region.

Crossing Points: Daimai(GB 26), Wushu(GB 27), and Weidao(GB 28).

5. Yin Link Vessel

The Course of the Vessel: It starts from the medial aspect of the leg, ascends along the medial aspect of the thigh to the abdomen to communicate with the

Spleen Meridian, then runs along the chest, and communicates with the Conception Vessel at the neck. (Fig. 1-18)

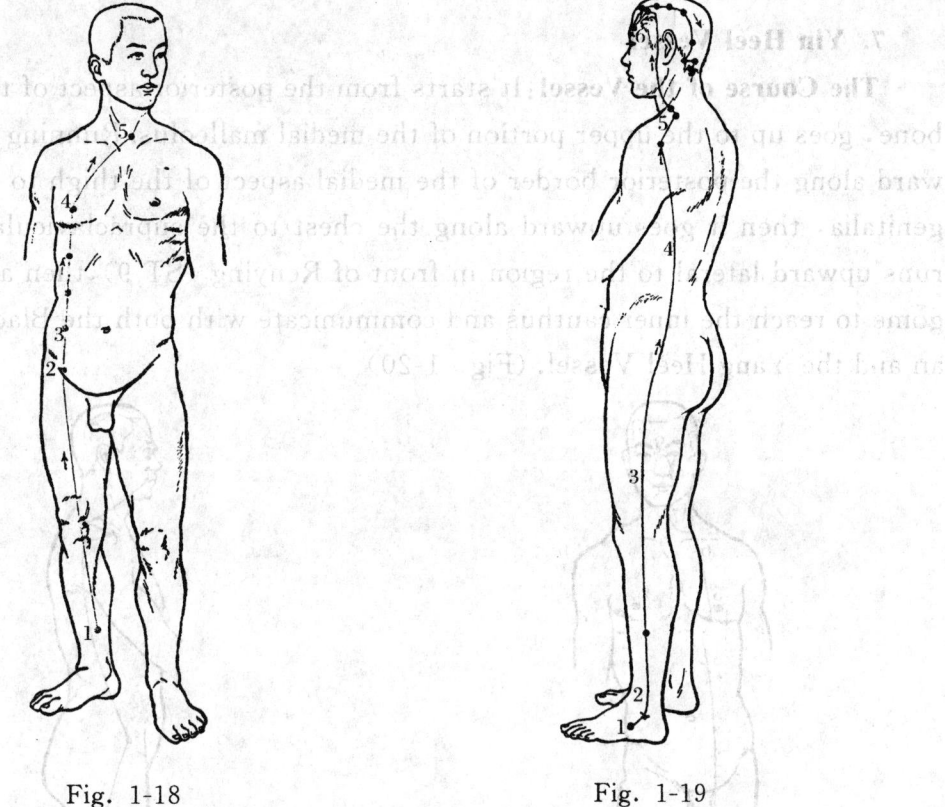

Fig. 1-18
The Yin Link Vessel

Fig. 1-19
The Yang Link Vessel

Principal Symptoms: Cardiac pain, melancholy.
Crossing points: Zhubin(KI 9), Fushe(SP 13), Daheng(SP 15), Fuai(SP 16), Qimen(LR 14), Tiantu(CV 22)and Lianquan(CV 23).

6. Yang Link Vessel

The Course of the Vessel: It starts from the lateral aspect of the heel, and runs upward along the external malleolus. Ascending along the Gallbladder Meridian, it passes through the hip region. It runs further upward along the posterior aspect of the hypochondriac and costal regions and posterior aspect of the axilla to the shoulder, and to the forehead. It then turns backward to the back of the neck to communicate with the Governor Vessel. (Fig. 1-19)

Principal Symptoms: Aversion to cold, fever, lumbar pain.
Crossing Points: Jinmen(BL 63), Yangjiao(GB 35), Naoshu(SI 10), Tianliao(ST 15), Jianjing(GB 21), Benshen(GB 13), Touwei(ST 8), Yangbai(GB

14), Toulinqi(GB 15), Muchuang(GB 16), Zhengying(GB 17), Chengling(GB 18), Naokong(GB 19), Fengchi(GB 20), Fengfu(GV16) and Yamen(GV 15).

7. Yin Heel Vessel

The Course of the Vessel: It starts from the posterior aspect of the navicular bone, goes up to the upper portion of the medial malleolus. Running straight upward along the posterior border of the medial aspect of the thigh to the external genitalia, then it goes upward along the chest to the supraclavicular fossa and runs upward lateral to the region in front of Renying (ST 9), then along the zygome to reach the inner canthus and communicate with both the Bladder Meridian and the Yang Heel Vessel. (Fig. 1-20)

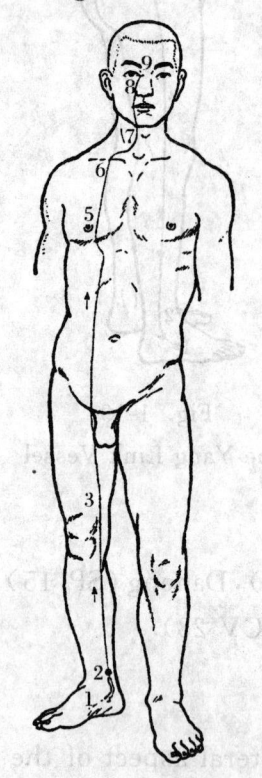

Fig. 1-20
The Yin Heel Vessel

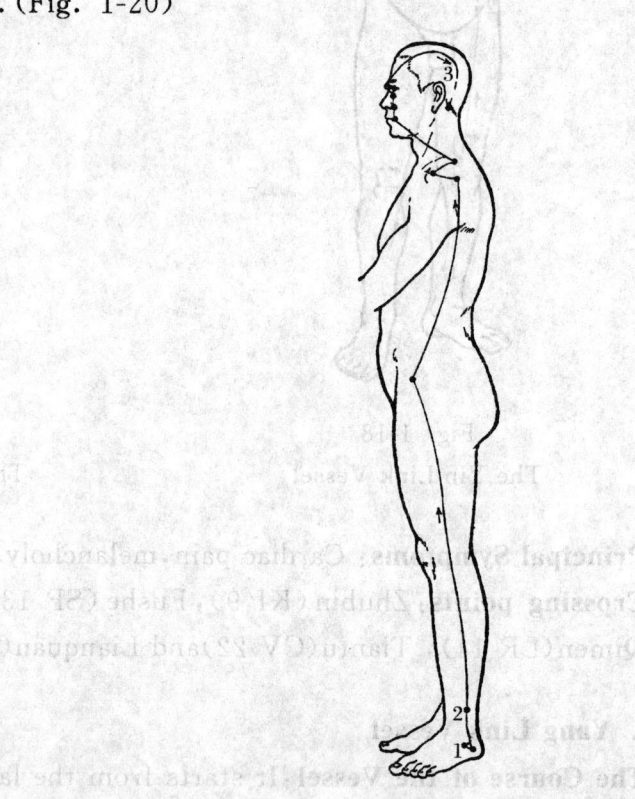

Fig. 1-21
The Yang Heel Vessel

Principal Symptoms: Somnolence, retention of urine and per varus.
Crossing points: Zhaohai(KI 6), Jiaoxin(KI 8) and Jingming (BL 1).

8. Yang Heel Vessel

The Course of the Vessel: It starts from the lateral side of the heel, runs upward along the external malleolus and passes the posterior border of the fibula, goes upward along the lateral side of the thigh and posterior side of the hypochondrium to the posterior axillary fold. Then, it runs over to the shoulder and ascends along the neck to the corner of the mouth. Then it enters the inner canthus to communicate with the Yin Heel Vessel. Running further upward along the Bladder Meridian to the forehead, it meets the Gallbladder Meridian at Fengchi(GB 20). (Fig. 1-21)

Principal Symptoms: Conjunctivitis from the inner canthus, insomnia, eversion of foot.

Crossing Points: Shenmai(BL 62), Pucan (LB 61), Fuyang(BL 59), Juliao (GB 29), Naoshu(SI 10), Jianju(LI 15), Jugu(LI 16), Tianliao(SI 15), Dicang (ST 4), Juliao(ST 3), Chengqi(ST 1), Jingming(BL 1) and Fengchi(GB 20).

Section 7 Acupoints, Courses, Principal Indications and Treatments of Fifteen Collaterals

The Collateral of Lung Meridian-Lieque(LU 7)

The Collateral of Lung Meridian takes Lieque(LU 7) as its acupoint. It starts parallel between the tendons of m. branchioradialis and m. abductor pollicis longus and runs parallel with the Lung Meridian into the palm of the hand and spreads over the thenar eminence.

Pathology:

Excessive Syndrome: Hot of carpal bones and palm.

Deficient Syndrome: Yawning, incontinence of urine, and pollakiuria.

Treatment: Lieque (LU 7) at 1.5 cun above the transverse crease of the wrist, connecting the Large Intestine Meridian.

The Collateral of Heart Meridian-Tongli(HT 5)

The Collateral of Heart Meridian takes Tongli as its acupoint. It branches out at Tongli(HT 5) 1 cun above the transverse crease of the wrist along the Heart Meridian, it enters the heart and runs to the root of the tongue and the eye.

Pathology:

Excessive Syndrome: Distressing fullness of the chest and hypochondrium.

Deficient Syndrome: Aphonia

Treatment: Tongli(HT 5) which connects with the Small Intestine Meridian.

The Collateral of Pericardium Meridian-Neiguan(PC 6)

The Collateral of Pericardium Meridian takes Neiguan(PC 6) as its acupoint. It begins from 2 cun above the wrist, disperses between the two tendons and runs along the Pericardium Meridian to the pericardium, and finally to the heart.

Pathology:

Excessive Syndrome: Cardiac pain.

Deficient Syndrome: Stiffness of neck.

Treatment: Neiguan(PC 6)

The Collateral of Small Intestine Meridian-Zhizheng(SI 7)

The Collateral of Small Intestine Meridian takes Zhizheng(SI 7)as its acupoint. It starts from 5 cun above the wrist and connects with the Heart Meridian. A branch runs upward, crosses the elbow and connects with Jianyu(LI 15).

Excessive Syndrome: Flaccid joints, dysfunction of elbow.

Deficient Syndrome: Flat wart, furuncle, and scabies.

Treatment: Zhizheng(SI 7).

The Collateral of Large Intestine Meridain-Pianli(LI 6)

The Collateral of Large Intestine Meridian takes Pianli(LI 6)as its acupoint. It starts from 3 cun above the wrist and connects with the Lung Meridian. A branch runs along the arm to Jianyu(LI 15), crosses the jaw and extends to the teeth. Another branch derives at the jaw and enters the ear to join the Triple Energizer, Gallbladder, Small Intestine and Stomach Meridians.

Pathology:

Excessive Syndrome: Tooth caries, deafness.

Deficient Syndrome: Sensitive teeth, and blockage.

Treatment: Pianli(LI 6)

The Collateral of Triple Energizer Meridian-Waiguan(TE 5)

The collateral of Triple Energizer Meridiana takes Waiguan(TE 5)as its acupoint. It starts from Waiguan(TE 5)2 cun above the dorsum of the wrist, travels up the posterior aspect of the arm and over the shoulder, disperses in the chest, to converge with the Pericardium Meridian.

Patholoy:

Excessive Syndrome: Spasm of elbow.

Deficient Syndrome: Flaccid elbow.

Treatment: Waiguan(TE 5)

The Collateral of Bladder Meridian-Feiyang(BL 58)

The Collateral of Bladder Meridian takes Feiyang(BL 58) as its acupoint. It arises from Feiyang(BL 58) 7 cun above the external malleolus, connects with the Kidney Meridian.

Pathology:

Excessive Syndrome: Stuffy nose, running nose, headache, back pain.

Deficient Syndrome: Running nose with bleeding.

Treatment: Feiyang(BL 58)

The Collateral of Gallbladder Meridian-Guangming(GB 37)

The Collateral of Gallbladder Meridian takes Guangming(GB 37) as its acupoint. It begins from Guangming(GB 37) 5 cun above the external malleolus, joins the Liver Meridian and runs downward, then disperses over the dorsum of foot.

Patheology:

Excessive Syndrome: Coldness of foot and leg.

Deficient Syndrome: Muscular atrophy, weak lower limbs.

Treatment: Guangming(GB 37)

The Collateral of Stomach Meridian-Fenglong(ST 40)

The Collateral of Stomach Meridian takes Fenglong (ST 40) as its acupoint. It starts from Fenglong (ST 40) 8 cun above the external malleolus, connects with the Spleen Meridian. A branch runs along the lateral aspect of the tibia upward to the top of the head to accept Qi from other meridians and then runs downward to the throat.

Pathology: Sore throat with hoarseness and sudden aphonia due to regurgitation of Qi.

Excessive Syndrome: Maciacinsanity.

Deficient Syndrome: Weak feet, muscular atrophy of the leg.

Treatment: Fenglong(ST 40)

The Collateral of Spleen Meridian-Gongsun(SP 4)

The Collateral of Spleen Meridian takes Gongsun(SP 4) as its acupoint. It branches out at Gongsun (SP 4), 1 cun posterior to the base of the first metatarsal bone, and then goes to join the Stomach Meridian. A branch runs upward in the abdomen and distributes to the stomach and intestine.

Pathology: Cholera due to regurgitation of Qi.

Excessive Syndrome: Severe pain in the intestines.

Deficient Syndrome: Drum-belly.

Treatment: Gongsun(SP 4)

The Collateral of Kidney Meridian-Dazhong(KI 4)

The Collateral of Kidney Meridian takes Dazhong (KI 4) as its ascupoint. It originates from Dazhong(KI 4) on the posterior aspect of internal malleolus, crosses the heel and joins the Bladder Meridian. A branch follows the Kidney Meridian upward to a point below the pericardium, and then pierces through the lumbar vertebrae.

Pathology: Dysphoria due to regurgitation of Qi.

Excessive Syndrome: Dysuria

Deficient Syndrome: Lumbar.

Treatment: Dazhong(KI 4).

The Collateral of Liver Meridian-Ligou(LR 5)

The Collateral of Liver Meridian takes Ligou(LR 5) as its acupoint. It starts from Ligou(LR 5) 5 cun above the inter malleolus and connects with the Gallbladder Meridian. A branch runs up the leg to the genitals.

Pathology: Swelling of testis because of regurgitation of Qi, sudden hernia.

Excessive Syndrome: Prolapse of genitalia, or abnormal erection of penis.

Deficient Syndrome: Itching of genital area.

Treatment: Ligou(LR 5).

The Collateral of Conception Vessel-Weiyi (Juiwei) (CV 15)

The collateral of Conception Vessel takes Weiyi(CV 15) as its acupoint. It separates at the lower end of the sternum, and spreads over the abdomen.

Pathology:

Excessive Syndrome: Sensitive skin in the abdominal region.

Deficient Syndrome: Pruritus of skin.

Treatment: Weiyi(CV 15)

The Collateral of Governor Vessel-Changqiang (GV 1)

The Collateral of Governor Vessel takes Changqiang(GV 1) as its acupoint. It arises from Changqiang(GV 1) in the perineum, runs upward along both sides of the spine to the nape, and spreads over the top of the head. It runs further downward to the scapular region and on the left side or the right side to connect with the Bladder Meridian, then it pierces through the spine.

Pathology:

Excessive Syndrome: Stiffness of spine, difficulty in prone and supine position.

Deficient Syndrome: Heaviness of head making the upper parts of the body unstable, diseases of the meridian along the spine.

Treatment: Changqiang(GV 1)

The Major Collateral of Spleen Meridian-Dabao(SP 21)

The Major Collateral of Spleen Meridian takes Dabao(SP 21) as its acupoint. It emerges at 3 cun below Yuanye(GB 22) and spreads through the chest and hypochondriac region.

Pathology:

Excessive Syndrome: Pain over the whole body.

Deficient Syndrome: Weakness of joints.

Like a network, this collateral spreads over the entire body. When there appears the stagnation of blood, select Dabao(SP 21) for treatment.

Chapter 2
An Introduction to Acupoints

Section 1 The Essential Concept of Acupoints

Acupoints are the sites through which the Qi of the Zang-Fu organs and meridians is transported to the body surface. These sites are not isolated points on the body surface, but they are connected with the internal Zang-Fu organs, and located in depression of muscles or bones. They function to commute the interior and the exterior and their positions are mainly holes. So, they are also called "Shuxue" (Acupoints). "Shu" means transportation; "Xue" means hole. Acupoints refer the sites where acupuncture treatment is applied. They include acupoints of the fourteen meridians, extraordianary points and Ashi points. In the ancient medical literature, acupoints have other terms such as "Qi point", "Qi Fu", "Jie", "Hui", "Gugong", "the origin of meridian Qi", "the sites where treatment with the flint needle and moxa can be applied" and "acupuncture points".

Section 2 The Development and Classification of Acupoints

Development of Acupoints: Acupoints were discovered individually and accumulated gradually in long experience against diseases by ancient Chinese. Its development experienced three stages: the stage of needling, the location on the body surface where pain or other abnormal sensation is left; the stage of localization and nomenclature of acupoints; and the stage of classification and meridian-tropism of acupoints. At the beginning of acupuncture treatment, there were no fixed acupoints. Acupuncture was applied only in the local regions affected by pain and diseases. This is the so-called "needling the location on the body surface where pain or other abnormal sensation is left". Through the accumulation of experience, the position of acupoints and their therapeutic effects have been confirmed, then acupoints have been defined and named to facilitate practice. That is the stage of localization and nomenclature. Later on acupuncture was developing continuously, practical acupoints increased, the scope of indications enlarged. Hence, people classified acupoints which had the similar therapeutic effects and the courses of sensation and transportation. So this entered the stage of classification and meridian-tropism. The acupoints in this book belong to this classification.

Classification of Acupoints:

Acupoints can be divided into three categories: acupoints of the fourteen meridians, extraordinary points and Ashi points. Acupoints of the fourteen meridians, also known as the "regular points", are distributed along the twelve regular meridians and the Governor and the Conception Vessels. They are the major acupoints, and have 361 regular names. Extraordinary points are named "extra points". In short, they are not attributed to the fourteen meridians but are especially effective in the treatment of certain diseases. Besides, in clinical practice, tender spots can be used as acupoints. These points which belong to neither the regular points nor extra points are named Ashi points, reflexing points or unfixed points. These points have no specific names and definite locations, and the tender spots and other sensitive spots are places for needling and moxibustion. Ashi points are located mainly in the affected area, sometimes in the distal area.

Section 3 Nomenclature of Acupoints

The names of acupoint have medical significance, and also one portion of brilliant culture in ancient China. *Precious Supplementary Prescriptions* points out, "Each point is named with profound significance", to understand the meanings of the acupoint names is helpful to know their locations, functions and indications.

Points named according to anatomical terms: Wangu (SI 4) on the lateral side of wrist, Rugen (ST 18), below the nipple, and Jizhong (GV 6) in the middle of the spinous process. Points named according to their therapeutic properties: Jingming (BL 1) and Guangming (GB 37) for curing disease of eyes; Shuifen (CV 9) and Shuidao (ST 28) for edema; Feishu (BL 13), Xinshu (BL 15) and Ganshu (BL 18) for treatment of diseases of Zang-Fu organs. Points named according to the theory of Traditional Chinese Medicine: Yangxi (LI 5), Yangchi (TE 4), and Yanggu (SI 5) on the lateral side of the upper limbs; Yinxi (HT 6) on the medial side of the upper limbs; Pohu (BL 42) and Shentang (BL 44) beside Feishu

(BL 13)and Xinshu(BL 15); Sanyinjiao(SP 6), Baihui(GV 20), Qihai(CV 6)and Xuehai(SP 10). Points named according to astronomical and meteorological phenomena and mountains and valleys: Chengshan(BL 57), Daling(PC 7), Shangqiu (SP 5), Shuigou(GV 26), Shangxing(GV 23), Riyue (GB 24)and Taiyi (ST 23). Points named according to analogy to animals or plants: Dubi(ST 35)below the knee, Jiuwei(CV 15)in the thoracic and abdominal regions and Cuanzhu (BL 2)at the end of eyebrow. Points named according to analogy to architectural structure: Shenque(CV 8), Yintang(EX-HN3), Zhishi(BL 52)and Kufang(ST 14).

Section 4 The Properties of Acupoints

Diagnostic Properties:

When the human body is under pathological conditions, there are reflexes on the acupoints which can be used as the basis for clinical diagnosis of acupuncture. For instance, there appears tenderness at Zusanli (ST 36)and Diji (SP 8)of the patient with disorder of stomach and intestines, meanwhile soft nodule can be felt in the region near the 5th and 8th vertebrae. There appear tenderness, allergic sensation, and subcutaneous nodules at Feishu (BL 13)and Zhongfu (LU 1)of the patient with the lung disorder. Thus in clinical practice, doctors use fingers to palpate the Back-Shu points, the Front-Shu points, the Xi-points and the Yuan points and observe tenderness, allergic sensation, swelling, hard nodules, cooling, heat, eminence of local muscles, the extent of firmness and softness of depression, the color of skin, petechia, papule and desquamation along above-mentioned points for diagnosis.

In recent years, there is new development with the help of applying acupoints in diagnosis. For instance, the test of auricular points in the auricle, the test of conductibility applied by the Yuan point, and the test of thermosensation applied by the twelve Jing Points. To certain degree, we know pathological changes reflected from meridians and collaterals, Zang-Fu organs and tissue, by testing these acupoints with the instruments, and all these add something new to diagnosis.

Therapeutic properties:

(1)**Local and Adjacent Therapeutic Properties:** All the points in the body share the common feature in their therapeutic properties. Each point located on a particular site is able to treat disorder of this area and of nearby tissues and organs. For instance, the diseases of eye can be treated by the points in eye region such as Jingming (BL 1),Chengqi(ST 1),Sibai(ST 2)and Tongziliao(GB 1). The diseases of ear can be treated by the points in ear region such as Tinggong(SI 19),Tinghui(GB 2),and Yifeng(TE 17). The diseases of the stomach can be treated by the points in stomach region, such as Zhongwan(CV 12),Jianli(CV 11) and Liangmen(ST 21).

(2)**Remote Therapeutic Properties**: This is the basic rule of the therapeutic properties of the points of the fourteen meridians. The points of the fourteen meridians, especially those of the Twelve Regular Meridians located below the elbow and knee joints, are effective not only for local disorders but also for disorder of the tissues and Zang-Fu organs so far as the meridians can reach. Some even have systemic therapeutic properties. For instance, Hegu(LI 4)is not only for disorders of the wrist, but also the disorder of the neck, the head and facial area, even fever caused by exogenous pathogens. Zusanli(ST 36)is not only for disorders of the lower limbs, but also for the whole digestive system, even with certain effect on immunity.

Special Therapeutic Properties: Clinical practice has proved that needling certain points may bring forth biphasic beneficial regulation on functional abnormalities. For instance, puncturing Tianshu(ST 25)relieves both diarrhea and constipation. In addition to this, the therapeutic properties of some points show relative specificity, for instance, Dazhui(GV 14),which has an antipyretic effect, and Zhiyin(BL 67), helps correct the malposition of a fetus.

Section 5 The Concept and Classification of Specific Points

Specific points refer to those points that have special therapeutic properties. They have their special names given after their indications and functions. There are ten categories of these points.

1. Five Shu Points

Five Shu Points refer the collective name of five specific points namely, Jing-(Well), Ying-(Spring), Shu-(Stream), Jing-(River) and He-(Sea), which are located below the elbow or knees on the twelve regular meridians. Their orders are arranged according to the theory of Biao,Ben, Gen and Jie. They are situated from the distal ends of the extremities to the elbow or knee. The ancient doctors gave the names of the Five Shu Points in analogy between the Qi flow in meridian and the flow of water in the nature to illustrate the origin and the direction of the Qi flow, the depth of the regions where the meridian Qi passed by, and their different functions. For instance, the Jing-(Well)Point is situated in the place where the meridian Qi starts to bubble; the Ying-(Spring)Point is where the meridian Qi starts to gush; the Shu-(Stream) Points is where the meridian Qi flourishes; the Jing-(River) Point is where the meridian Qi is pouring abundantly; and finally, the He-(Sea) signifies the confluence of rivers into the sea, where the meridian Qi meets in the Zang or Fu organs.

Chapter 68 of Book *Classic on Medical Problems* says: "The Jing-(Well) Point is generally indicated in epigastric fullness; the Ying-(Spring) Point in febrile diseases; the Shu-(Stream)Point, in heaviness and joint pain, the Jing-(River)Point, in asthma and coughing with fever; the He-(Sea)Point, in Qi rebellion with diarrhea." which summaries the scope of the indications of the Five Shu Point. Each of the Twelve Regular Meridians has one Jing-(Well) Point. They locate mainly at the junction of white and red skin. So the Jing-(Well) points have the function of communicating with Yin and Yang, Qi and blood, they are mainly used in emergency and have the properties of opening the heart blockage to awaken coma. They are also used for alleviating pain and inflammation. The Shu-(Stream) Points are applied for relieving pain, and heaviness in the body due to water retention. The Jing-(River) Points are for diseases caused by exogenous pathogen, cough and asthma. The He-(Sea) Points are mostly for the disorders of the six Fu-organs, such as vomiting, diarrhea, dizziness, headache and conduct the perversive Qi downward.

The Jing-(Well) Points in Diagnosis: The Jing-(Well) Points are the points of "Gen" of each meridian. Acupuncturists of Japan analysed the heat sensation of the Jing-(Well) Points by fuming the Jing-(Well) points with burning stick incense to check the excess or deficiency of each meridian. This is called the method of testing heat sensation.

Ancient Chinese analogized Zang and Fu organs to five elements on the basis of their different functions. That is, the liver and gallbladder pertain to wood, the heart and small intestine to water, the spleen and stomach to earth, the lung and large intestine to metal, and the kidney and bladder to water, then, Five Shu Points pertain to five elements. Chapter 64 of the book *Classic on Medical Problems* points out: "The Jing-(Well) points of Yin meridian pertains to wood, and the Jing-(Well)point of Yang meridian to metal; the Ying-(Spring) point of Yin meridian to fire, and the Ying-(Spring) point of Yang meridian to water; the Shu-(Stream) point of Yin meridian to earth, the Shu-(Stream) point of Yang meridian to wood; the Jing-(River) point of Yin meridian to metal, and the Jing-(River) point of Yang meridian to water; the He-(Sea) point of Yin meridian to water and the He-(Sea) point of Yang meridian to earth." Thus, according to the rule of mutual promotion of five elements and different manifestations of diseases, the treatment principle of "reducing the son for excess syndrome","reinforcing the mother for deficiency syndrome,"were made. This method is known as reinforcing the mother or reducing the son. In practice, there are the methods of reinforcing or reducing the affected meridians, the method of midnight-noon ebb-flow receiving the son and the method of reinforcing the mother and reducing the son of the related meridian (Table 2-5, 2-6)

Table 2-5 The Five-Shu Points of Six Yin Meridians Corresponding to Five Elements

Six Yin	Jing-(Well) (Wood)	Ying-(Spring) (Fire)	Shu-(Stream) (Earth)	Jing-(River) (Metal)	He-(sea) (Water)
Lung Meridian (Metal)	Shaoshang (LU 11)	Yuji (LU 10)	Taiyuan (LU 9)	Jingqu (LU 8)	Chize (LU 5)
Kidney Meridian (Water)	Yongquan (KI 1)	Rangu (KI 2)	Taixi (KI 3)	Fuliu (KI 7)	Yingu (KI 10)
Liver Meridian (Wood)	Dadun (LR 1)	Xingjian (LR 2)	Taichong (LR 3)	Zhongfeng (LR 4)	Ququan (LR 8)
Heart Meridian (Fire)	Shaochong (HT 9)	Shaofu (HT 8)	Shenmen (HT 7)	Lingdao (HT 4)	Shaohai (HT 3)
Spleen Meridian (Earth)	Yinbai (SP 1)	Dadu (SP 2)	Taibai (SP 3)	Shangqiu (SP 5)	Yinlingquan (SP 9)
Pericardium Meridian (The premier Fire)	Zhongchong (PC 9)	Laogong (PC 8)	Daling (PC 7)	Jianshi (PC 5)	Quze (PC 3)

Table 2-6 The Five-Shu Points of Six Yang Meridians Corresponding to Five Elements

Six Yang Meridians	Jing-(Well) (Metal)	Ying-(Spring) (Water)	Shu-(Stream) (Wood)	Ying-(River) (Fire)	He-(Sea) (Earth)
Large Intestine Meridian (Metal)	Shangyang (LI 1)	Erjian (LI 2)	Sanjian (LI 3)	Yangxi (LI 5)	Quchi (LI 11)
Bladder Meridian (Water)	Zhiyin (BL 67)	Zutonggu (BL 66)	Shugu (BL 65)	Kunlun (BL 60)	Weizhong (BL 40)
Gallbladder Meridian (Wood)	Zuqiaoyin (GB 44)	Xiaxi (GB 43)	Zulinqi (GB 41)	Yangfu (GB 38)	Yanglingquan (GB 34)
Small Intestine Meridian (Fire)	Shaoze (SI 1)	Qiangu (SI 2)	Houxi (SI 3)	Yanggu (SI 5)	Xiaohai (SI 8)
Stomach Meridian (Earth)	Lidui (ST 45)	Neiting (ST 44)	Xiangu (ST 43)	Jiexi (ST 41)	Zusanli (ST 36)
Triple Energizer Meridian (The Premier Fire)	Guanchong (TE 1)	Yemen (TE 2)	Zhongzhu (TE 3)	Zhigou (TE 6)	Tianjing (TE 10)

2. Yuan-(Primary) Points and Luo-Connecting Points

"Yuan" means the origin, the primary Qi. Yuan-(Primary) Point is the site where the Yuan(Primary) Qi of Zang-Fu organs passes and stays. Each of the twelve regular meridians has a Yuan-(Primary) Point on the limbs, also termed "twelve Yuan-(Primary) Points." In the Yin meridians, the Yuan-(Primary) Points overlap with the Shu-(Stream) Points of the Five Shu Points. Each Yang meridian, however, has its Yuan-(Primary) Point other than the Shu-(Stream) Points which are arranged behind the Shu-(Stream) Points.

Luo means connecting. Each of the twelve regular meridians has a collateral on the limbs. The point on each collateral is named Luo-(Connecting) Point which links its exteriorly-interiorly related Yin and Yang meridians. The Luo-(Connecting) Points of the twelve regular meridians are located below the elbow of knee joints. Jiuwei(CV 15), the Luo-(Connecting)Point of the Conception Vessel is situated in the abdomen region, Changqiang(GV 1), the Luo-(connecting)Point of the Governor Vessel in the sacrococcygeal region. Dabao(SP 21), the Luo-(Connecting)Point of the major collateral of the spleen in the hypochondriac region. There are all together fifteen points, so are termed "The Fifteen Luo-(Connecting)Points."

(1) Yuan-(Primary)Points

A. For Diagnosis:

The Chapter "Discussion on the Nine Needles and the Twelve Yuan (Primary)(Chapter 1) in *Miraculous Pivot* says: "Any disorder of Five Zang-organs are originated from the twelve Yuan (Primary) points, each of which has its origin. Once the sources are known and their corresponding reflexions are seen, the disorder of Five Zang-organs is identified." At present, we use meridian detector to measure the conductibility of the Luo-(Connecting) Points, to analyse the excess or deficiency of each meridian, and to diagnose the diseases of Zang-Fu organs. The reading varies reversely to that of heat sensation of the Jing-(Well) Points. The greater reading indicates the excess syndrome of Zang-Fu organs.

B. For Treatment:

The Chapter "Discussion on the Nine Needles and the Twelve Yuan (Primary) (Chapter I) in *Miraculous Pivot* says: "Select the Yuan-(Primary) Points of the twelve meridians for treating diseases of Five Zang-organs." Yuan (Primary) Point can regulate the functions of Zang-Fu organs and the meridians and collaterals. They can not only reinforce the deficience syndrome, but also reduce the excess syndrome. Yuan-(Primary)Points perform the better therapeutic effects on the disorders of Zang-Fu organs. They can be used solely or in combination with the exteriorly-interiorly related Luo-(Connecting) Points. So, this method is called the combined selection of Yuan-(Primary) Point and Luo-(Connecting) Point. Because in the method, the Yuan-(Primary) Points of the affected meridians are regarded primary, while Luo-(Connecting) Points of interior-exterior meridians regarded secondary. So this method is also called the combination of the primary Yuan-(Primary) Points and the secondary Luo-(Connecting) Points.

(2) Luo-(Connecting)Points

A. For Diagnosis:

The Chapter "Discussion on the meridians" (Chapter 10) in *Miraculous Pivot* says: "The Fifteen Collaterals become distincted in excess syndrome and faded in deficiency syndrome. If they are invisible, their location might be found a little upward or downward. The difference of a person's collaterals is the basis of what people differ from one another in collaterals." When diseases of the meridians appear at the Luo Points of the collaterals, there occur soreness, numbness, induration and changes of colour to help diagnosis.

B. For Treatment:

a. Luo-(Connecting)Points are mainly indicated for the diseases of collaterals. For instance, when the collateral of Heart meridian gets excessive, there appears chest congestion. While it gets deficient, there appears hoarseness. Select Tongli(HT 5) for treatment(See the syndromes of collaterals in detail).

b. One Luo-(Conecting)points can communicate with two meridians. That is, Luo-(Connecting)points indicated in diseases of the affected meridians, and their exteriorly-interiorly related meridians. For instance, Lieque(LU 7), the Luo-Connecting Point of Lung Meridian is indicated in the diseases of Lung meridian such as cough and asthma, meanwhile it is also for the diseases of the Large Intestine Meridian such as toothache, and pain and stiff neck.

c. Luo-(Connecting) point can be used to treat chronic diseases, especially chronic diseases of Zang-Fu organs. Ancient people said: "The primary diseases stay in the meridians, chronic diseases stay in the collaterals." which means when chronic diseases which is hard to be cured, the morbid Qi, blood and dampness-phlegm stay from meridians into collaterals. Thus, Luo-(Connecting) Points are selected to treat diseases due to endogenous pathogens and chronic diseases of Zang-Fu organs. Shallow insertion and bloodletting method are used to treat the excess syndrome of the collaterals. (Table 2-7)

Table 2-7 The Yuan-(Primary) Points and The Luo-(Connecting) Points of the Twelve Regular Meridians

Meridian	Yuan-(Primary)Point	Luo-(Connecting)Point
Lung Meridian	Taiyuan(LU 9)	Lieque(LU 7)
Large Intestine Meridian	Hegu(LI 4)	Painli(LI 6)
Stomach Meridian	Chongyang(ST 42)	Fenglong(ST 40)
Spleen Meridian	Taibai(SP 3)	Gongsun(SP 4)
Heart Meridian	Shenmen(HT 7)	Tongli(HT 5)
Small Intestine Meridian	Wangu(SI 4)	Zhizheng(SI 7)
Bladder Meridian	Jinggu(BL 64)	Feiyang(BL 58)
Kidney Meridian	Taixi(KI 3)	Dazhong(KI 4)
Pericardium Meridian	Daling(PC 7)	Neiguan(PC 6)
Triple Energizer Meridian	Yangchi(TE 4)	Waiguan(TE 5)
Gallbladder Meridian	Qiuxu(GB 40)	Guangming(GB 37)
Liver Meridian	Taichong(LR 3)	Ligou(LR 5)
Conception Vessel		Jiuwei(CV 15)
Governor Vessel		Changqiang(GV 1)
The Major Collateral of Spleen		Dabao(SP 21)

3. Back-(Shu) Points and Front-(Mu) Points

Back-(Shu) Points are corresponding points on the back and where the Qi of the respective Zang-Fu organs is infused; Front-(Mu) points are those on the chest and abdomen where the Qi of the respective Zang-Fu organs is infused and converged. Both Back-(Shu) points and Front-(Mu) Points are distributed over the trunk and closely related with Zang-Fu organs.

(1) Back-(Shu) Points

A. For Diagnosis

The Chapter "Discussion on the Back-(Shu) Points" in *Miraculous Pivot* says: "Then it is required to find it to check reflex. Upon pressing, pain is diminishing. This is its Back-(Shu) Point." The 67th Problem, a Chapter of *Classic on Medical Problems* says: "Yin diseases reflect on Yang. The Shu point is Yang." It refers if Five Zang-organs are diseased, abnormal reactions appear in Back-(Shu) Points of Yang (Back regarded as Yang). Pressing Back-(Shu) points is helpful for diagnosis.

B. For Treatment

Back-(Shu) Points are indicated in diseases of Five Zang-organs. "Chang Ci Jie Lun", a chapter of *Plain Questions*: "Back-(Shu) Point is a spot where the patient feels being punctured on back, while his organ is in trouble." which means puncturing Back-(Shu) Points has direct therapeutic effect on the diseases of Five Zang-organs. "The Principle of Yin-Yang Doctrine and Its Relation with Natural Things or Phenomena", Chapter 5 in *Plain Question* says: "Disease with symptoms on the Yin meridians is treated by needling on the points of Yang meridians." which illustrates the corresponding Back-(Shu) Points can be selected not only to treat diseases of Five Zang-organs, but also diseases of five sense organs, nine orifices, skin, muscle, tendon and bone. For instance, Ganshu(BL 18) for disorder of liver, the diseases of eye (The liver has its specific body opening in the eyes), and spasms of tendons (The condition of the liver determines the condition of the tendons, the liver constitutes a reservoir of blood.). Shenshu (BL 23) for disorder of kidney as well as deafness and tinnitus which connect with kidney. (The kidney has its specific body opening in the ears, sufficient essence of life gives a keen sense of hearing), importance (the kidney stores the essence of life, and is in charge of reproduction) and myelopathy (The condition of the kidney determines the condition of the bone, and marrow). Back-(Shu) points can be solely used or in combination with Front-(Mu) Point. So that is called combination of Back-(Shu) points and Front-(Mu) Points.

(2) Front-(Mu) Points

A. For Diagnosis

The 67th Problem, a Chapter of *Classic on Medical Problems* says: "Disorders of Yang (back side) reflected over Yin (front side) which shows the location of Front-(Mu) Point." which refers if Six Fu-organs are diseased, there appear abnormal reactions in Front-(Mu) Points in the chest and abdomen. Pressing Front-Mu points can help to make diagnosis, or Front-(Mu) points and Back-(Shu) Points are mutually conferred for diagnosis, it is so-called "Back-(Shu) can be observed by examining Front-(Mu) Point and observation on Back-(Shu) Point can lead to diagnosis of Front-(Mu) Point."

B. For Treatment

Front-(Mu) Points can be used to treat diseases of the affected Zang-Fu organs, and those of Yang meridians and collaterals. "The Principle of Yin-Yang

Doctrine and Its Relation with Natural Things or Phenomena", Chapter 5 in *Plain Questions* says: "Diseases with symptoms of the Yang meridians is treated by needling points of the Yin meridians."Front-(Mu) Points can be selected to treat diseases of Six Fu-organs and diseases of Yang meridians. For instance, Zhongwan(CV 12) for epigastric pain, Tianshu(ST 25) for abdominal pain and diarrhea and Zhongji(CV 3) of the Bladder Meridian for sciatica. (Table 2-8)

Table 2-8 The Back-(Shu) Points and Front-Mu Points of Zang-(Fu) Organs

Zang-(Fu) Organs	Back-(Shu) Point	Front-(Mu) Point
Lung	Feishu(BL 13)	Zhongfu(LU 1)
Large Intestine	Dachangshu(BL 25)	Tianshu(ST 25)
Stomach	Weishu(BL 21)	Zhongwan(CV 12)
Spleen	Pishu(BL 20)	Zhangmen(LR 13)
Heart	Xinshu(BL 15)	Juque(CV 14)
Small Intestine	Xiaochangshu(BL 27)	Guanyuan(CV 4)
Bladder	Pangguangshu(BL 28)	Zhongji(CV 3)
Kidney	Shenshu(BL 23)	Jingmen(GB 25)
Pericardium	Jueyinshu(BL 14)	Tanzhong(CV 17)
Triple Energizer	Sanjiaoshu(BL 22)	Shimen(CV 5)
Gallbladder	Danshu(BL 19)	Riyue(GB 24)
Liver	Ganshu(BL 18)	Qimen(LR 14)

4. Eight Converging Points

"Hui" means "join together". The Eight Converging Points are the eight points where the vital essence and energy of the Zang-organs, Fu-organs, Qi, blood, tendon, vessel, bone and bone join together. They're distributed over the trunk and the limbs.

For Treatment

The Eight Converging Points are closely related with physiological functions of their eight corresponding organs and tissues, and each of them is used for treating diseases linked with eight organs or tissues, especially chronic diseases, disorders of the feebleness and weakness. For instance, Zhangmen(LR 13), the

Converging Point of Zang-organs, for diseases of Five Zang-organs mainly disorders of liver and spleen. Zhongwan(CV 12), the Converging Points of Fu-organs for diseases of Six Fu-organs, especially disorders of the stomach and large intestine; Yanglingquan(GB 34), the Converging Point of tendon, for diseases of tendon, hemiparalysis, pain in shoulder and arm, spasms, paralysis, and obstruction; Xuanzhong(GB 39), the Converging Point of marrow for paralysis of the lower limbs, softness and weakness of the lower limbs, anaemia and pain. Dazhu(BL 11), the Converging Point of bone for disorders of bone, pain of all joints especially for ostalgia of neck, shoulder, back and the limbs. Geshu(BL 17), the Converging Point of bone, for diseases of blood, such as haematemesis, nose-bleeding, coughing blood, bloody stool, hemorrhoid bleeding, hematuria, metrorrhagia and metrostaxis; anemia, external hemorrhage and blood stasis. Tanzhong(CV 17), the Converging Point of Qi for diseases of Qi mechanism, such as chest, congestion dyspnea, hiccup, asthma, melancholy, regurgitation and eructation; Taiyuan(LU 9), the Converging Point of Vessel for diseases of vessel such vasculitis, pulseless syndrome, and arteriosclerosis.

5. Xi-(Cleft)Points

Xi means cleft. The Xi-(Cleft)Point is the site where the Qi of the meridian is deeply converged. Each of the Twelve Regular Meridians and the four extra meridians such as, Yin Heel Vessel, Yang Heel Vessel, Yin Link Vessel, Yang Link Vessel has a Xi-(Cleft)Point, amounting to sixteen in all. They are distributed below elbows and knees. (Table 2-9)

Table 2-9   The Sixteen Xi-(Cleft)Points

Yin Meridian	Xi-(Cleft)Points	Yang Meridian	Xi-(Cleft)Points
Lung Meridian	Kongzui(LU 6)	Large Intestine Meridian	Wenliu(LI 7)
Pericardium Meridian	Ximen(PC 4)	Triple Energizer Meridian	Huizong(TE 7)
Heart Meridian	Yinxi(HT 6)	Small Intestine Meridian	Yanglao(SI 6)
Spleen Meridian	Diji(SP 8)	Stomach Meridian	Liangqiu(ST 34)
Liver Meridian	Zhongdu(LR 6)	Gallbladder Meridian	Waiqiu(GB 36)
Kidney Meridian	Shuiquan(KI 5)	Bladder Meridian	Jinmen(BL 63)
Yin Link Vessel	Zhubin(KI 9)	Yang Link Vessel	Yangjiao(GB 35)
Yin Heel Vessel	Jiaoxin(KI 8)	Yang Heel Vessel	Fuyang(BL 59)

For Diagnosis

When Zang-Fu organs are diseased, Xi-(Cleft)point pressing is helpful for diagnosis.

For Treatment

Xi-(Cleft) Points are the site where Qi and blood are stored deeply, so, general speaking, the pathogens can't invade these points. If there appear abnormal reactions in Xi-(Cleft)Points, it shows that the pathogens have entered the deeper parts of Zang-Fu organs, the manifestation is acute and serious. Thus Xi-(Cleft)Points are used for acute, painful symptom, inflammation, protracted diseases of its pertaining meridian and Zang-Fu organs. The Xi-(Cleft) Points of Yin meridian have hemostatic function. For instance, Kongzui (LU 6) is effective to hemoptysis, Zhongdu(LR 6) is effective to metrorrhea, and Yinxi(HT 6) is effective to hemoptysis and rhinorrhea. The Xi-(Cleft) Points of Yang meridian can mainly relieve pain. For instance, Yanglao(SI 6) for acute lumbar pain and Liangqiu(ST 34) for epigastric pain. Xi-(Cleft) Point can be used solely or in combination with the Converging Points. This is called the combination of Xi-(Cleft) Points and the Converging Points. For instance, Liangqiu(ST 34) combined with Zhongwan(CV 12) can treat acute stomachache; Kongzui(LU 6) combined with Tanzhong(CV 17) can cure hemoptysis due to perversive flow of Qi.

6. Lower He-Sea Points

The lower He-(Sea)Points refer to the six points of the three Yang meridians of head and foot where the downward flowing Qi of the Six Fu-organs along the three Yang meridians of foot. Most of them are distributed around the knee joints.

Lower He-(Sea)Points are the main points for diseases of Six Fu-organs. The chapter "Discussion on the Pathogenic Factors, Zang-Fu and Syndromes" (Chapter 4)in *Miraculous Pivot* says: "Lower-He(Sea)points can be used for diseases of Six Fu-organs." For instance, Zusanli(ST 36) is effective to epigastric pain. Xiajuxu(ST 39)is effective to diarrhea, Shangjuxu(ST 37) is effective to intestine-carbuncle; Weiyang(BL 39)and Weizhong(BL 40)are effective to retention of urine and enuresis caused by dysfunction of Triple Energizer.

7. Eight Confluent Points and Crossing Points

The Eight Confluent Points refer to the eight points where the eight extra meridians communicate with the twelve regular meridians. They are distributed on the areas superior and inferior to the wrist joints and ankle joints. (Table 2-10)

Table 2-10 The Eight Confluent Points of the Eight Extra Meridian

Pertaining Meridian	Confluent Point	Extra Meridian	Region of Connection
Spleen Meridian	Gongsun(SP 4)	Thoroughfare Vessel	Stomach, Heart
Pericardium Meridian	Neiguan(PC 6)	Yin Link Vessel	Chest
Triple Energizer Meridian	Waiguan(TE 5)	Yang Link Vessel	Outer Canthus
Gallbladder Meridian	Zulinqi(GB 4)	Belt Vessel	Cheek, Neck, Posterior Ear, Shoulder
Small Intestine Meridian	Houxi(SI 3)	Governor Vessel	Inner Canthus, Nape, Ear
Bladder Meridian	Shenmai(BL 62)	Yang Heel Vessel	Shoulder Girdle
Lung Meridian	Lieque(LU 7)	Conception Vessel	Chest, Lung
Kidney Meridian	Zhaohai(KI 6)	Yin Heel Vessel	Diaphragm, Throat

Crossing Points are those at the intersections of two or more meridians. Most of them are distributed on trunk.

The Eight Confluent Points are widely used. In the book of *Elementary Course for Medicine*, Li Chan says: "Eight methods are mainly based on the eight points of extra meridians, and the eight points are the congregation of twelve meridians. There are three hundred and sixty points over the whole body, and sixty-six points of hand and foot are the conglomeration of them, while sixty-six points are conglomerated into the eight points." Because the Qi of both extra meridians and regular meridians meet at the Eight Confluent Points, they can be used to treat diseases of extra meridians and those of the regular meridian. For instance, Gongsun(SP 4) communicates with the Thoroughfare Vessel, as Gongsun(SP 4) is the point of Spleen Meridian, it can be used for diseases of the

Spleen Meridian and those of the Thoroughfare Vessel as well; Neiguan(PC 6) meets the Yin Link Vessel, and is also the point of the Pericardium Meridian. So Neiguan(PC 6)can be used for diseases of the Pericardium Meridian and the Yin Link Vessel, other points are on the analogus of this. In clinical practice, the combination of the upper points and lower points is taken in the application of the Eight Confluent Points while given acupuncture, points are often picked in pairs one with the other. Gongsun (SP 4)and Neiguan(PC 6)treat diseases of stomach, heart and chest and malaria; Houxi(SI 3)and Shenmai(BL 62)treat diseases of inner canthus, ear, nape and shoulder and fever due to aversion to cold; Waiguan(TE 5)and Zulinqi(GB 41)for diseases of outer canthus, ear, cheek and shoulder and alternate fever and chills; Lieque(LU 7)and Zhaohai(KI 6)for diseases of throat, chest, diaphragm and chest, and deficiency of Yin as the result of exhausted vital essence.

There are many crossing points over the whole body. They can be used to treat not only disorders of their affected meridians, but also those of the meridians which they communicate with. For instance, Zhongji(CV 3)and Guanyuan (CV 4)are the points of the Conception Vessel and meet three Yin Meridians of Foot as well, so these two points can be used for disorders of the Conception Vessel and three Yin Meridians of Foot; Dazhui(GV 14), the point of the Governor Vessel links with Three Meridians of Hand-Foot, so it can be used to treat diseases of Governor Vessel and disorders over the whole body caused by Yang meridians; Sanyinjiao(SP 6), the point of Spleen Meridian can be used to treat disorders of Spleen Meridian and those of Heart Meridian and Kidney Meridian.

Main Crossing Points of Meridians

1. Lung Meridian
Zhongfu(LU 1): The Crossing Point of Lung Meridian and Spleen Meridian.

2. Large Intestine Meridian
Jianyu(LI 15): The Crossing Point of Large Intestine Meridian and Yang Heel Vessel.

Yingxiang (LI 20): The Crossing Point of Large Intestine Meridian and Stomach Meridian.

3. Stomach Meridian
Chengqi(ST 1): The Crossing Point of Stomach Meridian, Yang Heel Vessel

and Conception Vessel.

Dicang (ST 4): The Crossing Points of Yang Heel Vessel, Large Intestine Meridian and Stomach Meridian.

Xiaguan (ST 7): The Crossing Points of Gallbladder Meridian and Stomach Meridian.

Touwei (ST 8): The Crossing Point of Gallbladder Meridian, Stomach Meridian and Yang Link Vessel.

4. Spleen Meridian

Sanyinjiao (SP 6): The Crossing Points of Spleen Meridian, Kidney Meridian, and Liver Meridian.

Daheng (SP 15): The Crossing Point of Spleen Meridian and Yin Link Vessel.

Fuai (SP 16): The Crossing Point of Spleen Meridian and Yang Link Vessel.

5. Small Intestine Meridian

Quanliao (SI 18): The Crossing Point of Small Intestine Meridian and Triple Energizer Meridian.

Tinggong (SI 19): The Crossing Point of Triple Energizer Meridian, Gallbladder Meridian and Small Intestine Meridian.

6. Bladder Meridian

Jingming (BL 1): The Crossing Point of Small Intestine Meridian, Bladder Meridian, Yin Heel Vessel and Yang Heel Vessel, Stomach Meridian.

Dazhu (BL 11): The Crossing Point of Small Intestine Meridian and Bladder Meridian.

Fengmen (BL 12): The Crossing Point of Governor Vessel and Bladder Meridian.

7. Kidney Meridian

Dahe (KI 12), Qixue (KI 13), Siman (KI 14), Zhongzhu (KI 15), Huangshu (KI 16), Shangqu (KI 17), Shiguan (KI 18), Yindu (KI 19), Futonggu (KI 20) and Youmen (KI 21): The Crossing Point of Kidney Meridian and Thoroughfare Vessel.

8. Pericardium Meridian

Tianchi(PC 1): The Crossing Point of Pericardium Meridian and Gallbladder Meridian.

9. Triple Energizer Meridian

Yifeng(TE 17): The Crossing Point of Triple Energizer Meridian and Gallbladder Meridian.

Jiaosun(TE 20): The Crossing Point of Triple Energizer Meridian, Gallbladder Meridian, and Large Intestine Meridian.

10. Gallbladder Meridian.

Tongziliao(GB 1): The Crossing Point of Small Intestine Meridian, Triple Energizer Meridian and Gallbladder Meridian.

Yangbai(GB 14): The Crossing Point of Gallbladder Meridian and Yang Link Vessel.

Toulinqi(GB 15): The Crossing Point of Bladder Meridian, Gallbladder Meridian and Yang Link Vessel.

Fengchi(GB 20): The Crossing Point of Gallbladder Meridian and Yang Link Vessel.

Jianjing(GB 21): The Crossing Point of Triple Energizer Meridian, Gallbladder Meridian and Yang Link Vessel.

Riyue(GB 24): The Crossing Point of Spleen Meridian and Gallbladder Meridian.

Daimai(BL 26): The Crossing Points of Gallbladder Meridian and Belt Vessel.

Huantiao(GB 30): The Crossing Point of Gallbladder Meridian and Bladder Meridan

11. Liver Meridian

Zhangmen (LR 13): The Crossing Point of Liver Meridian and Kidney Meridian.

Qimen(LR 14): The Crossing Point of Liver Meridian, Spleen Meridian and Yin Link Vessel.

12. The Conception Vessel

Chengjiang (CV 24): The Crossing Point of Stomach Meridian and Conception Vessel.

Lianquan (CV 23): The Crossing Point of Yin Link Vessel and Conception Vessel.

Tiantu (CV 22): The Crossing Point of Yin Link Vessel and Conception Vessel.

Shangwan (CV 13): The Crossing Point of Conception Vessel, Stomach Meridian and Lung Meridian.

Zhongwan (CV 12): The Crossing Point of Small Intestine Meridian, Triple Energizer Meridian, Stomach Meridian and Conception Vessel.

Xiawan (CV 10): The Crossing Point of Spleen Meridian and Conception Vessel.

Yinjiao (CV 7): The Crossing Point of Conception Vessel and Thoroughfare Vessel.

Guanyuan (CV 4): The Crossing Point of Spleen Meridian, Liver Meridian, Kidney Meridian and Conception Vessel.

Zhongji (CV 3): The Crossing Point of Spleen Meridian, Liver Meridian, Kidney Meridian and Conception Vessel.

Huiyin (CV 1): The Crossing Point of Conception Vessel, Governor Vessel and Thoroughfare Vessel.

13. The Governor Vessel

Shenting (GV 24): The Crossing Point of Governor Vessel, Bladder Meridian and Stomach Meridian.

Shuigou (GV 26): The Crossing Point of Governor Vessel, Large Intestine Meridian and Stomach Meridian.

Baihui (GV 20): The Crossing Point of Governor Vessel and Bladder Meridian.

Naohu (GV 17): The Crossing Point of Governor Vessel and Bladder Meridian.

Fengfu (GV 16): The Crossing Point of Governor Vessel and Yang Link Vessel.

Yamen (GV 15): The Crossing Point of Governor Vessel and Yang Link Vessel.

Dazhui(GV 14): The Crossing Point of Governor Vessel and the three Yang Meridians of Hand-Foot.

Taodao(GV 13): The Crossing Point of Governor Vessel and Bladder Meridian.

Source: Illustrated Manual on the Points for Acupuncture and Moxibustion as Found on the Bronze Figure; A classic of Acupuncture and Moxibustion, the words "hand" and "foot" omitted.

Section 6 Methods of Locating Acupoints

The methods of Locating acupoints are divided into three categories.

1. Anatomical Landmarks

The landmarks may be divided into two types: permanent lanmarks and impermanent landmarks. Fixed landmarks are those parts formed by eminence or depression consisting of bone joints and muscles, the contour of five sense organs, hairline, finger (toe) nails, nipple and umbilicus. For instance, Yanglingquan(GB 34) in the anterior and inferior side to the small head of the fibula; Binao (LI 14), in the region superior to the insertion of m. deltoideus; Cuanzhu (BL 2) in the depression on the medial end of eyebrow; Yintang(EX-HN 3) between the medial ends of the two eyebrows; Tanzhong(CV 17) between the two nipples. Impermanent landmarks refer to spaces, depression, wrinkles that appear while the joints, muscles, skin and others move voluntarily. For instance, Tinggong(SI 19) is located anterior to the tragus and posterior to the condyloid process of the mandible, in the depression formed when the mouth is open; Quchi (LI 11) is located at the lateral end of the transverse cubital cause, in the depression formed when elbow is bending.

2. Bone-Length Measurement

This is a method of locating acupoints in which the bone segments are taken as measurement markers to measure the width or length of various portions of the body, the measurements are converted proportionately into definite numbers of equal units as the standards. These standards are applicable on any patient of different sexes, ages, and body sizes. Standards for bone-length measurement as follows. (Table 2-11, Fig. 2-22)

Table 2-11 Standards for Bone-length Measurement

Body Part	Distance	Bonelength Measure	Method	Explanation
Head	From the midpoint of the anterior hairline to the midpoint of the posterior hairline	12 cun	Longitudinal Measurement	It is used to check longitudinal distances of the meridian points on the head.
	From the medial ends of the two eyebrows, (Yintang) (EX-HN 3) to the midpoint of the anterior hairline	3 cun	Longitudinal Measurement	It is used to check longitudinal distances of the meridian points on the anterior and posterior hairlines, and head.
	Below the spinous process of the seventh cervical vertebra (Dazhui) (GV 14) to the midpoint of the posterior hairline	3 cun	Longitudinal Measurement	
	From the medial ends of the two eyebrows (Yintang) (EX-HZ 3) to the midpoint of the posterior hairline, then to the spinous process of the seventh cervical vertebra (Dazhui) (GV 14)	18 cun	Longitudinal Measurement	
	Between the corners of the forehead (Touwei) (ST 8)	9 cun	Transverse Measurement	It is used to check the transverse distances of the meridian points of the anterior region of head.
	Between the two mastoid processes	9 cun	Transverse Measurement	It is used to check the transverse distances of the meridian points of the posterior region of head.

Body Part	Distance	Bonelength Measure	Method	Explanation
Chest and Abdomen	From the suprasternal fossa to the sternocostal angle	9 cun	Longitudinal Measurement	It is used to check the longitudinal distances of the points of Conception Vessel in the chest.
	From the sternocostal angle to the center of the umbilicus	8 cun	Longitudinal Measurement	It is used to check the longitudinal distances of the meridian points in the upper abdomen.
	From the center of the umbilicus to the upper of symphysis pubis	5 cun	Longitudinal Measurement	It is used to check the longitudinal distances of the meridian points in the lower abdomen.
	Between the two nipples	8 cun	Transverse Measurement	It is used to check the transverse distances of the meridian points in the chest and abdomen.
	From the end of axillary fold to the tip of the eleventh rib	12 cun	Longitudinal Measurement	It is used to check the longitudinal distances of the meridian points in hypochondria region.
Back	From the medial border of the scapula to the posterior midline	3 cun	Transverse Measurement	It is used to check the transverse distances of the meridian points in the back.
	From the lateral border of acromion to the posterior midline	8 cun	Transverse Measurement	It is used to check the transverse distances of the meridian points in the shoulder and back.
Upper Limbs	From the end of the axillary fold to the transverse cubital crease	9 cun	Longitudinal Measurement	Used to check the longitudinal distances of the meridian points of arm.
	From the transverse cubital crease and the transverse wrist crease	12 cun	Longitudinal Measurement	Used to check the longitudinal distances of the meridian points of forearm.

Body Part	Distance	Bonelength Measure	Method	Explanation
Lower limbs	From the level of the border of symphysis to the medial epicondyle of femur	18 cun	Longitudinal Measurement	Used to check the longitudinal distances of the points of the Three Foot Yin Meridians of the medial side of Lower Limbs.
	From the lower border of the medial condyle of tibia to the tip of medial malleolus	13 cun	Longitudinal Measurement	
	From the prominence of the great trochanter to the middle of patella	19 cun	Longitudinal Measurement	Used to check the longitudinal distances of the points of the Three Yang Meridians Foot of the lateral side of lower limbs (The distance from the gluteal crease to the center of patella is taken as 14 cun)
	From the center of patella to the tip of lateral malleolus	16 cun	Longitudinal Measurement	Used to check the longitudinal distances of the points of the Three Yang Meridians of Foot of the lateral side of lower limbs.

3. Finger Measurement

This refers to the length and width of the patient's fingers are taken as a standard for point location. (Fig. 2-23)

Thumb Measurement: The width of the interphalangeal joint of the patient's thumb is taken as one cun.

Middle Finger Measurement: When the patient's middle finger is flexed, the distance between the two medial ends of the creases of the interphalangeal joints is taken as one cun.

Four-Finger Measurement: The width of the four fingers (index, middle, ring and little) close together at the level of the dorsal skin crease of the proximal interphalangeal joint of the middle finger is taken as three cun. Location of acupoints should be based on the standard of bone-length measurement, and refers to the length and width of the patient, with the help of simple impermanent landmarks to ensure the standardized locations of acupoints.

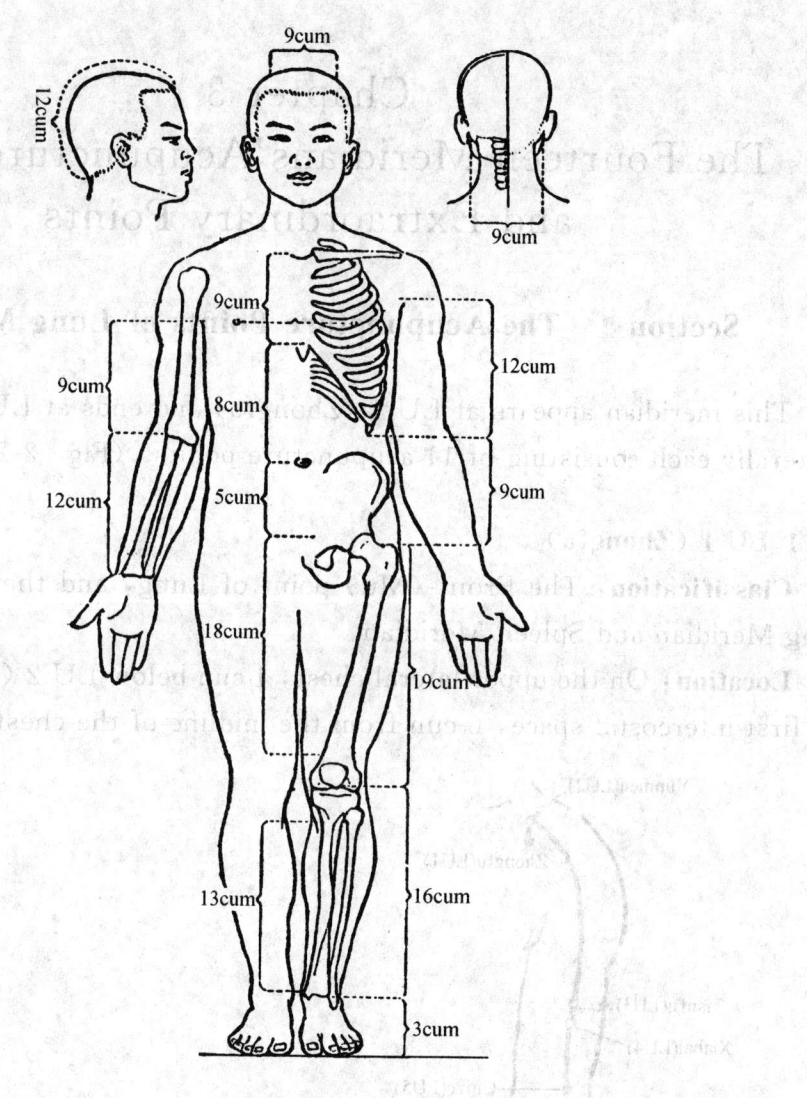

Fig. 1-22

Middle Finger Measurement

Thumb Measurement

Four-Finger Measurement

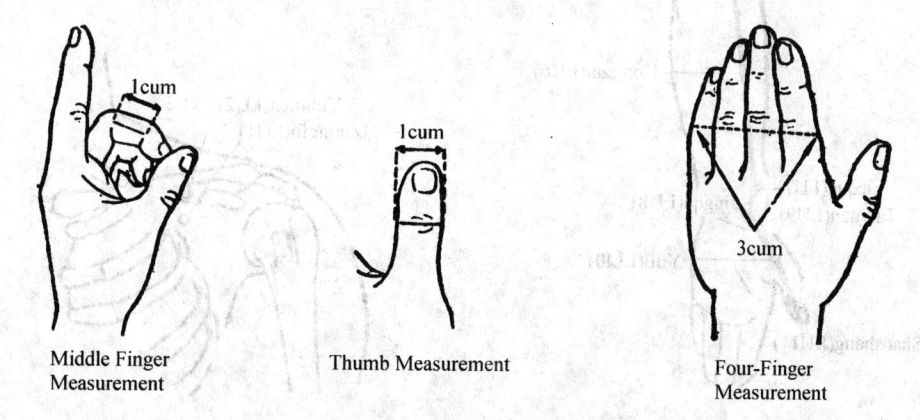

Fig 2-23 Four-Finger Measurement

69

Chapter 3
The Fourteen Meridians' Acupuncture Points and Extraordinary Points

Section 1 The Acupuncture Points of Lung Meridian

This meridian appears at LU 1 (Zhongfu) and ends at LU 11 (Shaoshang); bilaterally each consisting of 11 acupuncture points. (Fig. 2-24)

1. LU 1 (Zhongfu)

Classification: The Front-(Mu) point of Lung, and the Crossing point of Lung Meridian and Spleen Meridian.

Location: On the upper lateral chest, 1 cun below LU 2 (Yunmen), level in the first intercostal space, 6 cun from the midline of the chest. (Fig. 2-25)

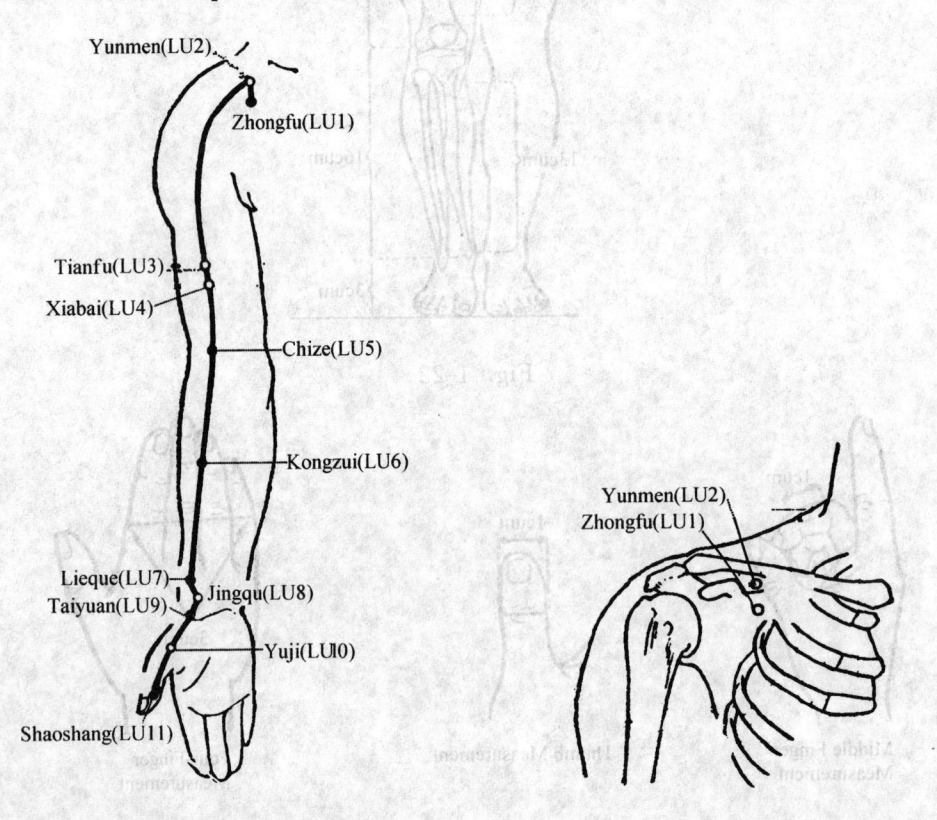

Fig. 2-24   Fig. 2-25

The Points of the Lung Meridian

Regional Anatomy: Skin→subcutaneous tissue→m. pectoralis major→m. pectoralis minor→thoracic cavity. The superficial layer (innervation and vasculature) contains intermediate supraclavicular nerve, the lateral cutaneous branch of the first intercostal nerve, cephalic vein, etc. Deep layer holds thoracoacromial artery and vein, and the anterior thoracic nerve.

Indications: (1) Cough, asthma, chest pain. (2) Shoulder and back pain. (3) Abdominal distention.

Needling and Moxibustion Method: Oblique insertion towards the lateral aspect of the chest or subcutaneous insertion 0.5—0.8 cun. Deep perpendicular insertion or toward the medial aspect are prohibited in order to avoid puncturing the lungs, causing pneumothorax. Mild moxibustion with moxa stick for 10—20 minutes is applicable.

Annotations: (1) This point is the Lung Front-(Mu) point which is one of the important points used in diagnosis and treatment of lung disease. Pulmonary tuberculosis and bronchial asthma patients often have a sensitive reaction at this point. Also, due to it being the Crossing Point of Lung Meridian and Spleen Meridian, this point can be used to strengthen the spleen, regulate the Qi and treat abdominal distentio.

(2) For every point hereafter, except for contraindicated points, the needling and moxibustion method stated is only a general introduction of the conventional needling method used in applying the filiform needle. For the moxibustion method, except for contraindicated points and use of special moxibustion techniques, normally, the points are warmed with the moxa stick for 10—20 minutes causing an area of the skin to become red. This will not be reiterated.

(3) For the regional anatomy, the order is from the superficial layer entering into the deeper layer. Differential layers are the skin→subcutaneous tissue→muscle (or tendon or fascia), blood vessel, and nerve. For every point hereafter, only the vasculature and innervation will be stated.

2. LU 2 (Yunmen)

Location: On the upper lateral chest, above the acromioscapula, in the depression below the acromial end of clavicle, 6 cun from the midline of the chest (Fig. 2-25)

Regional Anatomy: Deep layer, the axillary artery; the lateral cord of the brachial plexus.

Indications: (1) Cough, asthma. (2) Pain in the chest, pain in the shoulder and back.

Needling Method: Oblique insertion 0.5—0.8 cun toward the lateral aspect of the chest. Do not insert deeply toward the medial aspect to avoid puncturing the lungs.

3. LU (3 Tianfu)

Location: On the medial aspect of the upper arm, on the radial side of m. biceps brachii, 3 cun below the front end of the axillary fossa. (Fig. 2-26)

Regional Anatomy: The cephalic vein and muscular branches of the brachial artery and vein. The distribution of the lateral brachial cutaneous nerve.

Indications: (1) Epistaxis. (2) Cough, asthma. (3) Pain in the shoulder and medial aspect of the upper extremity.

Needling Method: Perpendicular insertion 0.5—1.0 cun.

Fig. 2-26   Fig. 2-27

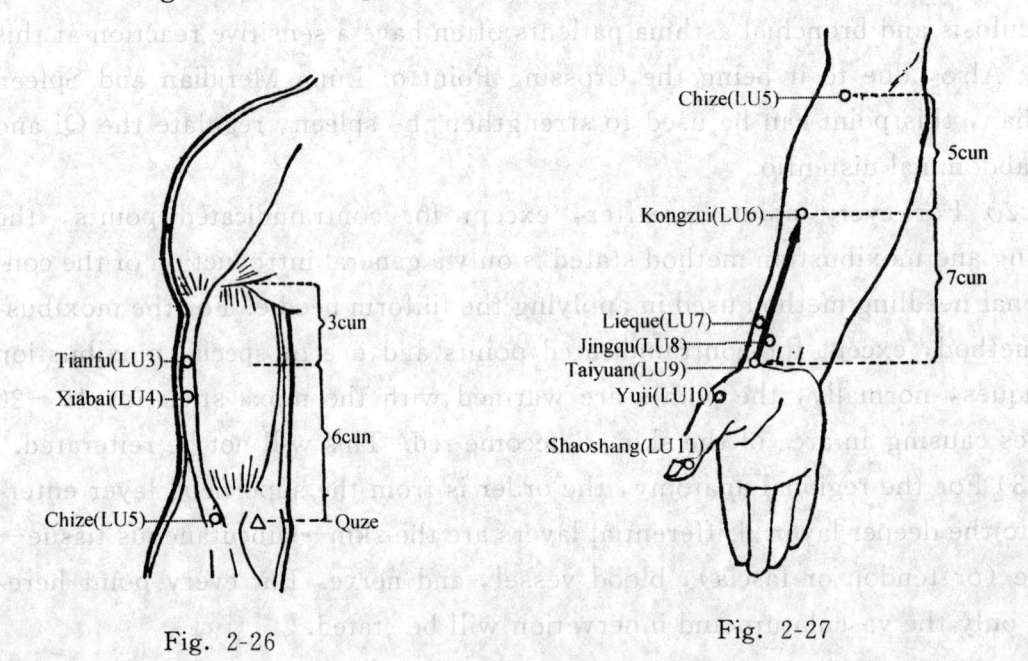

4. LU 4 (Xiabai)

Location: On the medial aspect of the upper arm, on the radial side of the m. biceps brachii, 4 cun below the front end of the axillary fossa, 5 cun above the cubital crease. (Fig. 2-26)

Regional Anatomy: Vasculature and innervation same as LU 3 (Tianfu).

Indications: (1) Cough, asthma, irritability, congestion (2) Nausea. (3) Pain in the medial aspect of the upper arm.

Needling Method: Perpendicular insertion 0.5—1.0 cun.

5. LU 5 (Chize)

Classification: He-(Sea) point.

Location: On the cubital crease, on the radial side of the tendon of m. biceps brachii. (Fig. 2-26)

Regional Anatomy: The cephalic vein; the radial nerve.

Indications: (1) Cough, asthma, hemoptysis, afternoon fever, chest congestion. (2) Sore throat. (3) Acute abdominal pain with vomiting and diarrhea. (4) Infantile convulsions. (5) Spasmodic pain of the elbow and arm.

Needling Method: (1) Perpendicular insertion 0.8-.2 cun. (2) When treating acute abdominal pain with vomiting and diarrhea, prick the cephalic vein on this point to make bleeding.

6. LU 6 (Kongzui)

Classification: Xi-(Cleft) point.

Location: On the radial palmar aspect of the forearm, on the line joining LU 5 (Chize) and LU 9 (Taiyuan), 7 cun above the transverse crease of the wrist. (Fig. 2-27)

Regional Anatomy: Cephalic vein, radial artery the superficial ramus of the radial nerve.

Indications: (1) Acute hemoptysis, bleeding hemorrhoids, epistaxis, cough and asthma. (2) Sore throat. (3) Febrile diseases without sweating. (4) Pain in the forearm.

Needling Method: Perpendicular insertion 0.5—1.0 cun.

7. LU 7 (Lieque)

Classification: Luo-(Connecting) point.

Location: On the radial margin of the forearm, superior to the styloid process of the radius, 1.5 cun above the transverse crease of the wrist. (Fig. 2-27) (Fig. 2-28)

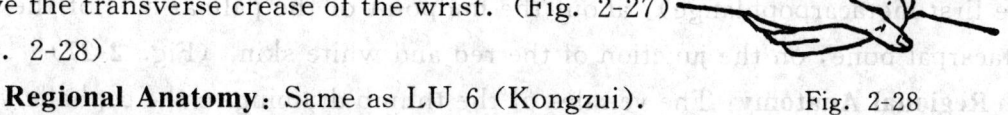

Fig. 2-28

Regional Anatomy: Same as LU 6 (Kongzui).

Indications: (1) Head and neck problem: migraine (central line and one-side) headache caused by exogenic pathogens, neck rigidity, wry face, toothache, sore throat, cough and asthma. (2) Urogenital system problems: pain in the penis, hematuria, spermatorrhea. (3) Abdominal distention. (4) Weakness of the thumb and index finger.

Needling Method: Insert obliquely upwards 0.3—0.5 cun.

8. LU 8 (Jingqu)

Classification: Jing-(River) point.

Location: On the radial palmar aspect of the forearm, in the depression between the styloid process of the radius and the radial artery, 1 cun above the transverse crease of the wrist (Fig. 2-27)

Regional Anatomy: Same as LU 6 (Kongzui).

Indications: (1) Cough, asthma, chest pain, sore throat. (2) Wrist pain.

Needling Method: Keep clear of radial artery. Perpendicular insertion 0.3—0.5 cun. *A-B Classic of Acupuncture and Moxibustion* says:"do not moxa."

9. LU 9 (Taiyuan)

Classification: Yuan-(Source) point, Shu-(Stream) point, One of the Eight Influential Points.

Location: On the radial end of the transverse crease of the wrist, where the radial artery pulsates. (Fig. 2-27)

Regional Anatomy: The radial artery; the superficial ramus of the radial nerve.

Indications: (1) Cough with large amount of phlegm, asthma with weakness. (2) Vascular problems: acrotism, headache, hemiplegia, cold, pain, and weakness in the lower extremity. (3) Wrist pain. (4) Hiccough.

Needling Method: Keep clear of artery. Perpendicular insertion 0.3—0.5 cun.

10. LU 10 (Yuji)

Classification: Ying-(Spring) point.

Location: In the depression behind the (thenar eminence) root of the thumb (the first metacarpophlange), about the midpoint of the palmar side of the first metacarpal bone, on the junction of the red and white skin. (Fig. 2-27)

Regional Anatomy: The venules of the thumb draining to the cephalic vein; the palmar cutaneous ramus of the median nerve, and superficial ramus of the radial nerve.

Indications: (1) Asthma. (2) Sore throat, fever, hoarseness. (3) Cough, hemoptysis.

Needling Method: Insert obliquely 0.5—0.8 cun toward center of palm.

11. LU 11 (Shaoshang)
Classification: Jing-(Well) point.
External Anatomical Location: On the radial side of the thumb, 0.1 cun (finger cun) distance from the corner of the nail. (Fig. 2-27)
Regional Anatomy: The arterial and venous network; the radial nerve and median nerve forming the terminal nerve network.
Indications: (1) Sore throat, cough, nose bleeding. (2) Fever. (3) Coma, manic disorders. (4) Numbness at fingertips.
Needling Method: Insert obliquely 0.1 cun towards upper direction, or prick the point to make bleeding.

Section 2 The Acupuncture Points of Large Intestine Meridian

This meridian starts at LI 1 (Shangyang) and goes to LI 20 (Yingxiang); bilaterally each consisting of 20 acupuncture points. (Fig. 2-29)

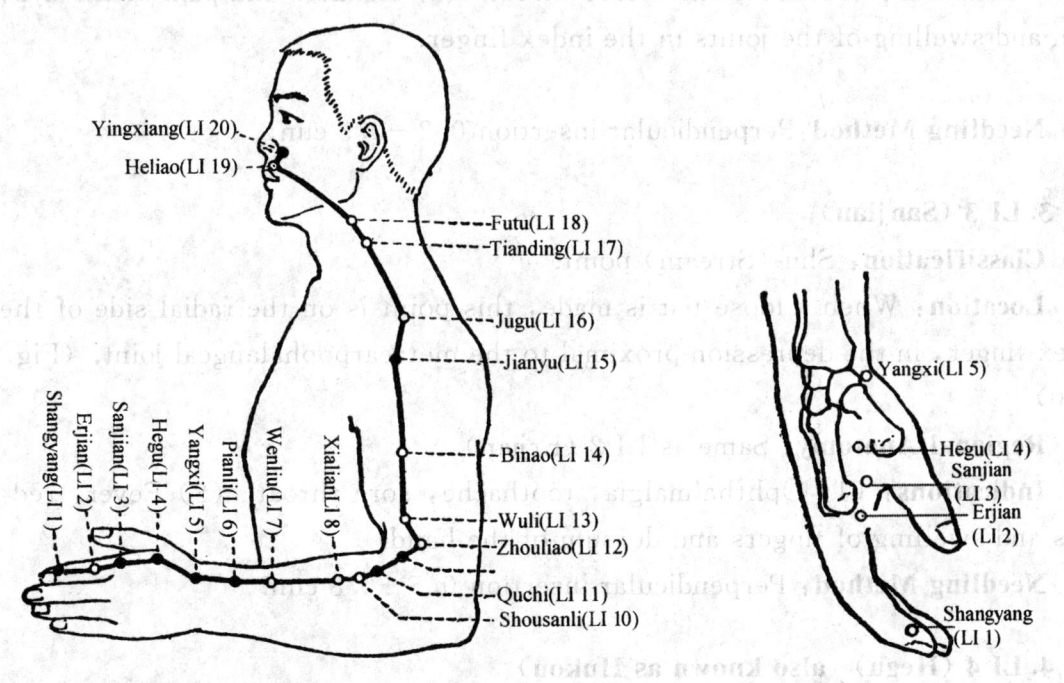

Fig. 2-29
Points of the Large Intestine Meridian

Fig. 2-30

1. **LI 1 (Shangyang)**

Classification: Jing-(Well) point.

Location: On the radial side of the distal phalanx of the index finger, 0.1 cun (finger cun) distance from the corner of the nail. (Fig. 2-30)

Regional Anatomy: Same as LU 11 (Shaoshang).

Indications: (1) Sore throat, toothache. (2) Coma caused by febrile disease. (3) Numbness at tip of index finger. (4) Deafness.

Needling Method: Shallow insertion 0.1 cun, or prick the point to make bleeding.

2. **LI 2 (Erjian)**

Classification: Ying-(Spring) point.

Location: When a loose fist is made, this point is on the radial side of the index finger, in the depression distal to the metacarpo-phalangeal joint. (Fig. 2-30)

Regional Anatomy: The dorsal digital and palmar digital arteries and veins. The distribution of the branches of the radial and median nerves.

Indications: (1) Toothache, sore throat. (2) Redness and pain of the eye, pain and swelling of the joints in the index finger.

Needling Method: Perpendicular insertion 0.2—0.3 cun.

3. **LI 3 (Sanjian)**

Classification: Shu-(Stream) point.

Location: When a loose fist is made, this point is on the radial side of the index finger, in the depression proximal to the metacarpophalangeal joint. (Fig. 2-30)

Regional Anatomy: Same as LI 2 (Erjian).

Indications: (1) Ophthalmalgia, toothache, sore throat. (2) Fever, redness and swelling of fingers and dorsum of the hand.

Needling Method: Perpendicular insertion 0.5—0.8 cun.

4. **LI 4 (Hegu) (also known as Hukou)**

Classification: Yuan-(Source) point.

Location: On the dorsum of the hand, between the 1st and 2nd metacarpal bones, in the middle of the 2nd metacarpal bone on the radial side. (Fig. 2-30)

Simple Technique: Using the transverse crease of the interphalangeal joint of the thumb, place on the margin of the web between the thumb and the index finger of the other hand. The point is where the tip of the thumb touches. (Fig. 2-31)

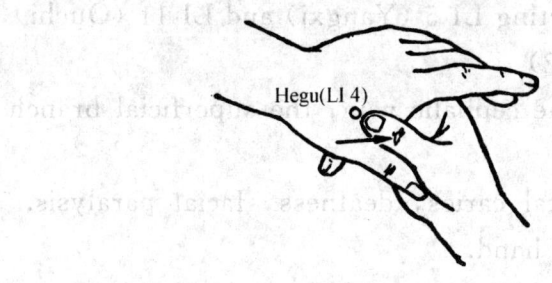

Fig. 2-31

Regional Anatomy: The venous network of the dorsum of the hand. The distribution of the superficial ramus of the radial nerve.

Indications: (1) Diseases of the head and face; i.e. external pathogenic headache and bodyache, dizziness, congestion, swelling and pain of the eye, nasosinusitis, epistaxis, toothache in the lower jaw, trismus, deafness, mumps, swelling of the face, facial paralysis, facial tic, swelling of the pharynx and aphonia. (2) Aversion to cold, fever, febrile disease, anhidrosis, hidrosis. (3) Dysmenorrhea, ammenorrhea, dystocia. (4) Gastric pain, abdominal pain, constipation, diarrhea, dysentery. (5) Hemiplegia, finger spasm, pain in the arm, infantile convulsion, manic psychosis and irritability. (6) Malignant sore, urticaria, scabies. (7) Every type of pain and psychogenic tense.

Needling Method: Perpendicular insertion 0.5—1.0 cun. This point is prohibited in pregnancy.

5. LI 5 (Yangxi)

Classification: Jing-(River) point.

Location: On the radial side of the dorsal crease of the wrist, when the thumb is pointed upwards, it is in the depression between the tendons of m. extensor pollicis longus and brevis. (Fig. 2-30)

Regional Anatomy: The cephalic vein, the radial artery the superficial ramus of the radial nerve.

Indications: (1) Frontal headache, congestion, swelling and pain of the eye, toothache. (2) Weakness of the wrist.

Needling Method: Perpendicular insertion 0.5—0.8 cun.

6. LI 6 (Pianli)

Classification: Luo-(Connecting) point.

Location: With the elbow flexed, the point is on the dorsal radial side of the forearm, on the line connecting LI 5 (Yangxi) and LI 11 (Quchi), 3 cun above the wrist crease. (Fig. 2-32)

Regional Anatomy: The cephalic vein; the superficial branch of the radial nerve.

Indications: (1) Dental caries, deafness, facial paralysis. (2) Edema, aching in the dorsum of the hand.

Needling Method: Perpendicular or oblique insertion 0.5—0.8 cun.

7. LI 7 (Wenliu)

Classification: Xi-(Cleft) point.

Location: With the elbow flexed, the point is on the dorsal radial side of the forearm, on the line connecting LI 5 (angxi) and LI 11 (Quchi), 5 cun above the wrist crease. (Fig. 2-32)

Regional Anatomy: The branch of the radial artery, the cephalic vein; the posterior antebrachial cutaneous nerve.

Indications: (1) Acute abdominal pain, borborygmus, aching of shoulders and back. (2) Facial paralysis, swelling of face.

Needling Method: Perpendicular insertion 0.5—1.0 cun.

8. LI 8 (Xialian)

Location: With the elbow flexed, the point is on the dorsal radial side of the forearm, on the line connecting LI 5 (Yangxi) and LI 11 (Quchi), 4 cun below the transverse cubital crease. (Fig. 2-32)

Regional Anatomy: Same as LI 7 (Wenliu).

Indications: (1) Abdominal distention, abdominal pain. (2) Pain in the elbow and arm.

Needling Method: Perpendicular insertion 0.5—1.0 cun.

9. LI 9 (Shanglian)

Location: With the elbow flexed, the point is on the dorsal radial side of the forearm, on the line connecting LI 5 (Yangxi) and LI 11 (Quchi), 3 cun below the transverse cubital crease. (Fig. 2-32)

Regional Anatomy: Same as LI 7 (Wenliu).

Indications: (1) Hemiplegia, aching of the shoulder and arm, numbness of the hand and arm. (2) Abdominal pain, borborygmus.

Needling Method: Perpendicular insertion 0.5—1.0 cun.

10. LI 10 (Shousanli)

Location: With the elbow flexed, the point is on the dorsal radial side of the forearm, on the line connecting LI 5 (Yangxi) and LI 11 (Quchi), 2 cun below the transverse cubital crease. (Fig. 2-32)

Regional Anatomy: The branches of the radial recurrent artery; the deep ramus of the radial nerve.

Indications: (1) Abdominal pain, diarrhea. (2) Paralysis of the upper extremities. (3) Pain. Tapping the needle on this point can stop aching and distention sensation caused by incorrect needling technique.

Needling Method: Perpendicular insertion 0.8—1.2 cun.

11. LI 11 (Quchi)

Classification: He-(Sea) point.

Location: When the elbow is flexed, the point is on the lateral end of the transverse cubital crease, at midpoint between LU 5 (Chize) and the lateral epicondyle of the humerus. (Fig. 2-32)

Regional Anatomy: The branches of the radial recurrent artery. The posterior antebrachial cutaneous nerve deeper, radial nerve.

Indications: (1) All febrile diseases, fever, sore throat, malaria. (2) Hemiplegia, pain and motor impairment of shoulder, swelling and pain of the knee. (3) Headache, dizziness, redness, swelling and pain of the eye, blurring vision, toothache. (4) Irregular menstruation, rubella, eczema, urticaria, erysipelas (5) Abdominal pain, vomiting, diarrhea. (6) Depressive psychosis and madness. (7) Scrofula.

Needling Method: Perpendicular insertion 1.0—1.5 cun. When treating scrofula, insert the needle tip subcutaneously up to LI 14 (Binao) point

12. LI 12 (Zhouliao)

Location: When the elbow is flexed, the point is on the lateral side of the arm, on the border of the humerus, 1 cun above LI 11 (Quchi). (Fig. 2-33)

Regional Anatomy: Radial collateral artery and posterior antebrachial cutaneous nerve; deeper on the medal side, radial nerve.

Indications: (1) Aching, numbness and spasm of the elbow and arm.

Needling Method: Perpendicular insertion 0.5—1.0 cun.

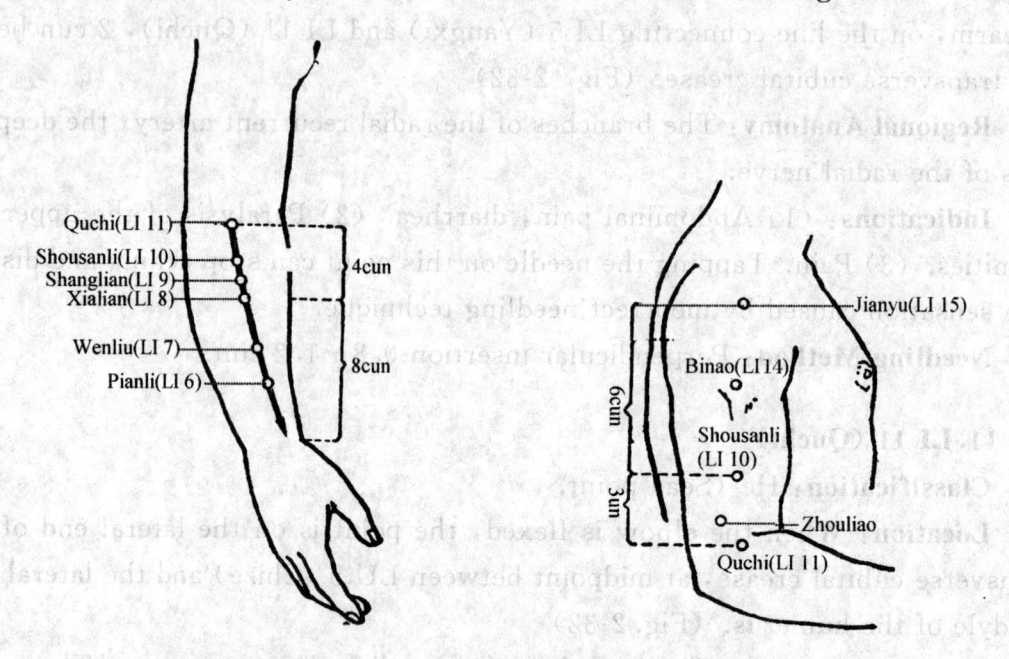

13. LI 13 (Shouwuli)

Location: On the lateral side of the arm, on the line connecting LI 11 (Quchi) and LI 15 (Jianyu), 3 cun above LI 11 (Quchi). (Fig. 2-33)

Fig. 2-32   Fig. 2-33

Regional Anatomy: Same as LI 12 (Zhouliao).

Indications: (1) Spasm and pain of the elbow and arm. (2) Scrofula.

Needling Method: Avoid injuring the artery. Perpendicular insertion 0.5—1.0 cun.

14. LI 14 (Binao)

Location: On the lateral side of the arm, superior to the insertion of m. deltoideus, on the line connecting LI 11 (Quchi) and LI 15 (Jianyu), 7 cun above LI 11 (Quchi). (Fig. 2-33)

Regional Anatomy: Deeper, deep brachial artery. Posterior brachial cutaneous nerve; deeper, radial nerve.

Indications: (1) Diseases of the eye: photophobia, burning pain, feeling of heaviness, redness, swelling and pain, diminishing vision, difficulty in differentiation of colors. (2) Scrofula, pain in shoulder and arm.

Needling Method: Perpendicular insertion or oblique insertion upwards 0.8—1.5 cun.

15. LI 15 (Jianyu)

Classification: The Crossing Point of Large Intestine Meridian and the Yang Heel Vessel.

Location: When the arm is abducted 90° laterally or forward, the point is on m. deltoideus of the shoulder, in the depression of the anterior superior portion of the shoulder. (Fig. 2-33, 2-34)

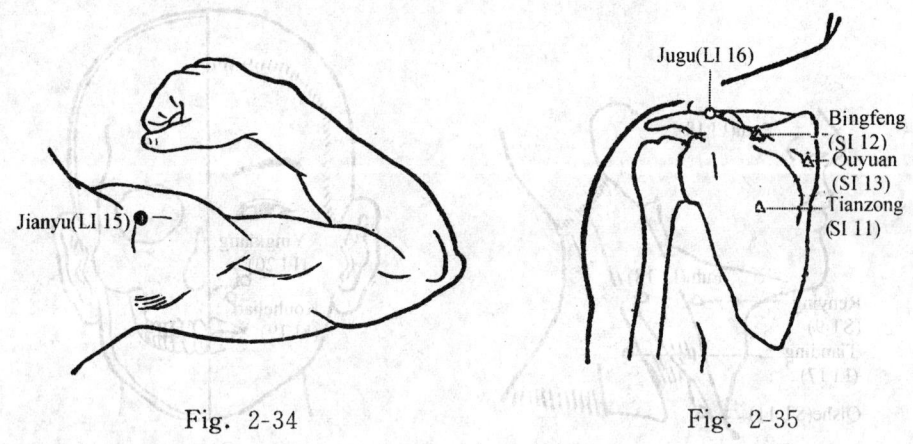

Fig. 2-34   Fig. 2-35

Regional Anatomy: The posterior circumflex humeral artery; the supraclavicular nerve.

Indications: (1) Paralysis of the upper extremities, pain and motor impairment of the shoulder. (2) Scrofula, rubella.

Needling Method: Perpendicular or oblique downward insertion 0.8—1.5 cun.

16. LI 16 (Jugu)

Classification: The Crossing Point of Large Intestine Meridian and Yang Heel Vessel.

Location: In the upper portion of the shoulder, in the depression between the acromial extremity of the clavicle and scapular spine. (Fig. 2-35)

Regional Anatomy: Deeper, the suprascapular artery and vein; the posterior branch of supraclavicular nerve.

Indications: (1) Pain of the shoulder and back, motor impairment of the upper extremities.

Needling Method: Perpendicular or slightly oblique laterally downwards insertion 0.5—1.0 cun.

17. LI 17 (Tianding)

Location: On the lateral side of the neck, on the posterior border of m. sternocleidomastoideus, lateral to Adam's apple, at the midpoint of the line connecting LI 18 (Futu) and ST 12 (Quepen). (Fig. 2-36)

Regional Anatomy: The external jugular vein; deeper, the phrenic nerve.

Indications: (1) Sudden loss of voice. (2) Sore throat, scrofula, goiter.

Needling Method: Perpendicular insertion 0.5—0.8 cun.

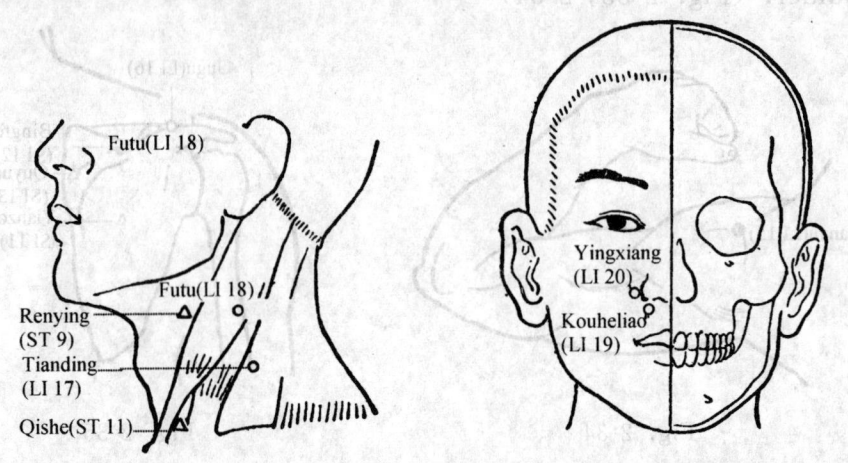

Fig. 2-36

Fig. 2-37

18. LI 18 (Futu)

Location: On the lateral side of the neck, on the side of the Adam's apple, between the sternal head and clavicular head of m. sternocleidomastoideus. (Fig. 2-36)

Regional Anatomy: Deeper, on the medial side, the ascending cervical artery; the phrenic nerve, the hypoglossus nerve.

Indications: (1) Hiccough. (2) Paralysis of the upper extremity, pain and limitation of the shoulder. (3) Sore throat, scrofula, goiter.

Needling Method: Perpendicular insertion 0.5—0.8 cun.

19. LI 19 (Kouheliao)

Location: On the upper lip, right below the lateral margin of the nostril, level with GV 26 (Shuigou). (Fig. 2-37)

Regional Anatomy: The superior labial branches of the facial artery and vein; the distribution of the anastomotic branch of facial and infraorbital nerves.

Indications: (1) Nasal congestion, epistaxis. (2) Trismus, wry face.
Needling Method: Perpendicular or oblique insertion 0.3—0.5 cun.

20. LI 20 (Yingxiang)

Classification: The Crossing Point of Stomach Meridian and Large Intestine Meridian.

Location: At the midpoint lateral to the border of the ala nasi, in the nasolabial groove. (Fig. 2-37)

Regional Anatomy: Same as LI 19 (Kouheliao).

Indications: (1) Nasal congestion, epistaxis. (2) Wry face, itching of the face. (3) Biliary ascariasis.

Needling Method: Oblique or subcutaneous insertion 0.3—0.5 cun. Moxibustion is not recommended.

Section 3 The Acupuncture Points of Stomach Meridian

This meridian appears at ST 1 (Chengqi) and goes to ST 45 (Lidui); bilaterally each consisting of 45 acupuncture points. (Fig. 2-38)

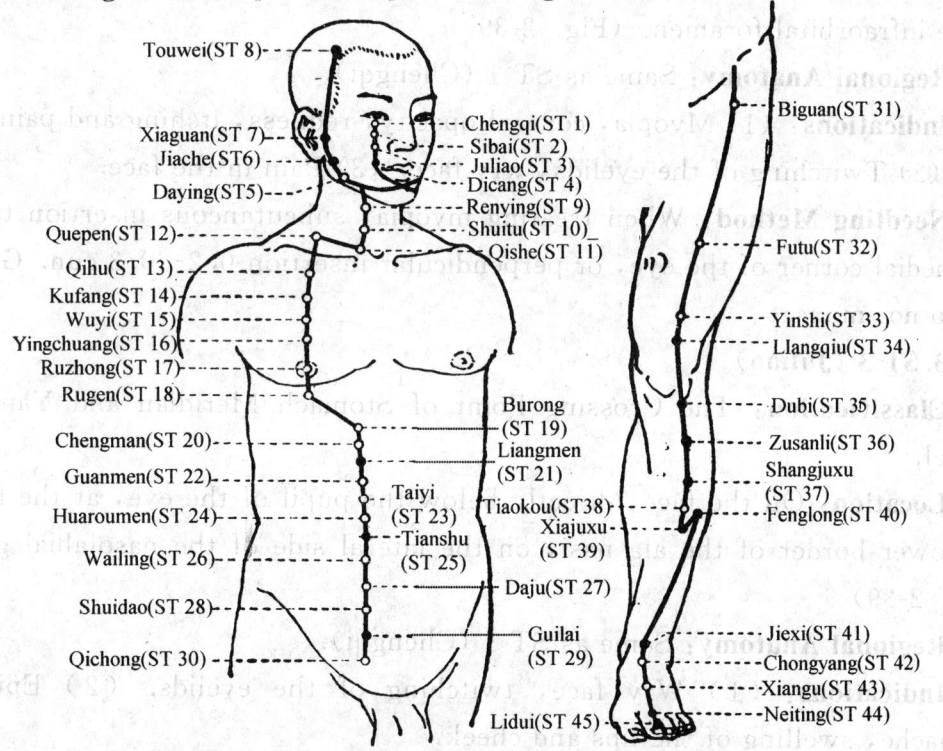

Fig. 2-38 The Points of the Stomach Meridian

1. ST 1 (Chengqi)

Classification: The Crossing Point of Stomach Meridian, Yang Heel Vessel, and Conception Vessel.

Location: On the face, the point is directly below the pupil of the eye, between the eyeball and the infraorbital ridge. (Fig. 2-39)

Regional Anatomy: The branches of the infraorbital and ophthalmic arteries and veins; branch of the infraorbital nerve, the inferior branch of the oculomotor nerve and the muscular branch of the facial nerve.

Indications: (1) Redness, swelling and pain of the eye, lacrimation, night blindness. (2) Twitch of the eyelids, wry face.

Needling Method: Push the eyeball upward slightly with the left thumb and puncture perpendicularly and slowly 0.5—1.5 cun along the infraorbital ridge. It is not advisable to manipulate the needle with large amplitude, to avoid injuring the blood vessel resulting in hematoma. Moxa is contraindicated.

2. ST 2 (Sibai)

Location: On the face, directly below the pupil of the eye, in the depression at the infraorbital foramen. (Fig. 2-39)

Regional Anatomy: Same as ST 1 (Chengqi).

Indications: (1) Myopia, corneal opacity, redness, itching and pain of the eye. (2) Twitching of the eyelids, wry face. (3) Pain in the face.

Needling Method: When treating myopia, subcutaneous insertion towards the medial corner of the eye, or perpendicular insertion 0.2—0.3 cun. Generally, do not moxa.

3. ST 3 (Juliao)

Classification: The Crossing Point of Stomach Meridian and Yang Heel Vessel.

Location: On the face, directly below the pupil of the eye, at the level of the lower border of the ala nasi, on the lateral side of the nasolabial groove. (Fig. 2-39)

Regional Anatomy: Same as ST 1 (Chengqi).

Indications: (1) Wry face, twitching of the eyelids. (2) Epistaxis, toothache, swelling of the lips and cheek.

Needling Method: Oblique or subcutaneous insertion 0.3—0.5 cun.

4. ST 4 (Dicang)

Classification: The Crossing Point of Large Intestine Meridian, Stomach Meridian and Yang Heel Vessel.

Location: On the face, lateral to the corner of the mouth, directly below the pupil of the eye. (Fig. 2-39)

Regional Anatomy: Deeper, the terminal branch of the buccal nerve.

Indications: (1) Wry mouth, salivation. (2) Twitching of the eyelids, twitching of the corner of the mouth.

Needling Method: Oblique or subcutaneous insertion 0.5—0.8 cun; or puncture towards ST 6 (Jiache).

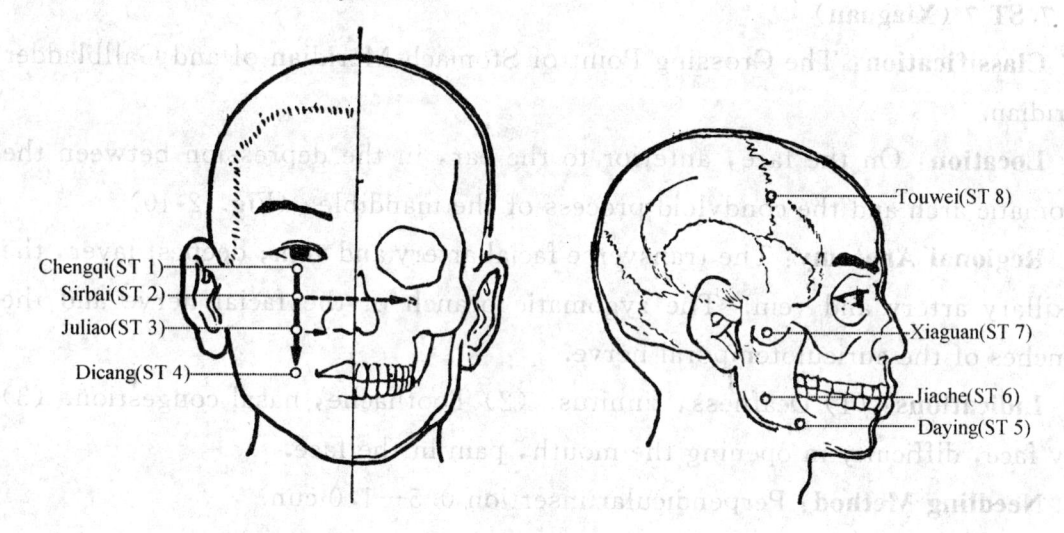

Fig. 2-39

Fig. 2-40

5. ST 5 (Daying)

Location: Anterior to the angle of the mandible, on the anterior border of the attached portion of m. masseter, where the facial artery pulsates. (Fig. 2-40)

Regional Anatomy: Anteriorly, the facial artery and vein; the facial and buccal nerves.

Indications: (1) Swelling of the cheek, toothache. (2) Wry mouth, trismus.

Needling Method: Avoid puncturing the artery. Oblique or subcutaneous insertion 0.3—0.5 cun.

6. ST 6 (Jiache)

Location: On the cheek, in the depression one finger-breadth (middle finger) anterior and superior to the lower angle of the mandible where m. masseter attaches, at the prominence of the muscle when the teeth are clenched. (Fig. 2-40)

Regional Anatomy: Masseteric artery; the great auricular nerve, facial nerve and masseteric nerve.

Indications: (1) Swelling of the cheek, wry mouth. (2) Toothache in the lower jaw, acute trismus, difficulty in opening the mouth.

Needling Method: Perpendicular insertion 0.3—0.5 cun, or subcutaneous insertion 0.5—1.0 cun. Or insert toward ST 4 (Dicang).

7. ST 7 (Xiaguan)

Classification: The Crossing Point of Stomach Meridian of and Gallbladder Meridian.

Location: On the face, anterior to the ear, in the depression between the zygomatic arch and the condyloid process of the mandible. (Fig. 2-40)

Regional Anatomy: The transverse facial artery and vein; deepest layer, the maxillary artery and vein. The zygomatic branch of the facial nerve and the branches of the auriculotemporal nerve.

Indications: (1) Deafness, tinnitus. (2) Toothache, nasal congestion. (3) Wry face, difficulty in opening the mouth, pain in the face.

Needling Method: Perpendicular insertion 0.5—1.0 cun.

8. ST 8 (Touwei)

Classification: The Crossing Point of Stomach Meridian, Gallbladder Meridian and Yang Link Vessel.

Location: On the both sides of scalp, 0.5 cun above the hairline at the corner of the forehead, 4.5 cun lateral from the midline of the head. (Fig. 2-40)

Regional Anatomy: The frontal branches of the superficial temporal artery and vein; the branch of the auriculotemporal nerve and the temporal branch of the facial nerve.

Indications: (1) Headache, dizziness and blurring vision. (2) Ophthalmalgia, lacrimation, twitching of the eyelids.

Needling Method: Subcutaneous insertion 0.5—1.0 cun. *Systematic Classic of Acupuncture and Moxibustion says*: " moxa is contraindicated."

9. ST 9 (Renying)

Classification: The Crossing point of Stomach Meridian and Gallbladder Meridian.

Location: On the neck, lateral to the Adam's apple, on the anterior border of m. sternocleidomastoideus, where the common carotid artery pulsates. (Fig. 2-41)

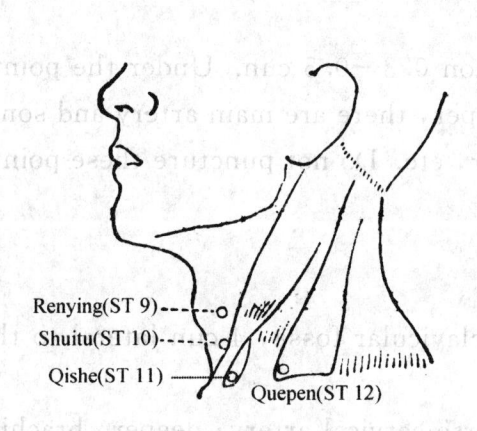

Fig. 2-41

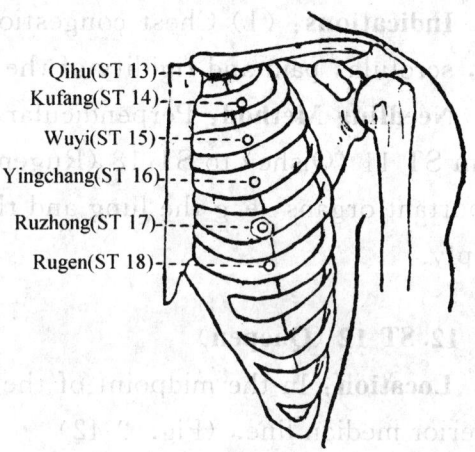

Fig. 2-42

Regional Anatomy: The bifurcation of the internal and the external carotid artery. Deeper, the cervical arterial bulbus and sympathetic trunk.

Indications: (1) Sore throat, scrofula, goiter. (2) Asthma, hemoptysis. (3) Hypertension, apoplexy, hemiplegia. (4) Arthralgia of the knee.

Needling Method: Keep away from the common carotid artery, perpendicular insertion 0.3—0.8 cun. *A-B Classic of Acupuncture and Moxibustion* says moxa is contraindicated. Notes to *the Familiar Conversation from the Emperor's Canon of Medicine* tell that puncturing deeply can cause fatal results.

10. ST 10 (Shuitu)

Location: On the neck, on the anterior border of m. sternocleidomastoideus, at the midpoint of the line joining ST 9 (Renying) and ST 11 (Qishe). (Fig. 2-41)

Regional Anatomy: Common carotid artery and sympathetic trunk.

Indications: (1) Sore throat. (2) Cough and asthma.

Needling Method: Perpendicular insertion 0.3—0.8 cun.

11. ST 11 (Qishe)

Location: On the neck, at the superior border of the sternal extremity of the clavicle, between the sternal head and clavicular head of m. sternocleidomastoideus. (Fig. 2-41)

Regional Anatomy: Deep, the common carotid artery; the anterior branch of the supraclavicular nerve.

Indications: (1) Chest congestion, cough and asthma, dyspnea. (2) Goiter, scrofula, pain and rigidity of the neck.

Needling Method: Perpendicular insertion 0.3—0.5 cun. Under the points from ST 11 (Qishe) to ST 18 (Rugen), deeper, there are main artery and some important organs, e.g the lung and the liver, etc. Do not puncture these points deeply.

12. ST 12 (Quepen)

Location: In the midpoint of the supraclavicular fossa, 4 cun lateral to the anterior median line. (Fig. 2-42)

Regional Anatomy: Superiorly, transverse cervical artery; deeper, brachial plexus.

Indications: (1) Cough, asthma, sore throat. (2) Pain in the supraclavicular fossa, scrofula.

Needling Method: Perpendicular or oblique insertion 0.3—0.5 cun. *Supplement to the Classic Fig. of Acupuncture and Moxibustion* says: "Needling is contraindicated in pregnancy."

13. ST 13 (Qihu)

Location: On the chest, at the lower border of the middle of the clavicle, 4 cun lateral to the anterior median line. (Fig. 2-42)

Regional Anatomy: The branches of the thoracoacromial artery and vein; the branches of the anterior thoracic nerve.

Indications: (1) Cough and asthma. (2) Pain and chest congestion.

Needling Method: Oblique or subcutaneous insertion 0.5—0.8 cun.

14. ST 14 (Kufang)

Location: On the chest, in the first intercostal space, 4 cun lateral to the anterior median line. (Fig. 2-42)

Regional Anatomy: Same as ST 13 (Qihu).

Indications: (1) Cough and asthma. (2) Distention and pain in the chest and hypochondria.

Needling Method: Oblique or subcutaneous insertion 0.5—0.8 cun.

15. ST 15 (Wuyi)

Location: On the chest, in the second intercostal space, 4 cun lateral to the anterior median line. (Fig. 2-42)

Regional Anatomy: Same as ST 13 (Qihu).

Indications: (1) Cough and asthma. (2) Distention and pain in the chest and hypochondria, acute mastitis.

Needling Method: Oblique or subcutaneous insertion 0.5—0.8 cun.

16. ST 16 (Yingchuang)

Location: On the chest, in the third intercostal space, 4 cun lateral to the anterior median line. (Fig. 2-42)

Regional Anatomy: Lateral thoracic artery and vein; the branch of the anterior thoracic nerve.

Indications: (1) Cough and asthma. (2) Distention and pain in the chest and hypochondria, acute mastitis.

Needling Method: Oblique or subcutaneous insertion 0.5—0.8 cun.

17. ST 17 (Ruzhong)

Location: On the chest, in the fourth intercostal space, 4 cun lateral to the anterior median line, in the center of the nipple. (Fig. 2-42)

Regional Anatomy: The anterior and lateral cutaneous branches of the fourth intercostal nerve.

Annotations: Acupuncture and moxibustion on this point are contraindicated. This point serves only as a landmark for locating points on the chest and abdomen.

18. ST 18 (Rugen)

Location: On the chest, directly below the nipple, at the base of the breast, in the fifth intercostal space, 4 cun lateral to the anterior median line. (Fig. 2-42)

Regional Anatomy: The branches of the intercostal artery and vein; the branch of the fifth intercostal nerve.

Indications: (1) Acute mastitis, insufficient lactation. (2) Chest pain, cough and asthma.

Needling Method: Oblique or subcutaneous insertion 0.5—0.8 cun.

19. ST 19 (Burong)

Location: On the upper abdomen, 6 cun above the center of the umbilicus, 2 cun lateral to the anterior median line. (Fig. 2-43)

Regional Anatomy: The branches of the seventh intercostal artery and vein; the branch of the seventh intercostal nerve.

Indications: (1) Gastric pain, vomiting. (2) Poor appetite, abdominal distention.

Needling Method: Perpendicular insertion 0.5—0.8 cun.

20. ST 20 (Chengman)

Location: On the upper abdomen, 5 cun above the center of the umbilicus, 2 cun lateral to the anterior median line. (Fig. 2-43)

Regional Anatomy: Same as ST 19 (Burong).

Indications: (1) Gastric pain, vomiting, (2) Poor appetite, abdominal distention.

Needling Method: Perpendicular insertion 0.5—0.8 cun.

21. ST 21 (Liangmen)

Location: On the upper abdomen, 4 cun above the center of the umbilicus, 2 cun lateral to the anterior median line. (Fig. 2-43)

Regional Anatomy: The branches of the eighth intercostal artery and vein; the branch of the eighth intercostal nerve.

Indications: (1) Gastric pain, vomiting, (2) Poor appetite, abdominal distention, diarrhea.

Needling Method: Perpendicular insertion 0.8—1.2 cun.

22. ST 22 (Guanmen)

Location: On the upper abdomen, 3 cun above the center of the umbilicus, 2 cun lateral to the anterior median line. (Fig. 2-43)

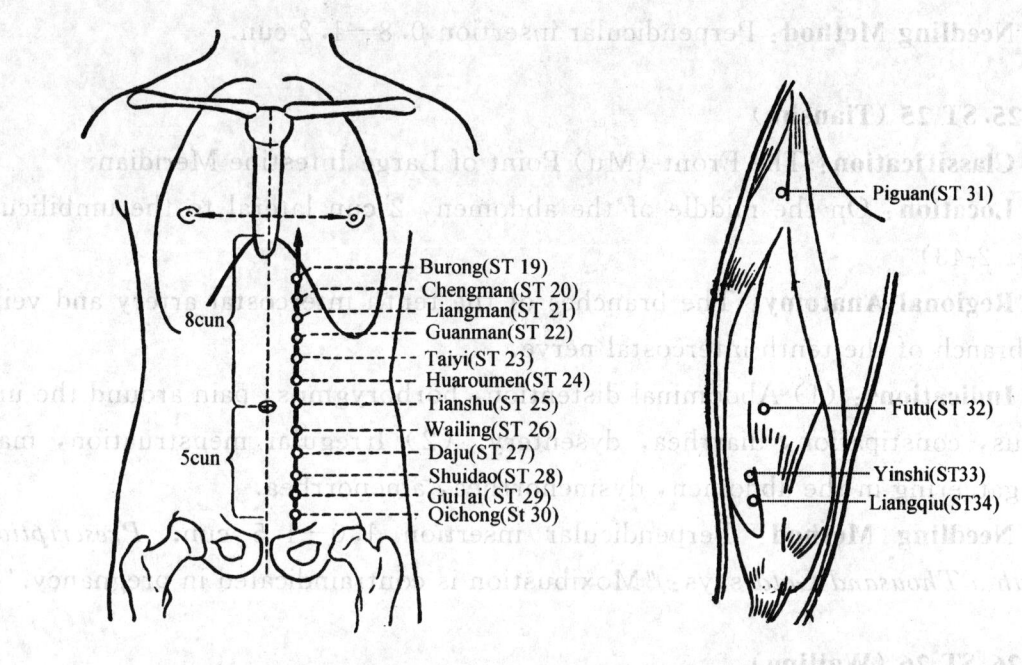

Fig. 2-43

Fig. 2-44

Regional Anatomy: Same as ST 21 (Liangmen).

Indications: (1) Abdominal distention and pain, borborygmus, diarrhea. (2) Edema.

Needling Method: Perpendicular insertion 0.8—1.2 cun.

23. ST 23 (Taiyi)

Location: On the upper abdomen, 2 cun above the center of the umbilicus, 2 cun lateral to the anterior median line. (Fig. 2-43)

Regional Anatomy: The branches of the eighth and ninth intercostal arteries and veins; the branches of the eighth and ninth intercostal nerves.

Indications: (1) Manic psychosis. (2) Irritability, protruding tongue.

Needling Method: Perpendicular insertion 0.8—1.2 cun.

24. ST 24 (Huaroumen)

Location: On the upper abdomen, 1 cun above the center of the umbilicus, 2 cun lateral to the anterior median line. (Fig. 2-43)

Regional Anatomy: The branches of the ninth intercostal artery and vein; the branch of the ninth intercostal nerve.

Indications: (1) Manic psychosis, vomiting. (2) Protruding tongue, stiff tongue.

Needling Method: Perpendicular insertion 0.8—1.2 cun.

25. ST 25 (Tianshu)
Classification: The Front-(Mu) Point of Large Intestine Meridian.
Location: On the middle of the abdomen, 2 cun lateral to the umbilicus. (Fig. 2-43)
Regional Anatomy: The branches of the tenth intercostal artery and vein; the branch of the tenth intercostal nerve.
Indications: (1) Abdominal distention, borborygmus, pain around the umbilicus, constipation, diarrhea, dysentery. (2) Irregular menstruation, mass and gathering in the abdomen, dysmenorrhea, amenorrhea.
Needling Method: Perpendicular insertion 1.0—1.5 cun. *Prescriptions Worth a Thousand Gold* says: "Moxibustion is contraindicated in pregnancy."

26. ST 26 (Wailing)
Location: On the lower abdomen, 1 cun below the center of the umbilicus, 2 cun lateral to the anterior median line. (Fig. 2-43)
Regional Anatomy: Same as ST 25 (Tianshu).
Indications: Abdominal pain, hernia, dysmenorrhea.
Needling Method: Perpendicular insertion 1.0—1.5 cun.

27. ST 27 (Daju)
Location: On the lower abdomen, 2 cun below the center of the umbilicus, 2 cun lateral to the anterior median line. (Fig. 2-43)
Regional Anatomy: The branches of the eleventh intercostal artery and vein; the branch of the eleventh intercostal nerve.
Indications: (1) Lower abdominal distention and pain, disuria. (2) Hernia. (3) Spermatorrhea, premature ejaculation.
Needling Method: Perpendicular insertion 1.0—1.5 cun.

28. ST 28 (Shuidao)
Location: On the lower abdomen, 3 cun below the center of the umbilicus, 2 cun lateral to the anterior median line. (Fig. 2-43)
Regional Anatomy: The branches of the subcostal artery and vein; the branch of the eleventh intercostal nerve.
Indications: (1) Lower abdominal distention, disuria. (2) Dysmenorrhea,

infertility, hernia. (3) Constipation.

Needling Method: Perpendicular insertion 1.0—1.5 cun.

29. ST 29 (Guilai)

Location: On the lower abdomen, 4 cun below the center of the umbilicus, 2 cun lateral to the anterior median line. (Fig. 2-43)

Regional Anatomy: The iliohypogastric nerve.

Indications: (1) Prolapse of uterus, irregular menstruation, amenorrhea, leukorrhea. (2) Hernia, abdominal pain.

Needling Method: Perpendicular insertion 1.0—1.5 cun.

30. ST 30 (Qichong)

Location: Above the inguinal groove, 5 cun below the center of the umbilicus, 2 cun lateral to the anterior median line. (Fig. 2-43)

Regional Anatomy: The branches of the superficial epigastric artery and vein; the pathway of the ilioinguinal nerve.

Indications: (1) Hernia. (2) Irregular menstruation, infertility. (3) Impotence, swelling of the vulva.

Needling Method: Perpendicular insertion 0.5—1.0 cun.

31. ST 31 (Biguan)

Location: On the anterior aspect of the thigh, on the line connecting the anterior superior iliac spine and the lower lateral border of the patella, level with the lower border of the symphysis pubis, in the depression on the lateral side of m. sartorius when the thigh is flexed. (Fig. 2-44)

Regional Anatomy: Deeper, the branches of the lateral circumflex femoral artery and vein; the lateral femoral cutaneous nerve.

Indications: (1) Muscular atrophy, weakness, numbness and pain of lower extremities, apoplexy, hemiplegia. (2) Coldness and pain of the lower back and knee.

Needling Method: Perpendicular insertion 1.0—2.0 cun.

32. ST 32 (Futu)

Location: On the anterior aspect of the thigh, on the line connecting the anterior superior iliac spine and the lower lateral border of the patella, 6 cun above the patella. (Fig. 2-44)

Regional Anatomy: The lateral femoral cutaneous nerve.

Indications: Paralysis or weakness of the lower extremities, coldness and pain of the lower back and knee.

Needling Method: Perpendicular insertion 1.0—2.0 cun.

33. ST 33 (Yinshi)

Location: On the anterior aspect of the thigh, on the line connecting the anterior superior iliac spine and the lower lateral border of the patella, 3 cun above the patella. (Fig. 2-44)

Regional Anatomy: The lateral femoral cutaneous nerve.

Indications: (1) Coldness and pain of the lower extremities and knee, limitation of the lower extremities. (2) Hernia, abdominal distention and pain.

Needling Method: Perpendicular insertion 1.0—1.5 cun.

34. ST 34 (Liangqiu)

Classification: Xi-(Cleft) point.

Location: When the knee is flexed, on the anterior aspect of the thigh, on the line connecting the anterior superior iliac spine and the lower lateral border of the patella, 2 cun above the patella. (Fig. 2-44)

Regional Anatomy: Same as ST 33 (Yinshi).

Indications: (1) Acute gastric pain, acute mastitis. (2) Swelling and pain of the knee joint, paralysis or weakness of the lower extremities.

Needling Method: Perpendicular insertion 0.5—1.0 cun. Moxibustion is applicable.

35. ST 35 (Dubi)

Location: When the knee is flexed, the point is at the knee, below the patella, in the depression lateral to the patella ligament. (Fig. 2-45)

Regional Anatomy: The arterial and venous network around the knee joint; the articular branch of the common peroneal nerve.

Indications: Swelling and pain of the knee joint, limitation of the knee.

Needling Method: Oblique insertion toward the medial back 0.5—1.0 cun.

36. ST 36 (Zusanli)

Classification: He-(Sea) Point. This point has a tonifying function. It is an important point for health maintenance.

Location: On the anterior aspect of the lower leg, 3 cun below ST 35 (Dubi), one finger-breadth (middle finger) from the anterior crest of the tibia. (Fig. 2-45)

Regional Anatomy: The anterior tibial artery and vein; the lateral sural cutaneous nerve and the cutaneous branch of the saphenous nerve, deeper, the deep peroneal nerve.

Indications: (1) Gastric pain, vomiting, dysphagia, abdominal distention, borborygmus, diarrhea, indigestion, dysentery, constipation, abdominal pain, acute mastitis. (2) Emaciation due to general deficiency, palpitation, shortness of breath, poor appetite, lassitude, dizziness, insomnia. (3) Cough and asthma. (4) Pain in the knee joint, apoplexy, hemiplegia, beriberi, edema. (5) Depressive psychosis and madness.

Needling Method: Perpendicular insertion 1.0—2.0 cun.

37. ST 37 (Shangjuxu)

Classification: The Lower He-(Sea) point of Large Intestine Meridian.

Location: On the anterior aspect of the lower leg, 6 cun below ST 35 (Dubi), one finger-breadth (middle finger) from the anterior crest of the tibia. (Fig. 2-45)

Regional Anatomy: Same as ST 36 (Zusanli).

Indications: (1) Acute appendicitis, abdominal pain, borborygmus, constipation, diarrhea. (2) Muscular atrophy, weakness, numbness and pain of lower extremities, beriberi.

Needling Method: Perpendicular insertion 1.0—1.5 cun.

38. ST 38 (Tiaokou)

Location: On the anterior aspect of the lower leg, 8 cun below ST 35 (Dubi), one finger-breadth (middle finger) from the anterior crest of the tibia. (Fig. 2-45)

Regional Anatomy: Same as ST 36 (Zusanli).

Indications: (1) Coldness, pain, and weakness of the shoulder. (2) Muscular atrophy, weakness, numbness and pain of lower extremities, swelling of the foot, spasm.

Needling Method: Perpendicular insertion 1.0—1.5 cun.

39. ST 39 (Xiajuxu)

Classification: The Lower He-(Sea) Point of Small Intestine Meridian.

Location: On the anterior aspect of the lower leg, 9 cun below ST 35 (Dubi), one finger-breadth (middle finger) from the anterior crest of the tibia. (Fig. 2-45)

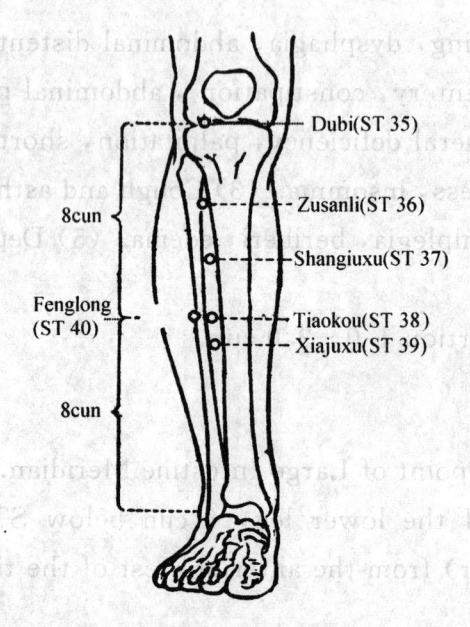

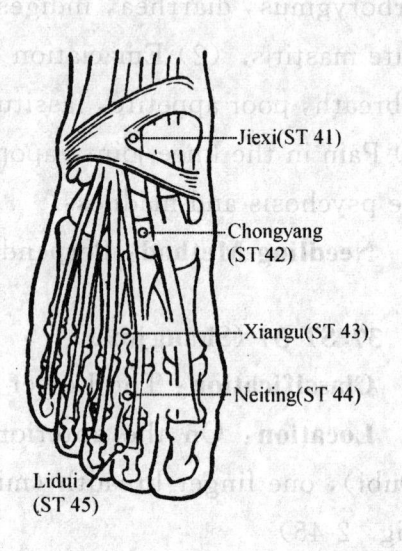

Fig. 2-45   Fig. 2-46

Regional Anatomy: The anterior tibial artery and vein; the distribution of the branches of the superficial peroneal nerve and the deep peroneal nerve.

Indications: (1) Lower abdominal pain, pain in the lower back referring to pain in the testicles. (2) Diarrhea, dysentery. (3) Muscular atrophy, weakness, numbness and pain of lower extremities.

Needling Method: Perpendicular insertion 1.0—1.5 cun.

40. ST 40 (Fenglong)

Classification: Luo-(Connecting) point.

Location: On the anterior aspect of the lower leg, 8 cun superior to the external malleolus, lateral to ST 38 (Tiaokou), two finger-breadth (middle finger) from the anterior crest of the tibia. (Fig. 2-45)

Regional Anatomy: The branches of the anterior tibial artery and vein; the distribution of the branches of the superficial peroneal nerve.

Indications: (1) Cough, excessive phlegm, asthma. (2) Manic psychosis, epilepsy. (3) Headache, dizziness. (4) Paralysis or weakness of the lower extremities.

Needling Method: Perpendicular insertion 1.0—1.5 cun.

41. ST 41 (Jiexi)

Classification: Jing-(River) point.

Location: At the junction of the dorsum of the foot and the lower leg, in the depression at the midpoint of the transverse crease of the ankle between the tendons of m. extensor hallucis longus and digitorum longus. (Fig. 2-46)

Regional Anatomy: The anterior tibial artery and vein; the distribution of the superficial and deep peroneal nerves.

Indications: (1) Pain of the ankle joint, weakness and muscular atrophy, numbness and pain of lower extremities. (2) Headache, dizziness, manic psychosis. (3) Abdominal distention, constipation.

Needling Method: Perpendicular insertion 0.5—1.0 cun.

42. ST 42 (Chongyang)

Classification: Yuan-(Source) point.

Location: At the highest point of the dorsum of the foot, between the tendons of m. extensor hallucis longus and digitorum longus, where the dorsal artery of the foot pulsates. (Fig. 2-46)

Regional Anatomy: The dorsal artery and vein of foot; deeper, the deep peroneal nerve.

Indications: (1) Gastric pain, abdominal distention. (2) Swelling and pain of the dorsum of the foot. (3) Swelling of the face, toothache, deviation of the mouth and eye.

Needling Method: Perpendicular insertion 0.2—0.5 cun.

43. ST 43 (Xiangu)

Classification: Shu-(Stream) point.

Location: On the dorsum of the foot, in the depression distal to the junction of the second and third metatarsal bones. (Fig. 2-46)

Regional Anatomy: The dorsal venous network of foot; the medial dorsal cutaneous nerve of foot.

Indications: (1) Myasthenia of the upper eyelid and difficult to open the eyes. (2) Facial and general edema, swelling and pain of the dorsum of the foot.

Needling Method: Perpendicular or oblique insertion 0.5—1.0 cun.

44. ST 44 (Neiting)
Classification: Ying-(Spring) point.
Location: On the dorsum of the foot, proximal to the web margin between the second and third toes, at the junction of the red and white skin. (Fig. 2-46)
Regional Anatomy: Same as ST 43 (Xiangu).
Indications: (1) Toothache in the upper jaw, sore throat, wry mouth, epistaxis. (2) Abdominal distention, constipation, gastric pain. (3) Swelling and pain of the dorsum of the foot.
Needling Method: Perpendicular or oblique insertion 0.5—0.8 cun.

45. ST 45 (Lidui)
Classification: Jing-(Well) point.
Location: On the foot, on the lateral side of the end of the second toe, 0.1 cun from the corner of the nail. (Fig. 2-46)
Regional Anatomy: The arterial and venous network formed by the dorsal digital artery and vein of foot; the distribution of the dorsal digital nerve derived from the superficial peroneal nerve.
Indications: (1) Swelling of the face, toothache, epistaxis, sore throat. (2) Nightmare, manic psychosis.
Needling Method: Subcutaneous insertion 0.1 cun.

Section 4 The Acupuncture Points of Spleen Meridian

The Spleen Meridian appears at SP 1(Yinbai) and goes to SP 21 (Dabao); bilaterally each consisting of 21 acupuncture points. (Fig. 2-47)

1. SP 1 (Yinbai)
Classification: Jing-(Well) Point.
Location: On the medial side of the big toe, 0.1 cun from the corner of the nail. (Fig. 2-52)
Regional Anatomy: The dorsal digital artery; the branches of the superficial peroneal nerve.
Indications: (1) Menorrhagia, metrorrhagia, bloody stools, hematuria. (2) Abdominal distention. (3) Manic psychosis, nightmares, convulsions.

Needling Method: Subcutaneous insertion 0.1 cun.

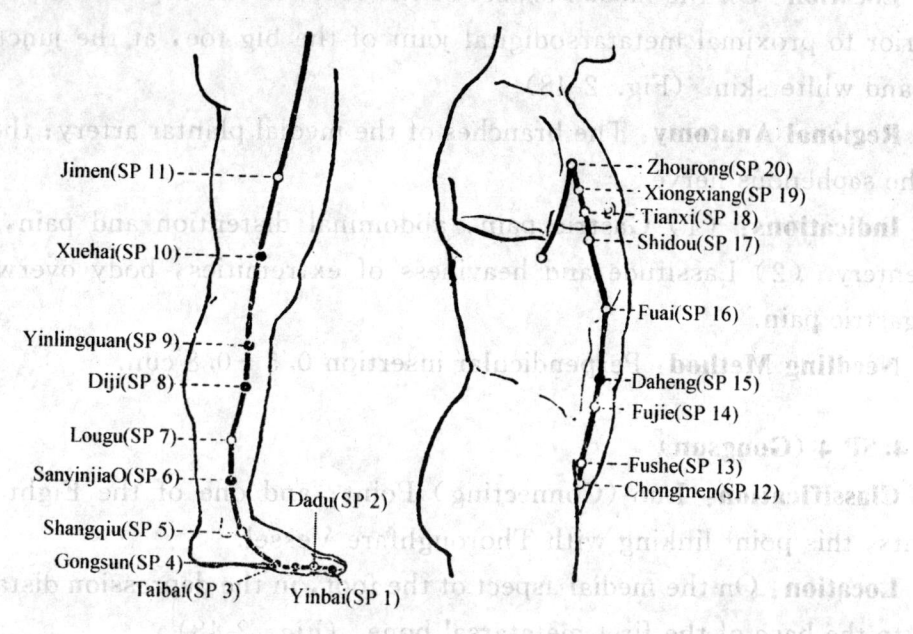

Fig. 2-47 The Points of the Spleen Meridian

2. SP 2 (Dadu)

Classification: Ying-(Spring) Point.

Location: On the medial aspect of the foot, in the depression anterior and inferior to proximal metatarsodigital joint of the big toe, at the junction of the red and white skin. (Fig. 2-48)

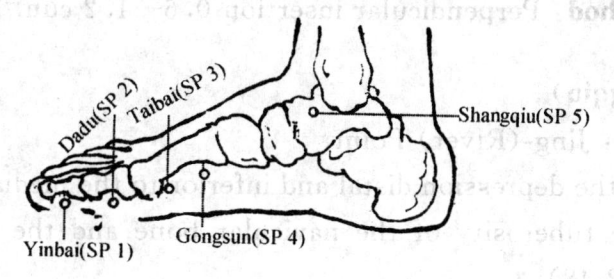

Fig. 2-48

Regional Anatomy: The branches of the medial plantar artery and vein; the plantar digital proprial nerve.

Indications: (1) Gastric pain, constipation. (2) Febrile diseases without sweating.

Needling Method: Perpendicular insertion 0.3—0.5 cun.

3. SP 3 (Taibai)

Classification: Shu-(Spring) Point and Yuan-(Source) Point.

Location: On the medial aspect of the foot, in the depression posterior and inferior to proximal metatarsodigital joint of the big toe, at the junction of the red and white skin. (Fig. 2-48)

Regional Anatomy: The branches of the medial plantar artery; the branches of the saphenous nerve.

Indications: (1) Gastric pain, abdominal distention and pain, diarrhea, dysentery. (2) Lassitude and heaviness of extremities, body overweight (3) Epigastric pain.

Needling Method: Perpendicular insertion 0.5—0.8 cun.

4. SP 4 (Gongsun)

Classification: Luo-(Connecting) Point; and one of the Eight Confluent Points, this point linking with Thoroughfare Vessel.

Location: On the medial aspect of the foot, in the depression distal and inferior to the base of the first metatarsal bone. (Fig. 2-48)

Regional Anatomy: The medial tarsal artery; the branch of the saphenous nerve.

Indications: (1) Acute gastric pain, gastric distention and stuffiness, poor appetite, pain around the umbilical region, diarrhea, bloody stools. (2) Epigastric pain, chest congestion, distention in the hypochondrium. (3) Irregular menstruation, retention of placenta, postpartum faintness.

Needling Method: Perpendicular insertion 0.6—1.2 cun.

5. SP 5 (Shangqiu)

Classification: Jing-(River) Point.

Location: In the depression distal and inferior to the medial malleolus, midpoint between the tuberosity of the navicular bone and the tip of the medial malleolus. (Fig. 2-48)

Regional Anatomy: The medial tarsal artery; the medial crural cutaneous nerve.

Indications: (1) Pain in the foot and ankle. (2) Hemorrhoids. (3) Abdominal distention, diarrhea, constipation.

Needling Method: Perpendicular insertion 0.5—0.8 cun.

6. SP 6 (Sanyinjiao)

Classification: The Crossing Point of Spleen Meridian, Kidney Meridian and Liver Meridian.

Location: On the medial aspect of the lower leg, 3 cun above the medial malleolus, on the posterior border of the medial aspect of the tibia. (Fig. 2-49)

Regional Anatomy: The great saphenous vein. The saphenous nerve; deeper, in the posterior aspect, the tibial nerve.

Indications: (1) Irregular menstruation, dysmenorrhea, metrorrhagia, leukorrhea, amenorrhea, mass and gathering in the abdomen, prolapse of uterus, dystocia, postpartum faintness, persistent lochia, infertility, nocturnal emission, spermatorrhea, impotence, premature ejaculation, pain in the penis, hernia, testicular atropy. (2) Enuresis, anuria, edema, dysuria. (3) Spleen and stomach deficiency, borborygmus, abdominal distention, diarrhea, paralysis of the foot, beriberi, muscular pain. (4) Disease of the skin, eczema, urticaria. (5) Insomnia, headache, dizziness, bilateral hypochondriac pain.

Needling Method: Perpendicular insertion 1.0—1.5 cun. This point is contraindicated to puncture in pregnancy.

7. SP 7 (Lougu)

Location: On the medial aspect of the lower leg, 6 cun above the medial malleolus on the line connecting the tip of the medial malleolus and SP 9 (Yinlingquan), on the posterior border of the medial aspect of the tibia. (Fig. 2-49)

Regional Anatomy: Same as SP 6 (Sanyinjiao).

Indications: (1) Borborygmus, abdominal distention. (2) Paralysis and numbness of the lower extremities.

Needling Method: Perpendicular insertion 1.0—1.5 cun.

8. SP 8 (Diji)

Classification: Xi-(Cleft) Point.

Location: On the medial aspect of the lower leg, 3 cun below SP 9 (Yinlingquan), on the line connecting the tip of the medial malleolus and SP 9 (Yinlingquan). (Fig. 2-49)

Regional Anatomy: Deeper, the posterior tibial artery and vein; innervation same as SP 6 (Sanyinjiao).

Indications: (1) Abdominal pain, diarrhea. (2) Dysuria, edema. (3) Irregular menstruation, dysmenorrhea, spermatorrhea, impotence, lumbar pain.

Needling Method: Perpendicular insertion 1.0—2.0 cun.

9. SP 9 (Yinlingquan)

Classification: He-(Sea) Point.

Location: On the medial aspect of the lower leg, in the depression of the lower border of the medial condyle of the tibia. (Fig. 2-49)

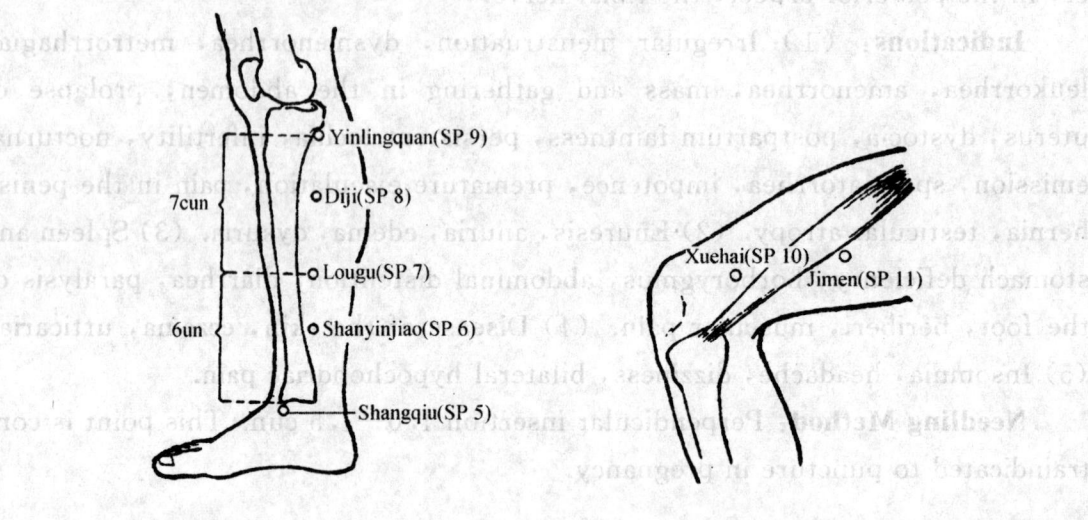

Fig. 2-49

Fig. 2-50

Regional Anatomy: Deeper, the posterior tibial artery and vein; the tibial nerve.

Indications: (1) Dysuria, incontinence of urine, edema. (2) Abdominal distention, diarrhea, jaundice. (3) Pain in the medial aspect of the knee. (4) Pain in the penis, dysmenorrhea, pain in the vulua.

Needling Method: Perpendicular insertion 1.0—2.0 cun.

10. SP 10 (Xuehai)

Location: When the knee is flexed, on the medial aspect of the thigh, the point is 2 cun above the mediosuperior border of the patella, on the bulge of the medial portion of m. quadriceps femoris. (Fig. 2-50)

Regional Anatomy: The muscular branches of the femoral artery and vein; the anterior femoral cutaneous nerve.

Indications: (1) Irregular menstruation, metrorrhagia, amenorrhea. (2) Urticaria, eczema, erysipelas.

Needling Method: Perpendicular insertion 1.0—1.5 cun.

11. SP 11 (Jimen)

Location: On the medial aspect of the thigh, 6 cun above SP 10 (Xuehai) on the line connecting SP 10 (Xuehai) and SP 12 (Chongmen). (Fig. 2-50)

Regional Anatomy: The great saphenous vein; deeper, the saphenous nerve.

Indications: (1) Swelling and pain of the inguinal region. (2) Dysuria, enuresis.

Needling Method: Keep away from the artery. Perpendicular insertion 0.5—1.0 cun.

12. SP 12 (Chongmen)

Classification: The Crossing Point of the Spleen Meridian and Liver Meridian.

Location: At the lateral end of the inguinal groove, 3.5 cun lateral to the midpoint of the upper margin of pubic symphsis, on the lateral side of the femoral artery. (Fig. 2-51)

Regional Anatomy: On the medial side, the femoral artery; the femoral nerve.

Indications: (1) Hernia, abdominal pain. (2) Metrorrhagia and metrostaxis, leukorrhea.

Needling Method: Keep away from the artery. Perpendicular insertion 0.5—1.0 cun.

13. SP 13 (Fushe)

Classification: The Crossing Point of Spleen Meridian, Liver Meridian and Yin Link Vessel.

Location: On the lower abdomen, 4 cun below the umbilicus, 0.7 cun laterosuperior to SP 12 (Chongmen), 4 cun from the anterior midline of the body. (Fig. 2-51)

Regional Anatomy: The ilioinguinal nerve.

Indications: Hernia, abdominal pain.

Needling Method: Perpendicular insertion 1.0—1.5 cun.

14. SP 14 (Fujie)

Location: On the lower abdomen, 1.3 cun below SP 15 (Daheng), 4 cun from the anterior midline of the body. (Fig. 2-51)

Regional Anatomy: The eleventh intercostal artery and vein; the eleventh intercostal nerve.

Indications: (1) Pain around the umbilical region, abdominal distention, diarrhea, constipation. (2) Hernia.

Needling Method: Perpendicular insertion 1.0—2.0 cun.

15. SP 15 (Daheng)

Classification: The Crossing Point of Spleen Meridian and Yin Link Vessel.

Location: On the middle of the abdomen, 4 cun lateral to the center of the umbilicus. (Fig. 2-51)

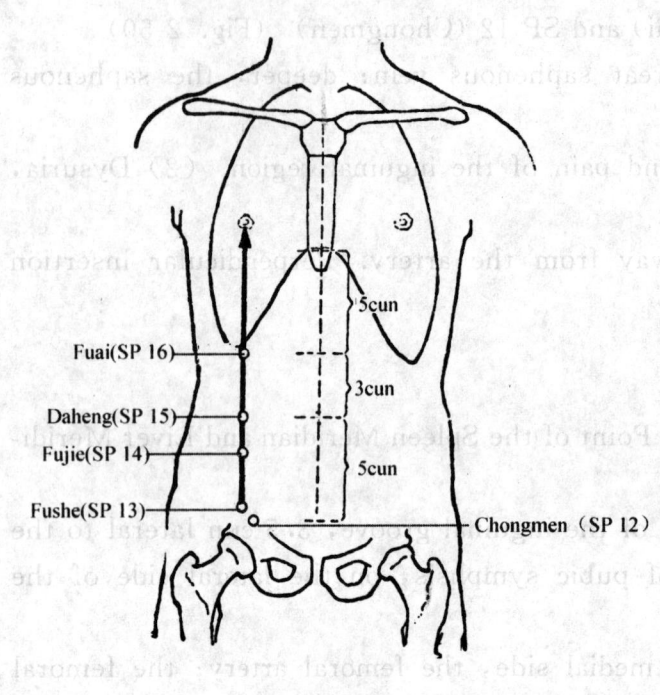

Fig. 2-51

Regional Anatomy: The tenth intercostal artery and vein; the tenth intercostal nerve.

Indications: Diarrhea, constipation, abdominal pain.

Needling Method: Perpendicular insertion 1.0—2.0 cun.

16. SP 16 (Fuai)

Classification: The Crossing Point of Spleen Meridian and Yin Link Vessel.

Location: On the upper abdomen, 3 cun above the center of the umbilicus, 4 cun from the anterior midline of the body. (Fig. 2-51)

Regional Anatomy: The eighth intercostal artery and vein; the eighth intercostal nerve.

Indications: Abdominal pain, borborygmus, dyspepsia.

Needling Method: Perpendicular insertion 1.0—1.5 cun.

17. SP 17 (Shidou)

Location: On the lateral aspect of the chest, in the fifth intercostal space, 6 cun from the anterior midline of the body. (Fig. 2-52)

Regional Anatomy: The thoracoepigastric vein; the distribution of the lateral cutaneous branch of the fifth intercostal nerve.

Indications: (1) Distention and pain in the chest and hypochondrium, nausea caused from gastric disorders, vomiting after eating. (2) Distention and edema in the abdomen, jaundice. (3) Fecal incontinence of elderly person.

Needling Method: Oblique or subcutaneous insertion toward the lateral direction 0.5—0.8 cun. Under the points from SP 17 (Shidou) to SP 21 (Dabao), deeper, there is the lung. Do not puncture these points deeply.

18. SP 18 (Tianxi)

Location: On the lateral aspect of the chest, in the fourth intercostal space, 6 cun from the anterior midline of the body. (Fig. 2-52)

Regional Anatomy: The fourth intercostal artery and vein; the lateral cutaneous branch of the fourth intercostal nerve.

Indications: (1) Pain in the chest and hypochondrium, cough. (2) Acute mastitis, insufficient lactation.

Needling Method: Oblique or subcutaneous insertion toward the lateral direction 0.5—0.8 cun.

19. SP 19 (Xiongxiang)

Location: On the lateral aspect of the chest, in the third intercostal space, 6 cun from the anterior midline of the body. (Fig. 2-52)

Regional Anatomy: The third intercostal artery and vein; the lateral cutaneous branch of the third intercostal nerve.

Indications: Distention and pain in the chest and hypochondrium.

Needling Method: Oblique or subcutaneous insertion toward the lateral direction 0.5—0.8 cun.

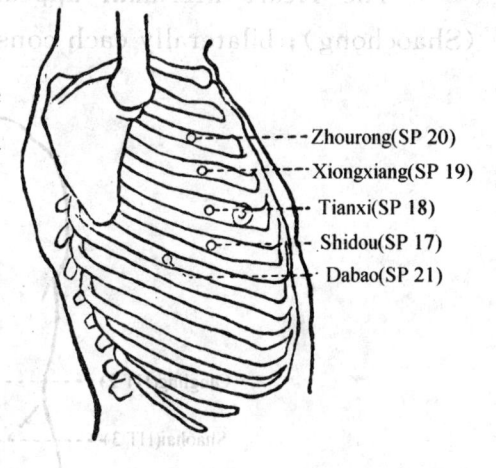

Fig. 2-52

20. SP 20 (Zhourong)

Location: On the lateral aspect of the chest, in the second intercostal space, 6 cun from the anterior midline of the body. (Fig. 2-52)

Regional Anatomy: The second intercostal artery and vein; the lateral cutaneous branch of the second intercostal nerve.

Indications: Cough, distention and pain in the chest and hypochondrium.

Needling Method: Oblique or subcutaneous insertion toward the lateral direction 0.5—0.8 cun.

21. SP 21 (Dabao)

Classification: Major Luo-(Connecting) Point of the Spleen.

Location: On the lateral aspect of the chest, on the mid-axillary line, in the sixth intercostal space. (Fig. 2-52)

Regional Anatomy: The seventh intercostal artery and vein; the seventh intercostal nerve.

Indications: (1) General aching and weakness of the limbs. (2) Asthma, pain in the chest and hypochondrium.

Needling Method: Oblique or subcutaneous insertion toward the posterior direction 0.5—0.8 cun.

Section 5 The Acupuncture Points of Heart Meridian

The Heart Meridian appears at HT 1 (Jiquan) and goes to HT 9 (Shaochong); bilaterally each consisting of 9 acupuncture points. (Fig. 2-53)

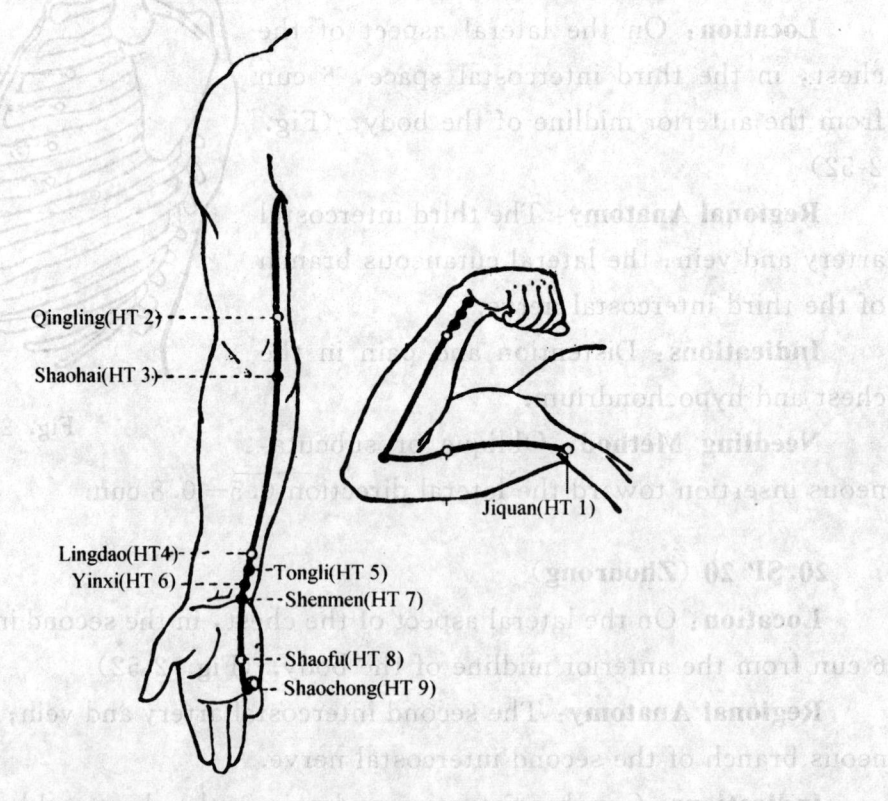

Fig. 2-53 The Points of the Heart Meridian

1. HT 1 (Jiquan)

Location: At the apex of the axillary fossa, where the axillary artery pulsates. (Fig. 2-53)

Regional Anatomy: Laterally, the axillary artery; below the point, the ulnar nerve and the median nerve.

Indications: (1) Chest congestion, shortness of breath, sad, anxious. (2) Apoplexy, hemiplegia, pain in the shoulder and arm, distention and pain in the chest and hypochondrium.

Needling Method: Keeping away from axillary artery, perpendicular or oblique insertion 0.3—0.5 cun.

2. HT 2 (Qingling)

Location: On the medial aspect of the upper arm, 3 cun above the transverse cubital crease on the line connecting HT 1 (Jiquan) and HT 3 (Shaohai), in the groove medial to m. biceps brachii. (Fig. 2-54)

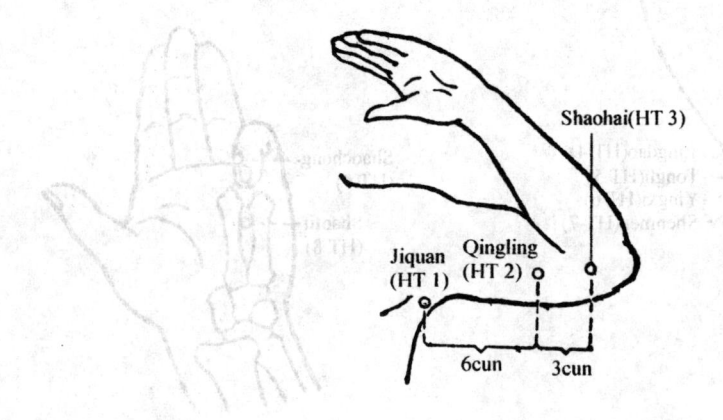

Fig. 2-54

Regional Anatomy: The basilic vein; the ulnar nerve.

Indications: Cardiac pain, pain in the hypochondrium, pain in the shoulder and arm.

Needling Method: Perpendicular insertion 0.5—1.0 cun.

3. HT 3 (Shaohai)

Classification: He-(Sea) Point.

Location: When the elbow is flexed, the point is at the midpoint of the line connecting the medial end of the transverse cubital crease and the medial epicondyle of the humerus. (Fig. 2-54)

Regional Anatomy: The basilic vein; the medial antebrachial cutaneous nerve.

Indications: (1) Cardiac pain, spasmodic pain and numbness of the elbow and arm, hand tremor. (2) Scrofula, pain in the axillary and hypochondrium.

Needling Method: Perpendicular insertion 0.5—1.0 cun.

4. HT 4 (Lingdao)

Classification: Jing-(River) Point.

Location: On the palmar aspect of the forearm, the point is on the radial side of the tendon of m. flexor carpi ulnaris, 1.5 cun above the transverse crease of the wrist. (Fig. 2-55)

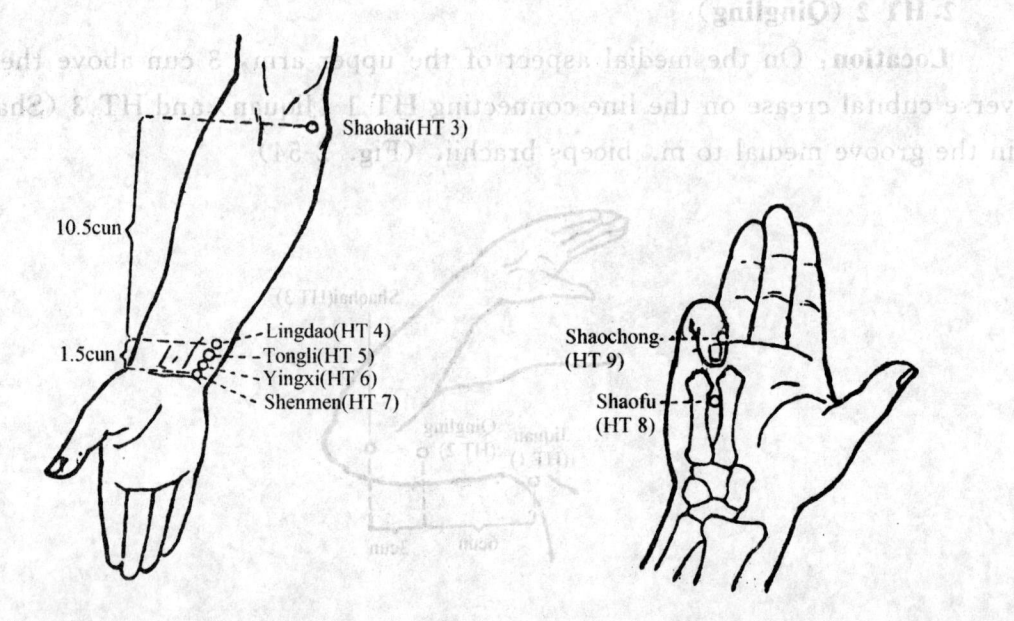

Fig. 2-55   Fig. 2-56

Regional Anatomy: The ulnar artery; the medial antebrachial cutaneous nerve.

Indications: Cardiac pain, sudden loss of voice.

Needling Method: Perpendicular insertion 0.3—0.5 cun.

5. HT 5 (Tongli)

Classification: Luo-Connecting Point.

Location: On the palmar aspect of the forearm, the point is on the radial side of the tendon of m. flexor carpi ulnaris, 1.0 cun above the transverse crease of the wrist. (Fig. 2-55)

Regional Anatomy: Same as HT 4 (Lingdao).

Indications: (1) Sudden loss of voice, stiffness of the tongue, pain in the wrist and arm. (2) Palpitation and severe palpitation.

Needling Method: Perpendicular insertion 0.3—0.5 cun.

6. HT 6 (Yinxi)

Classification: Xi-(Cleft) Point.

Location: On the palmar aspect of the forearm, the point is on the radial side of the tendon of m. flexor carpi ulnaris, 0.5 cun above the transverse crease of the wrist. (Fig. 2-55)

Regional Anatomy: Same as HT 4 (Lingdao).

Indications: (1) Cardiac pain, palpitation due to fright (2) Hectic fever and night sweat. (3) Hemoptysis, epistaxis, sudden loss of voice.

Needling Method: Perpendicular insertion 0.3—0.5 cun.

7. HT 7 (Shenmen)

Classification: Shu-(Stream) Point and Yuan-(Source) Point.

Location: On the wrist, at the ulnar end of the transverse crease of the wrist, in the depression on the radial side of the tendon of m. flexor carpi ulnaris. (Fig. 2-55)

Regional Anatomy: Same as HT 4 (Lingdao).

Indications: (1) Insomnia, amnesia. (2) Cardiac pain, palpitation due to fright, irritability, chest pain. (3) Manic, epilepsy, stupor.

Needling Method: Perpendicular insertion 0.3—0.5 cun.

8. HT 8 (Shaofu)

Classification: Ying-(Spring) Point.

Location: On the palm, between the fourth and fifth metacarpal bones. When a fist is made, the point is where the tip of the little finger touches. (Fig. 2-56)

Regional Anatomy: The common palmar digital artery and vein; the common palmar digital nerve.

Indications: (1) Pruritus and pain of the external genitalia. (2) Spasmodic pain of the little finger. (3) Palpitation, chest pain.

Needling Method: Perpendicular insertion 0.3—0.5 cun.

9. HT 9 (Shaochong)

Classification: Jing-(Well) Point.

Location: On the radial side of the distal phalanx of the little finger, 0.1 cun (finger cun) distance from the corner of the nail. (Fig. 2-56)

Regional Anatomy: The arterial and venous network formed by the palmar digital proprial artery and vein; the distribution of the palmar digital proprial nerve derived from the ulnar nerve.

Indications: (1) Palpitation, cardiac pain, pain in the chest and hypochondrium. (2) Manic psychosis, febrile diseases, loss of consciousness.

Needling Method: Subcutaneous insertion 0.1 cun, or prick to cause bleeding.

Section 6 The Acupuncture Points of Small Intestine Meridian

The Small Intestine Meridian appears at SI 1 (Shaoze) and goes to SI 19 (Tinggong); bilaterally each consisting of 19 acupuncture points. (Fig. 2-57)

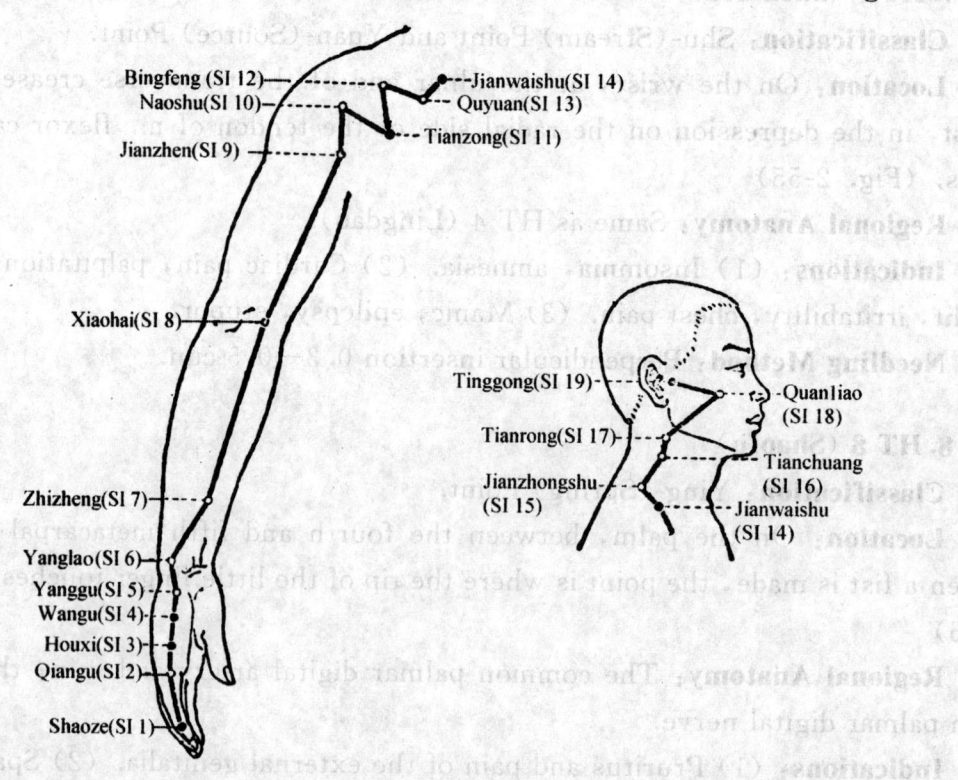

Fig. 2-57 The Points of the Small Intestine Meridian

1. SI 1 (Shaoze)

Classification: Jing-(Well) Point.

Location: On the ulnar side of the distal phalanx of the little finger, 0.1 cun (finger cun) distance from the corner of the nail. (Fig. 2-58)

Regional Anatomy: The arterial and venous network; the branches of the ulnar nerve.

Indications: (1) Febrile diseases, apoplexy, loss of consciousness. (2) Insufficient lactation, acute mastitis. (3) Sore throat, conjunctivitis, headache.

Needling Method: Subcutaneous insertion 0.1 cun, or prick to cause bleeding.

2. SI 2 (Qiangu)

Classification: Ying-(Spring) Point.

Location: When a loose fist is made, the point is on the ulnar aspect of the hand, distal to the fifth metacarpophalangeal joint, at the end of the transverse crease of the metacarpophalangeal joint, at the junction of the red and white skin. (Fig. 2-58)

Regional Anatomy: The dorsal digital artery and vein; the dorsal digital branch of the ulnar nerve.

Indications: (1) Numbness of the fingers. (2) Fever, headache, tinnitus. (3) Scanty dark urine.

Needling Method: Perpendicular insertion 0.3—0.5 cun.

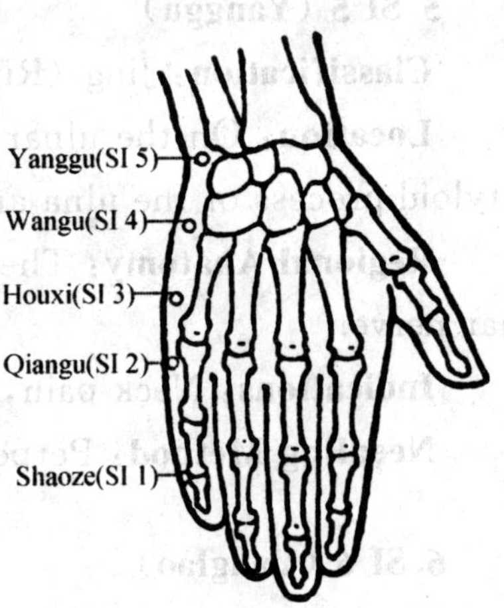

Fig. 2-58

3. SI 3 (Houxi)

Classification: Shu-(Stream) Point; and one of the Eight Confluent Points, this point linking with the Governor Vessel.

Location: When a loose fist is made, the point is on the ulnar aspect of the palm, proximal to the fifth metacarpophalangeal joint, at the end of the transverse crease of the palm, at the junction of the red and white skin. (Fig. 2-58)

Regional Anatomy: The dorsal digital artery and vein; the dorsal branch of the ulnar nerve.

Indications: (1) Pain and rigidity of the head and neck, malaria, pain in the lumbar and sacrum, acute spasm in the finger, elbow and arm. (2) Manic psychosis, epilepsy. (3) Deafness, eye congestion. (4) Night sweat.

Needling Method: Perpendicular insertion 0.5—1.0 cun.

4. SI 4 (Wangu)

Classification: Yuan-(Source) Point.

Location: On the ulnar aspect of the palm, in the depression between the fifth metacarpal bone and the hamate bone, at the junction of the red and white skin. (Fig. 2-58)

Regional Anatomy: The dorsal venous network of the hand; the dorsal branch of the ulnar nerve.

Indications: (1) Jaundice, diabetes. (2) Pain in the lumbar and leg, contracture of the fingers, pain in the wrist, weakness to hold things in the hand. (3) Pain and rigidity of the head and neck, tinnitus, conjunctivitis.

Needling Method: Perpendicular insertion 0.3—0.5 cun.

5. SI 5 (Yanggu)

Classification: Jing-(River) Point.

Location: On the ulnar aspect of the wrist, in the depression between the styloid process of the ulna and the triquetral bone. (Fig. 2-58)

Regional Anatomy: The posterior carpal artery; the dorsal branch of the ulnar nerve.

Indications: Neck pain, pain of the hand and wrist, febrile diseases.

Needling Method: Perpendicular insertion 0.3—0.5 cun.

6. SI 6 (Yanglao)

Classification: Xi-(Cleft) Point.

Location: On the dorsal ulnar aspect of the forearm, in the depression on the radial side of the styloid process of the ulna. (Fig. 2-59)

Regional Anatomy: The venous network of the wrist; the dorsal branch of the ulnar nerve.

Indications: (1) Blurring of the vision. (2) Aching of the shoulder, back, elbow and arm, acute lumbar pain.

Needling Method: Oblique insertion towards the elbow 0.5—0.8 cun.

7. SI 7 (Zhizheng)

Classification: Luo-(Connecting) Point.

Location: On the dorsal ulnar aspect of the forearm, 5 cun above the transverse crease of the wrist, on the line connecting SI 5 (Yanggu) and SI 8 (Xiaohai). (Fig. 2-59)

Regional Anatomy: The terminal branches of the posterior interosseous artery and vein; the dorsal branch of the ulnar nerve.

Indications: (1) Weakness of the joints, aching and dysfunction of the elbow. (2) Warts.

Needling Method: Perpendicular or oblique insertion 0.5—0.8 cun.

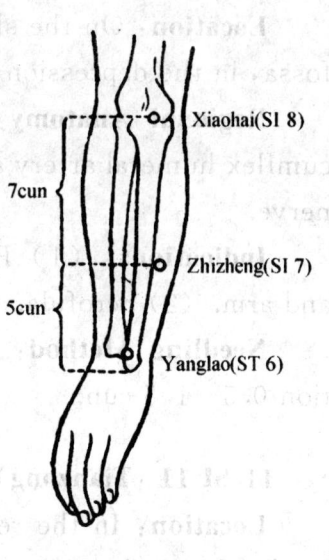

Fig. 2-59

8. SI 8 (Xiaohai)

Classification: He-(Sea) Point.

Location: On the medial aspect of the elbow, in the depression between the olecranon of the ulna and the medial epicondyle of the humerus. (Fig. 2-59)

Regional Anatomy: The superior and inferior ulnar collateral arteries and veins; the ulnar nerve.

Indications: (1) Pain in the elbow and arm. (2) Epilepsy.

Needling Method: Perpendicular insertion 0.3—0.5 cun.

9. SI 9 (Jianzhen)

Location: Posterior and inferior to the shoulder joint, when the arm is adducted, the point is 1 cun (finger inch) above the posterior end of the axillary fossa. (Fig. 2-60)

Regional Anatomy: The circumflex scapular artery and vein; deeper in the superior aspect, the radial nerve.

Indications: (1) Pain in the shoulder and arm. (2) Scrofula, tinnitus.

Needling Method: Perpendicular insertion 1.0—1.5 cun.

10. SI 10 (Naoshu)

Classification: The Crossing Point of Small Intestine Meridian, Bladder Meridian, Yang Link Vessel, and Yang Heel Vessel.

Location: On the shoulder, directly above the posterior end of the axillary fossa, in the depression inferior to the scapular spine. (Fig. 2-60)

Regional Anatomy: The posterior circumflex humeral artery and vein; the axillary nerve.

Indications: (1) Pain in the shoulder and arm. (2) Scrofula.

Needling Method: Perpendicular insertion 0.5—1.5 cun.

11. SI 11 (Tianzong)

Location: In the region of the scapula, in the depression in the center of the subscapular fossa, level with the fourth thoracic vertebra. (Fig. 2-60)

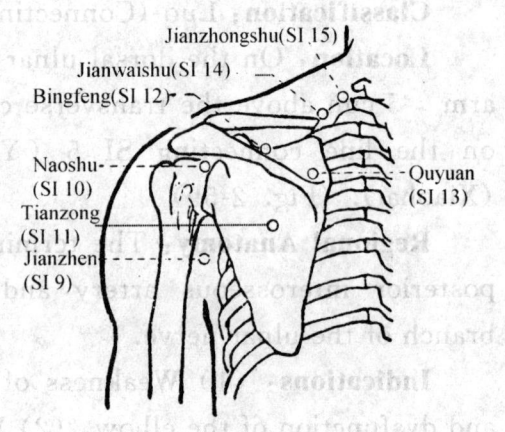

Fig. 2-60

Regional Anatomy: The muscular branches of the circumflex scapular artery and vein; the distribution of the suprascapular nerve.

Indications: (1) Pain in the shoulder and arm. (2) Asthma, acute mastitis.

Needling Method: Perpendicular or oblique insertion 0.5—1.0 cun.

12. SI 12 (Bingfeng)

Classification: The Crossing Point of the three Yang Meridians of Hand and Gallbladder Meridian.

Location: In the region of the scapula, in the center of the suprascapular fossa, directly above SI 11 (Tianzong), in the depression when the arm is lifted. (Fig. 2-60)

Regional Anatomy: The suprascapular artery and vein; deeper, the suprascapular nerve.

Indications: Pain in the shoulder and scapular region, aching and numbness of the upper extremities.

Needling Method: Perpendicular or oblique insertion 0.5—1.0 cun.

13. SI 13 (Quyuan)

Location: In the region of the scapula, on the medial extremity of the suprascapular fossa, midway between SI 10 (Naoshu) and the spinous process second thoracic vertebra. (Fig. 2-60)

Regional Anatomy: Deeper, the muscular branch of the suprascapular artery and vein; deeper, the muscular branch of the suprascapular nerve.

Indications: Pain in the shoulder and scapular region.

Needling Method: Perpendicular or oblique insertion 0.5—1.0 cun.

14. SI 14 (Jianwaishu)

Location: On the back, 3 cun lateral to the lower border of the spinous process of the first thoracic vertebra. (Fig. 2-60)

Regional Anatomy: Deeper, the transverse cervical artery and vein; deeper, the dorsal scapular nerve.

Indications: Pain in the shoulder and back, suddenly stiff neck.

Needling Method: Oblique insertion 0.5—0.8 cun.

15. SI 15 (Jianzhongshu)

Location: On the back, 2 cun lateral to the lower border of the spinous process of the seventh cervical vertebra. (Fig. 2-60)

Regional Anatomy: Same as SI 14 (Jianwaishu).

Indications: (1) Cough, asthma, hemoptysis. (2) Pain in the shoulder and back.

Needling Method: Oblique insertion 0.5—0.8 cun.

16. SI 16 (Tianchuang)

Location: On the lateral aspect of the neck, in the posterior border of m. sternocleidomastoideus, posterior to LI 18 (Futu), level with the Adam's apple. (Fig. 2-61)

Regional Anatomy: The ascending cervical artery; the emerging portion of the great auricular nerve.

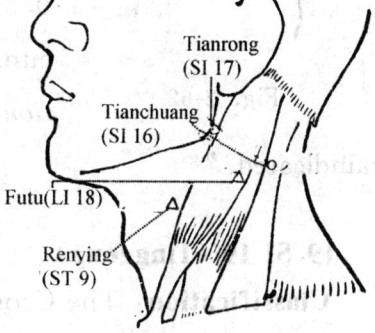

Fig. 2-61

Indications: (1) Sore throat, sudden loss of voice, pain and rigidity of the neck. (2) Tinnitus, deafness.

Needling Method: Perpendicular insertion 0.5—1.0 cun.

17. SI 17 (Tianrong)

Location: On the lateral aspect of the neck, posterior to the angle of mandible, in the depression on the anterior border of m. sternocleidomastoideus. (Fig. 2-61)

Regional Anatomy: Deeper, the internal carotid artery and internal jugular vein. The distribution of the anterior branch of the great auricular nerve; deeper, the sympathetic nerve chain passes.

Indications: Tinnitus, deafness, sore throat, swelling and pain of the neck.

Needling Method: Perpendicular insertion 0.5—1.0 cun.

18. SI 18 (Quanliao)

Classification: The Crossing Point of Triple Energizer Meridian and Small Intestine Meridian.

Location: On the face, directly below the outer canthus of the eye, in the depression on the lower border of zygoma. (Fig. 2-62)

Regional Anatomy: The branches of the transverse facial artery and vein; the distribution of the facial and infraorbital nerves.

Indications: (1) Wry face, twitching of eyelids. (2) Toothache, swelling of the cheek.

Needling Method: Perpendicular insertion 0.3—0.5 cun; oblique or subcutaneous insertion 0.5—1.0 cun. *"Supplement with Diagnosis to Sysematic Compilation of the Internal Classi"* says: "moxibustion is contraindicated."

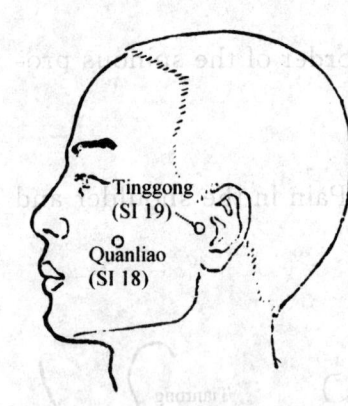

Fig. 2-62

19. SI 19 (Tinggong)

Classification: The Crossing Point of Triple Energizer Meridian, Gallbladder Meridian and Small Intestine Meridian.

Location: On the region of the face, anterior to the tragus and posterior to the condyloid process of the mandible, in the depression formed when the mouth is open. (Fig. 2-62)

Regional Anatomy: The auricular branches of the superficial temporal artery and vein; the distribution of the branch of the facial nerve, the auriculotemporal nerve.

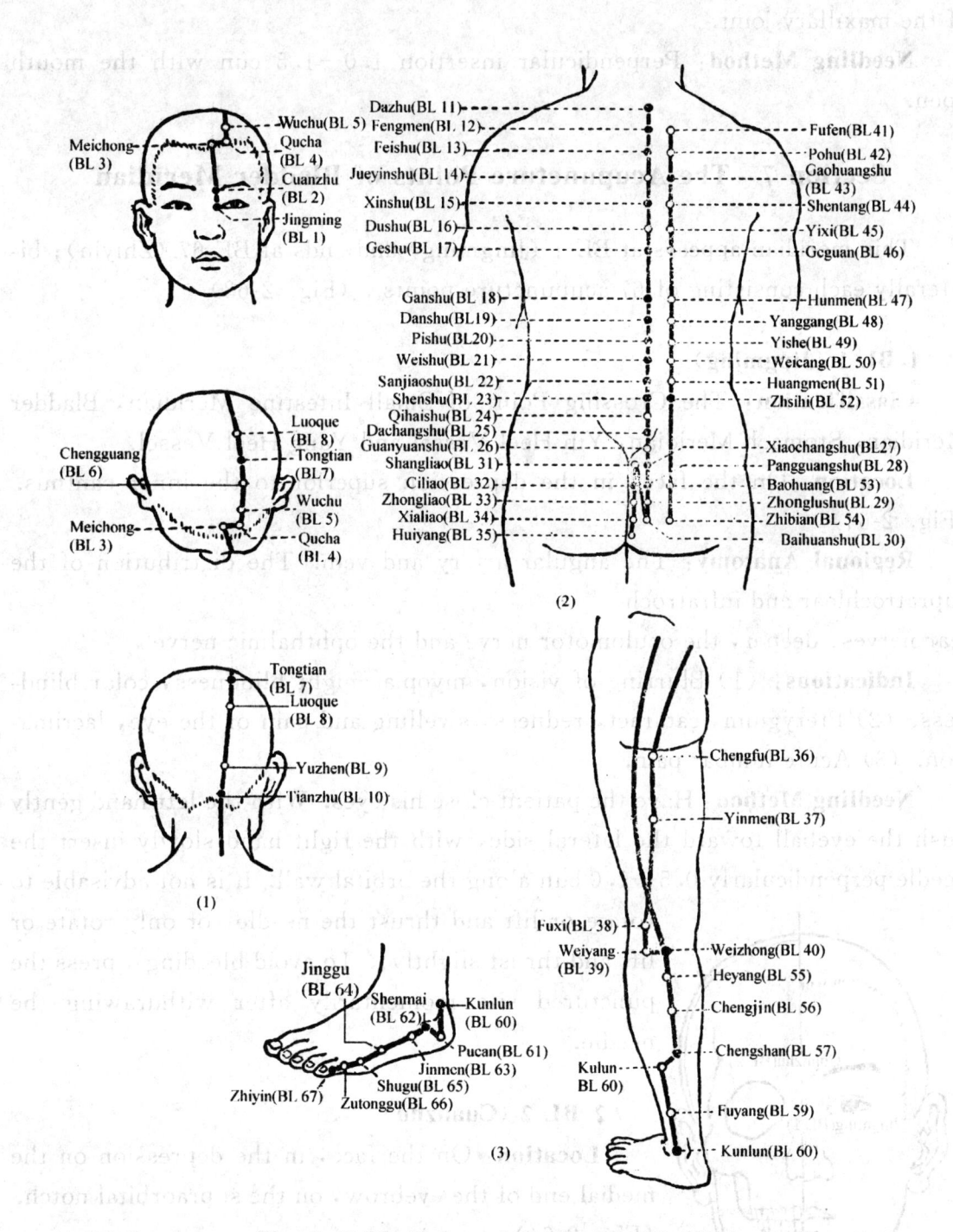

Fig. 2-63 The Points of the Bladder Meridian

Indications: (1) Tinnitus, deafness, otorrhea. (2) Toothache, dysfunction of the maxillary joint.

Needling Method: Perpendicular insertion 1.0—1.5 cun with the mouth open.

Section 7 The Acupuncture Points of Bladder Meridian

This meridian appears at BL 1 (Jingming) and ends at BL 67 (Zhiyin); bilaterally each consisting of 67 acupuncture points. (Fig. 2-63)

1. BL 1 (Jingming)

Classification: The Crossing Point of Small Intestine Meridian, Bladder Meridian, Stomach Meridian, Yin Heel Vessel and Yang Heel Vessel.

Location: On the face, in the depression superior to the inner canthus. (Fig. 2-64)

Regional Anatomy: The angular artery and vein. The distribution of the supratrochlear and infratrochlear nerves; deeper, the oculomotor nerve and the ophthalmic nerve.

Indications: (1) Blurring of vision, myopia, night blindness, color blindness. (2) Pterygium, cataract, redness, swelling and pain of the eye, lacrimation. (3) Acute lumbar pain.

Needling Method: Have the patient close his eyes. With the left hand gently push the eyeball toward the lateral side, with the right hand slowly insert the needle perpendicularly 0.5—1.0 cun along the orbital wall. It is not advisable to rotate or lift and thrust the needle (or only rotate or lift and thrust slightly). To avoid bleeding, press the punctured site momentarily after withdrawing the needle.

2. BL 2 (Cuanzhu)

Location: On the face, in the depression on the medial end of the eyebrow, on the supraorbital notch. (Fig. 2-64)

Regional Anatomy: The frontal artery and vein; the distributions of the medial branch of the frontal nerve.

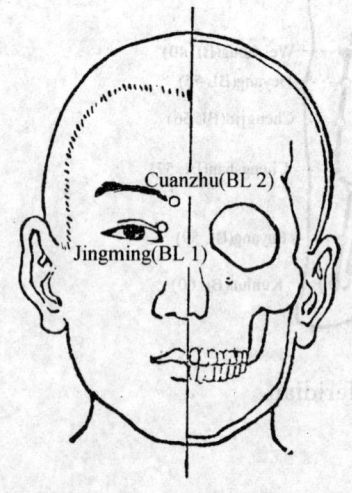

Fig. 2-64

Indications: (1) Pain in the supraorbital region, blurring of vision, redness, swelling and pain of the eye. (2) Hiccup. (3) Lumbar pain. (4) Spasm of the diaphragm.

Needling Method: Subcutaneous insertion 0.5—0.8 cun, or prick to cause bleeding. Moxibustion is contraindicated.

3. BL 3 (Meichong)

Location: On the scalp, directly above BL 1 (Cuanzhu), 0.5 cun within the anterior hairline, between GV 24 (Shenting) and BL 4 (Qucha). (Fig. 2-65)

Regional Anatomy: Same as BL 2 (Cuanzhu).

Indications: (1) Headache, vertigo, nasal congestion. (2) Epilepsy.

Needling Method: Subcutaneous insertion 0.3—0.5 cun.

4. BL 4 (Qucha)

Location: On the scalp, 0.5 cun within the anterior hairline, 1.5 cun lateral to the midline, at the junction of the medial third and lateral two-thirds of the distance from GV 24 (Shenting) to ST 8 (Touwei). (Fig. 2-65)

Regional Anatomy: The frontal artery and vein; the distribution of the lateral branch of the frontal nerve.

Indications: (1) Headache, nasal congestion, epistaxis. (2) Blurring of vision.

Needling Method: Subcutaneous insertion 0.5—0.8 cun.

5. BL 5 (Wuchu)

Location: On the scalp, 1.0 cun posterior to the anterior hairline, 1.5 cun lateral to the midline. (Fig. 2-65)

Regional Anatomy: Same as BL 4 (Qucha).

Indications: (1) Headache, dizziness. (2) Hemiplegia. (3) Epilepsy.

Needling Method: Subcutaneous insertion 0.5—0.8 cun.

6. BL 6 (Chengguang)

Location: On the scalp, 2.5 cun posterior to the anterior hairline, 1.5 cun lateral to the midline. (Fig. 2-65)

Regional Anatomy: The anastomotic network of the frontal, temporal and occipital artery and vein; the anastomotic branch of the lateral branch of the frontal nerve and the greater occipital nerve.

Indications: (1) Blurring of vision. (2) Hemiplegia, epilepsy. (3) Dizziness.

Needling Method: Subcutaneous insertion 0.3—0.5 cun.

7. BL 7 (Tongtian)

Location: On the scalp, 4.0 cun posterior to the anterior hairline, 1.5 cun lateral to the midline. (Fig. 2-65)

Regional Anatomy: The anastomotic network of the superficial temporal and the occipital artery and vein; the distribution of the branch of the greater occipital nerve.

Indications: (1) Nasal congestion, nasal polyps, nasal ulcers, rhinorrhea, epistaxis. (2) Headache, dizziness. (3) Hemiplegia, epilepsy.

Needling Method: Subcutaneous insertion 0.3—0.5 cun.

8. BL 8 (Luoque)

Location: On the scalp, 5.5 cun posterior to the anterior hairline, 1.5 cun lateral to the midline. (Fig. 2-65)

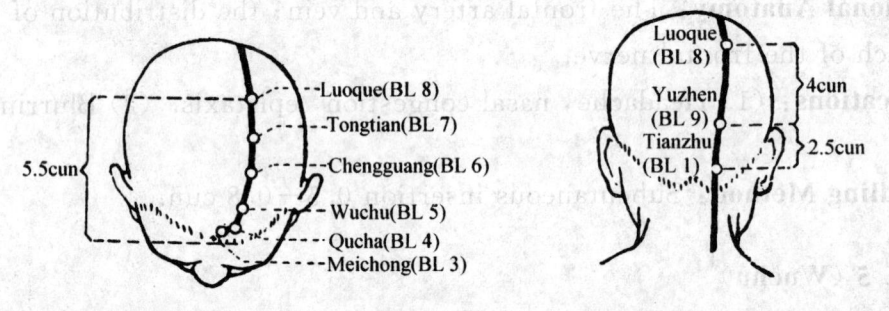

Fig. 2-65

Fig. 2-66

Regional Anatomy: The branches of the occipital artery and vein; the distribution of the branch of the greater occipital nerve.

Indications: (1) Blurring of vision. (2) Hemiplegia, epilepsy. (3) Tinnitus.

Needling Method: Subcutaneous insertion 0.3—0.5 cun.

9. BL 9 (Yuzhen)

Location: On the posterior aspect of the head, 2.5 cun superior to posterior hairline, 1.3 cun lateral to the midline, level with the superior border of the external occipital protuberance. (Fig. 2-66)

Regional Anatomy: The same as BL 8 (Luoque).
Indications: (1) Headache and neck pain, blurring of vision. (2) Nasal congestion. (3) Tinea pedis.
Needling Method: Subcutaneous insertion 0.3—0.5 cun.

10. BL 10 (Tianzhu)
Location: On the nape, in the depression on the lateral border of m. trapezius, within the posterior hairline, 1.3 cun lateral to the midline. (Fig. 2-66)
Regional Anatomy: Same as BL 8 (Luoque).
Indications: (1) Dizziness. (2) Headache, neck stiffness, pain in the shoulder and back. (3) Nasal congestion, sore throat.
Needling Method: Perpendicular or oblique insertion 0.5—0.8 cun. Do not insert the needle deeply medially upwards to avoid injuring medulla oblongata.

11. BL 11 (Dazhu)
Classification: The Converging Point of Bone. The Crossing Point of Small Intestine Meridian and Bladder Meridian.
Location: On the back, 1.5 cun lateral to the lower border of the spinous process of the first thoracic vertebra. (Fig. 2-67)
Regional Anatomy: The medial cutaneous branches of the posterior branches of the intercostal artery and vein. The distributions of the medial cutaneous branch of the posterior ramus of the first thoracic nerve; deeper, its lateral branch.
Indications: (1) All types of bone disease (including pain in the bone, joint pain in the shoulder, back, lumbar, sacrum, and knee). (2) Fever, cough, headache, nasal congestion.
Needling Method: Oblique insertion 0.5—0.8 cun.

12. BL 12 (Fengmen)
Classification: The Crossing Point of Bladder Meridian and Governor Vessel.
Location: On the back, 1.5 cun lateral to the lower border of the spinous process of the second thoracic vertebra. (Fig. 2-67)
Regional Anatomy: Vasculature is the same as BL 11 (Dazhu). The distribution of the medial cutaneous branches of the posterior rami of the second and third thoracic nerves; deeper, their lateral branches.

Indications: (1) Common cold, cough. (2) Fever, headache, neck stiffness, pain in the chest and back.

Needling Method: Oblique insertion 0.5—0.8 cun.

13. BL 13 (Feishu)

Classification: The Back Shu Point of Lung.

Location: On the back, 1.5 cun lateral to the lower border of the spinous process of the third thoracic vertebra. (Fig. 2-67)

Regional Anatomy: Vasculature is the same as BL 11 (Dazhu). The distributions of the medial cutaneous branches of the posterior rami of the third and fourth thoracic nerves; deeper, their lateral branches.

Indications: (1) Fever, cough, hemoptysis, night sweating, nasal congestion. (2) Alopecia, smallpox, rash, soreness, tinea.

Needling Method: Oblique insertion 0.5—0.8 cun.

14. BL 14 (Jueyinshu)

Classification: The Back Shu Point of Pericardium.

Location: On the back, 1.5 cun lateral to the lower border of the spinous process of the fourth thoracic vertebra. (Fig. 2-67)

Regional Anatomy: Vasculature is the same as BL 11 (Dazhu). The distribution of the medial cutaneous branches of the posterior rami of the fourth and fifth thoracic nerves; deeper, their lateral branches.

Indications: (1) Cardiac pain, palpitation. (2) Cough, chest congestion. (3) Toothache.

Needling Method: Oblique insertion 0.5—0.8 cun.

15. BL 15 (Xinshu)

Classification: The Back Shu Point of Heart.

Location: On the back, 1.5 cun lateral to the lower border of the spinous process of the fifth thoracic vertebra. (Fig. 2-67)

Regional Anatomy: Vasculature is the same as BL 11 (Dazhu). The distribution of the medial cutaneous branches of the posterior rami of the fifth and sixth thoracic nerves; deeper, their lateral branches.

Indications: (1) Cardiac pain, palpitation, chest congestion, shortness of breath. (2) Cough, hematemesis. (3) Insomnia, forgetful, epilepsy. (4) Nocturnal emission, night sweating.

Needling Method: Oblique insertion 0.5—0.8 cun.

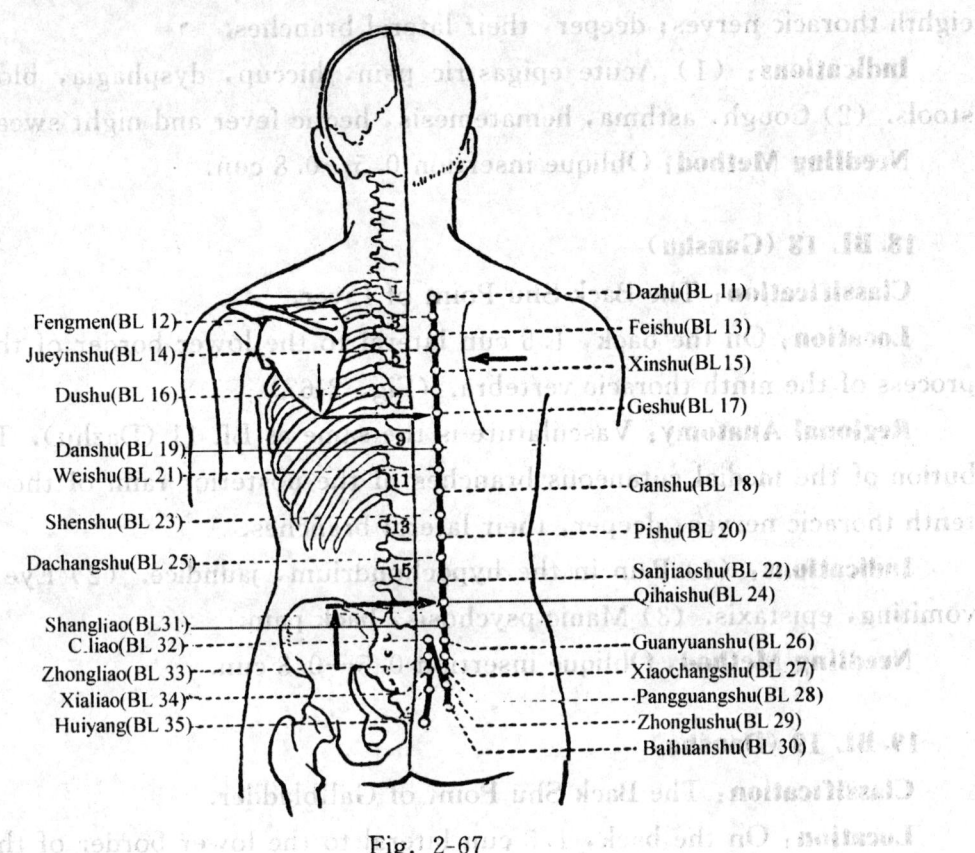

Fig. 2-67

Labels on figure:
- Fengmen(BL 12)
- Jueyinshu(BL 14)
- Dushu(BL 16)
- Danshu(BL 19)
- Weishu(BL 21)
- Shenshu(BL 23)
- Dachangshu(BL 25)
- Shangliao(BL 31)
- C.liao(BL 32)
- Zhongliao(BL 33)
- Xialiao(BL 34)
- Huiyang(BL 35)
- Dazhu(BL 11)
- Feishu(BL 13)
- Xinshu(BL 15)
- Geshu(BL 17)
- Ganshu(BL 18)
- Pishu(BL 20)
- Sanjiaoshu(BL 22)
- Qihaishu(BL 24)
- Guanyuanshu(BL 26)
- Xiaochangshu(BL 27)
- Pangguangshu(BL 28)
- Zhonglushu(BL 29)
- Baihuanshu(BL 30)

16. BL 16 (Dushu)

Location: On the back, 1.5 cun lateral to the lower border of the spinous process of the sixth thoracic vertebra. (Fig. 2-67)

Regional Anatomy: Vasculature is the same as BL 11 (Dazhu). The distribution of the medial cutaneous branches of the posterior rami of the sixth and seventh thoracic nerves; deeper, their lateral branches.

Indications: (1) Cardiac pain, chest congestion. (2) Gastric pain, abdominal pain. (3) Cough, asthma.

Needling Method: Oblique insertion 0.5—0.8 cun.

17. BL 17 (Geshu)

Classification: The Converging Point of Blood.

Location: On the back, 1.5 cun lateral to the lower border of the spinous process of the seventh thoracic vertebra. (Fig. 2-67)

Regional Anatomy: Vasculature is the same as BL 11 (Dazhu). The distri-

123

bution of the medial cutaneous branches of the posterior rami of the seventh and eighth thoracic nerves; deeper, their lateral branches.

Indications: (1) Acute epigastric pain, hiccup, dysphagia, blood in the stools. (2) Cough, asthma, hematemesis, hectic fever and night sweating.

Needling Method: Oblique insertion 0.5—0.8 cun.

18. BL 18 (Ganshu)

Classification: The Back Shu Point of Liver.

Location: On the back, 1.5 cun lateral to the lower border of the spinous process of the ninth thoracic vertebra. (Fig. 2-67)

Regional Anatomy: Vasculature is the same as BL 11 (Dazhu). The distribution of the medial cutaneous branches of the posterior rami of the ninth and tenth thoracic nerves; deeper, their lateral branches.

Indications: (1) Pain in the hypochondrium, jaundice. (2) Eye diseases, vomiting, epistaxis. (3) Manic psychosis, back pain.

Needling Method: Oblique insertion 0.5—0.8 cun.

19. BL 19 (Danshu)

Classification: The Back Shu Point of Gallbladder.

Location: On the back, 1.5 cun lateral to the lower border of the spinous process of the tenth thoracic vertebra. (Fig. 2-67)

Regional Anatomy: Vasculature same as BL 11 (Dazhu). The distribution of the medial cutaneous branches of the posterior rami of the tenth and eleventh thoracic nerves; deeper, their lateral branches.

Indications: (1) Jaundice, bitter taste in the mouth, pain in the hypochondrium. (2) Pulmonary tuberculosis, hectic fever.

Needling Method: Oblique insertion 0.5—0.8 cun.

20. BL 20 (Pishu)

Classification: The Back Shu Point of Spleen.

Location: On the back, 1.5 cun lateral to the lower border of the spinous process of the eleventh thoracic vertebra. (Fig. 2-67)

Regional Anatomy: Vasculature is the same as BL 11 (Dazhu). The distribution of the medial cutaneous branches of the posterior rami of the eleventh and twelfth thoracic nerves; deeper, their lateral branches.

Indications: (1) Abdominal distention, jaundice, vomiting, diarrhea, dysentery, blood in the stools. (2) Edema.

Needling Method: Oblique insertion 0.5—0.8 cun.

21. BL 21 (Weishu)

Classification: The Back Shu Point of Stomach.

Location: On the back, 1.5 cun lateral to the lower border of the spinous process of the twelfth thoracic vertebra. (Fig. 2-67)

Regional Anatomy: The medial branches of the posterior branches of the subcostal artery and vein. The distribution of the medial cutaneous branch of the posterior ramus of the twelfth thoracic nerve; deeper, its lateral branches.

Indications: (1) Epigastric pain, vomiting. (2) Abdominal distention, borborygmus.

Needling Method: Oblique insertion 0.5—0.8 cun.

22. BL 22 (Sanjiaoshu)

Classification: The Back Shu Point of Triple Energizer.

Location: On the lower back, 1.5 cun lateral to the lower border of the spinous process of the first lumbar vertebra. (Fig. 2-67)

Regional Anatomy: The posterior branches of the first and second lumbar arteries and veins; the posterior rami of the first and second lumbar nerves.

Indications: (1) Edema, dysuria. (2) Abdominal distention, borborygmus, diarrhea, dysentery. (3) Weak knee.

Needling Method: Perpendicular insertion 0.5—1.0 cun.

23. BL 23 (Shenshu)

Classification: The Back Shu Point of Kidney.

Location: On the lower back, 1.5 cun lateral to the lower border of the spinous process of the second lumbar vertebra. (Fig. 2-67)

Regional Anatomy: The posterior branches of the second and third lumbar arteries and veins; the distribution of the muscular branches of the posterior rami of the second and third lumbar nerves.

Indications: (1) Enuresis, dysuria, edema. (2) Spermatorrhea, impotence, irregular menstruation, leukorrhea. (3) Deafness, tinnitus, cough, asthma. (4) Hemiplegia, lumbar pain, bone disease.

Needling Method: Perpendicular insertion 0.5—1.0 cun.

24. BL 24 (Qihaishu)

Location: On the lower back, 1.5 cun lateral to the lower border of the spinous process of the third lumbar vertebra. (Fig. 2-67)

Regional Anatomy: The posterior branches of the third and fourth lumbar arteries and veins; the muscular branches of the posterior rami of the third and fourth lumbar nerves.

Indications: (1) Abdominal distention, borborygmus, anal fistula. (2) Dysmenorrhea, lumbar pain.

Needling Method: Perpendicular insertion 0.5—1.0 cun.

25. BL 25 (Dachangshu)

Classification: The Back Shu Point of Large Intestine.

Location: On the lower back, 1.5 cun lateral to the lower border of the spinous process of the fourth lumbar vertebra. (Fig. 2-67)

Regional Anatomy: The third and fourth lumbar arteries and veins; the muscular branches of the posterior rami of the fourth and fifth lumbar nerves.

Indications: (1) Abdominal distention, diarrhea, constipation, bleeding hemorrhoids. (2) Lumbar pain. (3) Urticaria.

Needling Method: Perpendicular insertion 0.8—1.2 cun.

26. BL 26 (Guanyuanshu)

Location: On the lower back, 1.5 cun lateral to the lower border of the spinous process of the fifth lumbar vertebra. (Fig. 2-67)

Regional Anatomy: The fifth lumbar and the first sacral arteries and veins; the muscular branch of the posterior ramus of the fifth lumbar nerve.

Indications: (1) Pain in the lumbosacral region. (2) Abdominal distention, diarrhea. (3) Frequent urination or dysuria, enuresis.

Needling Method: Perpendicular insertion 0.8—1.2 cun.

27. BL 27 (Xiaochangshu)

Classification: The Back Shu Point of Small Intestine.

Location: In the region of the sacrum, 1.5 cun lateral to the middle sacral crest, at the level of the first posterior sacral foramen. (Fig. 2-67)

Regional Anatomy: The posterior branches of the lateral sacral artery and vein; the distribution of the lateral branch of the posterior ramus of the first sacral nerve.

Indications: (1) Pain in the lumbosacral region and knee. (2) Lower abdominal distention and pain, dysuria. (3) Spermatorrhea, leukorrhea.

Needling Method: Perpendicular or oblique insertion 0.8—1.2 cun.

28. BL 28 (Pangguangshu)

Classification: The Back Shu Point of Bladder.

Location: In the region of the sacrum, 1.5 cun lateral to the middle sacral crest, at the level of the second posterior sacral foramen. (Fig. 2-67)

Regional Anatomy: Vasculature is the same as BL 27 (Xiaochangshu). The distribution of the lateral branches of the posterior rami of the first and second sacral nerves.

Indications: (1) Dysuria, enuresis. (2) Stiffness and pain of lower back, leg pain. (3) Diarrhea, constipation.

Needling Method: Perpendicular or oblique insertion 0.8—1.2 cun.

29. BL 29 (Zhonglushu)

Location: In the region of the sacrum, 1.5 cun lateral to the middle sacral crest, at the level of the third posterior sacral foramen. (Fig. 2-67)

Regional Anatomy: The posterior branches of the lateral sacral artery and vein, the branches of the inferior gluteal artery and vein; the distribution of the lateral branches of the posterior rami of the third and fourth sacral nerves.

Indications: (1) Diarrhea. (2) Hernia, lower back pain and stiffness.

Needling Method: Perpendicular insertion 1.0—1.5 cun.

30. BL 30 (Baihuanshu)

Location: In the region of the sacrum, 1.5 cun lateral to the middle sacral crest, at the level of the fourth posterior sacral foramen. (Fig. 2-67)

Regional Anatomy: The inferior gluteal artery and vein; deeper, the internal pudendal artery and vein. The distribution of the lateral branches of the posterior rami of the third and fourth sacral nerves, the inferior gluteal nerve.

Indications: (1) Spermatorrhea, leukorrhea, irregular menstruation, enuresis. (2) Lumbosacral pain, hernia.

Needling Method: Perpendicular insertion 1.0—1.5 cun.

31. BL 31 (Shangliao)

Location: In the region of the sacrum, between the posterior superior iliac spine and the midline of the back, in the first posterior sacral foramen. (Fig. 2-67)

Regional Anatomy: The posterior branches of the lateral sacral artery and vein; the posterior ramus of the first sacral nerve.

Indications: (1) Irregular menstruation, bloody leukorrhea, prolapse of uterus. (2) Spermatorrhea, impotence. (3) Constipation, dysuria, lumbosacral pain.

Needling Method: Perpendicular insertion 1.0—1.5 cun.

32. BL 32 (Ciliao)

Location: In the region of the sacrum, medial and inferior to the posterior superior iliac spine, in the second posterior sacral foramen. (Fig. 2-67)

Regional Anatomy: Vasculature is the same as BL 31 (Shangliao). The posterior ramus of the second sacral nerve.

Indications: (1) Spermatorrhea, impotence. (2) Irregular menstruation, bloody leukorrhea. (3) Lumbosacral pain, pain, weakness, and numbness of the lower extremities.

Needling Method: Perpendicular insertion 1.0—1.5 cun.

33. BL 33 (Zhongliao)

Location: In the region of the sacrum, medial and inferior to BL 32 (Ciliao), in the third posterior sacral foramen. (Fig. 2-67)

Regional Anatomy: Vasculature is the same as BL 31 (Shangliao). The posterior ramus of the third sacral nerve.

Indications: (1) Irregular menstruation, leukorrhea. (2) Dysuria, constipation, diarrhea. (3) Lumbosacral pain.

Needling Method: Perpendicular insertion 1.0—1.5 cun.

34. BL 34 (Xialiao)

Location: In the region of the sacrum, medial and inferior to BL 33 (Zhongliao), in the fourth posterior sacral foramen. (Fig. 2-67)

Regional Anatomy: The branches of the inferior gluteal artery and vein; the posterior ramus of the fourth sacral nerve.

Indications: (1) Lumbosacral pain, lower abdominal pain. (2) Dysuria, bloody leukorrhea.

Needling Method: Perpendicular insertion 1.0—1.5 cun.

35. BL 35 (Huiyang)

Location: In the region of the sacrum, 0.5 cun lateral to the tip of the coccyx. (Fig. 2-67)

Regional Anatomy: The branches of the inferior gluteal artery and vein; the distribution of the coccygeal nerve.

Indications: (1) Incontinence of feces, diarrhea, blood in the stools, hemorrhoids. (2) Impotence. (3) Bloody leukorrhea.

Needling Method: Perpendicular insertion 1.0—1.5 cun.

36. BL 36 (Chengfu)

Location: On the posterior aspect of the thigh, in the middle of the transverse gluteal fold. (Fig. 2-68)

Regional Anatomy: The artery and vein along the sciatic nerve; deeper, the sciatic nerve.

Indications: Pain in the lumbar, sacral, gluteal and femoral regions, hemorrhoids.

Needling Method: Perpendicular insertion 1.0—2.0 cun.

37. BL 37 (Yinmen)

Location: On the posterior aspect of the thigh, 6 cun below BL 36 (Chengfu), on the line connecting BL 36 (Chengfu) and BL 40 (Weizhong). (Fig. 2-68)

Regional Anatomy: Laterally, the third perforating branches of the deep femoral artery and vein; deeper, the sciatic nerve.

Indications: Lumbar pain, pain, numbness and weakness of the lower extremities.

Needling Method: Perpendicular insertion 1.0—2.0 cun.

38. BL 38 (Fuxi)

Location: At the lateral end of the popliteal transverse crease, 1 cun above BL 39 (Weiyang), on the medial side of the tendon of m. biceps femoris. (Fig. 2-68)

Regional Anatomy: The superolateral genicular artery and vein; the distribution of the common peroneal nerve.

Indications: Pain, numbness and spasm in the popliteal fossa.

Needling Method: Perpendicular insertion 1.0—1.5 cun.

39. BL 39 (Weiyang)

Classification: The Lower He-(Sea) Point of Triple Energizer.

Location: At the lateral end of the popliteal transverse crease, on the medial side of the tendon of m. biceps femoris. (Fig. 2-68)

Regional Anatomy: Vasculature and innervation are the same as BL 38 (Fuxi).

Indications: (1) Stiffness and pain of waist, lower abdominal distention, dysuria. (2) Spasm and pain of the leg and foot, faint and syncope.

Needling Method: Perpendicular insertion 1.0—1.5 cun.

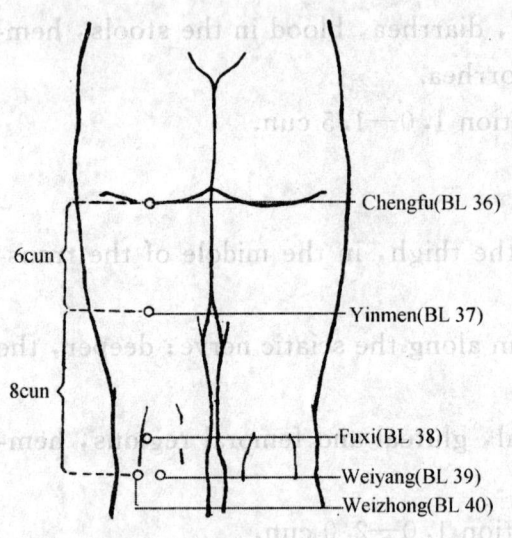

Fig. 2-68

40. BL 40 (Weizhong)

Classification: He-(Sea) Point.

Location: Midpoint of the transverse crease of the popliteal fossa, between the tendons of m. biceps femoris and m. semitendinous. (Fig. 2-68)

Regional Anatomy: The femoropopliteal vein; deeper, the popliteal artery. The tibial nerve.

Indications: (1) Lumbar pain, spasm of the popliteal tendons, hemiplegia, pain, numbness and weakness of the lower extremities. (2) Erysipelas, rash, general pruritus, furuncle, carbuncle on the back. (3) Abdominal pain, vomiting, diarrhea. (4) Enuresis, dysuria.

Needling Method: Perpendicular insertion 1.0—1.5 cun, or prick the popliteal vein with the three-edged needle to cause bleeding.

41. BL 41 (Fufen)

Classification: The Crossing Point of Bladder Meridian and Small Intestine Meridian.

Location: On the back, 3.0 cun lateral to the lower border of the spinous process of the second thoracic vertebra. (Fig. 2-69)

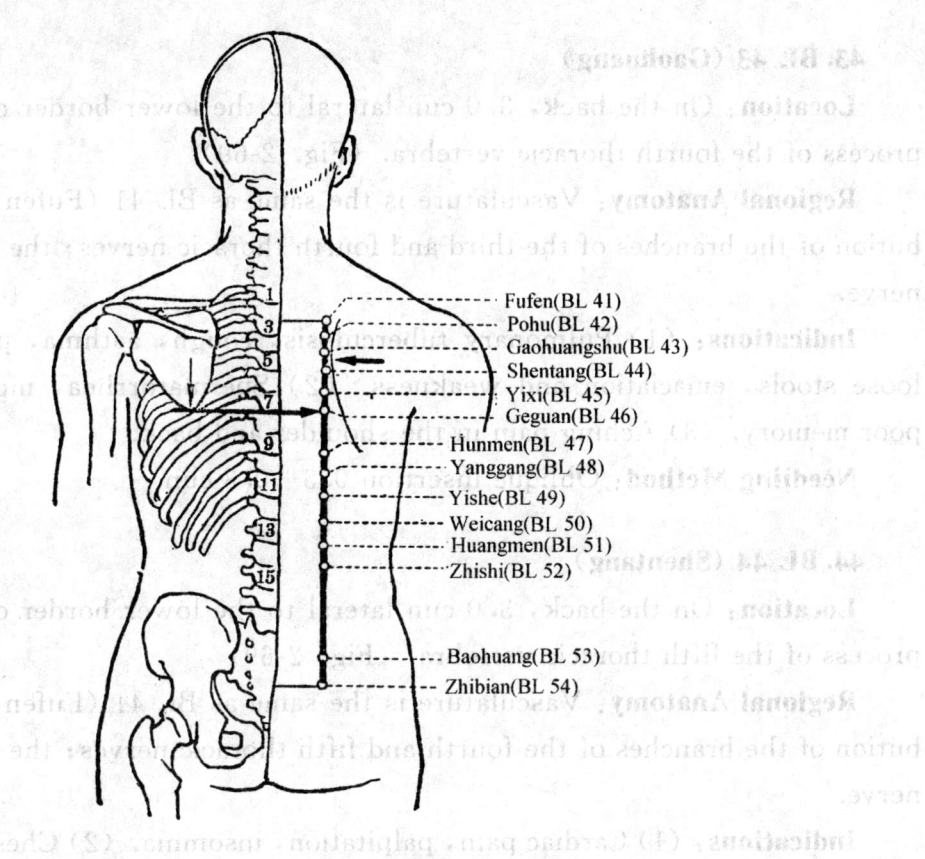

Fig. 2-69

Regional Anatomy: The branches of the intercostal artery and vein. The distribution of the branches of the first and second thoracic nerves; deeper, the dorsoscapular nerve.

Indications: Rigidity and pain of the neck, spasm of the shoulder and back, numbness of the elbow and arm.

Needling Method: Oblique insertion 0.5—0.8 cun.

42. BL 42 (Pohu)

Location: On the back, 3.0 cun lateral to the lower border of the spinous process of the third thoracic vertebra. (Fig. 2-69)

Regional Anatomy: Vasculature is the same as BL 41 (Fufen). The distribution of the branches of the second and third thoracic nerves; the dorsoscapular nerve.

Indications: (1) Cough, asthma, pulmonary tuberculosis. (2) Neck stiff-

131

ness, pain in the shoulder and back.

Needling Method: Oblique insertion 0.5—0.8 cun.

43. BL 43 (Gaohuang)

Location: On the back, 3.0 cun lateral to the lower border of the spinous process of the fourth thoracic vertebra. (Fig. 2-69)

Regional Anatomy: Vasculature is the same as BL 41 (Fufen). The distribution of the branches of the third and fourth thoracic nerves; the dorsoscapular nerve.

Indications: (1) Pulmonary tuberculosis, cough, asthma, poor appetite, loose stools, emaciation and weakness. (2) Spermatorrhea, night sweating, poor memory. (3) Aching pain in the shoulder and back.

Needling Method: Oblique insertion 0.5—0.8 cun.

44. BL 44 (Shentang)

Location: On the back, 3.0 cun lateral to the lower border of the spinous process of the fifth thoracic vertebra. (Fig. 2-69)

Regional Anatomy: Vasculature is the same as BL 41 (Fufen). The distribution of the branches of the fourth and fifth thoracic nerves; the dorsoscapular nerve.

Indications: (1) Cardiac pain, palpitation, insomnia. (2) Chest congestion, cough, asthma. (3) Pain of the shoulder and back.

Needling Method: Oblique insertion 0.5—0.8 cun.

45. BL 45 (Yixi)

Location: On the back, 3.0 cun lateral to the lower border of the spinous process of the sixth thoracic vertebra. (Fig. 2-69)

Regional Anatomy: The posterior branches of the intercostal artery and vein. The distribution of the branches of the fifth and sixth thoracic nerves.

Indications: (1) Cough, asthma. (2) Pain of the shoulder and back.

Needling Method: Oblique insertion 0.5—0.8 cun.

46. BL 46 (Geguan)

Location: On the back, 3.0 cun lateral to the lower border of the spinous process of the seventh thoracic vertebra. (Fig. 2-69)

Regional Anatomy: Vasculature is the same as BL 45 (Yixi). The distribution of the branches of the posterior rami of the sixth and seventh thoracic nerves.

Indications: (1) Dysphagia, hiccup, vomiting. (2) Stiffness and pain of the back.

Needling Method: Oblique insertion 0.5—0.8 cun.

47. BL 47 (Hunmen)

Location: On the back, 3.0 cun lateral to the lower border of the spinous process of the ninth thoracic vertebra. (Fig. 2-69)

Regional Anatomy: Vasculature is the same as BL 45 (Yixi). The distribution of the branches of the eighth and ninth thoracic nerves.

Indications: (1) Chest congestion and hypochondrium distention, vomiting, diarrhea. (2) Back pain.

Needling Method: Oblique insertion 0.5—0.8 cun.

48. BL 48 (Yanggang)

Location: On the back, 3.0 cun lateral to the lower border of the spinous process of the tenth thoracic vertebra. (Fig. 2-69)

Regional Anatomy: Vasculature is the same as BL 45 (Yixi). The distribution of the branches of the ninth and tenth thoracic nerves.

Indications: (1) Jaundice, abdominal pain, borborygmus, diarrhea. (2) Diabetes.

Needling Method: Oblique insertion 0.5—0.8 cun.

49. BL 49 (Yishe)

Location: On the back, 3.0 cun lateral to the lower border of the spinous process of the eleventh thoracic vertebra. (Fig. 2-69)

Regional Anatomy: Vasculature is the same as BL 45 (Yixi). The distribution of the branches of the tenth and eleventh thoracic nerves.

Indications: Abdominal distention, borborygmus, vomiting, diarrhea.

Needling Method: Oblique insertion 0.5—0.8 cun.

50. BL 50 (Weicang)

Location: On the back, 3.0 cun lateral to the lower border of the spinous process of the twelfth thoracic vertebra. (Fig. 2-69)

Regional Anatomy: The branches of the costal artery and vein. The distribution of the branch of the eleventh thoracic nerve.

Indications: (1) Epigastric pain, abdominal distention. (2) Infantile dyspepsia. (3) Edema.

Needling Method: Oblique insertion 0.5—0.8 cun.

51. BL 51 (Huangmen)

Location: On the lower back, 3.0 cun lateral to the lower border of the spinous process of the first lumbar vertebra. (Fig. 2-69)

Regional Anatomy: The posterior branches of the first lumbar artery and vein. The distribution of the branch of the twelfth thoracic nerve.

Indications: (1) Abdominal pain, constipation. (2) Abdominal mass, breast disease.

Needling Method: Oblique insertion 0.5—0.8 cun.

52. BL 52 (Zhishi)

Location: On the lower back, 3.0 cun lateral to the lower border of the spinous process of the second lumbar vertebra. (Fig. 2-69)

Regional Anatomy: The posterior branches of the second lumbar artery and vein. The distribution of the branches of the twelfth thoracic and first lumbar nerves.

Indications: (1) Spermatorrhea, impotence. (2) Dysuria, edema. (3) Lumbar stiffness and pain.

Needling Method: Oblique insertion 0.5—0.8 cun.

53. BL 53 (Baohuang)

Location: In the region of the sacrum, 3.0 cun lateral to the middle sacral crest, at the level of the second posterior sacral foramen. (Fig. 2-69)

Regional Anatomy: The superior gluteal artery and vein. The distribution of the superior gluteal nerve; deeper, the superior gluteal nerve.

Indications: (1) Anuria, swelling of vulva. (2) Lumbar pain. (3) Borborygmus, abdominal distention.

Needling Method: Perpendicular insertion 1.0—1.5 cun.

54. BL 54 (Zhibian)

Location: In the region of the sacrum, 3.0 cun lateral to the middle sacral crest, at the level of the fourth posterior sacral foramen. (Fig. 2-69)

Regional Anatomy: The inferior gluteal artery and vein. The distribution of the inferior gluteal nerve and the sciatic nerve.

Indications: (1) Lumbosacral pain, muscular atrophy, pain, numbness and motor impairment of the lower extremities. (2) Dysuria, constipation, hemorrhoids.

Needling Method: Perpendicular insertion 1.0—2.0 cun.

55. BL 55 (Heyang)

Location: On the posterior aspect of the lower leg, 2 cun below BL 40 (Weizhong), on the line connecting BL 40 (Weizhong) and BL 57 (Chengshan). (Fig. 2-70)

Regional Anatomy: The small saphenous vein; deeper, the popliteal artery and vein. Deeper, the tibial nerve.

Indications: (1) Lumbar stiffness and pain, pain, numbness and weakness of the lower extremities. (2) Hernia. (3) Metrorrhagia and metrostaxis and metrostaxis.

Needling Method: Perpendicular insertion 1.0—2.0 cun.

56. BL 56 (Chengjin)

Location: On the posterior aspect of the lower leg, 5 cun below BL 40 (Weizhong), on the line connecting BL 40 (Weizhong) and BL 57 (Chengshan), in the center of the belly of m. gastrocnemius. (Fig. 2-70)

Regional Anatomy: Vasculature and innervation are the same as BL 55 (Heyang).

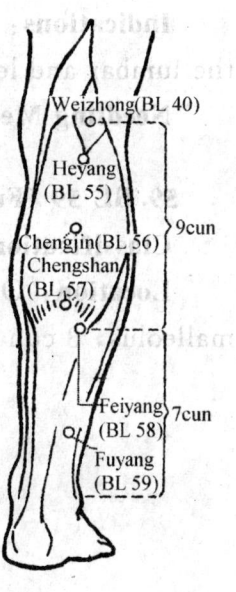

Fig. 2-70

Indications: (1) Hemorrhoids. (2) Spasm and pain of the lumbar and leg.

Needling Method: Perpendicular insertion 1.0—1.5 cun.

57. BL 57 (Chengshan)

Location: On the posterior midline of the lower leg between BL 40 (Weizhong) and BL 60 (Kunlun), when extending the toes straight or lifting the heel, the point is below the belly of m. gastrocnemius in the apex of the depression. (Fig. 2-70)

Regional Anatomy: Vasculature and innervation are the same as BL 55 (Heyang).

Indications: (1) Hemorrhoids, constipation. (2) Spasm and pain of the lumbar and leg. (3) Beriberi.

Needling Method: Perpendicular insertion 1.0—2.0 cun.

58. BL 58 (Feiyang)

Classification: Luo-(Connecting) Point.

Location: On the posterior aspect of the lower leg, behind the external malleolus, 7 cun directly above BL 60 (Kunlun), 1 cun inferior and lateral to BL 57 (Chengshan). (Fig. 2-70)

Regional Anatomy: The posterior tibial artery. The distribution of the lateral sural cutaneous nerve.

Indications: (1) Headache, dizziness, epistaxis. (2) Pain and weakness of the lumbar and leg. (3) Hemorrhoids.

Needling Method: Perpendicular insertion 0.7—1.0 cun.

59. BL 59 (Fuyang)

Classification: Xi-(Cleft) Point of the Yang Heel Vessel.

Location: On the posterior aspect of the lower leg, behind the external malleolus, 3 cun directly above BL 60 (Kunlun). (Fig. 2-70, 2-71)

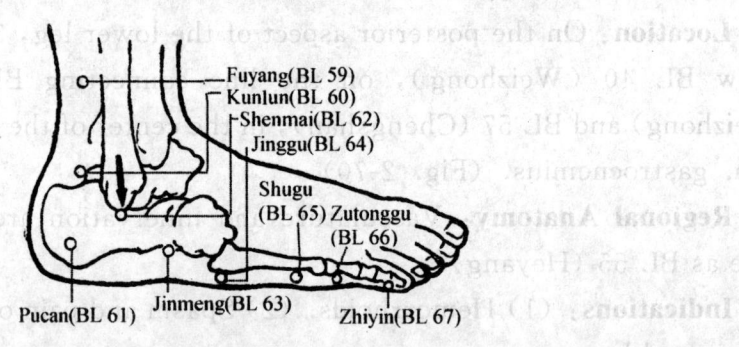

Fuyang(BL 59)
Kunlun(BL 60)
Shenmai(BL 62)
Jinggu(BL 64)
Shugu (BL 65)
Zutonggu (BL 66)
Pucan(BL 61) Jinmeng(BL 63) Zhiyin(BL 67)

Fig. 2-71

Regional Anatomy: The small saphenous vein; deeper, the terminal branch of the peroneal artery. The sural nerve.

Indications: (1) Headache, heavy sensation of the head. (2) Lumbosacral pain, pain, numbness and weakness of the lower extremities, swelling and pain of the external malleolus.

Needling Method: Perpendicular insertion 0.8—1.2 cun.

60. BL 60 (Kunlun)

Classification: Jing-(River) Point.

Location: On the foot, behind the external malleolus, in the depression between the tip of the external malleolus and tendo calcaneus. (Fig. 2-71)

Regional Anatomy: The small saphenous vein, the posteroexternal malleolar artery and vein. The distribution of the sural nerve.

Indications: (1) Acute lumbar pain, swelling and pain of the heel. (2) Difficult labor. (3) Headache, neck stiffness, dizziness, epistaxis. (4) Infantile convulsion.

Needling Method: Perpendicular insertion 0.5—1.0 cun.

61. BL 61 (Pucan)

Location: On the lateral aspect of the foot, posterior and inferior to the external malleolus, directly below BL 60 (Kunlun), lateral to the calcaneum at the junction of the red and white skin. (Fig. 2-71)

Regional Anatomy: The branches of the peroneal artery and vein. The distribution of the branch of the sural nerve.

Indications: (1) Pain, numbness and weakness of the lower extremities, pain in the heel. (2) Epilepsy.

Needling Method: Perpendicular insertion 0.3—0.5 cun.

62. BL 62 (Shenmai)

Classification: One of the Eight Confluent Points, this point linking with the Yang Heel Vessel.

Location: On the lateral aspect of the foot, in the depression directly below the external malleolus. (Fig. 2-71)

Regional Anatomy: The external malleolar arterial network. The distribution of the sural nerve.

Indications: (1) Epilepsy, manic psychosis. (2) Insomnia, extroversion of foot. (3) Headache, neck rigidity, pain of the lumbar and leg. (4) Blepharoptosis.

Needling Method: Perpendicular insertion 0.3—0.5 cun.

63. BL 63 (Jinmen)

Classification: Xi-(Cleft) Point.

Location: On the lateral aspect of the foot, directly below the anterior border of the external malleolus, lateral to the lower border of the cuboid bone. (Fig. 2-71)

Regional Anatomy: The lateral plantar artery and vein. The distribution of the lateral dorsal cutaneous nerve of the foot; deeper, the lateral plantar nerve.

Indications: (1) Manic psychosis, epilepsy, infantile convulsion. (2) Headache, lumbar pain, pain, numbness and weakness of the lower extremities, pain in the external malleolus.

Needling Method: Perpendicular insertion 0.3—0.5 cun.

64. BL 64 (Jinggu)

Classification: Yuan-(Source) Point.

Location: On the lateral aspect of the foot, below the tuberosity of the fifth metatarsal bone, at the junction of the red and white skin. (Fig. 2-71)

Regional Anatomy: Vasculature and innervation are the same as BL 63 (Jinmen).

Indications: (1) Headache, neck rigidity, nebula. (2) Pain of the lumbar and leg. (3) Epilepsy.

Needling Method: Perpendicular insertion 0.3—0.5 cun.

65. BL 65 (Shugu)

Classification: Shu-(Stream) Point.

Location: On the lateral aspect of the foot, posterior to the fifth metatarsophalangeal joint, at the junction of the red and white skin. (Fig. 2-71)

Regional Anatomy: The fourth common plantar digital artery and vein. The distribution of the fourth common plantar digital nerve and the lateral dorsal cutaneous nerve of the foot.

Indications: (1) Manic psychosis, headache, neck rigidity. (2) Pain of the lumbar and leg, anal pain.

Needling Method: Perpendicular insertion 0.3—0.5 cun.

66. BL 66 (Zutonggu)

Classification: Ying-(Spring) Point.

Location: On the lateral aspect of the foot, anterior to the fifth metatarsophalangeal joint, at the junction of the red and white skin. (Fig. 2-71)

Regional Anatomy: The plantar digital artery and vein. The distribution of the plantar digital proprial nerve, the lateral dorsal cutaneous nerve of the foot.

Indications: (1) Headache, neck rigidity, dizziness, epistaxis. (2) Manic psychosis.

Needling Method: Perpendicular insertion 0.2—0.3 cun.

67. BL 67 (Zhiyin)

Classification: Jing-(Well) Point.

Location: On the lateral side of the end of the small toe, 0.1 cun from the corner of the nail. (Fig. 2-71)

Regional Anatomy: The arterial network. Innervation is the same as BL 66 (Zutonggu).

Indications: (1) Malposition of fetus, difficult labor. (2) Headache, eye pain, nasal congestion, epistaxis.

Needling Method: Superficial insertion 0.1 cun. Use moxibustion for malposition of fetus.

Appendage: BL 67 (Zhiyin) is the Jing-(Well) Point which is the beginning point of the five transporting points. Because this point is the place where the Bladder Meridian and Kidney Meridian connect, it can regulate the Kidney and tonify Qi. *Simple Questions from Emperor's Canon of Medicine in the Chapter of Unusual Diseases* says: "The uterus is related with the kidney." If the Kidney Qi is not sufficient, it is difficult to maintain the fetus in the correct position. The deficiency of Kidney Qi also causes lack of strength, making the labor difficult. BL 67 (Zhiyin) regulates and tonifies Kidney Qi; thus, it can be used to treat the above-mentioned two syndromes.

Section 8 The Acupuncture Points of Kidney Meridian

This meridian appears at KI 1 (Yongquan) and ends at KI 27 (Shufu); bilaterally each consisting of 27 acupuncture points. (Fig. 2-72)

1. KI 1 (Yongquan)

Classification: Jing-(Well) Point.

Location: On the sole, in the depression when the foot is in plantar flexion, approximately at the anterior third and the posterior two thirds of the line from the web between the second and third toes to the back of the heel. (Fig. 2-73)

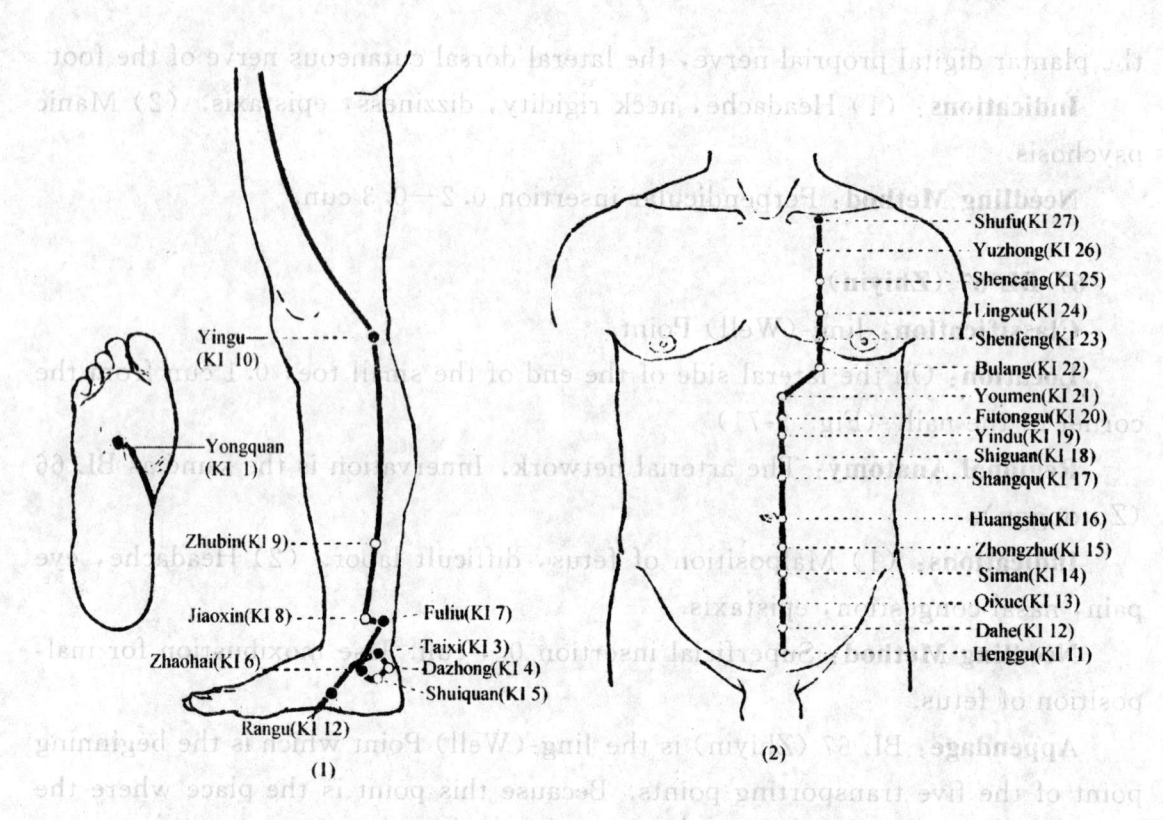

Fig. 2-72 The Points of the Kidney Meridian

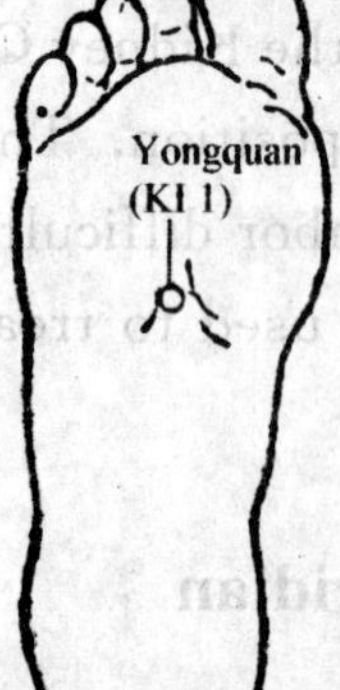

Fig. 2-73

Regional Anatomy: Deeper, the plantar arterial arch of the anterior tibial artery. The distribution of the second common plantar digital nerve.

Indications: (1) Loss of consciousness, headache, pain of the neck, dizziness, infantile convulsion, manic psychosis. (2) Nausea, vomiting. (3) Swelling of pharynx, dryness of the tongue, dysuria, constipation. (4) Hot sensation in the sole.

Needling Method: Perpendicular insertion 0.5—1.0 cun.

2. KI 2 (Rangu)

Classification: Ying-(Spring) Point.

Location: On the medial aspect of the foot, below the tuberosity of the navicular bone, at the junction of the red and white skin. (Fig. 2-74)

Regional Anatomy: The branches of the medial plantar and medial tarsal arteries. The distribution of the terminal branch medial crural cutaneous nerve, the medial plantar nerve.

Indications: (1) Prolapse of uterus, pruritus vulvae, irregular menstruation, bloody leukorrhea. (2) Acute infantile omphalitis, trismus. (3) Spermatorrhea, diabetes, swelling and pain of the dorsum of foot.

Needling Method: Perpendicular insertion 0.5—1.0 cun.

3. KI 3 (Taixi)

Classification: Yuan-(Source) Point and Shu-(Stream) Point.

Location: On the medial aspect of the foot, posterior to the medial malleolus, in the depression between the tip of the medial malleolus and tendo calcaneus. (Fig. 2-74)

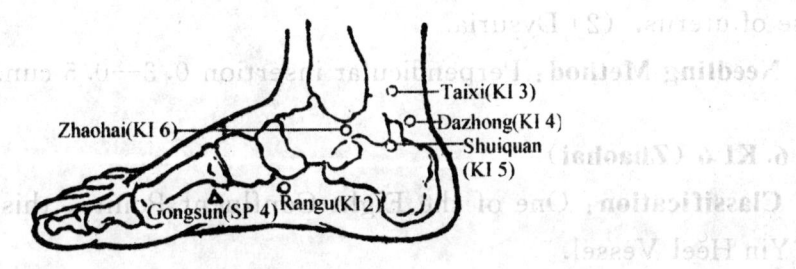

Fig. 2-74

Regional Anatomy: The posterior tibial artery and vein. The distribution of the branch of the tibial nerve.

Indications: (1) Impotence, spermatorrhea, frequent micturition, deafness, tinnitus, irregular menstruation, lumbar pain. (2) Headache, dizziness, blurring of vision, toothache, swelling of pharynx. (3) Cough, asthma, diabetes. (4) Insomnia.

Needling Method: Perpendicular insertion 0.5—1.0 cun.

4. KI 4 (Dazhong)

Classification: Luo-(Connecting) Point.

Location: On the medial aspect of the foot, posterior and inferior to the medial malleolus, in the depression anterior to the medial side of the attachment of tendo calcaneus. (Fig. 2-74)

Regional Anatomy: The medial calcaneal branch of the posterior tibial artery. The distribution of the medial crural cutaneous nerve and the medial calcaneal branch of the tibial nerve.

Indications: (1) Retention of urine, enuresis, constipation. (2) Hemoptysis, asthma. (3) Dementia, pain in the heel.

Needling Method: Perpendicular insertion 0.3—0.5 cun.

5. KI 5 (Shuiquan)

Classification: Xi-(Cleft) Point.

Location: On the medial aspect of the foot, posterior and inferior to the medial malleolus, 1 cun directly below KI 3 (Taixi), in the depression of the medial side of the tuberosity of the calcaneum. (Fig. 2-74)

Regional Anatomy: Vasculature and innervation are the same as KI 4 (Dazhong).

Indications: (1) Irregular menstruation, dysmenorrhea, amenorrhea, prolapse of uterus. (2) Dysuria.

Needling Method: Perpendicular insertion 0.3—0.5 cun.

6. KI 6 (Zhaohai)

Classification: One of the Eight Confluent Points, this point linking with the Yin Heel Vessel.

Location: On the medial aspect of the foot, in the depression below the tip of the medial malleolus. (Fig. 2-74)

Regional Anatomy: The posterior tibial artery and vein. The distribution of the medial crural cutaneous nerve; deeper, the tibial nerve.

Indications: (1) Dryness and soreness of throat, constipation, retention of urine. (2) Irregular menstruation, bloody leukorrhea, prolapse of uterus, pruritus vulvae. (3) Epilepsy.

Needling Method: Perpendicular insertion 0.3—0.5 cun.

7. KI 7 (Fuliu)

Classification: Jing-(River) Point.

Location: On the medial aspect of the lower leg, 2 cun directly above KI 3 (Taixi), anterior to tendo calcaneus. (Fig. 2-75)

Regional Anatomy: Deeper, anteriorly, the posterior tibial artery and vein. Deeper, the tibial nerve.

Indications: (1) Edema, abdominal distention, diarrhea. (2) Febrile disease without sweat or ceaselessly sweating, night sweating. (3) Weakness, numbness and pain of lower extremities.

Needling Method: Perpendicular insertion 0.6—1.0 cun.

8. KI 8 (Jiaoxin)

Classification: Xi-(Cleft) Point of the Yinqiao Meridian.

Location: On the medial aspect of the lower leg, 2 cun directly above KI 3 (Taixi), 0.5 cun anterior to KI 7 (Fuliu), posterior to the medial border of the tibia. (Fig. 2-75)

Regional Anatomy: Deeper, the posterior tibial artery and vein. Deeper, the tibial nerve.

Indications: (1) Irregular menstruation, metrorrhagia and metrostaxis, prolapse of uterus. (2) Hernia. (3) Diarrhea, constipation.

Needling Method: Perpendicular insertion 0.6—1.2 cun.

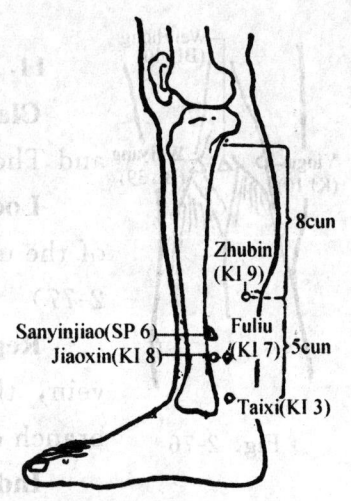

Fig. 2-75

9. KI 9 (Zhubin)

Classification: The Xi-(Cleft) Point of Yin Link Vessel.

Location: On the medial aspect of the lower leg, 5 cun above KI 3 (Taixi), on the line connecting KI 3 (Taixi) and KI 10 (Yingu), at the medial and inferior end of the belly of m. gastrocnemius. (Fig. 2-75)

Regional Anatomy: Deeper, the posterior tibial artery and vein. Deeper, the tibial nerve.

Indications: (1) Manic psychosis. (2) Hernia. (3) Pain of the lower leg.

Needling Method: Perpendicular insertion 1.0—1.5 cun.

10. KI 10 (Yingu)

Classification: He-(Sea) Point.

Location: When the knee is flexed, the point is on the medial side of the popliteal fossa, between the tendons of m. semitendinosus and semimembranosus. (Fig. 2-76)

Regional Anatomy: The medial superior genicular artery and vein. The distribution of the medial femoral cutaneous nerve.

Indications: (1) Impotence, hernia, metrorrhagia and metrostaxis. (2) Dysuria. (3) Pain in the knee and popliteal fossa.

Needling Method: Perpendicular insertion 1.0—1.5 cun.

Fig. 2-76

11. KI 11 (Henggu)

Classification: The Crossing Point of Kidney Meridian and Thoroughfare Vessel.

Location: On the lower abdomen, 5 cun below the center of the umbilicus, 0.5 cun lateral to the anterior midline. (Fig. 2-77)

Regional Anatomy: The inferior epigastric artery and vein, the external pudendal artery. The distribution of the branch of the iliohypogastric nerve.

Indications: (1) Lower abdominal distention and pain, dysuria, enuresis. (2) Spermatorrhea, impotence. (3) Hernia, pain of genitalia.

Needling Method: Perpendicular insertion 1.0—1.5 cun.

12. KI 12 (Dahe)

Classification: The Crossing Point of Kidney Meridian and Thoroughfare Vessel.

Location: On the lower abdomen, 4 cun below the center of the umbilicus, 0.5 cun lateral to the anterior midline. (Fig. 2-77)

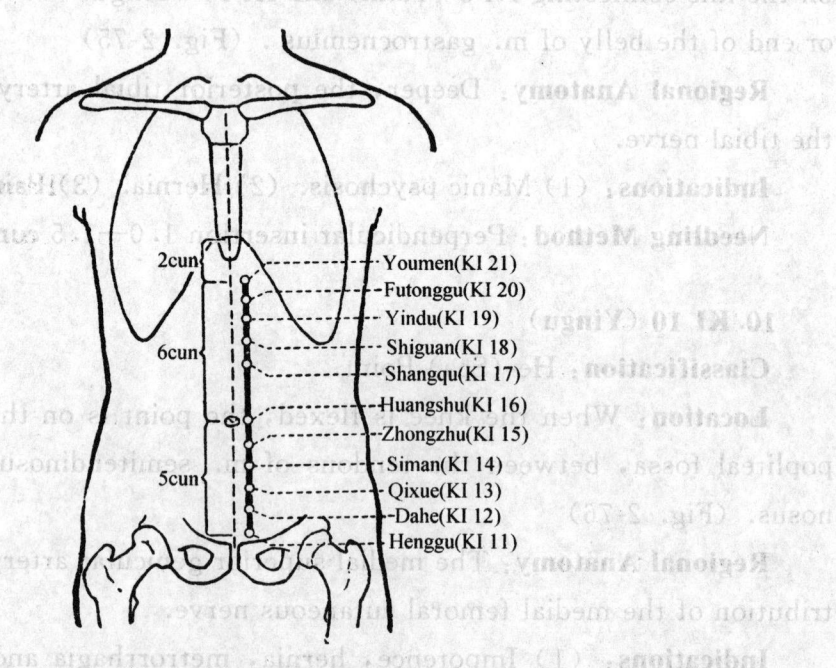

Fig. 2-77

Regional Anatomy: The muscular branches of the inferior epigastric artery and vein. The distribution of the branch of the iliohypogastric nerve.

Indications: (1) Spermatorrhea, impotence. (2) Prolapse of uterus, morbid leukorrhea.

Needling Method: Perpendicular insertion 1.0—1.5 cun.

13. KI 13 (Qixue)

Classification: The Crossing Point of Kidney Meridian and Thoroughfare Vessel.

Location: On the lower abdomen, 3 cun below the center of the umbilicus, 0.5 cun lateral to the anterior midline. (Fig. 2-77)

Regional Anatomy: Vasculature is the same as KI 12 (Dahe). The twelfth intercostal nerve.

Indications: (1) Irregular menstruation, morbid leukorrhea. (2) Dysuria. (3) Diarrhea.

Needling Method: Perpendicular insertion 1.0—1.5 cun.

14. KI 14 (Siman)

Classification: The Crossing Point of Kidney Meridian and Thoroughfare Vessel.

Location: On the lower abdomen, 2 cun below the center of the umbilicus, 0.5 cun lateral to the anterior midline. (Fig. 2-77)

Regional Anatomy: Vasculature is the same as KI 12 (Dahe). The eleventh intercostal nerve.

Indications: (1) Abdominal pain and distention, diarrhea, edema. (2) Irregular menstruation, dysmenorrhea.

Needling Method: Perpendicular insertion 1.0—1.5 cun.

15. KI. 15 (Zhongzhu)

Classification: The Crossing Point of Kidney Meridian and Thoroughfare Vessel.

Location: On the middle of the abdomen, 1 cun below the center of the umbilicus, 0.5 cun lateral to the anterior midline. (Fig. 2-77)

Regional Anatomy: Vasculature is the same as KI 12 (Dahe). The tenth intercostal nerve.

Indications: (1) Irregular menstruation, dysmenorrhea. (2) Abdominal pain, constipation, diarrhea.

Needling Method: Perpendicular insertion 1.0—1.5 cun.

16. KI 16 (Huangshu)

Classification: The Crossing Point of Kidney Meridian and Thoroughfare Vessel.

Location: On the middle of the abdomen, 0.5 cun lateral to the center of the umbilicus. (Fig. 2-77)

Regional Anatomy: Vasculature and innervation are the same as KI 15 (Zhongzhu).

Indications: Abdominal pain and distention, vomiting, constipation, diarrhea.

Needling Method: Perpendicular insertion 1.0—1.5 cun.

17. KI 17 (Shangqu)

Classification: The Crossing Point of Kidney Meridian and Thoroughfare Vessel.

Location: On the upper abdomen, 2 cun above the center of the umbilicus, 0.5 cun lateral to the anterior midline. (Fig. 2-77)

Regional Anatomy: The superior and inferior epigastric arteries and veins. The ninth intercostal nerve.

Indications: Abdominal pain, diarrhea, constipation.

Needling Method: Perpendicular insertion 1.0—1.5 cun.

18. KI 18 (Shiguan)

Classification: The Crossing Point of Kidney Meridian and Thoroughfare Vessel.

Location: On the upper abdomen, 3 cun above the center of the umbilicus, 0.5 cun lateral to the anterior midline. (Fig. 2-77)

Regional Anatomy: Vasculature is the same as KI 17 (Shangqu). The eighth intercostal nerve.

Indications: (1) Vomiting, abdominal pain, constipation. (2) Infertility.

Needling Method: Perpendicular insertion 1.0—1.5 cun.

19. KI 19 (Yindu)

Classification: The Crossing Point of Kidney Meridian and Thoroughfare Vessel.

Location: On the upper abdomen, 4 cun above the center of the umbilicus, 0.5 cun lateral to the anterior midline. (Fig. 2-77)

Regional Anatomy: Vasculature and innervation are the same as KI 18 (Shiguan).

Indications: (1) Abdominal pain and distention, constipation. (2) Infertility.

Needling Method: Perpendicular insertion 1.0—1.5 cun.

20. KI 20 (Futonggu)

Classification: The Crossing Point of Kidney Meridian and Thoroughfare Vessel.

Location: On the upper abdomen, 5 cun above the center of the umbilicus, 0.5 cun lateral to the anterior midline. (Fig. 2-77)

Regional Anatomy: Vasculature and innervation are the same as KI 18 (Shiguan).

Indications: Abdominal distention and pain, vomiting.

Needling Method: Perpendicular insertion 0.5—1.0 cun.

21. KI 21 (Youmen)

Classification: The Crossing Point of Kidney Meridian and Thoroughfare Vessel.

Location: On the upper abdomen, 6 cun above the center of the umbilicus, 0.5 cun lateral to the anterior midline. (Fig. 2-77)

Regional Anatomy: Vasculature is the same as KI 18 (Shiguan). The seventh intercostal nerve.

Indications: Abdominal pain and distention, vomiting, diarrhea.

Needling Method: Perpendicular insertion 0.5—1.0 cun, do not puncture deeply to avoid injuring the liver.

22. KI 22 (Bulang)

Location: On the chest, in the fifth intercostal space, 2.0 cun lateral to the anterior midline. (Fig. 2-78)

Regional Anatomy: The fifth intercostal artery and vein. Deeper, the fifth intercostal nerve.

Indications: (1) Cough, asthma, distention and fullness of the chest and hypochondrium. (2) Vomiting.

Fig. 2-78

Needling Method: Oblique or subcutaneous insertion 0.5—0.8 cun. These points on the chest should not be inserted deeply to avoid injuring the heart and lungs.

23. KI 23 (Shenfeng)

Location: On the chest, in the fourth intercostal space, 2.0 cun lateral to the anterior midline. (Fig. 2-78)

Regional Anatomy: The fourth intercostal artery and vein. Deeper, the fourth intercostal nerve.

Indications: (1) Cough, asthma, distention and fullness of the chest and hypochondrium. (2) Nodules in the breast.

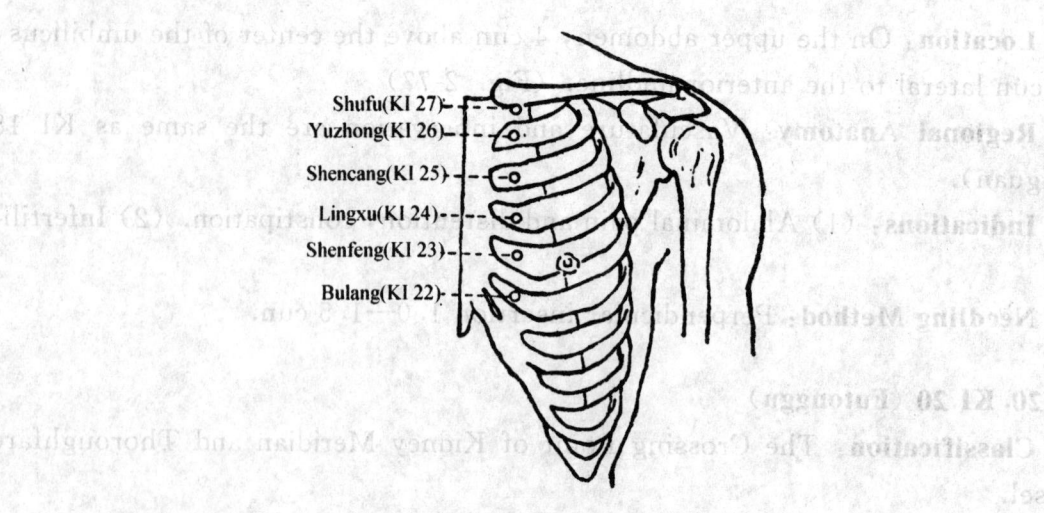

Needling Method: Oblique or Subcutaneous insertion 0.5—0.8 cun.

24. KI 24 (Lingxu)

Location: On the chest, in the third intercostal space, 2.0 cun lateral to the anterior midline. (Fig. 2-78)

Regional Anatomy: The third intercostal artery and vein. Deeper, the third intercostal nerve.

Indications: (1) Cough, asthma, distention of the chest and hypochondrium. (2) Nodules in the breast.

Needling Method: Oblique or subcutaneous insertion 0.5—0.8 cun.

25. KI 25 (Shencang)

Location: On the chest, in the second intercostal space, 2.0 cun lateral to the anterior midline. (Fig. 2-78)

Regional Anatomy: The second intercostal artery and vein. Deeper, the second intercostal nerve.

Indications: (1) Cough, asthma, chest pain. (2) Vomiting.

Needling Method: Oblique or subcutaneous insertion 0.5—0.8 cun.

26. KI 26 (Yuzhong)

Location: On the chest, in the first intercostal space, 2.0 cun lateral to the anterior midline. (Fig. 2-78)

Regional Anatomy: The first intercostal artery and vein. The anterior branch of the supraclavicular nerve; deeper, the first intercostal nerve.

Indications: Cough, asthma, distention of the chest and hypochondrium.

Needling Method: Oblique or subcutaneous insertion 0.5—0.8 cun.

27. KI 27 (Shufu)

Location: On the chest, on the lower border of the clavicle, 2.0 cun lateral to the anterior midline. (Fig. 2-78)

Regional Anatomy: The branches of the internal mammary artery and vein. The anterior branch of the supraclavicular nerve.

Indications: (1) Cough, asthma, chest pain. (2) Vomiting.

Needling Method: Oblique or subcutaneous insertion 0.5—0.8 cun.

Section 9 The Acupuncture Points of Pericardium Meridian

This meridian appears at PC 1 (Tianchi) and ends at PC 9 (Zhongchong); bilaterally each consisting of 9 acupuncture points. (Fig. 2-79)

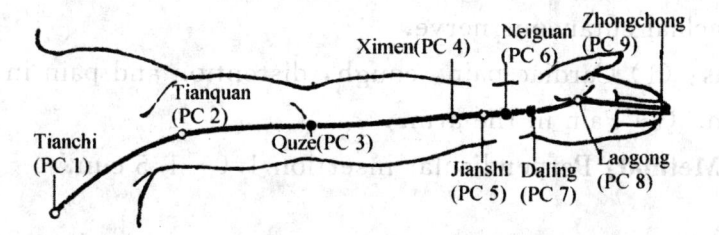

Fig. 2-79 The Points of the Pericardium Meridian

1. PC 1 (Tianchi)

Classification: The Crossing Point of Pericardium Meridian and Gallbladder Meridian.

Location: On the chest, in the fourth intercostal space, 1.0 cun lateral to the nipple, 5.0 cun lateral to the anterior midline. (Fig. 2-80)

Regional Anatomy: The branches of the lateral thoracic artery and vein. The fourth intercostal nerve.

Indications: (1) Mastitis, pain in the hypochondrium, scrofula. (2) Cough, asthma, chest congestion.

Needling Method: Oblique or Subcutaneous insertion 0.3—0.5 cun, do not puncture deeply to avoid injuring the lung.

2. PC 2 (Tianquan)

Location: On the medial aspect of the arm, 2 cun below the anterior axillary fossa, between the heads of m. biceps brachii longus and brevis. (Fig. 2-81)

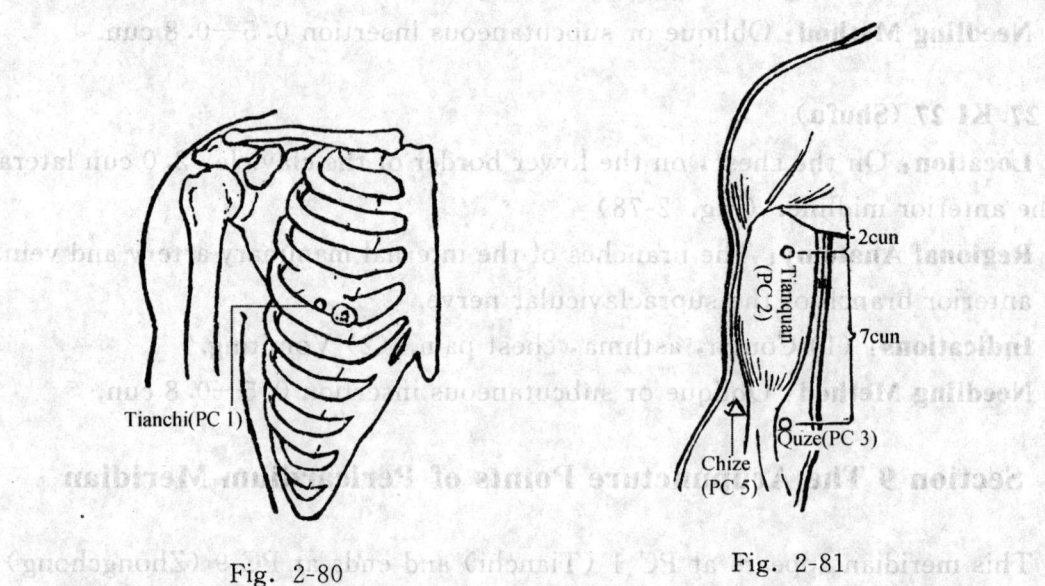

Fig. 2-80

Fig. 2-81

Regional Anatomy: The muscular branches of the brachial artery and vein. The medial brachial cutaneous nerve.

Indications: (1) Cardiac pain, cough, distention and pain in the chest and hypochondrium. (2) Pain in the arm.

Needling Method: Perpendicular insertion 1.0—1.5 cun.

3. PC 3 (Quze)

Classification: He-(Sea) Point.

Location: On the transverse crease of elbow, on the ulnar side of the tendon of m. biceps brachii. (Fig. 2-81)

Regional Anatomy: The brachial artery and vein. The median nerve.

Indications: (1) Cardiac pain, palpitation. (2) Gastric pain, vomiting, diarrhea. (3) Spasm and pain in the elbow and arm.

Needling Method: Perpendicular insertion 1.0—1.5 cun, or prick to cause bleeding.

4. PC 4 (Ximen)

Classification: Xi-(Cleft) Point.

Location: On the palmar aspect of the forearm, 5.0 cun above the transverse crease of the wrist, on the line connecting PC 3 (Quze) and PC 7 (Daling). (Fig. 2-82)

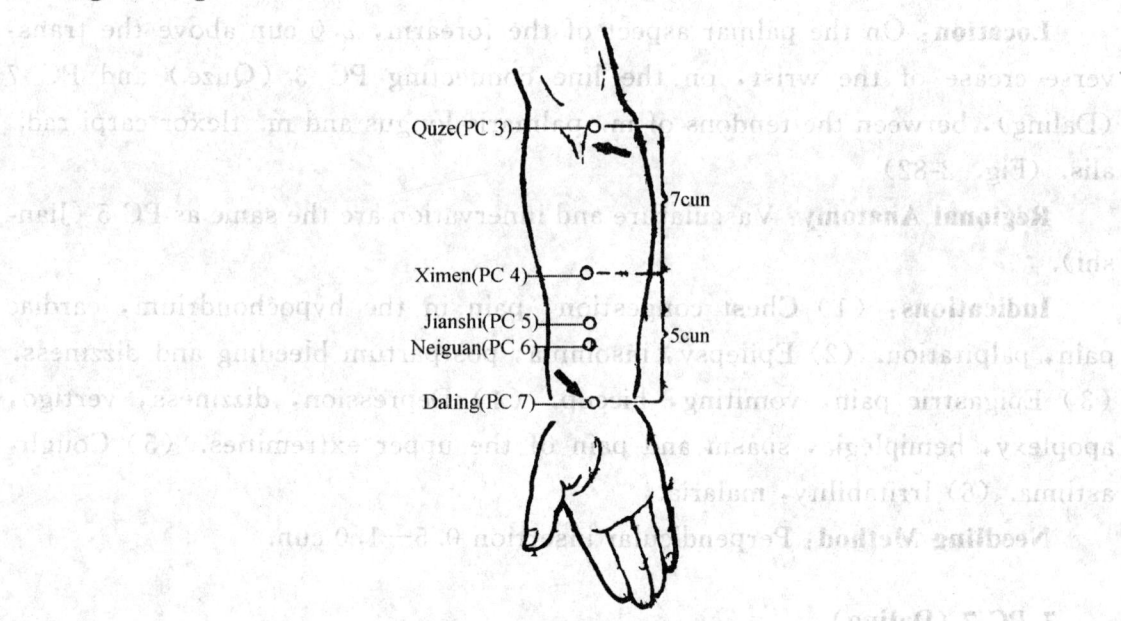

Fig. 2-82

Regional Anatomy: The median antebrachial artery and vein. Deeper, the median nerve.

Indications: (1) Cardiac pain, palpitation. (2) Hematemesis, hemoptysis. (3) Furuncle. (4) Epilepsy.

Needling Method: Perpendicular insertion 0.5—1.0 cun.

5. PC 5 (Jianshi)

Classification: Jing-(River) Point.

Location: On the palmar aspect of the forearm, 3.0 cun above the transverse crease of the wrist, on the line connecting PC 3 (Quze) and PC 7 (Daling), between the tendons of m. palmaris longus and m. flexor carpi radialis. (Fig. 2-82)

Regional Anatomy: Vasculature is the same as PC 4 (Ximen). The branches of the median nerve.

Indications: (1) Cardiac pain, palpitation. (2) Gastric pain, vomiting. (3) Febrile disease, malaria. (4) Manic psychosis, epilepsy.

Needling Method: Perpendicular insertion 0.5—1.0 cun.

6. PC 6 (Neiguan)

Classification: Luo-(Connecting) Point. One of the Eight Confluent Points, this point linking with the Yin Link Vessel.

Location: On the palmar aspect of the forearm, 2.0 cun above the transverse crease of the wrist, on the line connecting PC 3 (Quze) and PC 7 (Daling), between the tendons of m. palmaris longus and m. flexor carpi radialis. (Fig. 2-82)

Regional Anatomy: Vasculature and innervation are the same as PC 5 (Jianshi).

Indications: (1) Chest congestion, pain in the hypochondrium, cardiac pain, palpitation. (2) Epilepsy, insomnia, postpartum bleeding and dizziness. (3) Epigastric pain, vomiting, hiccup. (4) Depression, dizziness, vertigo, apoplexy, hemiplegia, spasm and pain of the upper extremities. (5) Cough, asthma. (6) Irritability, malaria.

Needling Method: Perpendicular insertion 0.5—1.0 cun.

7. PC 7 (Daling)

Classification: Yuan-(Source) Point and Shu-(Stream) Point.

Location: In the middle of the transverse crease of the wrist, between the tendons of m. palmaris longus and m. flexor carpi radialis. (Fig. 2-82)

Regional Anatomy: The palmar arterial and venous network of the wrist. Deeper, the median nerve.

Indications: (1) Cardiac pain, palpitation, pain in the chest and hypochondrium. (2) Gastric pain, vomiting. (3) Manic psychosis. (4) Pain of the heel.

Needling Method: Perpendicular insertion 0.5—0.8 cun.

8. PC 8 (Laogong)

Classification: Ying-(Spring) Point.

Location: In the center of the palm, between the second and third metacarpal bones, closer to the third metacarpal bone. When a fist is made, the point is where the tip of the middle finger touches. (Fig. 2-83)

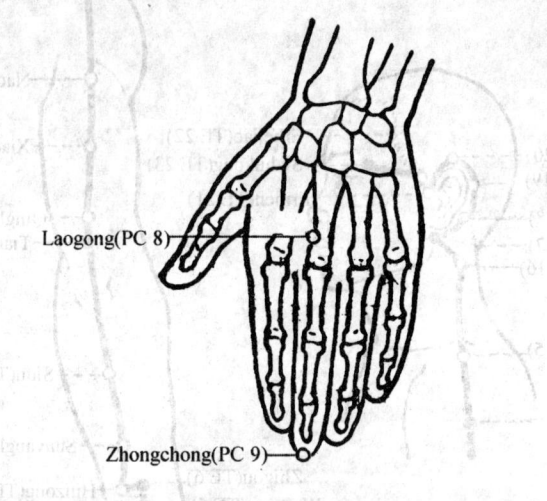

Fig. 2-83

Regional Anatomy: The common palmar digital artery. The second common palmar digital nerve of the median nerve.

Indications: (1) Aphtha, halitosis. (2) Coma, fungal infection of the hand. (3) Cardiac pain, vomiting.

Needling Method: Perpendicular insertion 0.3—0.5 cun.

9. PC 9 (Zhongchong)

Classification: Jing-(Well) Point.

Location: In the center of the tip of the distal phalanx of the middle finger. (Fig. 2-83)

Regional Anatomy: The arterial and venous network formed by the palmar digital proprial artery and vein. The palmar digital proprial nerve of the median nerve.

Indications: (1) Coma, heat stroke. (2) Cardiac pain, irritability, stiffness, swelling and pain of the tongue.

Needling Method: Superficial insertion 0.1 cun, or prick to cause bleeding.

Section 10 The Acupuncture Points of Triple Energizer Meridian

This meridian appears at TE 1 (Guanchong) and ends at TE 23 (Sizhukong); bilaterally each consisting of 23 acupuncture points. (Fig. 2-84)

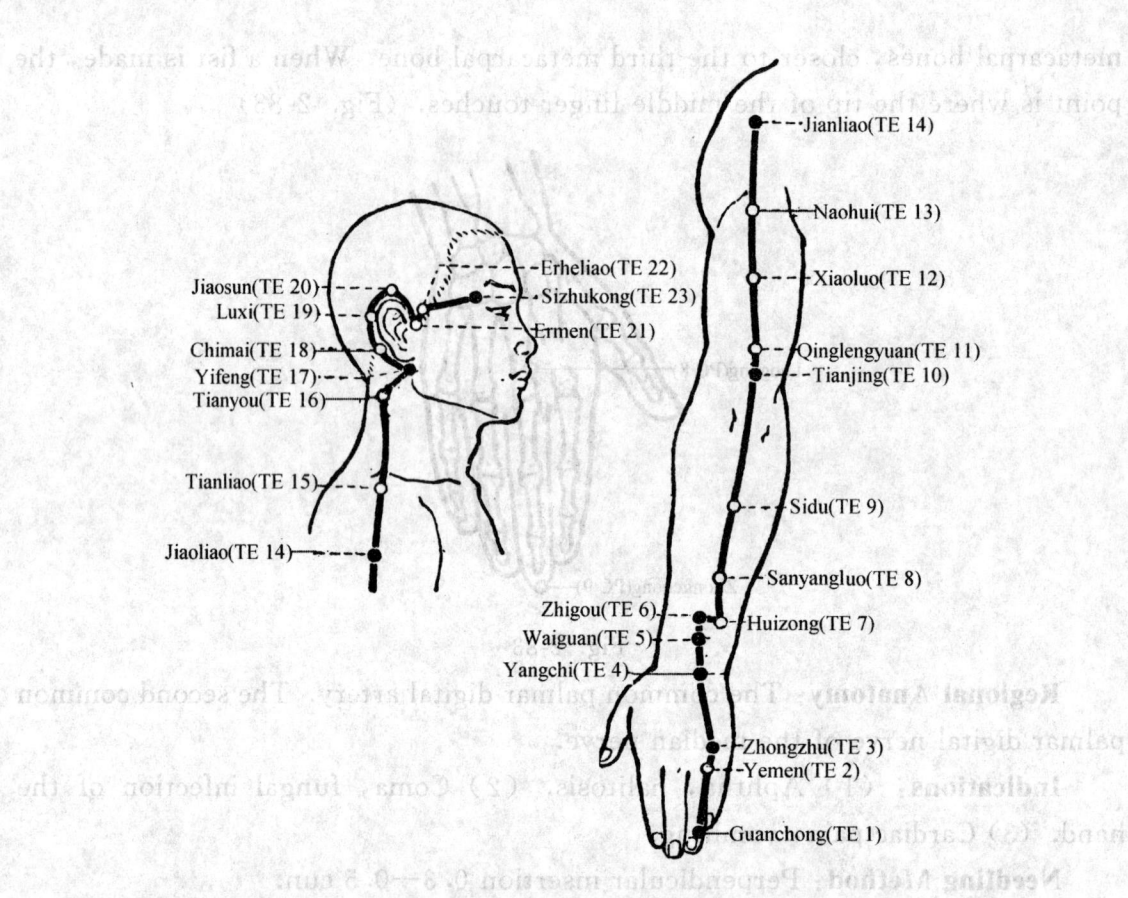

Fig. 2-84 The Points of the Triple Energizer Meridian

1. TE 1 (Guanchong)

Classification: Jing-(Well) Point.

Location: On the ulnar side of the distal phalanx of the ring finger, 0.1 cun distance from the nail. (Fig. 2-85)

Regional Anatomy: The palmar digital arterial and venous network. The branch of the ulnar nerve.

Indications: (1) Febrile disease, loss of consciousness. (2) Sore throat. (3) Headache, redness of the eye, deafness.

Needling Method: Superficial insertion 0.1 cun, or prick to cause bleeding.

2. TE 2 (Yemen)

Classification: Ying-(Spring) Point.

Location: On the dorsum of the hand, proximal to the margin of the web between the fourth and fifth fingers, at the junction of the red and white skin. (Fig. 2-85)

Regional Anatomy: The dorsal digital artery. The dorsal branch of the ulnar nerve.

Indications: (1) Malaria. (2) Sore throat. (3) Headache, redness of the eye, deafness.

Needling Method: Perpendicular insertion 0.3—0.5 cun.

3. TE 3 (Zhongzhu)

Classification: Shu-(Stream) Point.

Location: On the dorsum of the hand, in the depression between the fourth and fifth metacarpal bones, proximal to the fourth metacarpophalangeal joint. (Fig. 2-85)

Regional Anatomy: The dorsal venous network of hand and the fourth dorsal metacarpal artery. The dorsal branch of the ulnar nerve.

Indications: (1) Headache, redness of the eye. (2) Tinnitus, deafness. (3) Sore throat. (4) Pain in the scapular region, pain of the leg, fingers unable to extend.

Needling Method: Perpendicular insertion 0.3—0.5 cun.

4. TE 4 (Yangchi)

Classification: Yuan-(Source) Point.

Location: On the transverse crease of the dorsum of the wrist, in the depression on the ulnar side of the tendon of m. extensor digitorum communis. (Fig. 2-85)

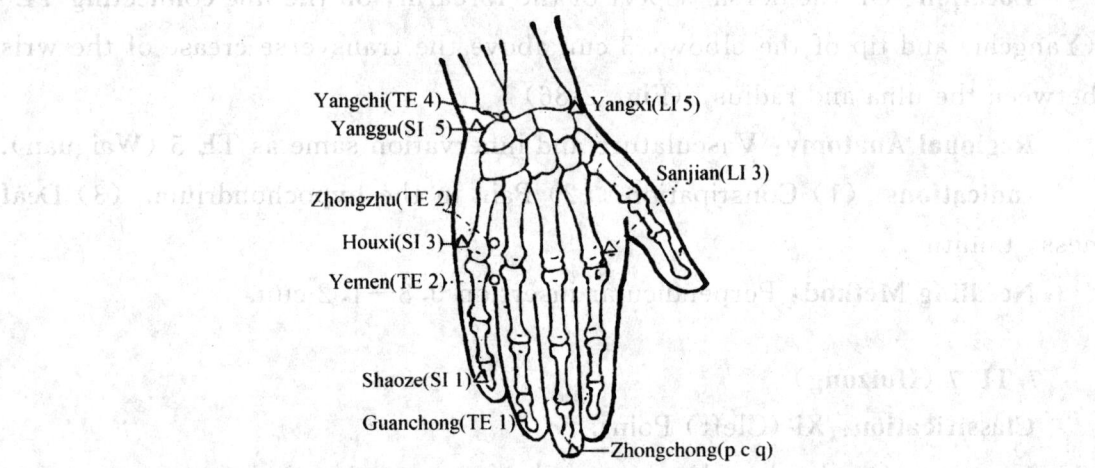

Fig. 2-85

Regional Anatomy: The dorsal venous network of the wrist and the carpal artery. The dorsal branch of the ulnar nerve.

Indications: (1) Diabetes. (2) Malaria. (3) Pain in the wrist. (4) Deafness.

Needling Method: Perpendicular insertion 0.3—0.5 cun.

5. **TE 5 (Waiguan)**

Classification: Luo-(Connecting) Point. One of the Eight Confluent Points. This point linking with the Yang Link Vessel.

Location: On the dorsal aspect of the forearm, on the line connecting TE 4 (Yangchi) and tip of the elbow, 2 cun above the transverse crease of the wrist between the ulna and radius. (Fig. 2-86)

Regional Anatomy: Deeper, the posterior and anterior antebrachial interosseous arteries and veins. The branches of the radial and median nerves.

Indications: (1) Febrile disease, headache, redness, swelling and pain of the eye. (2) Tinnitus, deafness. (3) Pain in the hypochondrium, spasm and pain of the upper extremities.

Needling Method: Perpendicular insertion 0.5—1.0 cun.

6. **TE 6 (Zhigou)**

Classification: Jing-(River) Point.

Location: On the dorsal aspect of the forearm, on the line connecting TE 4 (Yangchi) and tip of the elbow, 3 cun above the transverse crease of the wrist between the ulna and radius. (Fig. 2-86)

Regional Anatomy: Vasculature and innervation same as TE 5 (Waiguan).

Indications: (1) Constipation. (2) Pain in the hypochondrium. (3) Deafness, tinnitus.

Needling Method: Perpendicular insertion 0.8—1.2 cun.

7. **TE 7 (Huizong)**

Classification: Xi-(Cleft) Point.

Location: On the dorsal aspect of the forearm, 3 cun above the transverse crease of the wrist, on the ulnar side of TE 6 (Zhigou) and on the radial side of the ulna. (Fig. 2-86)

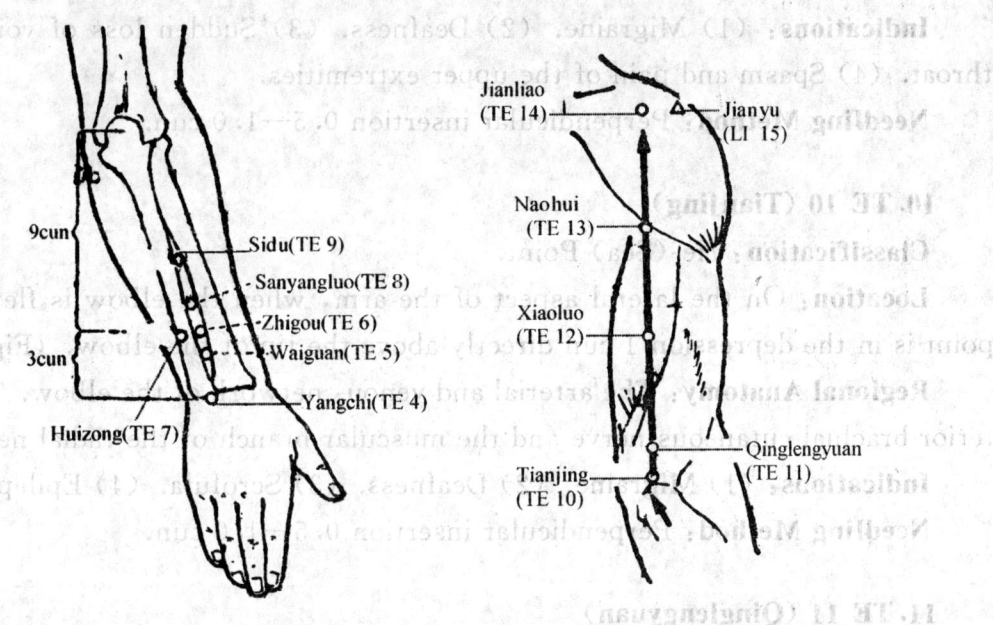

Fig. 2-86　　　　　　　Fig. 2-87

Regional Anatomy: The posterior antebrachial interosseous artery and vein. The posterior antebrachial cutaneous nerve.

Indications: (1) Deafness. (2) Epilepsy. (3) Spasm and pain of the upper extremities

Needling Method: Perpendicular insertion 0.5—1.0 cun.

8. TE 8 (Sanyangluo)

Location: On the dorsal aspect of the forearm, 4 cun above the transverse crease of the wrist between the ulna and radius. (Fig. 2-86)

Regional Anatomy: Vasculature and innervation are the same as TE 7 (Huizong).

Indications: (1) Deafness, sudden loss of voice. (2) Toothache. (3) Spasm and pain of the upper extremities.

Needling Method: Perpendicular insertion 0.8—1.2 cun.

9. TE 9 (Sidu)

Location: On the dorsal aspect of the forearm, on the line connecting TE 4 (Yangchi) and tip of the elbow, 5 cun below the tip of the elbow between the ulna and radius. (Fig. 2-86)

Regional Anatomy: Vasculature and innervation are the same as TE 7 (Huizong).

Indications: (1) Migraine. (2) Deafness. (3) Sudden loss of voice, sore throat. (4) Spasm and pain of the upper extremities.

Needling Method: Perpendicular insertion 0.5—1.0 cun.

10. TE 10 (Tianjing)

Classification: He-(Sea) Point.

Location: On the lateral aspect of the arm, when the elbow is flexed, the point is in the depression 1 cun directly above the tip of the elbow. (Fig. 2-87)

Regional Anatomy: The arterial and venous network of the elbow. The posterior brachial cutaneous nerve and the muscular branch of the radial nerve.

Indications: (1) Migraine. (2) Deafness. (3) Scrofula. (4) Epilepsy.

Needling Method: Perpendicular insertion 0.5—1.0 cun.

11. TE 11 (Qinglengyuan)

Location: On the lateral aspect of the arm, when the elbow is flexed, the point is 2 cun directly above the tip of the elbow, 1 cun above TE 10 (Tianjing). (Fig. 2-87)

Regional Anatomy: The terminal branches of the median collateral artery and vein. Innervation is the same as TE 10 (Tianjing).

Indications: (1) Headache, yellowness of the eye. (2) Spasm and pain of the upper extremities.

Needling Method: Perpendicular insertion 0.8—1.2 cun.

12. TE 12 (Xiaoluo)

Location: On the lateral aspect of the arm, at the midpoint of the line connecting TE 11 (Qinglengyuan) and TE 13 (Naohui). (Fig. 2-87)

Regional Anatomy: Vasculature and innervation are the same as TE 11 (Qinglengyuan).

Indications: Headache, neck rigidity, pain of the shoulder and back.

Needling Method: Perpendicular insertion 1.0—1.5 cun.

13. TE 13 (Naohui)

Location: On the lateral aspect of the arm, on the line connecting the olecranon and TE 14 (Jianliao), 3 cun below TE 14 (Jianliao), on the posterior and inferior border of m. deltoideus. (Fig. 2-87)

Regional Anatomy: Vasculature and innervation are the same as TE 11

(Qinglengyuan).

Indications: (1) Goiter, scrofula. (2) Spasm and pain of the upper extremities.

Needling Method: Perpendicular insertion 1.0—1.5 cun.

14. TE 14 (Jianliao)

Location: On the region of the shoulder, when the arm is abducted, the point is posterior to LI 15 (Jianyu), in the depression posterior and inferior to the acromion. (Fig. 2-87)

Regional Anatomy: The muscular branch of the posterior circumflex humeral artery. The muscular branch of the axillary nerve.

Indications: Pain and limitation of the shoulder and arm.

Needling Method: Perpendicular insertion toward the shoulder joint 1.0—1.5 cun.

15. TE 15 (Tianliao)

Classification: The Crossing Point of Triple Energizer Meridian and Yang Link Vessel.

Location: On the region of the scapula, midway between GB 21 (Jianjing) and SI 13 (Quyuan), on the superior angle of the scapula. (Fig. 2-88)

Regional Anatomy: The descending branch of the transverse cervical artery. The accessory nerve and the branch of the suprascapular nerve.

Indications: Pain of the shoulder and arm, acute neck rigidity.

Needling Method: Perpendicular insertion 0.5—0.8 cun.

16. TE 16 (Tianyou)

Location: On the side of the neck, directly inferior to the posterior aspect of the mastoid process, at the level of the angle of the mandible, on the posterior border of m. sternocleidomastoideus. (Fig. 2-89)

Regional Anatomy: The posterior auricular artery. The minor occipital nerve.

Indications: (1) Headache, neck rigidity. (2) Eye pain, deafness. (3) Scrofula.

Needling Method: Perpendicular insertion 0.5—1.0 cun.

17. TE 17 (Yifeng)

Classification: The Crossing Point of Triple Energizer Meridian and Gallbladder Meridian.

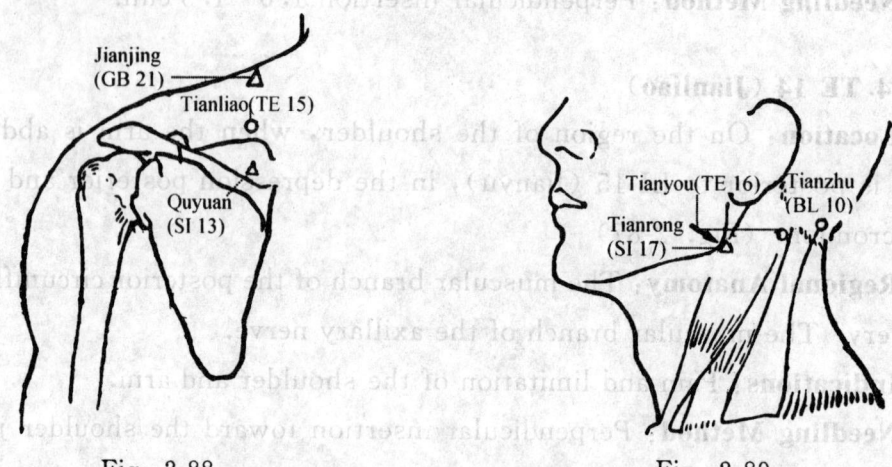

Fig. 2-88   Fig. 2-89

Location: Posterior to the lobule of the ear, in the depression between the angle of the mandible and the mastoid process. (Fig. 2-90)

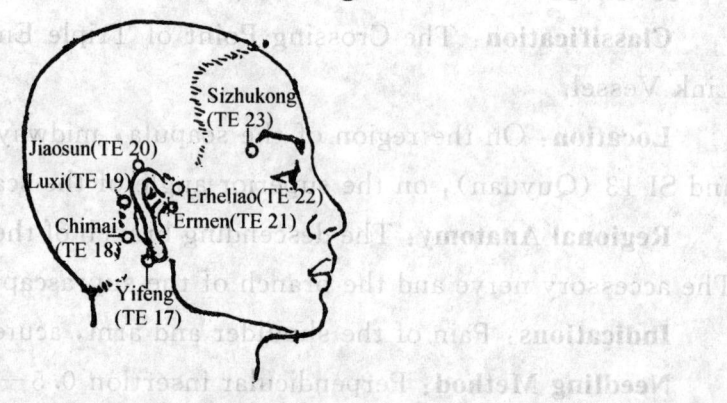

Fig. 2-90

Regional Anatomy: The posterior auricular artery and vein. The great auricular nerve; deeper, the site where the facial nerve emerges out of the stylomastoid foramen.

Indications: (1) Tinnitus, deafness. (2) Wry face, swelling of the cheek. (3) Toothache. (4) Scrofula.

Needling Method: Perpendicular insertion 0.8—1.2 cun.

18. TE 18 (Chimai)

Location: On the head, posterior to the ear in the center of the mastoid process, at the junction of the middle and lower third of the curve connecting TE 20

160

(Jiaosun) and TE 17 (Yifeng) posterior to the helix. (Fig. 2-90)

Regional Anatomy: The posterior auricular artery and vein. The posterior auricular branch of the great auricular nerve.

Indications: (1) Infantile convulsion. (2) Headache, tinnitus, deafness.

Needling Method: Sbucutaneous insertion 0.3—0.5 cun, or prick to cause bleeding.

19. TE 19 (Luxi)

Location: On the head, at the junction of the upper and middle third of the curve connecting TE 20 (Jiaosun) and TE 17 (Yifeng) posterior to the helix. (Fig. 2-90)

Regional Anatomy: The posterior auricular artery and vein. The anastomotic branch of the great auricular nerve and the major occipital nerve.

Indications: (1) Headache, tinnitus, deafness. (2) Infantile convulsion.

Needling Method: Subcutaneous insertion 0.3—0.5 cun.

20. TE 20 (Jiaosun)

Classification: The Crossing Point of Triple Energizer Meridian, Gallbladder Meridian and Large Intestine Meridian.

Location: On the head, bending the auricle forward, the point is directly above the apex of the auricle, within the hairline. (Fig. 2-90)

Regional Anatomy: The branches of the superficial temporal artery and vein. The branches of the auriculotemporal nerve.

Indications: (1) Mumps. (2) Nebula. (3) Toothache. (4) Neck rigidity.

Needling Method: Subcutaneous insertion 0.3—0.5 cun.

21. TE 21 (Ermen)

Location: On the face, in the depression anterior to the supra-tragus notch and on the posterior border of the condyloid process of the mandible. (Fig. 2-90)

Regional Anatomy: The superficial temporal artery and vein. The branches of the auriculotemporal nerve and facial nerve.

Indications: (1) Tinnitus, deafness, otitis media. (2) Toothache.

Needling Method: Perpendicular insertion 0.5—1.0 cun with the mouth open.

22. TE 22 (Erheliao)

Classification: The Crossing Point of Triple Energizer Meridian, Gallbladder Meridian and Small Intestine Meridian.

Location: On the side of the head, on the posterior border of the hairline of the temple, at the level with the root of the auricle, posterior to the superficial temporal artery. (Fig. 2-90)

Regional Anatomy: Vasculature and innervation are the same as TE 21 (Ermen).

Indications: (1) Headache, tinnitus. (2) Trismus, wry mouth.

Needling Method: Avoiding the artery, oblique or subcutaneous insertion 0.3—0.5 cun.

23. TE 23 (Sizhukong)

Location: On the face, in the depression at the lateral end of the eyebrow. (Fig. 2-90)

Regional Anatomy: The superficial temporal artery and vein. The zygomatic branch of the facial nerve and the branch of the auriculotemporal nerve.

Indications: (1) Redness, swelling and pain of the eye, twitching of the eyelid. (2) Manic psychosis, epilepsy.

Needling Method: Subcutaneous insertion 0.5—1.0 cun.

Section 11 The Acupuncture Points of Gallbladder Meridian

This meridian appears at GB 1 (Tongziliao) and ends at GB 44 (Zuqiaoyin); bilaterally each consisting of 44 acupuncture points. (Fig. 2-91)

1. GB 1 (Tongziliao)

Classification: The Crossing Point of Small Intestine Meridian, Triple Energizer Meridian and Gallbladder Meridian.

Location: On the region of the face, lateral to the outer canthus on the lateral side of the orbit. (Fig. 2-92)

Regional Anatomy: The zygomaticoorbital artery and vein. The temporal branch of the facial nerve.

Indications: Headache, redness, swelling and pain of the eye, nebula, glaucoma.

Needling Method: Subcutaneous insertion 0.3—0.5 cun.

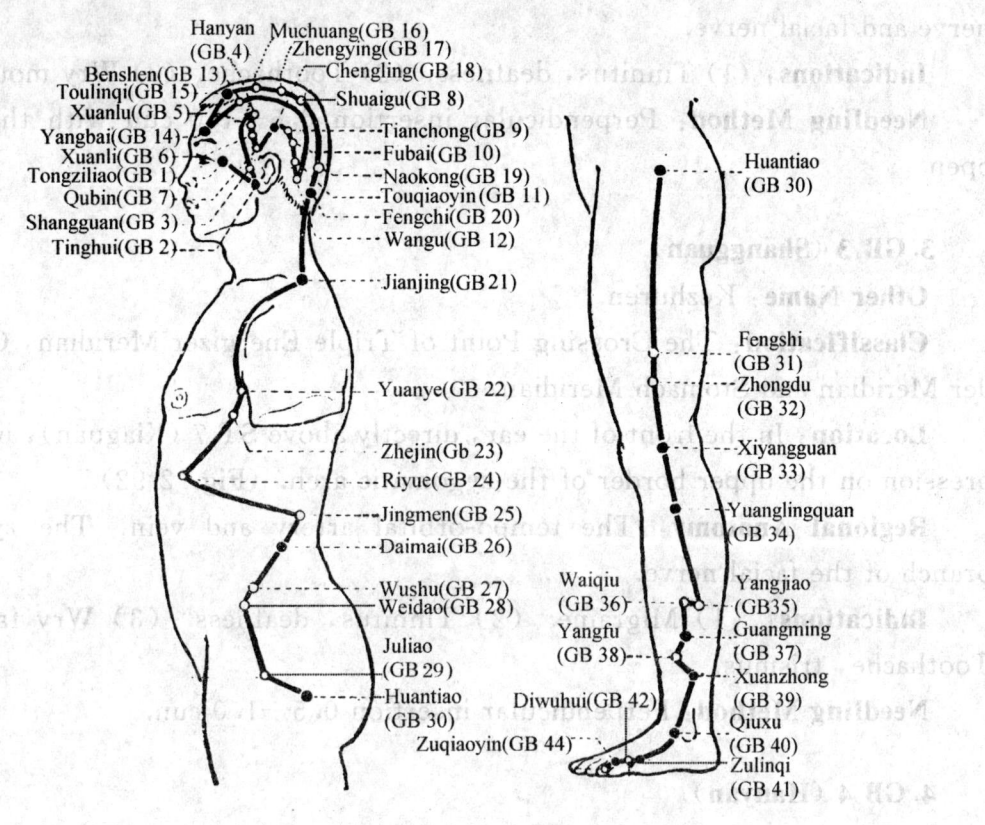

Fig. 2-91 The Points of the Gallbladder Meridian

2. GB 2 (Tinghui)

Location: On the face, anterior to the inter-tragus notch, at the posterior border of the condyloid process of the mandible. When the mouth is open, the point is in the depression. (Fig. 2-92)

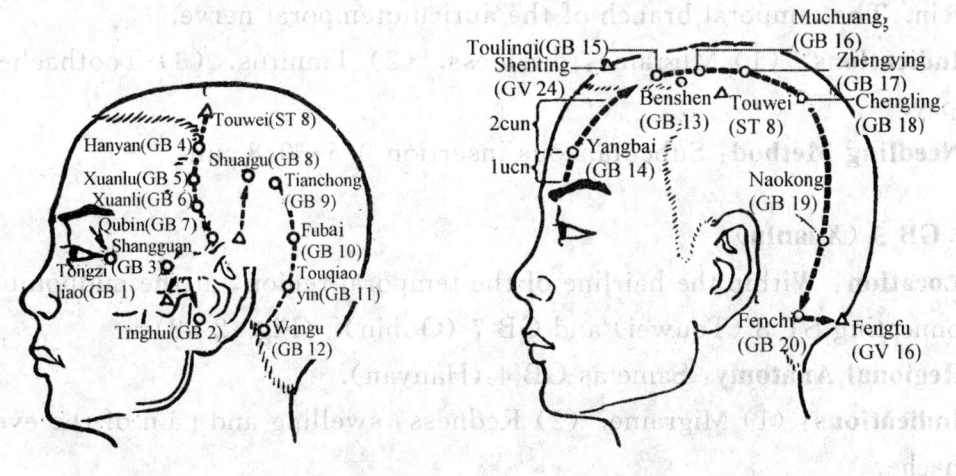

Fig. 2-92   Fig. 2-93

163

Regional Anatomy: The superficial temporal artery. The great auricular nerve and facial nerve.

Indications: (1) Tinnitus, deafness. (2) Toothache. (3) Wry mouth.

Needling Method: Perpendicular insertion 0.5—1.0 cun with the mouth open.

3. GB 3 (Shangguan)

Other Name: Kezhuren.

Classification: The Crossing Point of Triple Energizer Meridian, Gallbladder Meridian and Stomach Meridian.

Location: In the front of the ear, directly above ST 7 (Xiaguan), in the depression on the upper border of the zygomatic arch. (Fig. 2-92)

Regional Anatomy: The tempo-orbital artery and vein. The zygomatic branch of the facial nerve.

Indications: (1) Migraine. (2) Tinnitus, deafness. (3) Wry face. (4) Toothache, trismus.

Needling Method: Perpendicular insertion 0.5—1.0 cun.

4. GB 4 (Hanyan)

Classification: The Crossing Point of Triple Energizer Meridian, Gallbladder Meridian and Stomach Meridian.

Location: Within the hairline of the temporal region, at the junction of the upper one-fourths and lower three-four ths of the arc connecting ST 8 (Touwei) and GB 7 (Qubin). (Fig. 2-92)

Regional Anatomy: The parietal branches of the superficial temporal artery and vein. The temporal branch of the auriculotemporal nerve.

Indications: (1) Migraine, dizziness. (2) Tinnitus. (3) Toothache. (4) Epilepsy.

Needling Method: Subcutaneous insertion 0.5—0.8 cun.

5. GB 5 (Xuanlu)

Location: Within the hairline of the temporal region, at the midpoint of the arc connecting ST 8 (Touwei) and GB 7 (Qubin). (Fig. 2-92)

Regional Anatomy: Same as GB 4 (Hanyan).

Indications: (1) Migraine. (2) Redness, swelling and pain of the eye. (3) Toothache.

Needling Method: Subcutaneous insertion 0.5—0.8 cun.

6. GB 6 (Xuanli)

Classification: The Crossing Point of Triple Energizer Meridian, Gallbladder Meridian and Stomach Meridian.

Location: Within the hairline of the temporal region, at the junction of the upper 3/4 and lower 1/4 of the arc connecting ST 8 (Touwei) and GB 7 (Qubin). (Fig. 2-92)

Regional Anatomy: Same as GB 4 (Hanyan).

Indications: (1) Migraine. (2) Redness, swelling and pain of the eye. (3) Tinnitus.

Needling Method: Subcutaneous insertion 0.5—0.8 cun.

7. GB 7 (Qubin)

Classification: The Crossing Point of Gallbladder Meridian and Bladder Meridian.

Location: On the head, the point is where the vertical line of the posterior hairline anterior to the ear and the horizontal line level with the apex of the auricle intersect. (Fig. 2-92)

Regional Anatomy: Vasculature and innervation are the same as GB 4 (Hanyan).

Indications: (1) Headache. (2) Toothache, trismus, acute aphonia.

Needling Method: Subcutaneous insertion 0.5—0.8 cun.

8. GB 8 (Shuaigu)

Classification: The Crossing Point of Gallbladder Meridian and Bladder Meridian.

Location: On the head, directly above the apex of the auricle and TE 20 (Jiaosun), 1.5 cun within the hairline. (Fig. 2-92)

Regional Anatomy: The parietal branches of the superficial temporal artery and vein. The anastomotic branch of the auriculotemporal nerve and occipital nerve.

Indications: (1) Migraine, vertigo. (2) Infantile convulsion.

Needling Method: Subcutaneous insertion 0.5—0.8 cun.

9. GB 9 (Tianchong)

Classification: The Crossing Point of Gallbladder Meridian and Bladder Meridian.

Location: On the head, directly above the posterior border of the auricle, 2 cun within the hairline, 0.5 cun posterior to GB 8 (Shuaigu). (Fig. 2-92)

Regional Anatomy: The posterior auricular artery and vein. The branch of the major occipital nerve.

Indications: (1) Headache. (2) Deafness, tinnitus. (3) Mania. (4) Swelling and pain of the gums.

Needling Method: Subcutaneous insertion 0.5—0.8 cun.

10. GB 10 (Fubai)

Classification: The Crossing Point of Gallbladder Meridian and Bladder Meridian.

Location: On the head, posterior to the auricle, posterior and superior to the mastoid process, at the junction of the middle third and upper third of the arc connecting GB 9 (Tianchong) and GB 12 (Wangu). (Fig. 2-92)

Regional Anatomy: Same as GB 9 (Tianchong).

Indications: (1) Headache. (2) Tinnitus, deafness. (3) Eye pain. (4) Goiter.

Needling Method: Subcutaneous insertion 0.5—0.8 cun.

11. GB 11 (Touqiaoyin)

Classification: The Crossing Point of Gallbladder Meridian and Bladder Meridian.

Location: On the head, posterior to the auricle, posterior and superior to the mastoid process, at the junction of the middle third and lower third of the arc connecting GB 9 (Tianchong) and GB 12 (Wangu). (Fig. 2-92)

Regional Anatomy: The branches of the posterior auricular artery and vein. The anastomotic branch of the major and minor occipital nerves.

Indications: (1) Headache. (2) Tinnitus, deafness, ear pain.

Needling Method: Subcutaneous insertion 0.5—0.8 cun.

12. GB 12 (Wangu)

Classification: The Crossing Point of Gallbladder Meridian and Bladder

Meridian.

Location: On the head, posterior to the auricle, in the depression posterior and inferior to the mastoid process. (Fig. 2-92)

Regional Anatomy: The posterior auricular artery and vein. The minor occipital nerve.

Indications: (1) Headache, stiffness and pain of the neck. (2) Toothache, swelling of the cheek. (3) Wry face.

Needling Method: Oblique insertion 0.5—0.8 cun.

13. **GB 13 (Benshen)**

Classification: The Crossing Point of Gallbladder Meridian and Yang Link Vessel.

Location: On the head, 0.5 cun within the anterior hairline of the forehead, 3 cun lateral to GV 24 (Shenting), at the junction of the medial two-thirds and the lateral one-third of the line connecting GV 24 (Shenting) and ST 8 (Touwei). (Fig. 2-93)

Regional Anatomy: The frontal branches of the superficial temporal artery and vein. The lateral branch of the frontal nerve.

Indications: (1) Headache, dizziness. (2) Epilepsy. (3) Infantile convulsion.

Needling Method: Subcutaneous insertion 0.5—0.8 cun.

14. **GB 14 (Yangbai)**

Classification: The Crossing Point of Gallbladder Meridian and Yang Link Vessel.

Location: On the forehead, directly above the pupil of the eye, 1.0 cun superior to the eyebrow. (Fig. 2-93)

Regional Anatomy: The frontal artery and vein. The lateral branch of the frontal nerve.

Indications: (1) Facial paralysis, ptosis of the lower eyelid, difficulty in closing eyes. (2) Blurring of vision, eye pain. (3) Forehead pain, vertigo.

Needling Method: Subcutaneous insertion 0.3—0.5 cun.

15. **GB 15 (Toulinqi)**

Classification: The Crossing Point of Gallbladder Meridian, Bladder Meridian and Yang Link Vessel.

Location: On the head, directly above the pupil of the eye, 0.5 cun within the anterior hairline, at the midpoint of the line connecting GV 24 (Shenting) and ST 8 (Touwei). (Fig. 2-93)

Regional Anatomy: The frontal artery and vein. The anastomotic branch of the medial and lateral branches of the frontal nerve.

Indications: (1) Headache, nasal congestion. (2) Dizziness, lacrimation. (3) Infantile convulsion.

Needling Method: Subcutaneous insertion 0.3—0.5 cun.

16. GB 16 (Muchuang)

Classification: The Crossing Point of Gallbladder Meridian and Yang Link Vessel.

Location: On the head, 1.5 cun posterior to the anterior hairline, 2.25 cun lateral to the midline of the head. (Fig. 2-93)

Regional Anatomy: Same as GB 15 (Toulinqi).

Indications: (1) Blurring of vision, glaucoma, redness, swelling and pain of the eye. (2) Headache, nasal congestion, swelling of facial region. (3) Epilepsy.

Needling Method: Subcutaneous insertion 0.3—0.5 cun.

17. GB 17 (Zhengying)

Classification: The Crossing Point of Gallbladder Meridian and Yang Link Vessel.

Location: On the head, 2.25 cun posterior to the anterior hairline, 2.25 cun lateral to the midline of the head. (Fig. 2-93)

Regional Anatomy: The anastomotic plexus formed by the parietal branches of the superficial temporal artery and vein and the occipital artery and vein. The anastomotic branch of the frontal and major occipital nerves.

Indications: (1) Headache, dizziness, acute stiffness of the lips. (2) Toothache.

Needling Method: Subcutaneous insertion 0.3—0.5 cun.

18. GB 18 (Chengling)

Classification: The Crossing Point of Gallbladder Meridian and Yang Link Vessel.

Location: On the head, 4.0 cun posterior to the anterior hairline, 2.25 cun lateral to the midline of the head. (Fig. 2-93)

Regional Anatomy: The branches of the occipital artery and vein. The branch of the major occipital nerve.

Indications: (1) Headache, dizziness, eye pain. (2) Nasal congestion, epistaxis.

Needling Method: Subcutaneous insertion 0.3—0.5 cun.

19. GB 19 (Naokong)

Classification: The Crossing Point of Gallbladder Meridian and Yang Link Vessel.

Location: On the region of the head, on the lateral side of the superior border of the external occipital protuberance, 2.25 cun lateral to the midline of the head. (Fig. 2-93)

Regional Anatomy: Same as GB 18 (Chengling).

Indications: (1) Headache, dizziness. (2) Rigidity and pain of the neck. (3) Manic psychosis, epilepsy.

Needling and Moxibustion Method: Subcutaneous insertion 0.3—0.5 cun.

20. GB 20 (Fengchi)

Classification: The Crossing Point of Gallbladder Meridian and Yang Link Vessel.

Location: On the nape, below the occiput, at the level of GV 16 (Fengfu), in the depression between the upper portion of m. sternocleidomastoideus and m. trapezius. (Fig. 2-93)

Regional Anatomy: The branches of the occipital artery and vein. The branch of the minor occipital nerve.

Indications: (1) Common cold, nasal congestion, headache, redness, swelling and pain of the eye, rhinorrhea, epistaxis, rigidity and pain of the neck, pain and limitation of the shoulder. (2) Dizziness, vertigo, hemiplegia, epilepsy.

Needling Method: Oblique insertion 0.8—1.2 cun towards the tip of the nose with the tip of the needle slightly downwards, or subcutaneous insertion through GV 16 (Fengfu). Towards the middle in the deeper layer, is the medulla oblongata; the angle and depth of the needle must be strictly controlled.

21. GB 21 (Jianjing)

Classification: The Crossing Point of Triple Energizer Meridian, Gallbladder Meridian, Stomach Meridian and Yang Link Vessel.

Location: On the shoulder, directly above the nipple, at the midpoint of the line connecting GV 14 (Dazhui) and the acromion. (Fig. 2-94)

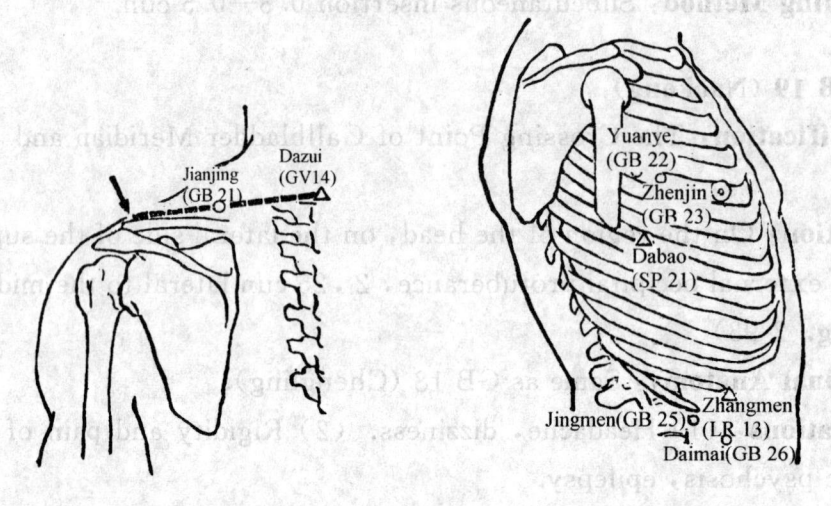

Fig. 2-94   Fig. 2-95

Regional Anatomy: The transverse cervical artery and vein. The posterior branch of the supraclavicular nerve, the accessory nerve.

Indications: (1) Mastitis, insufficient lactation. (2) Dizziness, headache, rigidity and pain of the neck, limitation of the upper extremities. (3) Difficult labor, scrofula.

Needling Method: Perpendicular insertion 0.5—0.8 cun. Below this point is the apex of the lung, do not puncture deeply. Needling this point is contraindicated in pregnancy.

22. GB 22 (Yuanye)

Location: On the lateral side of the chest, when the arm is raised, the point is on the mid-axillary line, 3 cun below the axilla, in the fourth intercostal space. (Fig. 2-95)

Regional Anatomy: The fourth intercostal artery and vein. The lateral cutaneous branch of the fourth intercostal nerve.

Indications: (1) Chest congestion, pain in the hypochondrium. (2) Spasm and pain in the upper extremities.

Needling Method: Oblique or Subcutaneousinsertion 0.5—0.8 cun. On this

Meridian, do not puncture deeply all points from GB 22 (Yuanye) to GB 25 (Jingmen) to avoid injuring important internal organs.

23. GB 23 (Zhejin)

Location: On the lateral side of the chest, 1 cun anterior to GB 22 (Yuanye), at the level of the nipple, in the fourth intercostal space. (Fig. 2-95)

Regional Anatomy: Same as GB 22 (Yuanye).

Indications: (1) Chest congestion, pain in the hypochondrium. (2) Asthma.

Needling Method: Oblique or Subcutaneous insertion 0.5—0.8 cun.

24. GB 24 (Riyue)

Classification: Front-Mu Point. The Crossing Point of Gallbladder Meridian and Bladder Meridian.

Location: On the upper abdomen, directly below the nipple, in the seventh intercostal space, 4 cun lateral to the anterior midline. (Fig. 2-96)

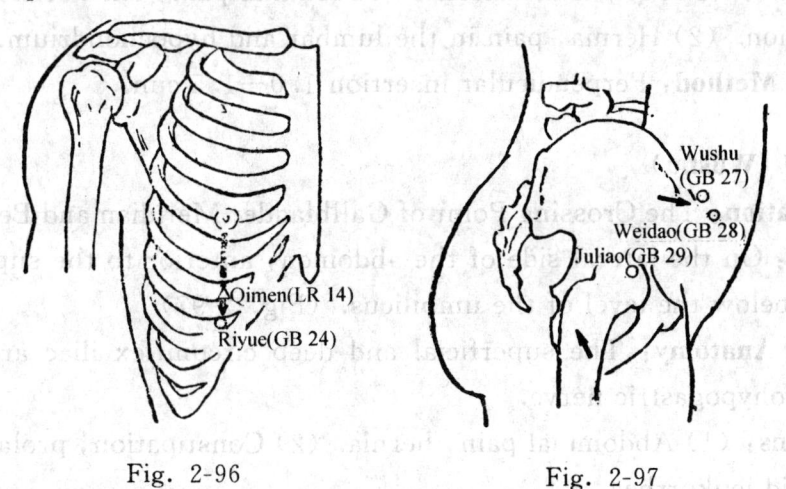

Fig. 2-96   Fig. 2-97

Regional Anatomy: The seventh intercostal artery and vein. The seventh intercostal nerve.

Indications: (1) Swelling and pain in the hypochondrium. (2) Jaundice. (3) Vomiting, hiccup, acid regurgitation.

Needling Method: Oblique or Subcutaneous insertion 0.5—0.8 cun.

25. GB 25 (Jingmen)

Classification: The Front-Mu Point of Kidney.

Location: On the lateral side of the abdomen, 1.8 cun posterior to LR 13 (Zhangmen), on the lower border of the free end of the twelfth floating rib. (Fig. 2-95)

Regional Anatomy: The eleventh intercostal artery and vein. The eleventh intercostal nerve.

Indications: (1) Dysuria, edema, lumbar pain. (2) Pain in the hypochondrium, abdominal pain, diarrhea.

Needling Method: Perpendicular insertion 0.5—1.0 cun.

26. GB 26 (Daimai)

Classification: The Crossing Point of Gallbladder Meridian and Belt Vessel.

Location: On the lateral side of the abdomen, 1.8 cun below LR 13 (Zhangmen), where the vertical line of the free end of the eleventh rib and the horizontal line of the umbilicus intersect. (Fig. 2-95)

Regional Anatomy: The twelfth intercostal artery and vein. The twelfth intercostal nerve.

Indications: (1) Morbid leukorrhea, abdominal pain, amenorrhea, irregular menstruation. (2) Hernia, pain in the lumbar and hypochondrium.

Needling Method: Perpendicular insertion 1.0—1.5 cun.

27. GB 27 (Wushu)

Classification: The Crossing Point of Gallbladder Meridian and Belt Vessel.

Location: On the lateral side of the abdomen, anterior to the superior iliac spine, 3 cun below the level of the umbilicus. (Fig. 2-97)

Regional Anatomy: The superficial and deep circumflex iliac arteries and veins. The iliohypogastric nerve.

Indications: (1) Abdominal pain, hernia. (2) Constipation, prolapse of the uterus, morbid leukorrhea.

Needling Method: Perpendicular insertion 1.0—1.5 cun.

28. GB 28 (Weidao)

Classification: The Crossing Point of Gallbladder Meridian and Belt Vessel.

Location: On the lateral side of the abdomen, anterior and inferior to the superior iliac spine, 0.5 cun anterior and inferior to GB 27 (Wushu). (Fig. 2-97)

Regional Anatomy: Vasculature is the same as GB 27 (Wushu). The ilioinguinal nerve.

Indications: (1) Abdominal pain, hernia. (2) Prolapse of the uterus. (3) Morbid leukorrhea.

Needling Method: Perpendicular or oblique insertion towards the anterior inferior direction 1.0—1.5 cun.

29. GB 29 (Juliao)

Classification: The Crossing Point of Gallbladder Meridian and Yang Heel Vessel.

Location: On the region of the hip, at the midpoint of the line connecting the anterior iliac spine and the great trochanter of the femur. (Fig. 2-97)

Regional Anatomy: The branches of the superficial circumflex iliac artery and vein, the ascending branches of the lateral circumflex femoral artery and vein. The lateral femoral cutaneous nerve.

Indications: Lumbar pain, difficulty in rotation of the body, weakness, numbness and pain of lower extremities.

Needling Method: Perpendicular insertion 1.0—1.5 cun.

30. GB 30 (Huantiao)

Classification: The Crossing Point of Gallbladder Meridian and Bladder Meridian.

Location: On the lateral side of the buttocks, when the patient is in the lateral recumbent position and the thigh is flexed, this point is at the junction of the lateral one-third and medial one-third of the line connecting the greater trochanter and the hiatus of the sacrum. (Fig. 2-98)

Regional Anatomy: The inferior gluteal cutaneous nerve, the inferior gluteal nerve; deeper, the sciatic nerve.

Indications: Weakness, numbness and pain of lower extremities, pain of the lumbar and leg, hemiplegia.

Needling Method: Perpendicular insertion 2.0—3.0 cun.

31. GB 31 (Fengshi)

Location: On the midline of the lateral aspect of the thigh, 7 cun above the transverse popliteal crease. When the patient is standing erect with the hands are hanging down close to the sides, the point is where the tip of the middle finger touches. (Fig. 2-99)

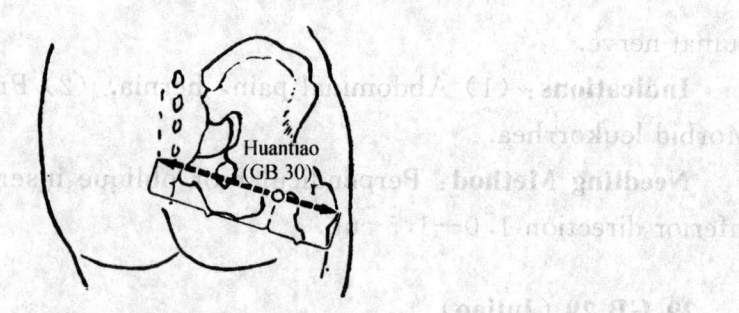

Fig. 2-98

Regional Anatomy: The lateral femoral cutaneous nerve and the muscular branch of the femoral nerve.

Indications: (1) Weakness, numbness and pain of lower extremities, beriberi. (2) General pruritus. (3) Sudden deafness.

Needling Method: Perpendicular insertion 1.0—2.0 cun.

32. **GB 32 (Zhongdu)**

Location: On the lateral aspect of the thigh, 2 cun below GB 31 (Fengshi), 5 cun above the transverse popliteal crease, between m. vastus lateralis and m. biceps femoris. (Fig. 2-99)

Regional Anatomy: Same as GB 31 (Fengshi).

Indications: Weakness, numbness and pain of lower extremities, hemiplegia.

Needling Method: Perpendicular insertion 1.0—2.0 cun.

33. **GB 33 (Xiyangguan)**

Location: On the lateral aspect of the thigh, 3 cun above GB 34 (Yanglingquan), in the depression anterior to the lateral epicondyle of the femur. (Fig. 2-99)

Regional Anatomy: Same as GB 31 (Fengshi).

Indications: Coldness and pain of the knee, spasm of the tendons in popliteal fossa, numbness of the lower leg.

Needling Method: Perpendicular insertion 1.0—1.5 cun.

34. **GB 34 (Yanglingquan)**

Classification: He-(Sea) Point. The Converging Point of Tendon.

Location: On the lateral aspect of the lower leg, in the depression anterior and inferior to the head of the fibula. (Fig. 2-100)

Regional Anatomy: The inferior lateral genicular artery and vein. The site where the common peroneal nerve bifurcates into the superficial and deep peroneal nerves.

Indications: (1) Hemiplegia, pain of the shoulder, weakness, numbness and pain of lower extremities, swelling and pain of the knee, beriberi. (2) Pain in the hypochondrium, bitter taste in the mouth, vomiting, jaundice. (3) Infantile convulsion.

Needling Method: Perpendicular insertion 1.0—1.5 cun.

35. GB 35 (Yangjiao)

Classification: The Xi-(Cleft) Point of Yang Link Vessel.

Location: On the lateral aspect of the lower leg, 7 cun above the tip of the external malleolus, on the posterior border of the fibula. (Fig. 2-100)

Regional Anatomy: The branches of the peroneal artery and vein. The lateral sural cutaneous nerve.

Indications: (1) Distention and fullness of the chest and hypochondrium. (2) Weakness, numbness and pain of lower extremities.

Needling Method: Perpendicular insertion 1.0—1.5 cun.

36. GB 36 (Waiqiu)

Location: On the lateral aspect of the lower leg, 7 cun above the tip of the external malleolus, on the anterior border of the fibula, at the level of GB 35 (Yangjiao). (Fig. 2-100)

Regional Anatomy: The muscular branches of the anterior tibial artery and vein. The superficial peroneal nerve.

Indications: (1) Distention and pain of the chest and hypochondrium, neck pain. (2) Weakness, numbness and pain of lower extremities. (3) Rabies.

Needling Method: Perpendicular insertion 1.0—1.5 cun.

37. GB 37 (Guangming)

Classification: Luo-(Connecting) Point.

Location: On the lateral aspect of the lower leg, 5 cun above the tip of the external malleolus, on the anterior border of the fibula. (Fig. 2-100)

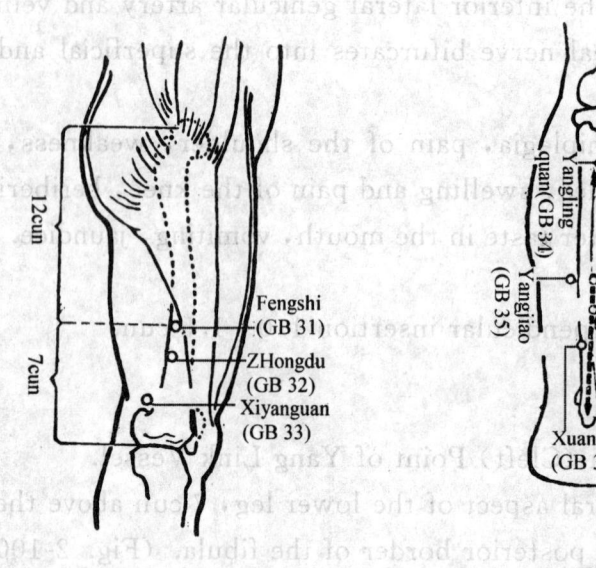

Fig. 2-99 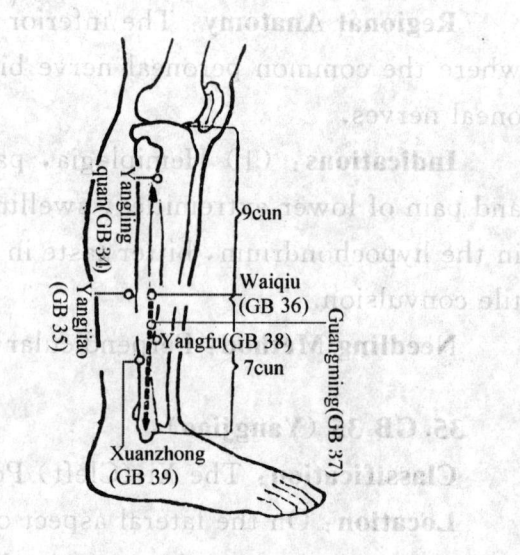   Fig. 2-100

Regional Anatomy: Same as GB 36 (Waiqiu).

Indications: (1) Eye pain, night blindness, blurring of vision. (2) Weakness, numbness and pain of lower extremities. (3) Distention and pain of the breast.

Needling Method: Perpendicular insertion 1.0—1.5 cun.

38. GB 38 (Yangfu)

Classification: Jing-(River) Point.

Location: On the lateral aspect of the lower leg, 4 cun above the tip of the external malleolus, slightly anterior to the anterior border of the fibula. (Fig. 2-100)

Regional Anatomy: Same as GB 36 (Waiqiu).

Indications: (1) Migraine, pain of the outer canthus. (2) Swelling and pain in the axillary region. (3) Distention and pain in the chest and hypochondrium, weakness, numbness and pain of lower extremities.

Needling Method: Perpendicular insertion 1.0—1.5 cun.

39. GB 39 (Xuanzhong)

Other Name: Juegu.

Classification: The Converging Point of Marrow.

Location: On the lateral aspect of the lower leg, 3 cun above the tip of the external malleolus, on the anterior border of the fibula. (Fig. 2-100)

Regional Anatomy: Same as GB 36 (Waiqiu).

Indications: (1) Hemiplegia, rigidity and pain of the neck, weakness, numbness and pain of lower extremities, beriberi. (2) Pain in the hypochondrium.

Needling Method: Perpendicular insertion 1.0—1.5 cun.

40. GB 40 (Qiuxu)

Classification: Yuan-(Source) Point.

Location: On the foot, anterior and inferior to the external malleolus, in the depression on the lateral side of the tendon of m. extensor digitorum longus. (Fig. 2-101)

Regional Anatomy: The branches of the anterior lateral malleolar artery and vein. The superficial peroneal nerve.

Indications: (1) Distention and pain in the chest and hypochondrium. (2) Weakness, numbness and pain of lower extremities, swelling and pain of the external malleolus. (3) Malaria.

Needling Method: Perpendicular insertion 0.5—0.8 cun.

41. GB 41 (Zulinqi)

Classification: Shu-(Stream) Point. One of the Eight Confluent Points. This point linking with the Belt Vessel.

Location: On the lateral side of the dorsum of the foot, proximal to the fourth metatarsophalangeal joint, in the depression lateral to the tendon of m. extensor digiti minimi of the foot. (Fig. 2-101)

Regional Anatomy: The dorsal arterial and venous network of foot. The branch of the intermediate dorsal cutaneous nerve of the foot.

Indications: (1) Migraine, redness and pain of the eye, pain in the hypochondrium, spasm and pain of the foot and toe. (2) Mastitis, breast distention, irregular menstruation. (3) Scrofula, malaria.

Needling Method: Perpendicular insertion 0.3—0.5 cun.

42. GB 42 (Diwuhui)

Location: On the lateral side of the dorsum of the foot, proximal to the fourth metatarsophalangeal joint, between the fourth and fifth metatarsal bones, on the medial side of the tendon of m. extensor digiti minimi of the foot. (Fig. 2-101)

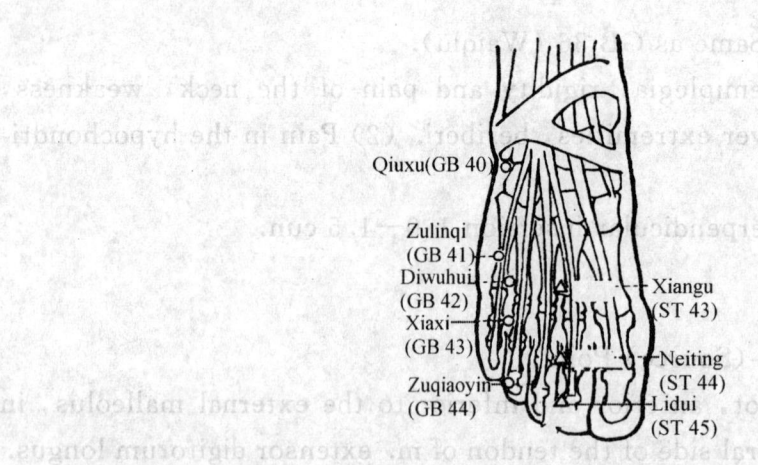

Fig. 2-101

Regional Anatomy: Same as GB 41 (Zulinqi).

Indications: (1) Mastitis, breast distention. (2) Headache, eye pain, tinnitus, deafness. (3) Pain in the hypochondrium, swelling and pain of the dorsum of foot.

Needling Method: Perpendicular insertion 0.3—0.5 cun.

43. GB 43 (Xiaxi)

Classification: Ying-(Spring) Point.

Location: On the lateral side of the dorsum of the foot, proximal to the margin of the web between the fourth and fifth toes, at the junction of the red and white skin. (Fig. 2-101)

Regional Anatomy: The digital artery and vein. The dorsal digital nerve.

Indications: (1) Headache, dizziness, redness, swelling and pain of the eye. (2) Tinnitus, deafness. (3) Mastitis, pain in the hypochondrium. (4) Febrile disease.

Needling Method: Perpendicular insertion 0.3—0.5 cun.

44. GB 44 (Zuqiaoyin)

Classification: Jing-(Well) Point.

Location: On the foot, on the lateral side of the end of the fourth toe, 0.1 cun (finger cun) from the corner of the nail. (Fig. 2-101)

Regional Anatomy: The arterial and venous network. The dorsal digital nerve.

Indications: (1) Migraine, redness and pain of the eye, pain in the chest and hypochondrium. (2) Tinnitus, deafness. (3) Hemiplegia.

Needling Method: Perpendicular insertion 0.1—0.3 cun.

Section 12 The Acupuncture Points of Liver Meridian

This meridian appears at LR 1 (Dadun) and ends at LR 14 (Qimen); bilaterally each consisting of 14 acupuncture points. (Fig. 2-102)

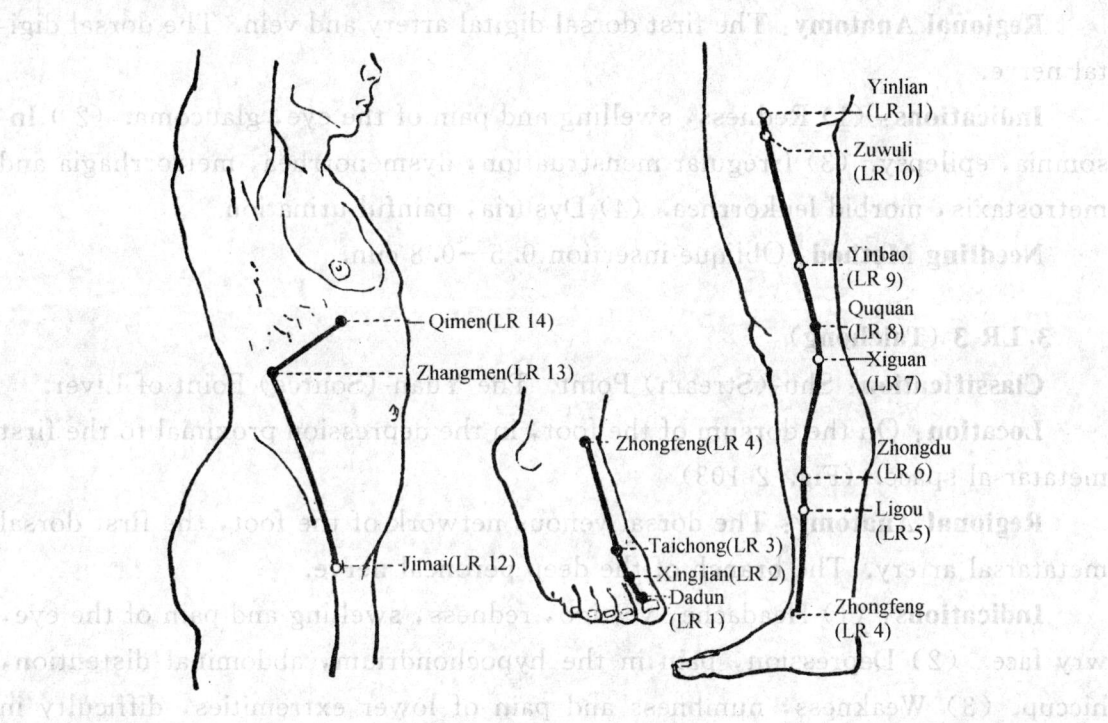

Fig. 2-102 The Points of the Liver Meridian

1. LR 1 (Dadun)

Classification: Jing-(Well) Point.

Location: On the foot, on the lateral side of the end of the great toe, 0.1 cun from the corner of the nail. (Fig. 2-103)

Regional Anatomy: The dorsal digital artery and vein. The dorsal digital nerve.

Indications: (1) Hernia. (2) Enuresis. (3) Metrorrhagia and metrostaxis, prolapse of uterus, amenorrhea. (4) Epilepsy.

Needling Method: Oblique insertion 0.1—0.2 cun, or prick to cause bleeding. *Supplement with Diagnosis to Systematic Compilation of the Internal Classic* says: " moxibustion is contraindicated in pregnancy and postpartum."

2. LR 2 (Xingjian)

Classification: Ying-(Spring) Point.

Location: On the dorsum of the foot, proximal to the margin of the web between the first and second toes, at the junction of the red and white skin. (Fig. 2-103)

Regional Anatomy: The first dorsal digital artery and vein. The dorsal digital nerve.

Indications: (1) Redness, swelling and pain of the eye, glaucoma. (2) Insomnia, epilepsy. (3) Irregular menstruation, dysmenorrhea, metrorrhagia and metrostaxis, morbid leukorrhea. (4) Dysuria, painful urination.

Needling Method: Oblique insertion 0.5—0.8 cun.

3. LR 3 (Taichong)

Classification: Shu-(Stream) Point. The Yuan-(Source) Point of Liver.

Location: On the dorsum of the foot, in the depression proximal to the first metatarsal space. (Fig. 2-103)

Regional Anatomy: The dorsal venous network of the foot, the first dorsal metatarsal artery. The branch of the deep peroneal nerve.

Indications: (1) Headache, vertigo, redness, swelling and pain of the eye, wry face. (2) Depression, pain in the hypochondrium, abdominal distention, hiccup. (3) Weakness, numbness and pain of lower extremities, difficulty in walking. (4) Irregular menstruation, metrorrhagia and metrostaxis, hernia, enuresis. (5) Epilepsy, infantile convulsion.

Needling Method: Perpendicular insertion 0.5—0.8 cun.

4. LR 4 (Zhongfeng)

Classification: Jing-(River) Point.

Location: On the dorsum of the foot, between SP 5 (Shangqiu) and ST 41 (Jiexi), in the depression on the medial side of the tendon of m. tibialis anterior. (Fig. 2-103)

Regional Anatomy: The anterior medial malleolar artery. The saphenous nerve.

Indications: (1) Hernia, abdominal pain. (2) Spermatorrhea. (3) Dysuria.

Needling Method: Perpendicular insertion 0.5—0.8 cun.

Fig. 2-103

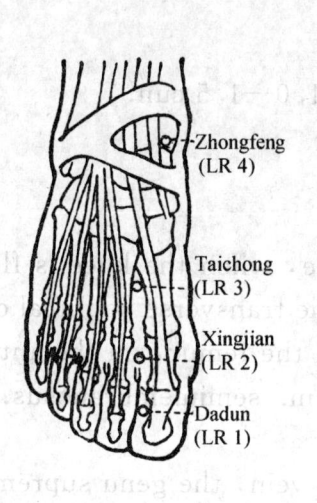

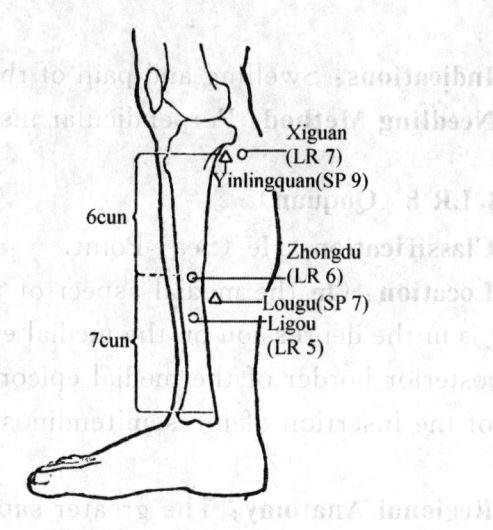

Fig. 2-104

5. LR 5 (Ligou)

Classification: Luo-(Connecting) Point.

Location: On the medial aspect of the lower leg, 5 cun above the tip of the medial malleolus, on the middle of the medial aspect of the tibia. (Fig. 2-104)

Regional Anatomy: The branch of the saphenous nerve.

Indications: (1) Pruritus vulva, persistent erection. (2) Irregular menstruation, morbid leukorrhea. (3) Dysuria, hernia, swelling and pain of the foot.

Needling Method: Subcutaneous insertion 0.5—0.8 cun.

6. LR 6 (Zhongdu)

Classification: Xi-(Cleft) Point.

Location: On the medial aspect of the lower leg, 7 cun above the tip of the medial malleolus, on the middle of the medial aspect of the tibia. (Fig. 2-104)

Regional Anatomy: Same as LR 5 (Ligou).

Indications: (1) Pain in the hypochondrium, abdominal distention and pain, diarrhea. (2) Prolonged lochia. (3) Hernia.

Needling Method: Subcutaneous insertion 0.5—0.8 cun.

7. LR 7 (Xiguan)

Location: On the medial aspect of the lower leg, posterior and inferior to the medial condyle of the tibia, in the upper portion of the medial head of m. gastrocnemius, 1 cun posterior to SP 9 (Yinlingquan). (Fig. 2-104)

Regional Anatomy: Deeper, the posterior tibial artery. Deeper, the tibial nerve.

Indications: Swelling and pain of the knee.

Needling Method: Perpendicular insertion 1.0—1.5 cun.

8. LR 8 (Ququan)

Classification: He-(Sea) Point.

Location: On the medial aspect of the knee, when the knee is flexed, the point is in the depression on the medial end of the transverse popliteal crease, on the posterior border of the medial epicondyle of the femur, on the anterior portion of the insertion of m. semitendinosus and m. semimembranosus. (Fig. 2-105)

Regional Anatomy: The greater saphenous vein, the genu suprema artery. The saphenous nerve.

Indications: (1) Lower abdominal pain, dysuria. (2) Spermatorrhea, prolapse of uterus, pruritus vulva, pain in the external genitalia. (3) Irregular menstruation, morbid leukorrhea, dysmenorrhea. (4) Pain in the medial aspect of the knee and thigh.

Needling Method: Perpendicular insertion 1.0—1.5 cun.

9. LR 9 (Yinbao)

Location: On the medial aspect of the thigh, 4 cun above the medial epicondyle of the femur, between m. vastus medialis and m. sartorius. (Fig. 2-105)

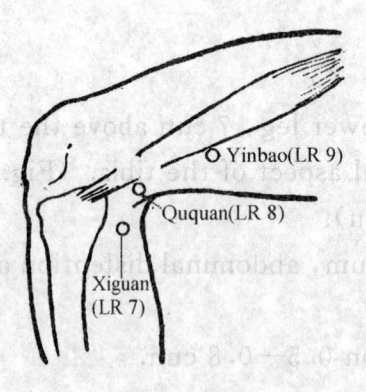

Fig. 2-105

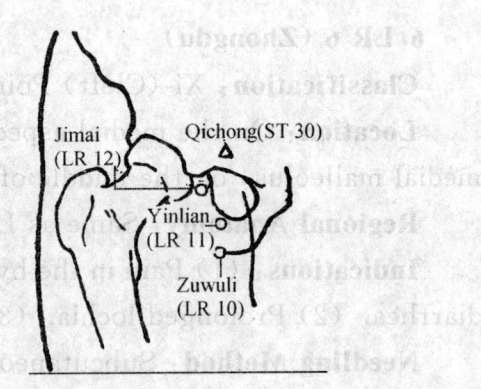

Fig. 2-106

Regional Anatomy: The superficial branch of the medial circumflex femoral artery. The anterior branch of the obturator nerve.

Indications: (1) Lumboscaral pain, lower abdominal pain, dysuria, enuresis. (2) Irregular menstruation.

Needling Method: Perpendicular insertion 1.0—2.0 cun.

10. LR 10 (Zuwuli)

Location: On the medial aspect of the upper thigh, 3 cun directly below ST 30 (Qichong), inferior to the pubictubercle, on the lateral border of m. abductor longus. (Fig. 2-106)

Regional Anatomy: The superficial branches of the medial circumflex femoral artery and vein. The genitofemoral nerve.

Indications: (1) Lower abdominal distention and pain, dysuria. (2) Prolapse of uterus, swelling and pain of the testicle. (3) Scrofula.

Needling Method: Perpendicular insertion 1.0—2.0 cun.

11. LR 11 (Yinlian)

Location: On the medial aspect of the upper thigh, 2 cun directly below ST 30 (Qichong), inferior to the pubictubercle, on the lateral border of m. abductor longus. (Fig. 2-106)

Regional Anatomy: The branches of the medial circumflex femoral artery and vein. The genitofemoral nerve.

Indications: (1) Irregular menstruation, morbid leukorrhea. (2) Lower abdominal distention and pain.

Needling Method: Perpendicular insertion 1.0—2.0 cun.

12. LR 12 (Jimai)

Location: On the lateral side of the pubictubercle, lateral and inferior to ST 30 (Qichong), at the inguinal groove where the fermoral artery pulsates. (Fig. 2-106)

Regional Anatomy: The branches of the external pudendal artery and vein. The ilioinguinal nerve.

Indications: (1) Hernia, abdominal pain. (2) Pain in the external genitalia, dysmenorrhea, prolapse of uterus, pruritus vulva.

Needling Method: Avoid the artery, perpendicular insertion 0.5—0.8 cun.

Annotations: Note to *Simple Questions by* Dr. Wang : Moxibustion can be used; do not needle.

13. LR 13 (Zhangmen)

Classification: The Front-Mu Point of Spleen; The Converging Point of

Zang Organs. The Crossing Point of Liver Meridian and the Gallbladder Meridian.

Location: On the lateral side of the abdomen, below the free end of the eleventh floating rib. (Fig. 2-107)

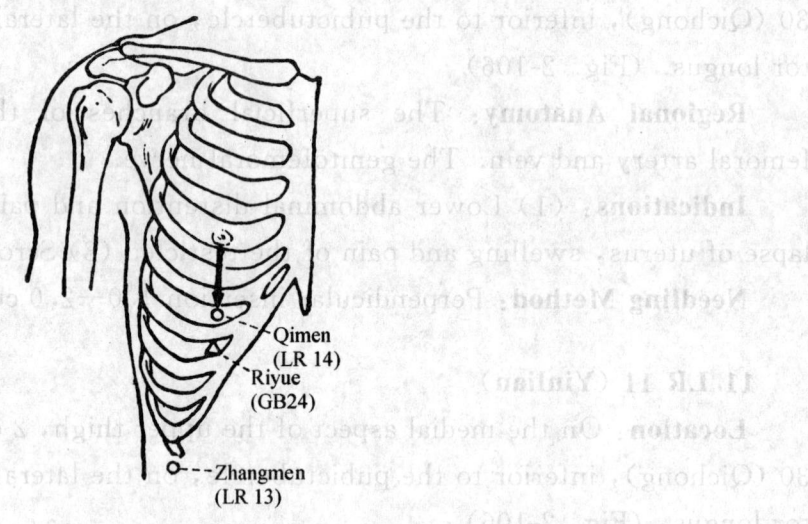

Fig. 2-107

Regional Anatomy: The terminal branch of the tenth intercostal artery. The tenth and eleventh intercostal nerves.

Indications: (1) Abdominal distention, diarrhea. (2) Pain in the hypochondrium, abdominal mass.

Needling Method: Perpendicular insertion 0.8—1.0 cun.

14. LR 14 (Qimen)

Classification: Front-Mu Point. The Crossing Point of Liver Meridian, Spleen Meridian and Yin Link Vessel.

Location: On the chest, directly below the nipple, in the sixth intercostal space, 4 cun lateral to the anterior midline. (Fig. 2-107)

Regional Anatomy: The sixth intercostal artery and vein. The sixth intercostal nerve.

Indications: (1) Depression. (2) Distention and pain of the chest and hypochondrium. (3) Abdominal distention, hiccup, acid regurgitation.

Needling Method: Oblique or subcutaneous insertion 0.5—0.8 cun.

Section 13 The Acupuncture Points of Governor Vessel

This meridian appears at GV 1 (Changqiang) and ends at GV 28 (Yinjiao);

consisting of a total of 28 acupuncture points. (Fig. 2-108)

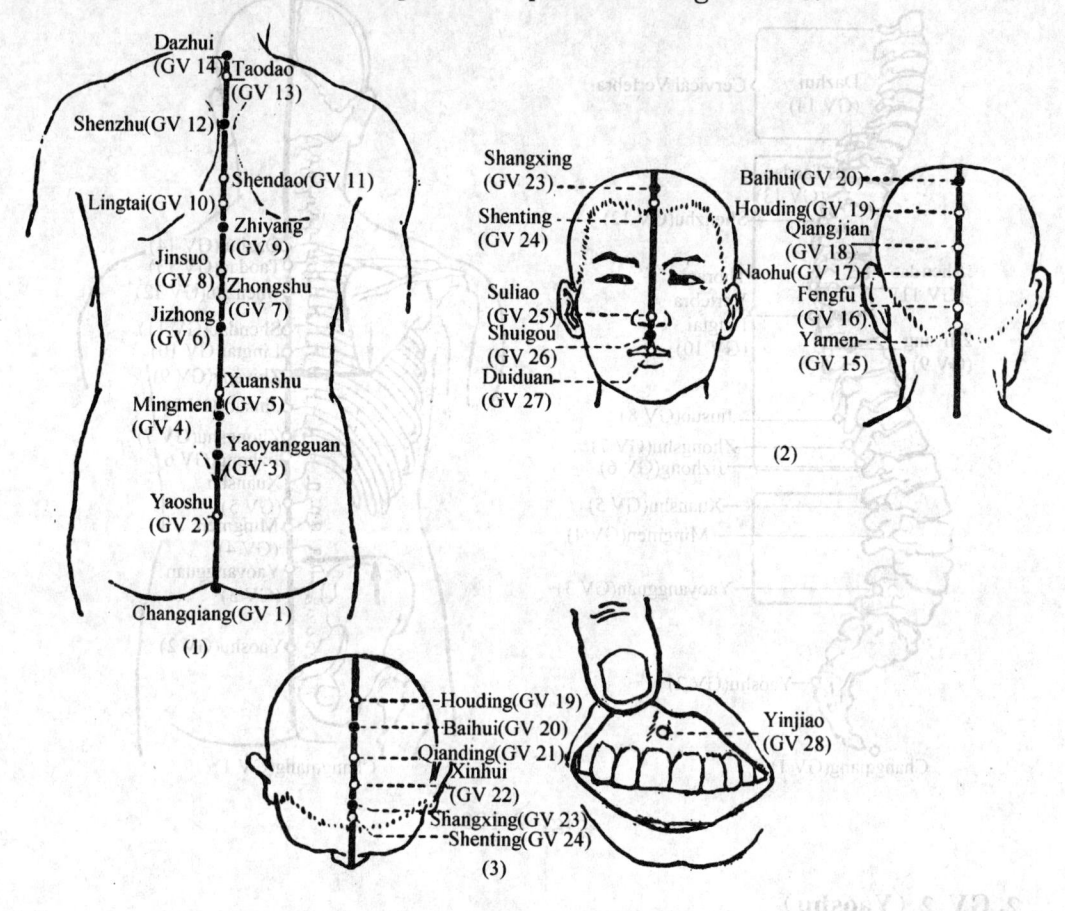

Fig. 2-108 the Points of the Governor Vessel

1. GV 1 (Changqiang)

Classification: The Crossing Point of Governor Vessel, Kidney Meridian and Spleen Meridian. Luo-(Connecting) Point.

Location: Below the tip of the coccyx, at the midpoint between the tip of the coccyx and the anus. (Fig. 2-109)

Regional Anatomy: The branches of the anal artery and vein. The posterior ramus of the coccygeal nerve, the anal nerve.

Indications: (1) Diarrhea, blood in the stools, constipation, hemorrhoids, prolapse of the rectum. (2) Manic psychosis, epilepsy.

Needling Method: Oblique insertion 0.8—1.0 cun right in front of the coccyx. Perpendicular insertion can easily injure the rectum.

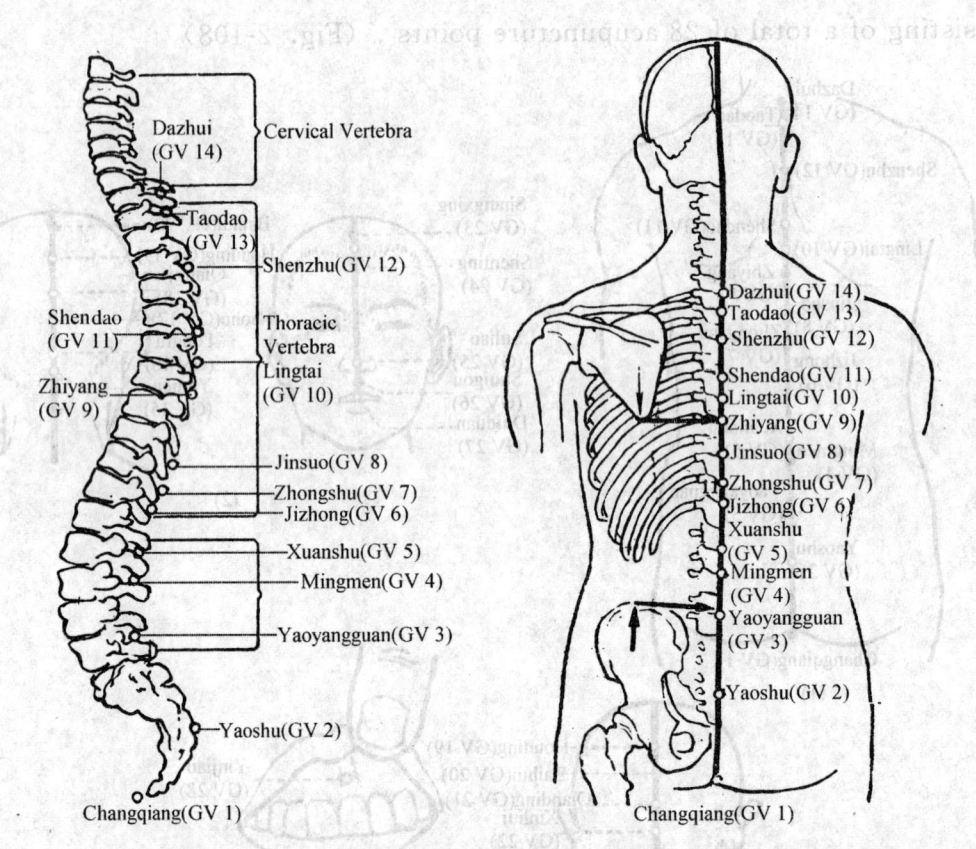

Fig. 2-109

2. GV 2 (Yaoshu)

Location: On the sacrum, on the posterior median line in the hiatus of the sacrum. (Fig. 2-109)

Regional Anatomy: The branches of the median sacral artery and vein. The branch of the coccygeal nerve.

Indications: (1) Mania, epilepsy. (2) Hemorrhoids. (3) Stiffness and pain of the lumbar, pain, numbness and weakness of the lower extremities. (4) Irreular menstruation.

Needling Method: Oblique insertion upward 0.5—1.0 cun.

3. GV 3 (Yaoyangguan)

Location: On the lumbar region, on the posterior median line, in the depression below the spinous process of the fourth lumbar vertebra. (Fig. 2-109)

Regional Anatomy: The posterior branch of the lumbar artery. The medial branch of the posterior ramus of the lumbar nerve.

Indications: (1) Irregular menstruataion, spermatorrhea, impotence. (2)

Lumbosacral pain, pain, numbness and weakness of the lower extremities.

Needling Method: Oblique insertion upward 0.5—1.0 cun.

4. GV 4 (Mingmen)

Location: On the lumbar region, on the posterior median line, in the depression below the spinous process of the second lumbar vertebra. (Fig. 2-109)

Regional Anatomy: Same as GV 3 (Yaoyangguan).

Indications: (1) Spermatorrhea, impotence. (2) Irregular menstruation, leukorrhea. (3) Diarrhea. (4) Stiffness and pain of the lumbar.

Needling Method: Oblique insertion upward 0.5—1.0 cun.

5. GV 5 (Xuanshu)

Location: On the lumbar region, on the posterior median line, in the depression below the spinous process of the first lumbar vertebra. (Fig. 2-109)

Regional Anatomy: Same as GV 3 (Yaoyangguan).

Indications: (1) Stiffness and pain of the lumbar. (2) Diarrhea, abdominal pain.

Needling Method: Oblique insertion upward 0.5—1.0 cun.

6. GV 6 (Jizhong)

Location: On the back, on the posterior median line, in the depression below the spinous process of the eleventh thoracic vertebra. (Fig. 2-109)

Regional Anatomy: Same as GV 3 (Yaoyangguan).

Indications: (1) Diarrhea. (2) Jaundice. (3) Hemorrhoids. (4) Epilepsy.

Needling Method: Oblique insertion upward 0.5—1.0 cun.

7. GV 7 (Zhongshu)

Location: On the back, on the posterior median line, in the depression below the spinous process of the tenth thoracic vertebra. (Fig. 2-109)

Regional Anatomy: The posterior branch of the tenth intercostal artery. The medial branch of the posterior ramus of the tenth thoracic nerve.

Indications: (1) Jaundice, hiccup, vomiting, distention of the abdomen. (2) Stiffness and pain of the lumbar.

Needling Method: Oblique insertion upward 0.5—1.0 cun.

8. GV 8 (Jinsuo)

Location: On the back, on the posterior median line, in the depression below the spinous process of the ninth thoracic vertebra. (Fig. 2-109)

Regional Anatomy: The posterior branch of the ninth intercostal artery. The medial branch of the posterior ramus of the ninth thoracic nerve.

Indications: (1) Epilepsy. (2) Stiffness of the back. (3) Gastric pain.

Needling Method: Oblique insertion upward 0.5—1.0 cun.

9. GV 9 (Zhiyang)

Location: On the back, on the posterior median line, in the depression below the spinous process of the seventh thoracic vertebra. (Fig. 2-109)

Regional Anatomy: The posterior branch of the seventh intercostal artery. The medial branch of the posterior ramus of the seventh thoracic nerve.

Indications: (1) Acute gastric pain. (2) Jaundice. (3) Distention and pain in the chest and hypochondrium, cough, back pain.

Needling Method: Oblique insertion upward 0.5—1.0 cun.

10. GV 10 (Lingtai)

Location: On the back, on the posterior median line, in the depression below the spinous process of the sixth thoracic vertebra. (Fig. 2-109)

Regional Anatomy: The posterior branch of the sixth intercostal artery. The medial branch of the posterior ramus of the sixth thoracic nerve.

Indications: (1) Acute gastric pain. (2) Furuncles. (3) Cough, asthma, stiffness and pain of the back.

Needling Method: Oblique insertion upward 0.5—1.0 cun.

11. GV 11 (Shendao)

Location: On the back, on the posterior median line, in the depression below the spinous process of the fifth thoracic vertebra. (Fig. 2-109)

Regional Anatomy: The posterior branch of the fifth intercostal artery. The medial branch of the posterior ramus of the fifth thoracic nerve.

Indications: (1) Palpitations, cardiac pain, insomnia, poor memory. (2) Coughing, choking. (3) Stiffness and pain of the back.

Needling Method: Oblique insertion upward 0.5—1.0 cun.

12. GV 12 (Shenzhu)

Location: On the back, on the posterior median line, in the depression below the spinous process of the third thoracic vertebra. (Fig. 2-109)

Regional Anatomy: The posterior branch of the third intercostal artery. The medial branch of the posterior ramus of the third thoracic nerve.

Indications: (1) Cough, asthma. (2) Epilepsy. (3) Back stiffness and pain.

Needling Method: Oblique insertion upward 0.5—1.0 cun.

13. GV 13 (Taodao)

Classification: The Crossing Point of Governor Vessel and Bladder Meridian.

Location: On the back, on the posterior median line, in the depression below the spinous process of the first thoracic vertebra. (Fig. 2-109)

Regional Anatomy: The posterior branch of the first intercostal artery. The medial branch of the posterior ramus of the first thoracic nerve.

Indications: (1) Febrile diseases, malaria. (2) Headache, stiffness of the back.

Needling Method: Oblique insertion upward 0.5—1.0 cun.

14. GV 14 (Dazhui)

Classification: The Crossing Point of the Three Yang Meridians of Hand and the Three Yang Meridians of Foot.

Location: On the posterior median line, in the depression below the spinous process of the seventh cervical vertebra. (Fig. 2-109)

Regional Anatomy: The branch of the transverse cervical artery. The posterior ramus of the eighth cervical nerve.

Indications: (1) Febrile diseases, malaria, hectic fever and night sweat. (2) Aversion to cold, common cold, redness, swelling and pain of the eye, neck rigidity and pain. (3) Epilepsy. (4) Cough.

Needling Method: Oblique insertion upward 0.5—1.0 cun.

15. GV 15 (Yamen)

Classification: The Crossing Point of Governor Vessel and Yang Link Vessel.

Location: On the back of the neck, 0.5 cun directly above the midpoint of the posterior hairline, below the spinous process of the first cervical vertebra. (Fig. 2-110)

Regional Anatomy: The branches of the occipital artery and vein. The third occipital nerve.

Indications: (1) Lack of vitality caused by emotional disturbance. (2) Deafness and mute. (3) Apoplexy, stiffness of the tongue and aphasia, sudden hoarseness of voice. (4) Manic psychosis, epilepsy. (5) Occipital headache, neck rigidity. (6) Epistaxis.

Needling Method: Perpendicular or oblique insertion downward 0.5— 1.0 cun, do not puncture obliquely upward or deep. Deeper is the medulla oblongata; strict attention must be paid to the needle angle and depth.

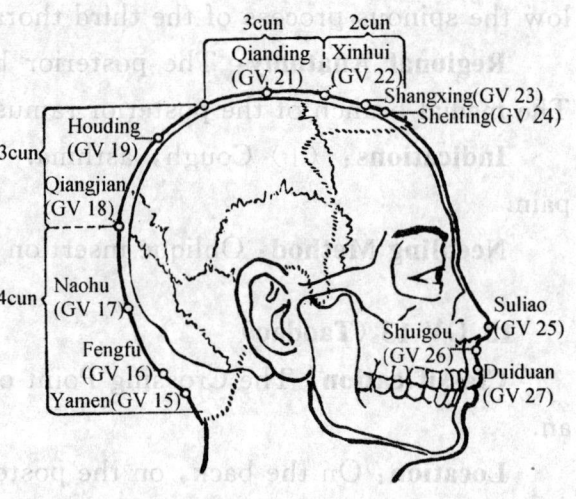

Fig. 2-110

16. GV 16 (Fengfu)

Classification: The Crossing Point of Governor Vessel and Yang Link Vessel.

Location: On the back of the neck, 1.0 cun directly above the midpoint of the posterior hairline, directly below the external occipital protuberance, in the depression between m. trapezius of both sides. (Fig. 2-110)

Regional Anatomy: Same as GV 15 (Yamen).

Indications: (1) Post-apoplexy aphasia, hemiplegia, manic psychosis. (2) Neck pain and rigidity, vertigo, sore throat.

Needling Method: Perpendicular or oblique insertion downward 0.5-.0 cun, do not puncture deeply. Deeper is the medulla oblongata; attention should be given to needling method.

17. GV 17 (Naohu)

Classification: The Crossing Point of Governor Vessel and Bladder Meridian.

Location: On the head, 2.5 cun directly above the midpoint of the posterior hairline, 1.5 cun above GV 16 (Fengfu), in the depression superior to the external occipital protuberance. (Fig. 2-110)

Regional Anatomy: The branches of the occipital arteries and veins of both sides. The branch of the greater occipital nerve.

Indications: (1) Dizziness, neck rigidity. (2) Epilepsy.

Needling Method: Subcutaneous insertion 0.5-0.8 cun.

18. GV 18 (Qiangjian)

Location: On the head, 4.0 cun directly above the midpoint of the posterior hairline, 1.5 cun above GV 17 (Naohu). (Fig. 2-110)

Regional Anatomy: Same as GV 17 (Naohu).

Indications: (1) Headache, vertigo. (2) Manic psychosis, epilepsy. (3) Apoplexy, hemiplegia.

Needling Method: Subcutaneous insertion 0.5—0.8 cun.

19. GV 19 (Houding)

Location: On the head, 5.5 cun directly above the midpoint of the posterior hairline, 3.0 cun above GV 17 (Naohu). (Fig. 2-110)

Regional Anatomy: Same as GV 17 (Naohu).

Indications: (1) Headache, vertigo. (2) Manic psychosis, epilepsy. (3) Apoplexy, hemiplegia.

Needling Method: Subcutaneous insertion 0.5—0.8 cun.

20. GV 20 (Baihui)

Classification: The Crossing Point of Governor Vessel and Bladder Meridian.

Location: On the head, 5.0 cun directly above the midpoint of the anterior hairline. Or, at the midpoint of the line connecting the apexes of the two auricles. (Fig. 2-110)

Regional Anatomy: The anastomotic network formed by the superficial temporal arteries and veins and the occipital arteries and veins on both sides. The branch of the major occipital nerve.

Indications: (1) Vertigo, dizziness. (2) Coma, apoplexy, hemiplegia, aphasia. (3) Prolapse of rectum, prolapse of uterus. (4) Manic psychosis, insomnia.

Needling Method: Subcutaneous insertion 0.5—0.8 cun.

21. GV 21 (Qianding)

Location: On the head, 3.5 cun directly above the midpoint of the anterior hairline, 1.5 cun anterior to GV 20 (Baihui). (Fig. 2-110)

Regional Anatomy: Same as GV 20 (Baihui).

Indications: (1) Headache, vertigo. (2) Rhinorrhea. (3) Apoplexy, hemiplegia, epilepsy.

Needling Method: Subcutaneous insertion 0.5—0.8 cun.

22. GV 22 (Xinhui)

Location: On the head, 2.0 cun directly above the midpoint of the anterior hairline, 3.0 cun anterior to GV 20 (Baihui). (Fig. 2-110)

Regional Anatomy: The anastomotic network formed by the superficial temporal artery and vein and the frontal artery and vein. The branch of the frontal nerve.

Indications: (1) Headache, vertigo. (2) Rhinorrhea. (3) Epilepsy. (4) Infantile convulsion.

Needling Method: Subcutaneous insertion 0.5—0.8 cun. Acupuncture is contraindicated in infants with unclosure of fontanel.

23. GV 23 (Shangxing)

Location: On the head, 1.0 cun directly above the midpoint of the anterior hairline. (Fig. 2-110)

Regional Anatomy: The branches of the frontal artery and vein. The branch of the frontal nerve.

Indications: (1) Headache, eye pain. (2) Rhinorrhea, epistaxis. (3) Manic psychosis. (4) Apoplexy, hemiplegia.

Needling Method: Subcutaneous insertion 0.5—1.0 cun.

24. GV 24 (Shenting)

Classification: The Crossing Point of Governor Vessel, Bladder Meridian and Stomach Meridian.

Location: On the head, 0.5 cun directly above the midpoint of the anterior hairline. (Fig. 2-110)

Regional Anatomy: Same as GV 23 (Shangxing).

Indications: (1) Insomnia, palpitation, epilepsy. (2) Headache, vertigo.

(3) Rhinorrhea.

Needling Method: Subcutaneous insertion 0.5—0.8 cun.

25. GV 25 (Suliao)

Location: On the region of the face, on the tip of the nose. (Fig. 2-110)

Regional Anatomy: The lateral nasal branches of the facial artery and vein. The branch of the ophthalmic nerve.

Indications: (1) Loss of consciousness, coma, asphyxia neonatorum. (2) Nasal congestion, epistaxis, rhinorrhea, rosacea. (3) Distention and pain in the eye, blurring of vision. (4) Heel pain.

Needling Method: Oblique insertion upward 0.3—0.5 cun.

26. GV 26 (Shuigou)

Classification: The Crossing Point of Governor Vessel, Large Intestine Meridian and Stomach Meridian.

Location: On the face, at the junction of the superior one-third and middle one-third of the philtrum. (Fig. 2-110)

Regional Anatomy: The superior labial artery and vein. The buccal branch of the facial nerve, and the branch of the infraorbital nerve.

Indications: (1) Syncope, heatstroke, coma, mental disorders, trismus. This point is used for emergency treatment. (2) Manic psychosis, epilepsy. (3) Acute lumbar pain. (4) Gastric pain, wry mouth, swelling of the face.

Needling Method: Oblique insertion upward 0.3—0.5 cun.

27. GV 27 (Duiduan)

Location: On the face, at the tip of the upper lip, where the skin of the philtrum and the upper lip join. (Fig. 2-110)

Regional Anatomy: Same as GV 26 (Shuigou).

Indications: (1) Manic psychosis. (2) Swelling and pain of the gums, wry mouth.

Needling Method: Oblique insertion upward 0.2—0.3 cun.

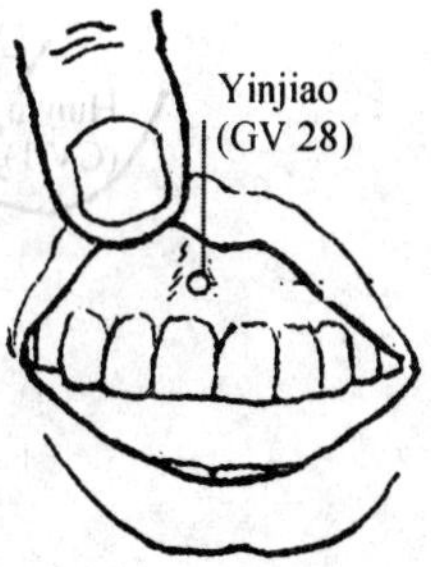

28. GV 28 (Yinjiao)

Location: On the inside of the upper lip, at the junction of the frenulum of the upper lip and the gum. (Fig. 2-111)

Fig. 2-111

Regional Anatomy: The superior labial artery and vein. The branch of the superior alveolar nerve.

Indications: (1) Acute lumbar pain. (2) Bleeding hemorrhoids, hemorrhoid pain. (3) Swelling and pain of the gums. (4) Rhinorrhea. (5) Manic psychosis.

Needling Method: Oblique insertion upward 0.2—0.3 cun, or prick to cause bleeding.

Section 14 The Acupuncture Points of Conception Vessel

This meridian appears at CV 1 (Huiyin) and ends at CV 24 (Chengjiang); consisting of a total of 24 acupuncture points. (Fig. 2-112)

1. CV 1 (Huiyin)

Classification: The Crossing Point of Conception Vessel, Governor Vessel and Thoroughfare Vessel.

Location: On the perineum, at the midpoint between the root of the scrotum and the anus in males, and at the midpoint between the posterior labial commissure and the anus in females. (Fig. 2-112)

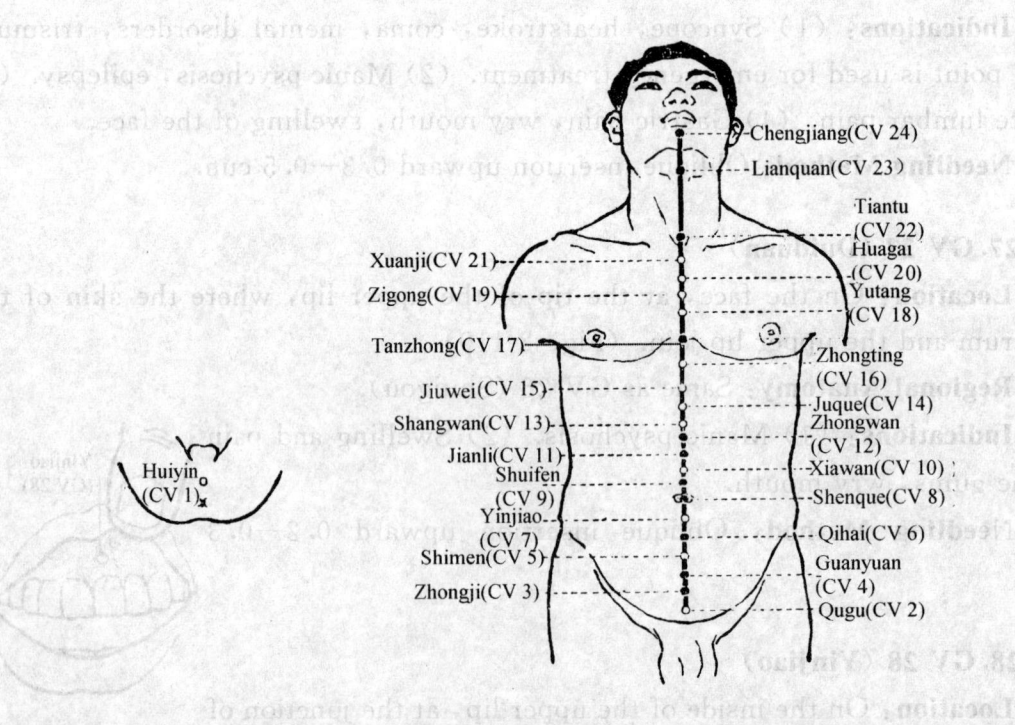

Fig. 2-112 The Points of the Ren Meridian

Regional Anatomy: The branches of the perineal artery and vein. The branch of the perineal nerve.

Indications: (1) Constipation and dysuria, or incontinence of feces and urine, hemorrhoids, prolapse of rectum. (2) Spermatorrhea, impotence, pruritus vulva. (3) Asphyxiation from drowning, loss of consciousness, manic psychosis.

Needling Method: Perpendicular insertion 0.5—1.0 cun.

2. CV 2 (Qugu)

Classification: The Crossing Point of Conception Vessel and Liver Meridian.

Location: On the anterior median line of the lower abdomen, at the midpoint of the upper border of the symphysis pubis. (Fig. 2-113)

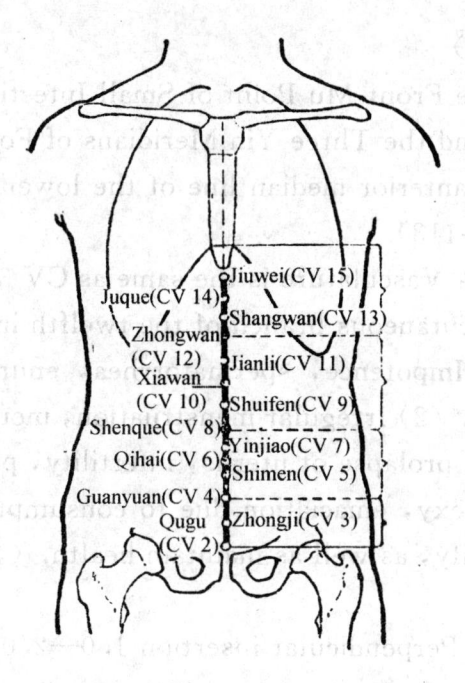

Fig. 2-113

Regional Anatomy: The branch of the inferior epigastric artery. The branch of the iliohypogastric nerve.

Indications: (1) Dysuria, enuresis. (2) Spermatorrhea, impotence. (3) Irregular menstruation, leukorrhea.

Needling Method: Perpendicular insertion 1.0—1.5 cun.

3. CV 3 (Zhongji)

Classification: The Front-Mu Point of Bladder. The Crossing Point of Conception Vessel and the Three Yin Meridians of Foot.

Location: On the anterior median line of the lower abdomen, 4 cun below the umbilicus. (Fig. 2-113)

Regional Anatomy: The branches of the superficial epigastric artery and vein, and the branches of the inferior epigastric artery and vein. The branch of the iliohypogastric nerve.

Indications: (1) Enuresis, dysuria. (2) Spermatorrhea, impotence. (3) Irregular menstruation, metrorrhagia, leukorrhea, prolapse of uterus, infertility. (4) Hernia.

Needling Method: Perpendicular insertion 1.0—1.5 cun.

4. CV 4 (Guanyuan)

Classification: The Front-Mu Point of Small Intestine. The Crossing Point of Conception Vessel and the Three Yin Meridians of Foot.

Location: On the anterior median line of the lower abdomen, 3 cun below the umbilicus. (Fig. 2-113)

Regional Anatomy: Vasculature is the same as CV 3 (Zhongji). The medial branch of the anterior cutaneous branch of the twelfth intercostal nerve.

Indications: (1) Impotence, spermatorrhea, enuresis, frequent micturition, retention of urine. (2) Irregular menstruation, metrorrhagia, morbid leukorrhea, dysmenorrhea, prolapse of uterus, infertility, postpartum hemorrhage. (3) Flaccidity of apoplexy, emaciation due to consumptive disease. This point has the function to tonify, as well as maintain health. (4) Diarrhea, prolapse of rectum, dyspepsia.

Needling Method: Perpendicular insertion 1.0—2.0 cun.

5. CV 5 (Shimen)

Classification: The Front-Mu Point of Triple Energizer.

Location: On the anterior median line of the lower abdomen, 2 cun below the umbilicus. (Fig. 2-113)

Regional Anatomy: Vasculature is the same as CV 3 (Zhongji). The anterior cutaneous branch of the eleventh intercostal nerve.

Indications: (1) Dysuria, edema. (2) Hernia, abdominal pain, diarrhea.

(3) Amenorrhea, morbid leukorrhea, metrorrhagia.

Needling Method: Perpendicular insertion 1.0—2.0 cun.

6. CV 6 (Qihai)

Location: On the anterior median line of the lower abdomen, 1.5 cun below the umbilicus. (Fig. 2-113)

Regional Anatomy: Vasculature and innervation are the same as CV 5 (Shimen).

Indications: (1) Abdominal pain, diarrhea, constipation. (2) Enuresis. (3) Hernia. (4) Spermatorrhea, impotence. (5) Irregular menstruation, amenorrhea. (6) Emaciation due to comsumptive disease. This point has the function to tonify, as well as maintain health.

Needling Method: Perpendicular insertion 1.0—2.0 cun.

7. CV 7 (Yinjiao)

Classification: The Crossing Point of Conception Vessel and Thoroughfare Vessel.

Location: On the anterior median line of the lower abdomen, 1 cun below the umbilicus. (Fig. 2-113)

Regional Anatomy: Same as CV 5 (Shimen).

Indications: (1) Dysuria, edema. (2) Hernia, abdominal pain. (3) Irregular menstruation, morbid leukorrhea, metrorrhagia, pruritus vulva, postpartum hemorrhage.

Needling Method: Perpendicular insertion 1.0—2.0 cun.

8. CV 8 (Shenque)

Location: In the middle of the abdomen, in the center of the umbilicus. (Fig. 2-113)

Regional Anatomy: The inferior epigastric artery and vein. The anterior cutaneous branch of the tenth intercostal nerve.

Indications: (1) Flaccidity of apoplexy, coldness of the four extremities. (2) Chronic diarrhea, hemihydrosis. (3) Edema.

Needling Method: Indirect moxibustion with moxa stick, or moxibustion on some type of material (salt, ginger, etc.).

9. CV 9 (Shuifen)

Location: On the anterior median line of the upper abdomen, 1 cun above the umbilicus. (Fig. 2-113)

Regional Anatomy: Vasculature are the same as CV 8 (Shenque). The anterior cutaneous branches of the eighth and ninth intercostal nerve.

Indications: (1) Edema, retention of urine. (2) Abdominal pain, diarrhea, regurgitation of food from stomach.

Needling Method: Perpendicular insertion 0.5—1.0 cun.

10. CV 10 (Xiawan)

Classification: The Crossing Point of Conception Vessel and Bladder Meridian.

Location: On the anterior median line of the upper abdomen, 2 cun above the umbilicus. (Fig. 2-113)

Regional Anatomy: Vasculature is the same as CV 8 (Shenque). The anterior cutaneous branch of the eighth intercostal nerve.

Indications: (1) Epigastric pain, abdominal distention, diarrhea, vomiting, hiccup.

Needling Method: Perpendicular insertion 1.0—2.0 cun.

11. CV 11 (Jianli)

Location: On the anterior median line of the upper abdomen, 3 cun above the umbilicus. (Fig. 2-113)

Regional Anatomy: The branches of the superior and inferior epigastric arteries. The anterior cutaneous branch of the eighth intercostal nerve.

Indications: (1) Gastric pain, vomiting. (2) Anorexia. (3) Abdominal distention, borborygmus.

Needling Method: Perpendicular insertion 1.0—2.0 cun.

12. CV 12 (Zhongwan)

Classification: The Front-Mu Point of Stomach. The Converging Point of the Fu-Organs. The Crossing Point of Conception Vessel, Small Intestine Meridian, Triple Energizer Meridian and Stomach Meridian.

Location: On the anterior median line of the upper abdomen, 4 cun above the umbilicus. (Fig. 2-113)

Regional Anatomy: The superior epigastric artery and vein. The anterior cutaneous branch of the eighth intercostal nerve.

Indications: (1) Epigastric pain, vomiting, hiccup, acid regurgitation. (2) Abdominal distention, diarrhea, dyspepsia. (3) Cough, copious phlegm. (4) Jaundice. (5) Insomnia.

Needling Method: Perpendicular insertion 1.0—1.5 cun.

13. CV 13 (Shangwan)

Classification: The Crossing Point of Conception Vessel, Stomach Meridian and Small Intestine Meridian.

Location: On the anterior median line of the upper abdomen, 5 cun above the umbilicus. (Fig. 2-113)

Regional Anatomy: Same as CV 12 (Zhongwan).

Indications: (1) Gastric pain, vomiting, abdominal distention. (2) Epilepsy.

Needling Method: Perpendicular insertion 1.0—1.5 cun.

14. CV 14 (Juque)

Classification: The Front-Mu Point of Heart.

Location: On the anterior median line of the upper abdomen, 6 cun above the umbilicus. (Fig. 2-113)

Regional Anatomy: Internally, the upper border of the liver, and the pylorus. Vasculature and innervation are the same as CV 12 (Zhongwan).

Indications: (1) Pain in the cardiac region and chest, palpitation. (2) Manic psychosis, epilepsy. (3) Gastric pain, vomiting.

Needling Method: Oblique insertion downward 0.5—1.0 cun.

15. CV 15 (Jiuwei)

Classification: The Luo-(Connecting) Point of Conception Vessel.

Location: On the anterior median line of the upper abdomen, 1 cun below the xiphisternal synchondroses. (Fig. 2-113)

Regional Anatomy: Same as CV 12 (Zhongwan).

Indications: (1) Manic depression, epilepsy. (2) Chest pain, palpitation, abdominal distention.

Needling Method: Oblique insertion downward 0.4—0.6 cun.

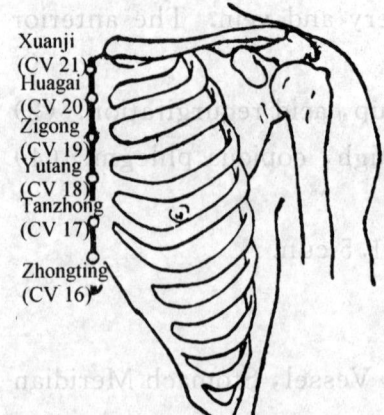

Xuanji (CV 21)
Huagai (CV 20)
Zigong (CV 19)
Yutang (CV 18)
Tanzhong (CV 17)
Zhongting (CV 16)

Fig. 2-114

16. CV 16 (Zhongting)

Location: On the anterior median line of the chest, at the level of the fifth intercostal space, near the xiphisternal synchondroses. (Fig. 2-114)

Regional Anatomy: The anterior perforating branches of the internal mammary artery and vein. The anterior cutaneous branch of the sixth intercostal nerve.

Indications: (1) Distention and fullness in the chest and costal region, cardiac pain. (2) Vomiting, infantile milk regurgitation.

Needling Method: Subcutaneous insertion 0.3—0.5 cun.

17. CV 17 (Tanzhong)

Classification: The Front-Mu Point of Pericardium. The Converging Point of Qi.

Location: On the anterior median line of the chest, at the level of the fourth intercostal space, at the midpoint between the two nipples. (Fig. 2-114)

Regional Anatomy: Vasculature same as CV 16 (Zhongting). The anterior cutaneous branch of the fourth intercostal nerve.

Indications: (1) Asthma, pain and oppression of the chest. (2) Cardiac pain, palpitation. (3) Insufficient lactation, hiccup, dysphagia.

Needling Method: Subcutaneous insertion 0.3—0.5 cun.

18. CV 18 (Yutang)

Location: On the anterior median line of the chest, at the level of the third intercostal space. (Fig. 2-114)

Regional Anatomy: Vasculature same as CV 16 (Zhongting). The anterior cutaneous branch of the third intercostal nerve.

Indications: (1) Cough, asthma. (2) Chest pain, pain of the breast.

Needling Method: Subcutaneous insertion 0.3—0.5 cun.

19. CV 19 (Zigong)

Location: On the anterior median line of the chest, at the level of the second intercostal space. (Fig. 2-114)

Regional Anatomy: Vasculature is the same as CV 16 (Zhongting). The anterior cutaneous branch of the second intercostal nerve.

Indications: Cough, asthma, chest pain.

Needling Method: Subcutaneous insertion 0.3—0.5 cun.

20. CV 20 (Huagai)

Location: On the anterior median line of the chest, at the level of the first intercostal space. (Fig. 2-114)

Regional Anatomy: Vasculature is the same as CV 16 (Zhongting). The anterior cutaneous branch of the first intercostal nerve.

Indications: Cough, asthma, distention and pain in the chest and hypochondrium.

Needling Method: Subcutaneous insertion 0.3—0.5 cun.

21. CV 21 (Xuanji)

Location: On the anterior median line of the chest, 1 cun below CV 22 (Tiantu). (Fig. 2-114)

Regional Anatomy: Vasculature is the same as CV 16 (Zhongting). The anterior cutaneous branch of the supraclavicular nerve.

Indications: (1) Cough, asthma. (2) Chest pain, sore throat.

Needling Method: Subcutaneous insertion 0.3—0.5 cun.

22. CV 22 (Tiantu)

Classification: The Crossing Point of Conception Vessel and Yin Link Vessel.

Location: On the anterior median line of the neck, in the center of the suprasternal fossa. (Fig. 2-115)

Regional Anatomy: Subcutaneously, the jugular venous arch and the branch of the inferior thyroid artery; deeper, the trachea; inferiorly, at the posterior aspect of the sternum, the innominate vein and the aortic arch. The anterior branch of the supraclavicular nerve.

Indications: (1) Cough, asthma, chest pain. (2) Sore throat, sudden hoarseness of the voice,

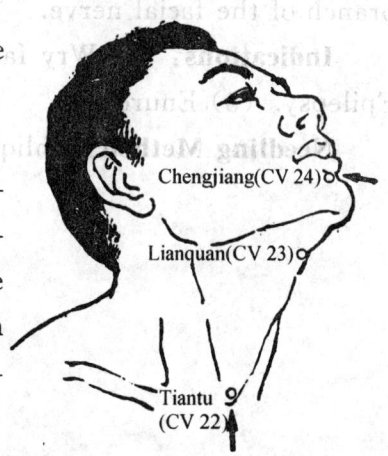

Fig. 2-115

goiter. (3) Plum pit sensation in the throat, dysphagia.

Needling Method: First, puncture perpendicularly 0.2 cun, then insert the needle tip downward along the posterior aspect of the sternum 1.0—1.5 cun. Strict attention must be paid to the needle angle and depth; the lung can easily be injured.

23. CV 23 (Lianquan)

Classification: The Crossing Point of Conception Vessel and Yin Link Vessel.

Location: On the anterior median line of the neck, above the throat prominence, in the depression above the upper border of the hyoid bone. (Fig. 2-115)

Regional Anatomy: The anterior jugular vein. The branches of the hypoglossal nerve and the glossopharyngeal nerve.

Indications: Swelling and pain of the subglossal region, salivation with flaccid tongue, aphasia with stiffness of tongue, sudden hoarseness of the voice, difficulty in swallowing.

Needling Method: Oblique insertion toward tongue root 0.5—0.8 cun.

24. CV 24 (Chengjiang)

Classification: The Crossing Point of Conception Vessel and Stomach Meridian.

Location: On the region of the face, in the depression in the center of the mentolabial groove. (Fig. 2-115)

Regional Anatomy: The branches of the inferior labial artery and vein. The branch of the facial nerve.

Indications: (1) Wry face, swelling and pain of the gums, salivation. (2) Epilepsy. (3) Enuresis.

Needling Method: Oblique insertion 0.3—0.5 cun.

Chapter 4
Extraordinary Points

Section 1 Region of the Head and Neck

1. EX-HN 1 (Sishencong)

Location: At the vertex of the head, a group of four points, 1 cun respectively anterior, posterior and lateral to GV 20 (Baihui). (Fig. 2-116)

Regional Anatomy: The anastomotic network formed by the occipital artery and vein, the parietal branches of the superficial temporal artery and vein, and the supraorbital artery and vein. The branches of the greater occipital nerve, the auriculotemporal nerve and the supraorbital nerve.

Indications: (1) Headache, vertigo. (2) Insomnia, poor memory. (3) Epilepsy.

Needling Method: Subcutaneous insertion 0.5—0.8 cun.

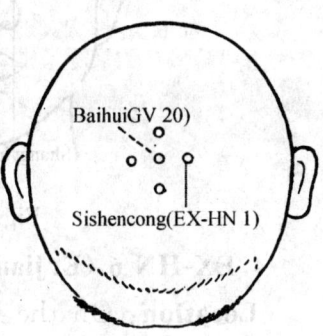

Fig. 2-116

2. EX-HN 3 (Yintang)

Location: On the forehead, at the midpoint between the two medial ends of the eyebrow. (Fig. 2-117)

Regional Anatomy: The branches of the medial frontal artery and vein. The supratrochlear nerve.

Indications: (1) Headache, heavy sensation of the head, vertigo. (2) Rhinorrhea, epistaxis. (3) Infantile convulsion. (4) Insomnia.

Needling Method: Subcutaneous insertion 0.3—0.5 cun.

3. EX-HN 5 (Taiyang)

Location: In the region of the temples, in the depression about one fingerbreadth posterior to the midpoint between the lateral end of the eyebrow and the outer canthus. (Fig. 2-118)

Regional Anatomy: The superficial temporal artery and vein. The second and third branches of the trigeminal nerve, the temporal branch of the facial nerve.

Indications: (1) Headache, redness, swelling and pain of the eye. (2) Toothache, facial pain.

Needling Method: Perpendicular or oblique insertion 0.3—0.5 cun, or prick to cause bleeding.

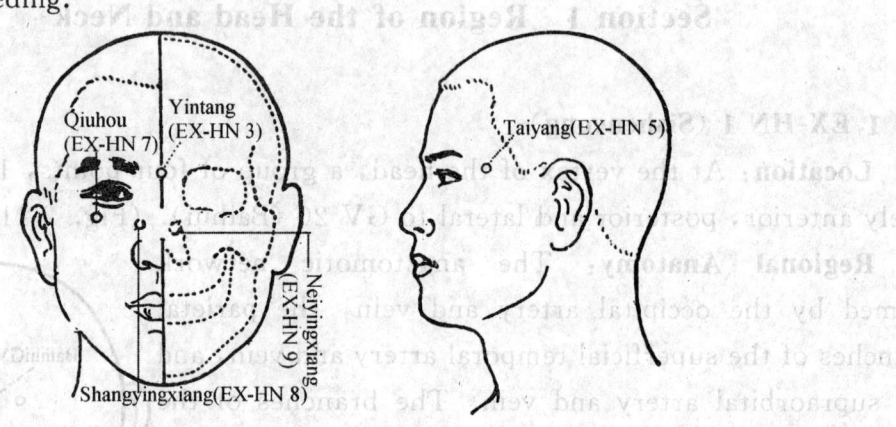

Fig. 2-117   Fig. 2-118

4. EX-HN 6 (Erjian)

Location: On the top region of the auricle, fold the auricle forward, the point is at the apex of the auricle. (Fig. 2-119)

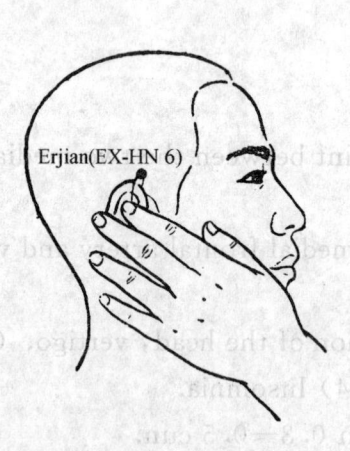

Fig. 2-119 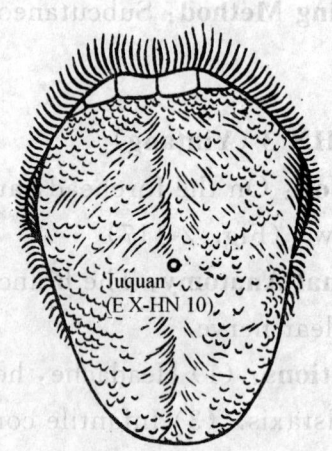   Fig. 2-120

Regional Anatomy: The artery and vein posterior to the auricle, the auriculotemporal nerve.

Indications: (1) Redness, swelling and pain of the eye, nebula, blurring of vision. (2) Spontaneous sweating, palpitation.

Needling Method: Prick to cause bleeding.

5. EX-HN 7 (Qiuhou)

Location: On the region of the face, at the junction of the lateral one-fourth and the medial three-fourths of the infraorbital margin. (Fig. 2-117)

Regional Anatomy: Deeper, the eye muscle. Superficial, the facial artery and vein. Deeper, the oculomotor nerve and the optic nerve.

Indications: Eye diseases such as optic neuritis, optic atrophy, pigmentary degeneration of retina, glaucoma, early stage of cataract, myopia.

Needling Method: Pushing the eyeball upward gently, perpendicularly insert the needle slowly 0.5—1.5 cun along the orbital margin; do not lift and thrust or rotate the needle. Moxibustion is contraindicated.

6. EX-HN 8 (Shangyingxiang)

Location: On the region of the face, at the junction of the cartilage of the ala nasi and the nasal concha, near the upper end of the nasolabial groove. (Fig. 2-117)

Regional Anatomy: The branches of the facial artery and vein. The preganglionic nerves.

Indications: Rhinorrhea, soreness and furuncle in the nasal region.

Needling Method: Subcutaneous insertion medially upward 0.3—0.5 cun.

7. EX-HN 9 (Neiyingxiang)

Location: Inside of the nostrils, on the mucosa membrane at the junction of the cartilage of the ala nasi and the nasal concha. (Fig. 2-117)

Regional Anatomy: On the mucosa membrane in the nasal cavity. The dorsal nasal branches of the facial artery and vein. The lateral nasal branch of the preganglionic nerve.

Indications: Redness, swelling and pain of the eye.

Needling Method: Prick the nasal mucosa membrane to let out 10—15 drops of blood.

8. EX-HN 10 (Juquan)

Location: In the mouth, at the midpoint on the median line of the dorsum of the tongue. (Fig. 2-120)

Regional Anatomy: The lingual artery. The branch of the third branch of the trigeminal nerve, the lingual nerve.

Indications: (1) Stiffness of the tongue, flaccidity of the tongue, diabetes. (2) Asthma. (3) Taste sensitivity reduced.

Needling Method: Stablize the tongue, then perpendicularly insert 0.1—0.2 cun; or use a three-edged needle, prick to cause bleeding. *Compendium of Acupuncture and Moxibustion* says:" If use moxibustion; generally, do not burn more than seven cones. Moxibustion method: using a fresh ginger slice, cut to the thickness of a coin, place on the point on top of the tongue and burn. When finished with moxibustion, to clear up ginger taste thoroughly chew tea leaves and ginger and swallow. To treat an abnormal tongue coating or stiffness of the tongue, use a small needle to cause bleeding."

9. EX-HN 12 (Jinjin)

Location: In the mouth, on the vein under the tongue on the left side of the frenulum of the tongue. (Fig. 2-121)

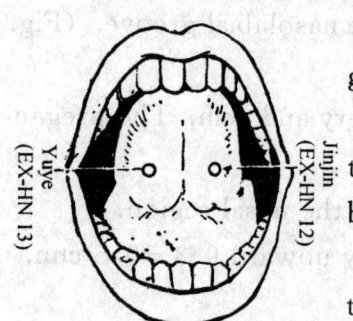

Regional Anatomy: The sublingual vein. The lingual nerve and the hypoglossal nerve.

Indications: (1) Ulcers in the mouth and on the tongue, swelling of the tongue. (2) Vomiting, diabetes.

Needling Method: Stablize the tongue, then prick to cause bleeding. Do not use moxibustion.

Fig. 2-121

10. EX-HN 13 (Yuye)

Location: In the mouth, on the vein under the tongue on the right side of the frenulum of the tongue. (Fig. 2-121)

Regional Anatomy: Same as EX-HN 12 (Jinjin).

Indications: Same as EX-HN 12 (Jinjin).

Needling Method: Same as EX-HN 12 (Jinjin).

11. EX-HN 14 (Yiming)

Location: On the neck, 1 cun posterior to TE 17 (Yifeng). (Fig. 2-122)

Regional Anatomy: The posterior auricular artery and vein. The great auricular nerve and the lesser occipital nerve.

Indications: (1) Eye diseases. (Myopia, hyperopia, night blindness, optic atrophy, early stage of cataract.) (2) Tinnitus, deafness. (3) Insomnia.

Needling Method: Perpendicular insertion 0.5—1.0 cun.

12. EX-HN 15 (Jingbailao)

Location: On the neck, 2 cun above GV 14 (Dazhui), 1 cun lateral to the posterior median line. (Fig. 2-122)

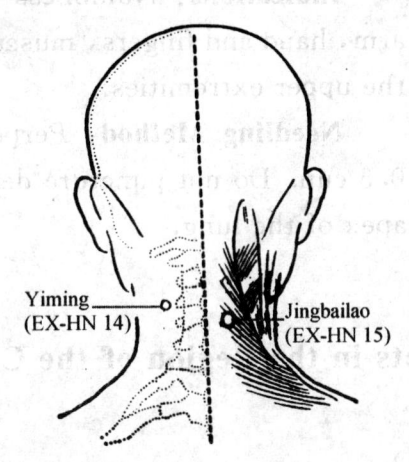

Fig. 2-122

Regional Anatomy: The occipital artery and vein and the vertebral artery and vein. The branches of the greater and lesser occipital nerves.

Indications: (1) Steaming bone hectic fever, night sweating, spontaneous sweating. (2) Scrofula. (3) Swelling of the pharynx, cough. (4) Stiffness and pain of the neck.

Needling Method: Perpendicular insertion 0.5—1.0 cun.

13. EX-HN (Shanglianquan)

Location: Sitting straight with the chin up and the head tilted back, the point is in the center of the upper region of the neck, in the depression between the lower border of the lower mandible and the hyoid bone. (Fig. 2-123)

Regional Anatomy: The lingual artery and vein. The hypoglossal nerve.

Indications: Stiffness of the tongue, mute, unclear speech, aphasia, salivation, sore throat, ulcers on the tongue.

Needling Method: Oblique insertion toward the tongue root 0.5—0.8 cun.

14. EX-HN (Jingbi)

Location: Lying in the supine position without using a pillow, have the patient turn his head to the side. The point is 1 cun directly above the junction of the medial one-third and lateral two-thirds of the clavicle, at the posterior border of the sternal head of m. sternocleidomastoideus. (Fig. 2-124)

Regional Anatomy: The branches of the external jugular artery and vein. The brachial nerve.

Indications: Numbness or pain of the shoulder, arm, hand and fingers, muscular atrophy, weakness of the upper extremities.

Needling Method: Perpendicular insertion 0.3—0.5 cun. Do not puncture deeply to avoid injuring the apex of the lung.

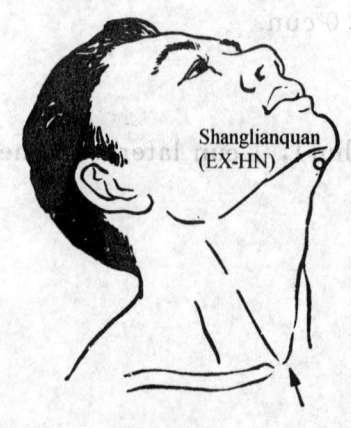

Fig. 2-123

Section 2 The Points in the Region of the Chest and Abdomen

1. EX-CA (Weishang)

Location: 2 cun above the umbilicus, 4 cun lateral to the anterior median line. (Fig. 2-125)

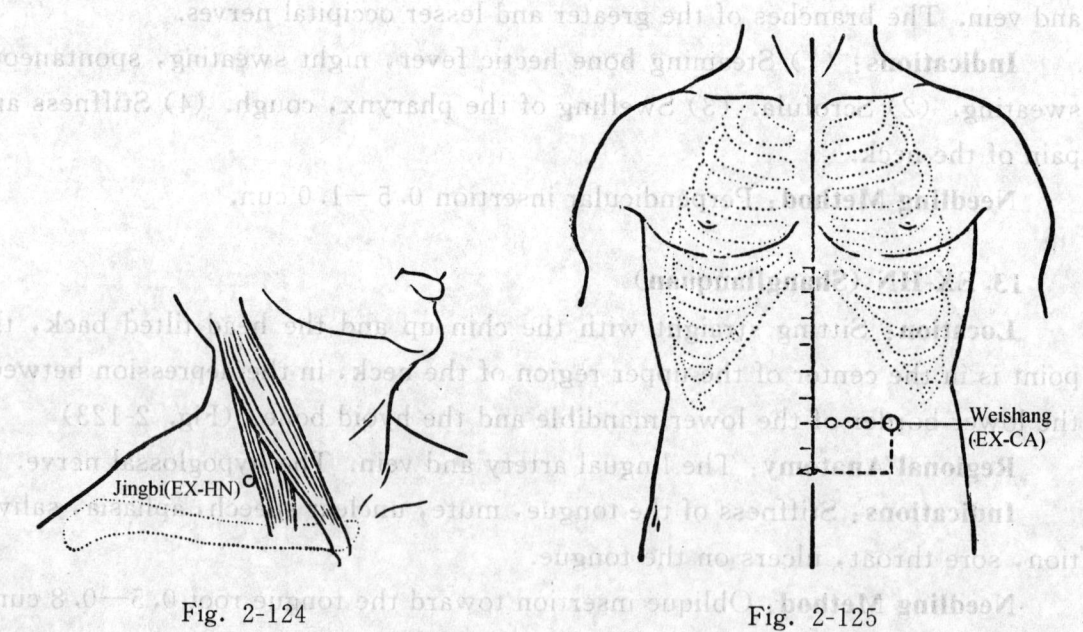

Fig. 2-124

Fig. 2-125

Regional Anatomy: The superficial epigastric vein. The lateral branches of the ninth and tenth intercostal nerves.

Indications: Gastroptosis, gastric pain, abdominal distention.

Needling Method: Oblique insertion toward the umbilicus or toward ST. 25

(Tianshu) 2.0—3.0 cun. Moxibustion is applicable.

2. EX-CA (Sanjiaojiu)

Location: Use the distance between the two corners of the mouth of the patient as the length of one side of an equilateral triangle. Place the apex of this equilateral triangle at the center of the umbilicus and the base line is horizontal. The points are located at the two bottom angles of the triangle. (Fig. 2-126)

Regional Anatomy: The muscular branches of the inferior epigastric artery and vein. The tenth intercostal nerve.

Indications: Hernia, borborygmus, pain around the umbilical region, infertility.

Needling Method: Moxibustion.

3. EX-CA (Liniaoxue)

Location: At the midpoint between CV 8 (Shenque) and the upper border of the symphysis pubis. (Fig. 2-127)

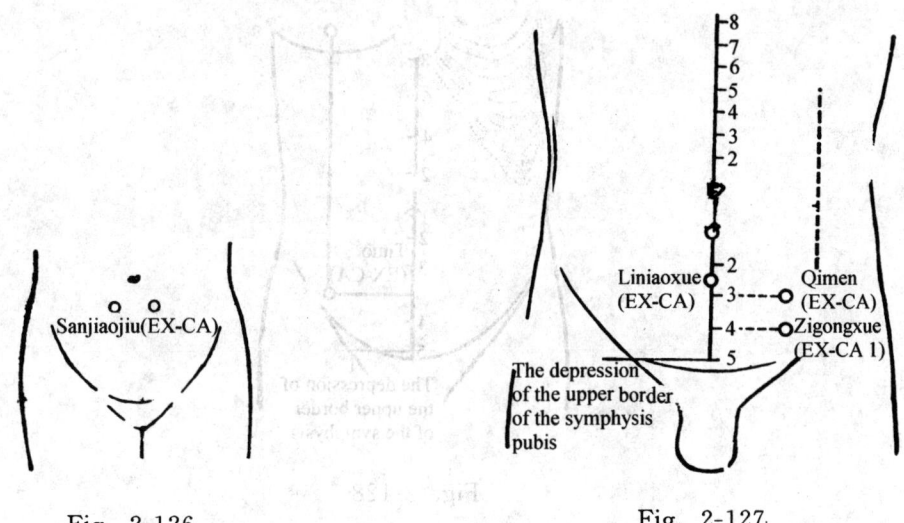

Fig. 2-126

Fig. 2-127

Regional Anatomy: The branches of the inferior epigastric artery and vein. The anterior cutaneous branch of the medial branch of the twelfth intercostal nerve.

Indications: Dysuria, dribbling of urine, hematuria, abdominal pain, diarrhea, prolapse of uterus, gastroptosis.

Needling Method: Perpendicular insertion 0.5—1.0 cun. Moxibustion or acupressure are applicable.

4. EX-CA (Qimen)

Location: 3 cun lateral to CV 4 (Guanyuan). (Fig. 2-127)

Regional Anatomy: Same as EX-CA (Liniaoxue.)

Indications: Infertility, prolonged lochia, metrorrhagia, dsyuria and other urinary disorders, lower abdominal pain.

Needling Method: Perpendicular insertion 0.5—1.0 cun. Moxibustion is applicable.

5. EX-CA (Tituo)

Location: 4 cun lateral to CV 4 (Guanyuan). (Fig. 2-128)

Regional Anatomy: The superficial circumflex iliac artery and vein. The iliohypogastric nerve.

Indications: Prolapse of uterus, dysmenorrhea, abdominal distention, hernia, renal ptosis.

Needling Method: Subcutaneous insertion toward 3.0—4.0 cun, or perpendicular insertion 0.5—1.0 cun. Moxibustion.

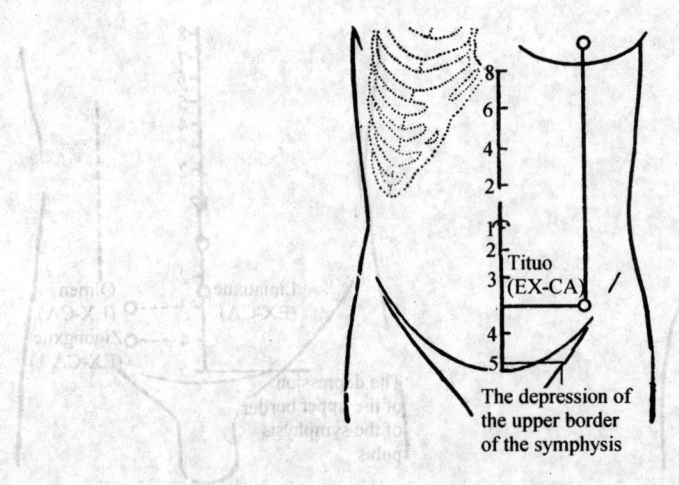

Fig. 2-128

6. EX-CA 1 (Zigongxue)

Location: On the lower abdomen, 4 cun below the umbilicus, 3 cun lateral to CV 3 (Zhongji). (Fig. 2-127)

Regional Anatomy: The superficial epigastric artery and vein. The iliohypogastric nerve.

Indications: (1) Prolapse of uterus, irregular menstruation, metrorrhagia, dysmenorrhea, amenorrhea, infertility. (2) Hernia, lumbar pain.

Needling Method: Perpendicular insertion 0.8—1.2 cun.

Section 3 The Points in the Region of the Back and Lumbar

1. EX-B 1 (Dingchuan)

Location: On the back, 0.5 cun lateral to the lower border of the spinous process of the seventh cervical vertebra. (Fig. 2-129)

Regional Anatomy: The transverse cervical artery and the branch of the superficial cervical artery. The posterior branches of the seventh and eighth cervical nerves.

Indications: (1) Asthma, cough, oppression of the chest, shortness of breath. (2) Sore throat.

Needling Method: Perpendicular insertion 0.5—0.8 cun.

2. EX-B 2 (Jiaji)

Location: On the back and lower back, 0.5 cun lateral to the lower border of each spinous process from the first thoracic vertebra to the fifth lumbar vertebra. One side has 17 points, both sides of the spinal column have a total of 34 points. (Fig. 2-129)

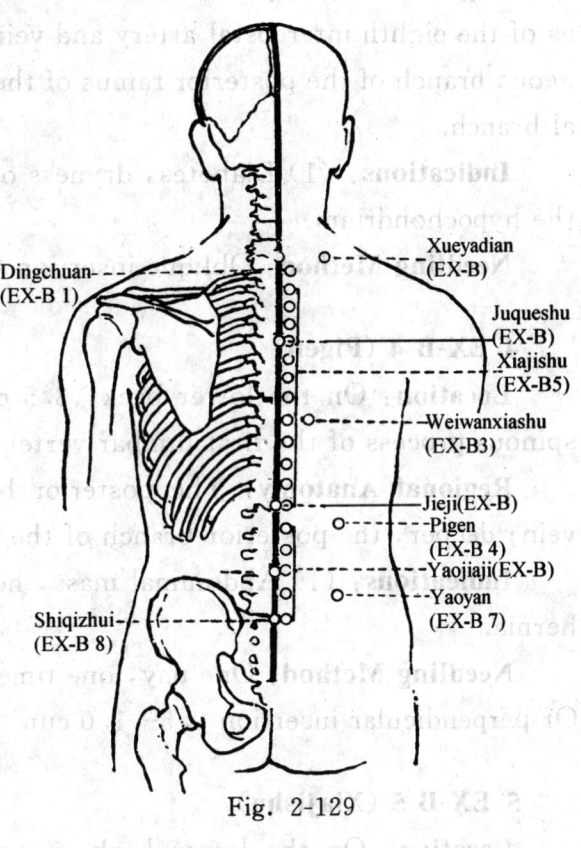

Fig. 2-129

Regional Anatomy: In the interspinous transverse ligaments and muscles. Each point has its related posterior branch of the spinal nerve starting from below the vertebra, and the accompanying artery and vein.

Indications: (1) The points on the upper portion of the thorax are used to treat diseases of the throat, heart, lung, and upper extremities. (2) The points on the lower portion of the thorax are used to treat diseases of the liver, gallbladder, spleen and stomach. (3) The points on the lumbar region are used to treat diseases of the urogenital system, the intestinal tract, the lumbosacral region and lower extremities.

Needling Method: Perpendicular insertion 0.3—0.5 cun, or use plum blossom needle for tapping.

3. EX-B 3 (Weiwanxiashu)

Other Names: Bashu, Yishu.

Location: On the back, 1.5 cun lateral to the lower border of the spinous process of the eighth thoracic vertebra. (Fig. 2-129)

Regional Anatomy: The medial cutaneous branches of the posterior branches of the eighth intercostal artery and vein. The distribution of the medial cutaneous branch of the posterior ramus of the first thoracic nerve; deeper, its lateral branch.

Indications: (1) Diabetes, dryness of the throat. (2) Gastric pain, pain in the hypochondrium.

Needling Method: Oblique insertion 0.3—0.5 cun.

4. EX-B 4 (Pigen)

Location: On the lower back, 3.5 cun lateral to the lower border of the spinous process of the first lumbar vertebra. (Fig. 2-129)

Regional Anatomy: The posterior branch of the first lumbar artery and vein; deeper, the posterior branch of the first lumbar nerve.

Indications: (1) Abdominal mass, hepatosplenomegaly. (2) Lumbar pain, hernia.

Needling Method: One day, one time; each time burn 10—20 moxa cones. Or perpendicular insertion 0.5—1.0 cun.

5. EX-B 5 (Xiajishu)

Location: On the lower back, on the posterior median line, below the spinous process of the third lumbar vertebra. (Fig. 2-129)

Regional Anatomy: The subcutaneous interspinal venous network. The medial branch of the posterior ramus of the lumbar nerve.

Indications: (1) Lumbar pain. (2) Abdominal pain, diarrhea.

Needling Method: Perpendicular insertion 0.5—1.0 cun.

6. EX-B 7 (Yaoyan)

Location: On the lower back, in the depression 3.5 cun lateral to the lower border of the spinous process of the fourth lumbar vertebra. (Fig. 2-129)

Regional Anatomy: The dorsal branches of the second lumbar artery and vein. The lateral branch of the first lumbar nerve.

Indications: (1) Lumbar pain, frequent micturition. (2) Emaciation due to consumptive disease. (3) Irregular menstruation, morbid leukorrhea.

Needling Method: Perpendicular insertion 1.5 cun.

7. EX-B 8 (Shiqizhui)

Location: On the lower back, on the posterior median line, below the spinous process of the fifth lumbar vertebra. (Fig. 2-129)

Regional Anatomy: The posterior branch of the lumbar artery, the subcutaneous interspinal venous network. The medial branch of the posterior ramus of the lumbar nerve.

Indications: (1) Pain of the lumbar region and leg, paralysis of the lower extremities. (2) Metrorrhagia, irregular menstruation.

Needling Method: Oblique insertion upward 1.0—1.5 cun.

8. EX-B (Xueyadian)

Location: The point is 2 cun lateral to the interspace between the spinous process of the sixth and seventh cervical vertebra, lateral to the posterior median line. (Fig. 2-129)

Regional Anatomy: The transverse cervical artery and the branch of the deep cervical artery. The posterior branch of the seventh cervical nerve.

Indications: Hypertension, hypotension.

Needling Method: Perpendicular insertion 0.5—1.0 cun. Moxibustion is applicable.

9. EX-B (Juqueshu)

Location: The point is in the depression between the spinous process of the fourth and fifth thoracic vertebra, on the posterior median line. (Fig. 2-129)

Regional Anatomy: The posterior branch of the fourth intercostal artery. The medial branch of the posterior ramus of the fourth intercostal nerve.

Indications: (1) Cardiac pain, insomnia. (2) Cough, asthma, pain of the chest and hypochondrium. (3) Pain of the shoulder and back.

Needling Method: Oblique insertion 0.5—1.0 cun. Moxibustion is applicable.

10. EX-B (Jieji)

Location: The point is in the depression between the spinous process of the twelfth thoracic vertebra and the first lumbar vertebra, on the posterior median line. (Fig. 2-129)

Regional Anatomy: The posterior branch of the twelfth intercostal artery. The medial branch of the posterior ramus of the twelfth intercostal nerve.

Indications: (1) Dysentery in children, prolapse of the rectum, abdominal pain, diarrhea, dyspepsia. (2) Epilepsy. (3) Hernia.

Needling Method: Oblique insertion 0.5—1.0 cun. Moxibustion is applicable.

Section 4 The Points in the Region of the Upper and Lower Extremities

1. EX-UE 1 (Zhoujian)

Location: On the posterior aspect of the elbow, with the elbow flexed, the point is on the tip of the ulnar olecranon. (Fig. 2-130)

Regional Anatomy: The arterial network of the elbow joint. The antebrachial cutaneous nerve.

Indications: (1) Scrofula, carbuncle and gangrene, furuncle, appendicitis. (2) Cholera.

Needling Method: Moxibustion is applicable.

Zhoujian(EX-UE)

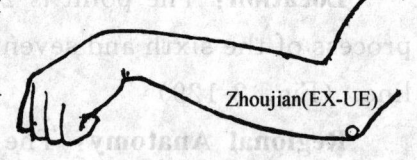

Fig. 2-130

2. EX-UE 2 (Erbai)

Location: On the palmar aspect of the forearm, 4 cun above the transverse crease of the wrist, on both sides of the tendon of m. flexor carpi radialis. Each side has one point, each arm has two points, both arms have a total of four points. (Fig. 2-131)

Regional Anatomy: The anterior interosseous artery and vein. The median nerve and radial nerve.

Indications: (1) Hemorrhoids, prolapse of the rectum. (2) Pain of the forearm, pain in the chest and hypochondrium.

Needling Method: Perpendicular insertion 0.5—0.8 cun.

3. EX-UE 3 (Zhongquan)

Location: On the middle of the transverse crease of the dorum of wrist, in the depression on the radial side of the tendon of m. extensor digitorum communis. (Fig. 2-132)

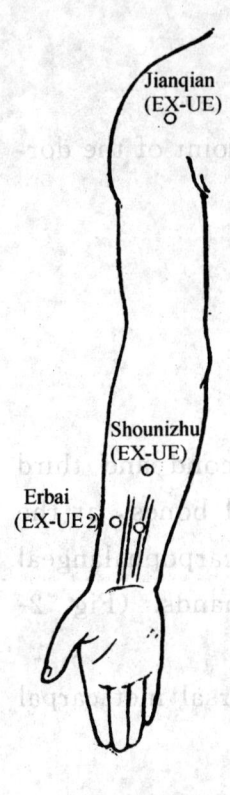

Regional Anatomy: The dorsal carpal branch of the radial artery, the dorsal carpal venous network. The superficial branch of the radial nerve.

Indications: (1) Distention and oppression of the chest and hypochondrium. (2) Epigastric pain, abdominal distention. (3) Cardiac pain.

Needling Method: Perpendicular insertion 0.3—0.5 cun.

4. EX-UE 4 (Zhongkui)

Location: On the midpoint of the proximal interphalangeal joint of the dorsum of the middle finger. (Fig. 2-133)

Regional Anatomy: The dorsal digital artery and nerve.

Indications: (1) Dsyphagia, regurgitation. (2) Vitiligo.

Needling and Moxibustion Method: Moxibustion is applicable.

5. EX-UE 5 (Dagukong)

Location: On the midpoint of interphalangeal joint of the dorsum of the thumb. (Fig. 2-133)

Fig. 2-131

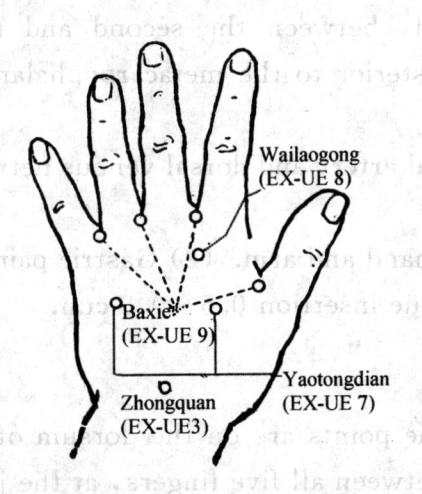

Fig. 2-132

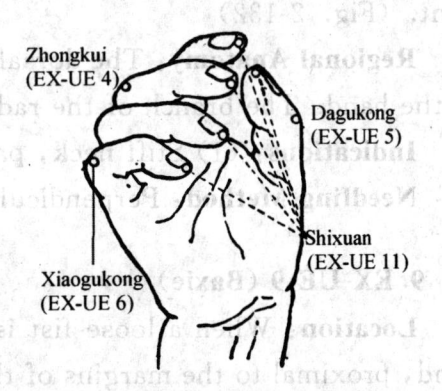

Fig. 2-133

Regional Anatomy: The dorsal digital artery and nerve.

Indications: (1) Eye pain, nebula, cataract. (2) Vomiting, epistaxis.

215

Needling Method: Moxibustion is applicable.

6. EX-UE 6 (Xiaogukong)

Location: On the midpoint of the proximal interphalangeal joint of the dorsum of the little finger. (Fig. 2-133)

Regional Anatomy: The dorsal digital artery and nerve.

Indications: Nebula, redness, swelling and pain of the eye.

Needling Method: Moxibustion is applicable.

7. EX-UE 7 (Yaotongdian)

Location: On the dorsum of the hand, between the second and third metacarpal bones, and between the fourth and fifth metacarpal bones, at the midpoint between the transverse crease of the wrist and the metacarpophalangeal joint. One hand has two points, a total of four points on both hands. (Fig. 2-132)

Regional Anatomy: The dorsal metacarpal artery. The dorsal metacarpal nerve, the common palmar digital nerve.

Indications: Acute lumbar strain.

Needling Method: Oblique insertion toward the center of the palm 0.5—0.8 cun from both sides.

8. EX-UE 8 (Wailaogong)

Location: On the dorsum of the hand, between the second and third metacarpal bones, 0.5 cun (finger inch) posterior to the metacarpophalangeal joint. (Fig. 2-132)

Regional Anatomy: The dorsal metacarpal artery and dorsal venous network of the hand. The branch of the radial nerve.

Indications: (1) Stiff neck, pain of the hand and arm. (2) Gastric pain.

Needling Method: Perpendicular or oblique insertion 0.5—0.8 cun.

9. EX-UE 9 (Baxie)

Location: When a loose fist is made, the points are on the dorsum of the hand, proximal to the margins of the webs between all five fingers, at the junction of the red and white skin. Both hands altogether have a total of eight points. (Fig. 2-132)

Regional Anatomy: The dorsal metacarpal artery and the dorsal venous network of the hand. The dorsal branches of the ulnar and radial nerves.

Indications: (1) Snake-bite, swelling and pain of the dorsum of the hand. (2) Excessive heat, eye pain.

Needling Method: Oblique insertion upward 0.5—0.8 cun; or prick to cause bleeding.

10. EX-UE 10 (Sifeng)

Location: On the palmar surface, in the midpoint of the transverse creases of the proximal interphalangeal joints of the index, middle, ring and little fingers. One hand has four points, both hands have a total of eight points. (Fig. 2-134)

Regional Anatomy: The branches of the proprial palmar digital artery and vein. The proprial palmar digital nerve.

Indications: (1) Malnutrition and indigestion syndrome in children. (2) Whooping cough.

Needling Method: Prick to cause bleeding; or prick, then squeeze out a small amount of yellowish viscous fluid.

Fig. 2-134

11. EX-UE 11 (Shixuan)

Location: On the tips of the ten fingers, 0.1 cun (finger inch) distal to the nails. Both hands altogether have ten points. (Fig. 2-133)

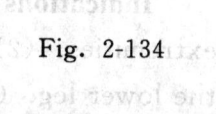

Regional Anatomy: The palmar digital arterial and venous network. A large number of algesireceptors.

Indications: (1) Coma, epilepsy. (2) High fever, sore throat.

Needling Method: Superficial insertion 0.1—0.2 cun; or prick to cause bleeding.

12. EX-UE (Wuhu)

Location: When a fist is made, on the dorsum of the hand at the high point of the small head of the second and fourth metacarpal bones. (Fig. 2-135)

Regional Anatomy: The dorsal digital artery and vein. The dorsal branch of the ulnar and radial nerve.

Indications: Contracture of the fingers.

Needling Method: Moxibustion is applicable.

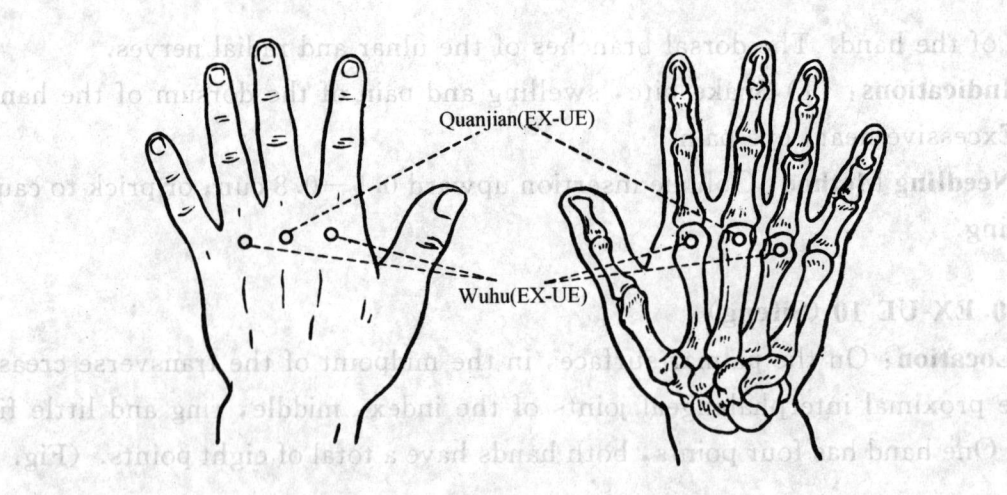

Fig. 2-135

13. EX-UE (Shounizhu)

Location: Extend arm palm facing upwards, between the tendons of m. palmaris longus and m. flexor carpi radialis, on the midpoint between the transverse crease of the wrist and the transverse cubital crease. (Fig. 2-131)

Regional Anatomy: The dorsal digital artery and vein. The dorsal digital branches of ulnar nerve and radial nerve.

Indications: (1) Pain of the forearm, paralysis or contracture of the upper extremities. (2) Mastitis, pain in the chest and hypochondrium. (3) Aching of the lower leg. (4) Hysteria.

Needling Method: Perpendicular insertion 0.5—0.8 cun. Moxibustion is applicable.

14. EX-UE (Jianqian)

Location: The midpoint between the end of the anterior axillary fold and LI 15 (Jianyu). (Fig. 2-131)

Regional Anatomy: The thoracoacromial artery and vein. Deeper, the axillary nerve.

Indications: Pain and limitation of the shoulder, paralysis of the upper extremities, disorders of the shoulder joint and the surrounding soft tissue.

Needling Method: Perpendicular insertion 0.5—1.0 cun. Moxibustion is applicable.

15. EX-LE 2 (Heding)

Location: Above the knee, in the depression of the midpoint of the superior patellar border. (Fig. 2-136)

Regional Anatomy: The arterial network of the knee. The anterior cutaneous branch and the muscular branch of the femoral nerve.

Indications: Aching of the knee joint, weakness of the leg and foot, arthroncus of knee, beriberi.

Needling Method: Perpendicular insertion 0.5—0.8 cun.

16. EX-LE (Baichongwo)

Location: When the knee is flexed, the point is on the medial aspect of the thigh, 3 cun superior to the medial end of the patella, 1 cun superior to Sp. 10 (Xuehai). (Fig. 2-136)

Regional Anatomy: The femoral artery and vein. The femoral nerve.

Indications: (1) Pruritus of the skin, rubella, skin ulcers on the lower portion of the body. (2) Ascariasis.

Needling Method: Perpendicular insertion 0.5—1.0 cun.

17. EX-LE 4 (Neixiyan)

Location: When the knee is flexed, the point is in the depression medial to the patellar ligament. (Fig. 2-136)

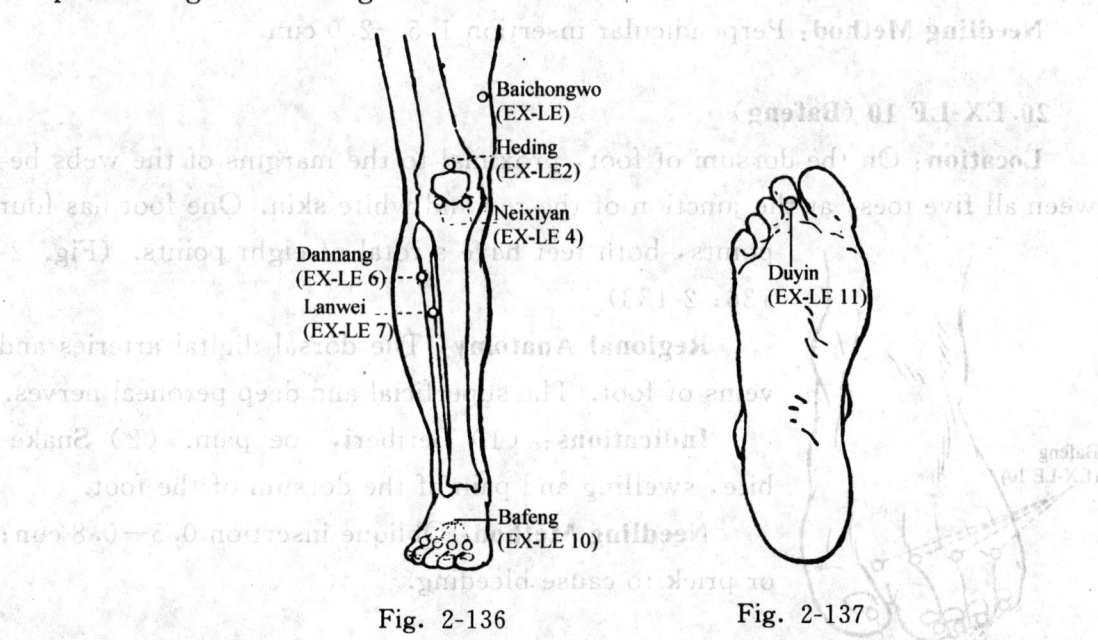

Fig. 2-136　　　Fig. 2-137

Regional Anatomy: The arterial and venous network of the knee. The branch of the saphenous nerve.

Indications: Swelling and pain of the knee joint.

Needling Method: Oblique insertion laterally upward 0.5—1.0 cun.

18. EX-LE 6 (Dannang)

Location: On the superior lateral aspect of the lower leg, 2 cun directly below the depression anterior and inferior to the head of the fibula, GB 34 (Yanglingquan). (Fig. 2-136)

Regional Anatomy: The branch of the anterior tibial artery and vein. The lateral cutaneous nerve of the calf, the deep peroneal nerve.

Indications: (1) Acute and chronic cholecystitis, cholelithiasis, biliary ascariasis. (2) Weakness, numbness and pain of lower extremities.

Needling Method: Perpendicular insertion 1.0—2.0 cun.

19. EX-LE 7 (Lanwei)

Location: On the superior anterior aspect of the lower leg, 5 cun below ST 35 (Dubi), one finger-breadth from the anterior crest of the tibia. (Fig. 2-136)

Regional Anatomy: The anterior tibial artery and vein. The lateral cutaneous nerve of the calf, the deep peroneal nerve.

Indications: (1) Acute and chronic appendicitis. (2) Dyspepsia. (3) Paralysis of the lower extremities.

Needling Method: Perpendicular insertion 1.5—2.0 cun.

20. EX-LE 10 (Bafeng)

Location: On the dorsum of foot, proximal to the margins of the webs between all five toes, at the junction of the red and white skin. One foot has four points, both feet have a total of eight points. (Fig. 2-136; 2-138)

Regional Anatomy: The dorsal digital arteries and veins of foot. The superficial and deep peroneal nerves.

Indications: (1) Beriberi, toe pain. (2) Snakebite, swelling and pain of the dorsum of the foot.

Needling Method: Oblique insertion 0.5—0.8 cun; or prick to cause bleeding.

Bafeng (EX-LE 10)
Qiduan (EX-LE 12)
Fig. 2-138

21. EX-LE 11 (Duyin)

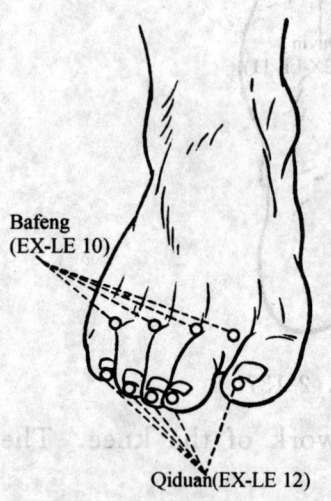

Location: On the foot, on the plantar aspect of the distal end of the second toe, in the midpoint of the interphalangeal joint. (Fig. 2-137)

Regional Anatomy: The proprial plantar digital artery artery and vein. The proprial plantar digital nerve.

Indications: (1) Acute cardiac pain, pain in the chest and hypochondrium. (2) Irregular menstruation, retention of afterbirth, stillbirth. (3) Hernia.

Needling Method: Perpendicular insertion 0.1—0.2 cun.

22. EX-LE 12 (Qiduan)

Location: On the foot, on the tips of the ten toes, 0.1 cun (finger inch) distal to the nails. Both feet altogether have ten points. (Fig. 2-138)

Regional Anatomy: The dorsal digital arteries and nerves of the toes.

Indications: (1) Emergency treatment for apoplexy, numbness of the toes. (2) Redness, swelling and pain of the instep of the foot.

Needling Method: Perpendicular insertion 0.1—0.2 cun; or use three-edged needle to cause bleeding.

Part II Acupuncture And Moxibustion Techniques

Acupuncture and moxibustion are two different therapeutic methods. Acupuncture also known as needling is a procedure by which diseases can be prevented and treated through proper insertion of needles into points accompanied by different manipulations. Clinically, the needles of common use are the filiform needle, the cutaneous needle, the intradermal needle, the three-edged needle, etc, among which, the filiform needle is the commonest.

Moxibustion treats and prevents diseases by applying heat to points or certain place of the human body. The material used is chiefly "moxa wool" in the form of a cone or stick. Since ancient time moxibustion and acupuncture have been used together very often in clinical practice.

Chapter 1 Filiform Needle

Section 1 The Structure and Specification

The filiform needles are widely adopted at present in clinic. It is mainly made of stainless steel. A filiform needle may be divided into five parts: the handle, the tail, the tip, the body, and the root. (Fig. 2-139)

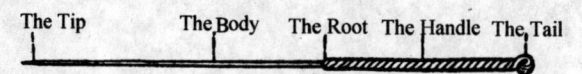

Fig 2-139 The Structure of a Filiform Needle

The filiform needles vary in length and diameter (Table 2-12); (Table 2-13).

Table 2-12 Length

cun	0.5	1	1.5	2	2.5	3	3.5	4	4.5	5
mm	15	25	40	50	65	75	90	100	115	125

Table 2-13 Gauge

No	26	28	30	32	34
Dia(cm)	0.45	0.38	0.32	0.26	0.22

Section 2 Needle Practice

As the filiform needle is fine and pliable, it is difficult to insert it into the skin without some strength exerted by the fingers and conduct manipulations. An appropriate finger force is the guarantee to minimize the pain and raise the therapeutic effects.

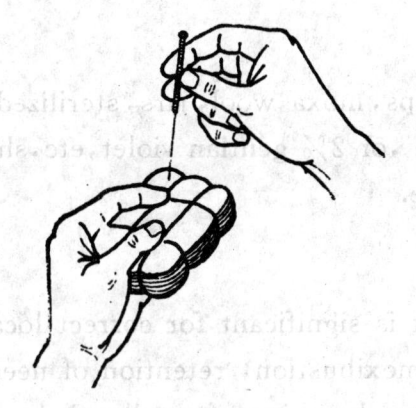

Fig. 2-140 Practising
Needling on Folded Paper

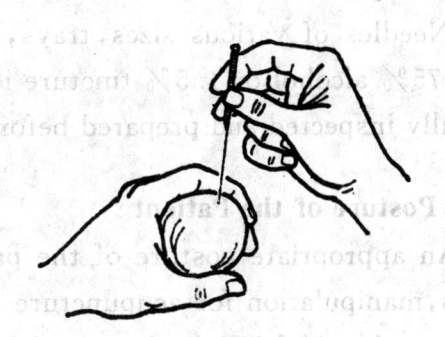

Fig. 2-141 Practising
Needling on Cotton Cushion

1. Practice with Sheets of Paper

Fold fine and soft tissue into a small packet about 5×8 cm in size and 2 cm in thickness, then find the packet with gause thread. Hold the paper packet in the left hand and the needle handle in the right hand. Rotate the needle into the packet and turn it out. Repeat the practice until you feel it is easy to do, then practice the rotating clockwise and counter-clockwise exercise as well as the lifting and thrusting manipulation. (Fig. 2-140)

2. Practice with a Cotton Cushion

Make a cotton cushion of about 6—7cm in diameter wrapped in gauze. The practice made on the paper packet can be also done on the cotton cushion. As the cushion is softer than the paper packet, more basic techniques of reinforcement and reduction, such as the manipulation of combining lifting, thrusting and rotating, can be practiced on it. (Fig. 2-141)

3. Practice on Your Own Body

This may follow the practice on the paper packet and cushion so as to have the personal experience of the needling sensation. This practice requires pian free no bent of the needle, and good needling sensation radiating to certain direction. Treatment can not be conducted on the patient unless you are able to insert the needle properly and skillfully.

Section 3 Preparations Prior to Acupuncture Treatment

1. Inspection of the Instruments

Needles of various sizes, trays, forceps, moxa wool, jars, sterilized cotton balls, 75% alcohol or 1.5% tincture iodine, or 2% gentian violet, etc, should be carefully inspected and prepared before use.

2. Posture of the Patient

An appropriate posture of the patient is significant for correct location of points, manipulation for acupuncture and moxibustion, retention of needle, and in prevention of fainting, bent, sticking and breaking of needle. Generally, the proper posture of the patient should be convenient for manipulation without hinderance, and comfortable to the patient. The common postures in the practice are as follows:

Supine Posture: Suitable for the points on the head and face, chest and abdomen and the four limbs. (Fig. 2-142)

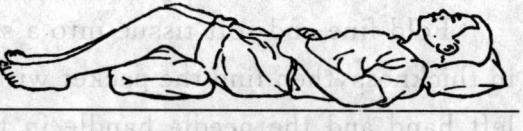

Fig. 2-142 Supine Posture

Lateral Recumbent: Suitable for the points at the lateral side of the body. (Fig. 2-143)

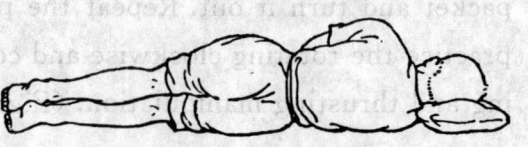

Fig 2-143 Lateral Recumbent

Prone Posture: Suitable for the points on the head, neck, back, lumbus, buttocks and the posterior aspect of the lower limbs. (Fig. 2-144)

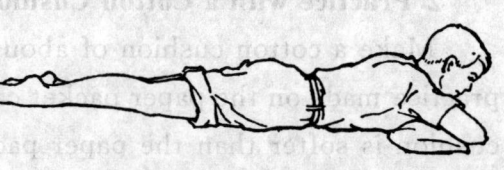

Fig. 2-144 Prone Posture

Straight-Sitting with the Back Leaning against the Chair: Suitable for the

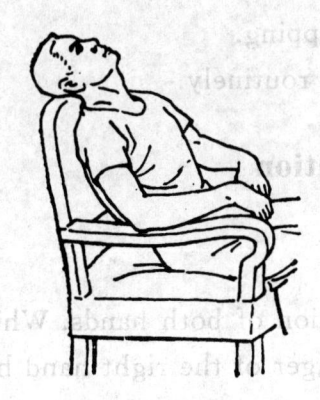

Fig. 2-145
Sitting Position on a Lazy Back

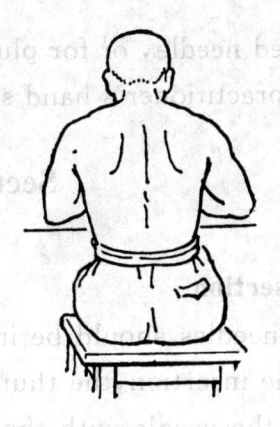

Fig. 2-146
Sitting in Flexion

points on the head, face, neck, chest and the four limbs. (Fig. 2-145)

Sitting in Flexion:
Suitable for the points on the head, neck and back. (Fig. 2-146)

Sitting with One Side of the Body Exposing the Practitioner: Suitable for the points on the vertex, the temple, the auricular place and the cheek. (Fig. 2-147)

Fig. 2-147 Sitting in Lateral Flexion

3. Sterilization:

(1) Needle sterilization

Autoclave sterilization

Needles should be sterilized in an autoclave at 1.5 atmospheric pressure and 125 degree for 30 minutes.

Boiling Sterilization

Needles and other instruments are boiled in water for 30 minutes. This method is easy and effective without need of special equipment.

Medicinal Sterilization

Soak the needles in 75% alcohol from 30 to 60 minutes. Then take them out and wipe off the liquid from the needles with a piece of sterile dry cloth. The needle tray and forceps which have directly contacted with the filiform needles should also be sterilized. Besides, needles used in infectious disease should be sterilized and stored in separately.

(2) Skin Disinfection

The locations on the body surface selected for treatment must be disinfected with 75% alcohol, or first with 2.5% tincture iodine, and then by an 75% alcohol cotton ball to remove the iodine. The later is suitable for blood-letting with three-edged needle, or for plumblossom needle tapping.

The practitioner's hand should be disinfected routinely.

Section 4 Manipulation

1. Insertion

The needles should be inserted by coordination of both hands. While conducting the insertion, the thumb and the index finger of the right hand hold the handle of the needle with the middle finger of the same hand being against the body of the needle, the tip of the needle is punctured rapidly into the point with a certain finger force, then the needle is rotated to a deep layer. The right hand is called "the puncturing hand". (Fig. 2-148) In the process, the left hand presses around the point to be punctured to fix the skin so that the needle can be punctured at the right spot. In case of inserting with a long needle, with the help of the left hand, the body of the needle will be kept unswayed. The proper manipulation of the left hand can minimize the pain during the insertion. As a result, it can enhance the therapeutic effects. The left hand therefore is known as the "pressing hand." In the book *Classic on Medical Problems*, it is said: "An experienced acupuncturist believes in the important function of the left hand, while an inexperienced believes in the important function of the right hand." It is further stated in *Lyrics of Standard Profundities* that: " Press heavily with the left hand to disperse Qi and insert the needle gently and slowly to avoid pain." These explanations show the importance of the coordination of the right and left hands on insertion. In the clinic, the common methods of insertion are as follows:

(1) Inserting the Needle Aided by the Pressure of the Finger of the Pressing Hand

Press beside the acupuncture point with the nail of the thumb or the index finger of the left hand and keep the needle tip closely to the nail, and then insert the needle into the point. This method is suitable for short needles. (Fig. 2-149)

(2) Inserting the Needle with the Help of Puncturing and Pressing Hands

Wrap the needle body with a cotton ball by the thumb and the index finger of the left hand, leaving

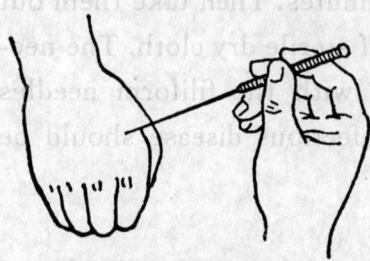

Fig. 2-148
Holding the Needle

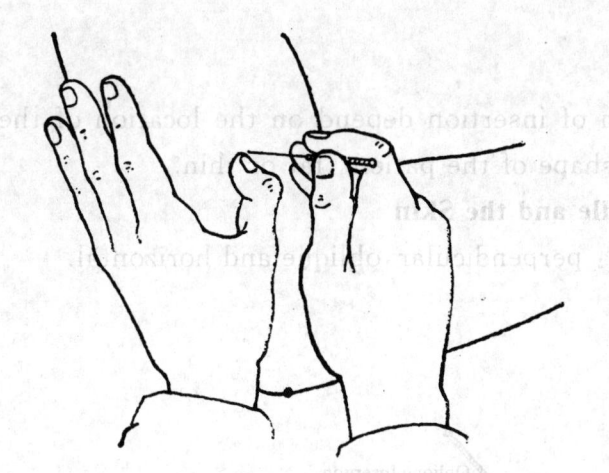

Fig. 2-149 Finger Press Insertion

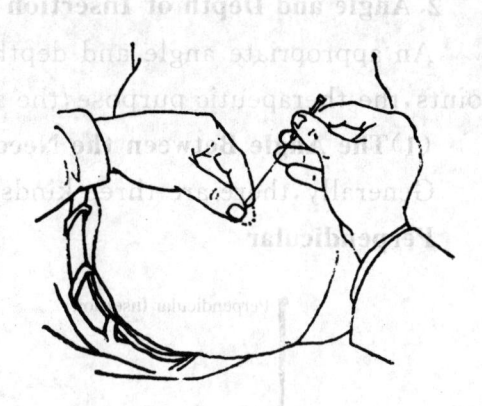

Fig. 2-150 Pinch Needle Method

0.2—0.3 cm of its tip exposed, and hold the needle handle with the thumb and index finger of the right hand. As the needle tip is directly over the selected point, insert the needle swiftly into the skin with the right hand. This method is suitable for long needles. (Fig. 2-150)

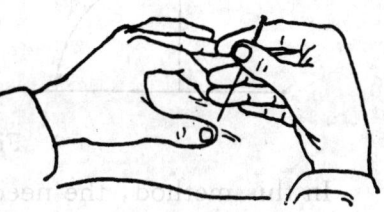

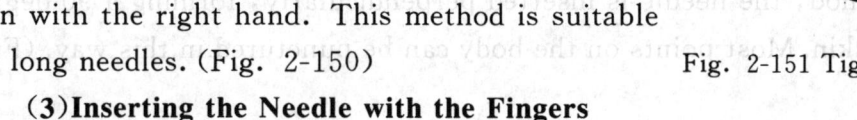

Fig. 2-151 Tight Skin Method

(3) Inserting the Needle with the Fingers Stretching the Skin

Stretch the skin where the point is located with the thumb and index finger of the left hand, hold the needle with the right hand and insert it into the point rapidly to a required depth. This method is suitable for the points on the abdomen where the skin is loose. (Fig. 2-151)

(4) Inserting the Needle by Pinching the Skin

Pinch the skin up around the point with the thumb and index finger of the left hand, insert the needle rapidly into the point with the right hand. This method is suitable for puncturing the points on the face, where the muscle and skin are thinnish. (Fig. 2-152)

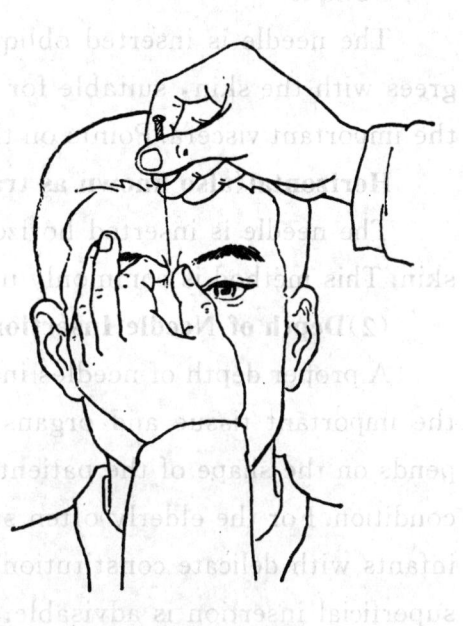

Fig. 2-152 Pinch Skin Method

227

2. Angle and Depth of Insertion

An appropriate angle and depth of insertion depend on the location of the points, the therapeutic purpose, the shape of the patient, fat or thin.

(1) The Angle Between the Needle and the Skin

Generally, there are three kinds: perpendicular, oblique and horizontal.

Perpendicular

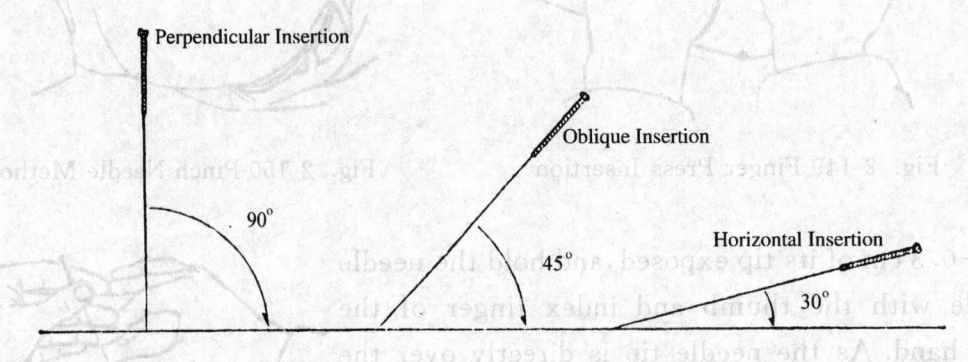

Fig. 2-153 Angle of Insertion

In this method, the needle is inserted perpendicularly, forming a 90 degree angle with the skin. Most points on the body can be punctured in this way. (Fig. 2-153)

Oblique

The needle is inserted obliquely to form an angle of approximately 45 degrees with the skin, suitable for the points where the muscle is thin or close to the important viscera. Points on the chest and back are often needled in this way.

Horizontal (also known as transverse insertion)

The needle is inserted horizontally to form a 15—25 degree angle with the skin. This method is commonly used in the places where the muscle is thinnish.

(2) Depth of Needle Insertion

A proper depth of needles induces better needling sensation without hurting the important tissue and organs. Clinically, the depth of insertion mostly depends on the shape of the patient, the location of the points and the pathological condition. For the elderly often suffering from deficiency of Qi and blood, or for infants with delicate constitution, and such places as the head, face, and back, superficial insertion is advisable. For the young and middle-aged with musculature or fatty shape, or for the points on the four extremities, buttocks, and abdomen, deep insertion is employed.

3. Manipulations and Arrival of Qi (needling sensation)

Manipulation here refers to the methods of needling to induce needling sensation.

The Arrival of Qi refers to the sensation of soreness, numbness of a distending feeling around the point when the needle is inserted to a certain depth. At the same time, the operator may feel tightness around the needle.

(1) The Fundamental Manipulation Techniques

A Lifting and Thrusting

The so-called lifting and thrusting is conducted by lifting the needle to a superficial layer after the needle is inserted to a desired depth, then thrust the needle to a deep layer, which is repeatedly performed as required. Generally, lifting and thrusting in a large degree and high-frequency may induce a strong stimulation, and in a small degree and low frequency lead to a weak stimulation. (Fig. 2-154)

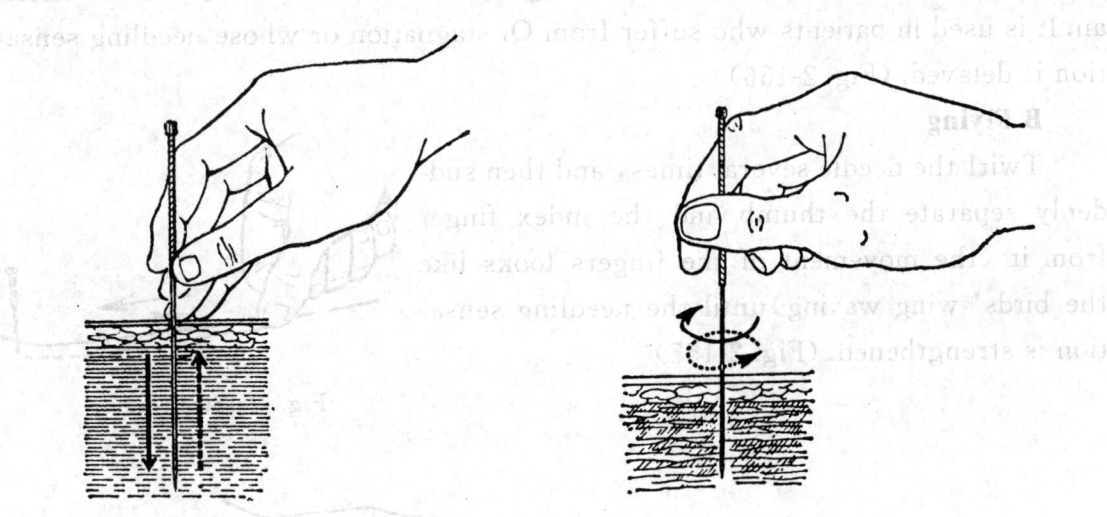

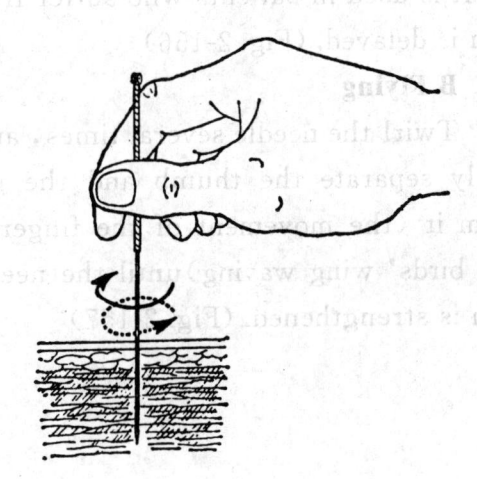

Fig. 2-154 Lifting and Thrusting   Fig. 2-155 Twirling or Rotating

B Twirling or Rotating

After the needle is inserted to a desired depth, twirl and rotate the needle clockwise and counter-clockwise continuously. Generally, the needle is rotated with an amplitude from 180° to 360°. Rotating clockwise or counter-clockwise alone may twine the muscle fibers and produce pain and difficulty in further manipulation. (Fig. 2-155)

(2) The Supplementary Manipulation Techniques

In the process of acupuncture, no matter what manipulation it is, the arrival of Qi must be achieved. In the first chapter of *Miraculous Pivot*, it is described that "Acupuncture therapy does not take effect until the arrival of Qi comes out." In *Ode of Golden Needle*, it is said: "Quick arrival of Qi suggests good effects in treatment; slow arrival of Qi shows retarded effects in treatment." It indicates that the arrival of Qi is especially important in acupuncture treatment. Acupuncturists in the past dynasties attached importance to the arrival of Qi, therefore, they summarized a number of manipulations for promoting the arrival of Qi (known as supplementary techniques). When there is no needling reaction, or the arrival of Qi is not apparent after needle is inserted, manipulations for promoting the Qi should be conducted. In clinic, following six kinds of technique are commonly applied.

A Pressing

Slightly press the skin along the course of the meridian, the point of which is punctured without sensation, for encouraging the movement of Qi in the meridian. It is used in patients who suffer from Qi stagnation or whose needling sensation is delayed. (Fig. 2-156)

B Flying

Twirl the needle several times, and then suddenly separate the thumb and the index finger from it (the movement of the fingers looks like the birds' wing waving) until the needling sensation is strengthened. (Fig. 2-157)

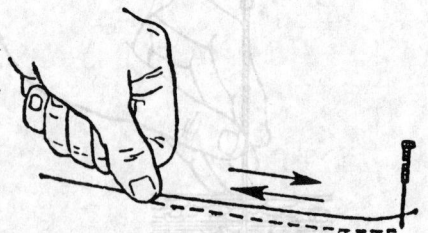

Fig. 2-156 Pressing

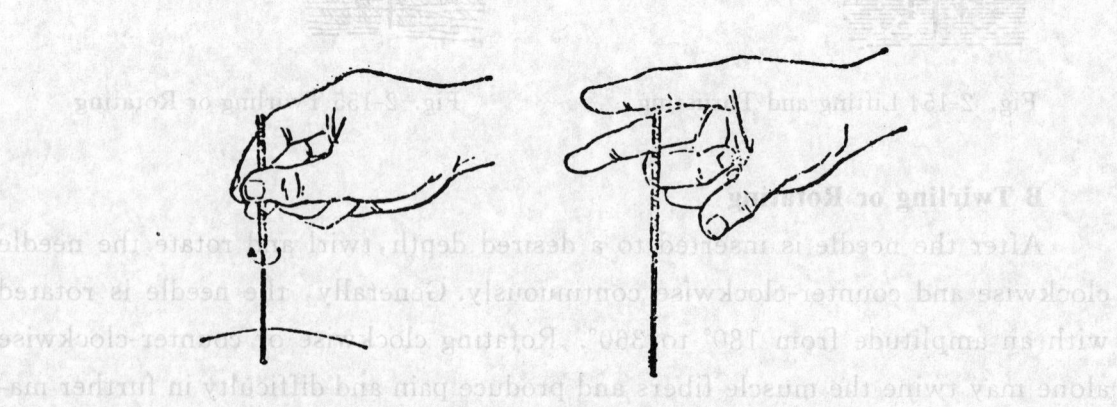

Fig 2-157 Flying

C Scraping

The thumb (the index finger or the middle finger) of the right hand is placed on the tail end to keep the needle steady, scrape the handle with the nail of the index finger (the middle finger or the thumb) of the right hand upward or downward for strengthening the needling sensation and promoting the dispersion of the sensation. (Fig. 2-158)

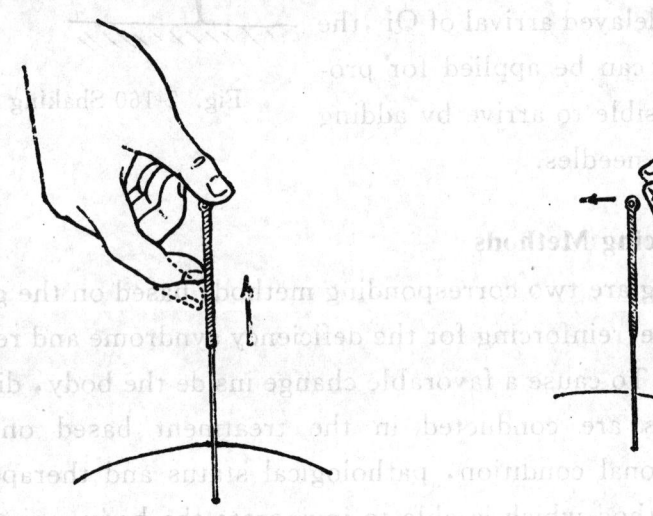

Fig. 2-158 Scraping   Fig. 2-159 Plucking

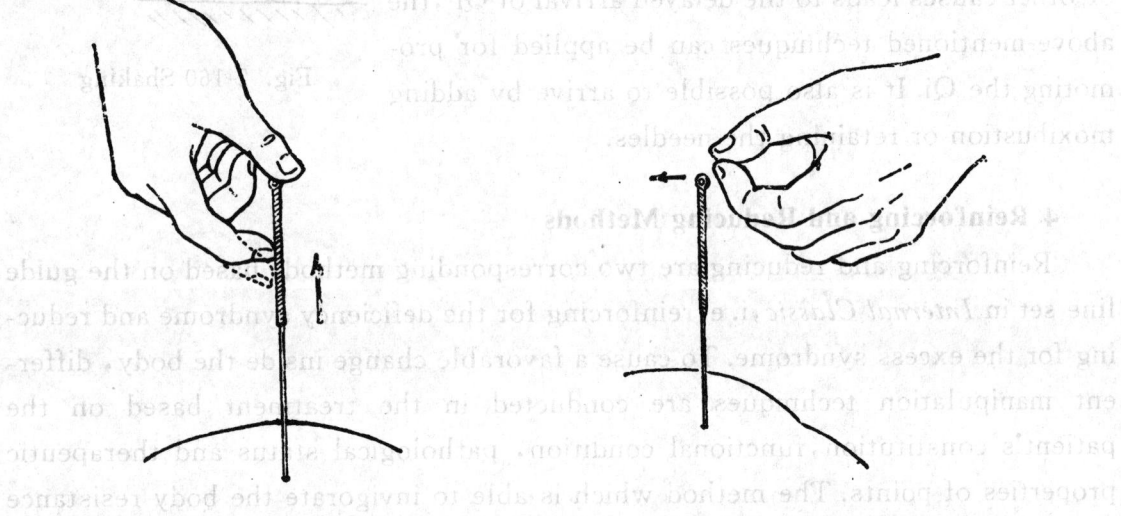

D Plucking

Pluck the handle of the needle lightly, causing it to tremble for the enhancement of the stimulation. It is used for the treatment which needs restimulating slightly during retention of the needles. (Fig. 2-159)

E Shaking

Hold the handle of the needle and shake the needle as the movement of a scull. For the purpose of reducing, shaking is combined with lifting at the withdrawal of the needle in perpendicular insertion. For the needles obliquely or transversely inserted, shake the needle by moving the handle left and right, but the needle body inside the point is kept at the same place. It is used to push the needling sensation in certain direction. (Fig. 2-160)

F Trembling

Hold the needle with the fingers of the right hand and apply quick lift-thrust or twirl movement in a small amplitude to cause vibration. It is for promoting the arrival of Qi or strengthening the needling sensation.

In the process of acupuncture, if the arrival of Qi is delayed, or no sensation is obtained, the factors influencing the arrival of Qi should be found out. It may be due to the inaccurate location of the points, improper depth, angle or direction of the needle insertion. Readjustment of the point location, depth, angle or direction of the insertion is necessary. If the weakness with Qi deficiency or other causes leads to the delayed arrival of Qi, the above-mentioned techniques can be applied for promoting the Qi. It is also possible to arrive by adding moxibustion or retaining the needles.

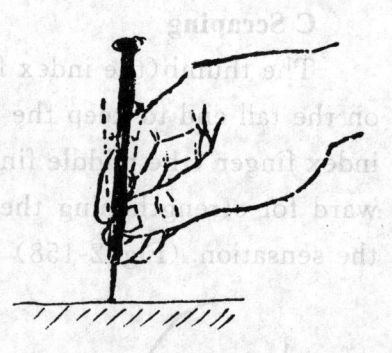

Fig. 2-160 Shaking

4. Reinforcing and Reducing Methods

Reinforcing and reducing are two corresponding methods based on the guide line set in *Internal Classic*, i. e. reinforcing for the deficiency syndrome and reducing for the excess syndrome. To cause a favorable change inside the body, different manipulation techniques are conducted in the treatment based on the patient's constitution, functional condition, pathological status and therapeutic properties of points. The method which is able to invigorate the body resistance and to strengthen the weakened physiological function is called reinforcing, while the other one which is able to eliminate the pathological functions is known as reducing. The reinforcing and reducing for the regulation of the functions of Zang-Fu organs and the balance of Yin and Yang are achieved by stimulating the points to activate the Qi of meridians.

The effects of reinforcing or reducing mainly depend upon the following factors:

(1) The Functioned Conditions of the Patient

Under different pathological conditions, acupuncture may produce different regulating functions, either reinforcing or reducing. If an individual is in a collapse condition, acupuncture functions to rescue Yang from collapse; when an individual is under a condition of internal pathogenic heat, acupuncture functions to expel the heat. Acupuncture can relax the stomach and intestine when they are in spasm and can strengthen the stomach and intestinal peristalsis when they are hypotomic. This dual regulating function is closely related to the defensive ability of human body. If it is vigorous, the meridian Qi is easy to be activated and the regulating function is good. On the contrary, if it is lowered, the meridian Qi is difficult to be excited and the regulating function is poor.

(2) Therapeutic Properties of the Points

Acupuncture points have relative specificity as far as the therapeutic properties are concerned; some points tend to reinforce the body resistance, such as Qihai(CV6), Guanyuan(CV4), Mingmen(GV4), Zusanli(ST36), Gaohuang(BL43) etc, which are mainly applied for deficiency syndromes; and some points such as Shaoshang(LU11) and Shixuan(EX-UE11), which have the property of clearing away heat and promoting the resuscitation are employed often for excessive heat syndromes.

(3) Needling Methods

Needling methods are important for reinforcing and reducing. In order to achieve reinforcing or reducing effects, ancient acupuncturists did create a considerable number of reinforcing and reducing methods of needling. The common reinforcing and reducing methods in clinic are introduced below.

A Reinforcing or Reducing by Twirling and Rotating the Needle

The reinforcing and reducing of this kind can be differentiated by the amplitude and speed used. When the needle is inserted to a certain depth and the Qi arrives, rotating the needle gently and slowly with small amplitude for relatively a short period is called reinforcing, on the contrary, rotating the needle rapidly and heavily with large amplitude for relatively a long period is known as the reducing. It is also considered that rotating the needle with the thumb forward forcefully in large amplitude is reinforcing, while rotating the needle with the index finger forward forcefully in large amplitude is reducing.

B Reinforcing and Reducing by Lifting and Thrusting the Needle

In this method, the reinforcing and reducing can be differentiated by the force and speed used. After the needle is inserted to a given depth and the needling sensation appears, the reinforcing is obtained by lifting the needle gently and slowly, while thrusting the needle heavily and rapidly. The reducing is achieved by lifting the needle forcefully and rapidly while thrusting the needle gently and slowly.

C The Reinforcing and Reducing Achieved by Rapid and Slow Insertion and Withdrawal of the Needle

This sort of reinforcing and reducing method is distinguished by the speed of insertion and withdrawal of the needle. During manipulations, the reinforcing method is conducted by inserting the needle to a given depth slowly and lifting it rapidly just beneath the skin, and a moment later withdrawing it. The reducing is performed by inserting the needle rapidly to the given depth in one step and withdrawing it slowly in a few steps.

D The Reinforcing and Reducing Achieved by Keeping the Hole Open or Close

On withdrawing of the needle, pressing the needling hole quickly to close it and prevent the vital Qi from escaping is called reinforcing. Shaking the needle to enlarge the hole while withdrawing it, and keeping the hole open is known as reducing.

E The Reinforcing and Reducing Achieved by the Direction the Needle Tip Pointing to

The needle tip pointing in the direction of the meridian is known as reinforcing, and the needle tip pointing against the meridian direction is considered as reducing.

F The Reinforcing and Reducing Achieved by Means of Respiration

In the method, the reinforcing is achieved by inserting the needle when the patient breathes in and withdrawing the needle when the patient breathes out. The reducing is achieved in an opposite way.

G Even Reinforcing and Reducing Movement

When the needle is inserted into the point and the needling sensation appears, lift, thrust and rotate the needle evenly, then withdraw the needle. Clinically, the above-mentioned methods can be applied alone or in combination. In addition, there are following comprehensive reinforcing and reducing methods.

a Setting the Mountain on Fire

This method is to insert the needle to the first 1/3 of the given depth (superficial layer), after the needling sensation appears, conduct heavy thrust and gentle lift at this layer for 9 times; then the needle is inserted to the middle 1/3 of the depth (medium layer), repeat the same procedure as done in the superficial layer; afterwards the needle is further inserted to the third 1/3 (deep layer) and manipulated same as that of in both the superficial and medium layers. When the whole process finishes and warm sensation has not appeared, repeat the process for two more times to produce warm sensation, then the needle is retained at the deep layer. In the process, the reinforcing can be achieved by combined use of breathing. This method is mainly used for cold Bi syndrome, stubborn numbness and deficient cold syndromes.

b Penetrating-Heaven Coolness

In this method, first insert the needle to the deep layer, the third 1/3 of a given depth, after needling sensation appears, lift the needle quickly and thrust the needle slowly at this layer for 6 times; then lift the needle to the middle 1/3 of the depth (medium layer), repeat the same procedure as that of in the deep layer, finally, lift the needle to the first 1/3 of the depth (superficial layer), repeat the same procedure as done in both the deep and medium layers. After the whole process, if no cool sensation is obtained, repeat the process for two more times to induce cool sensation. In the process, the reducing method achieved by means of respiration can be associated. This method is often employed for heat Bi syndrome and other heat syndromes, such as acute carbuncle with swelling.

5. Retaining and Withdrawing the Needle

(1). Retaining

Retaining means to keep the needle in place after it is inserted to a given depth below the skin and manipulated. The purpose of it is to prolong the needling sensation and for further manipulation. Pathological conditions decide the retaining and its duration. In general, the needle is retained for fifteen to twenty minutes after the arrival of Qi. But for some chronic, intractable, painful and spastic cases, the time of retaining the needle may be appropriately prolonged. For some diseases, the duration may be as long as several hours. Meanwhile, manipulations may be given at intervals in order to strengthen the therapeutic effects. For patients with a dull needling sensation, retaining the needle serves as a method to wait Qi to come.

(2) Withdrawing

On withdrawing the needle, press the skin around the point with the thumb and index finger of the pressing hand, rotate the needle gently and lift it slowly to the subcutaneous level, then withdraw it quickly and press the punctured point with a sterilized cotton ball for a while to prevent bleeding. Be sure not to leave any needle on the body.

Section 5 Management of Possible Accidents

Although acupuncture is safe, some accidents may take place owing to negligence of contraindications, imperfect manipulations, or lack of the knowledge of anatomy. The possible accidents are seen as follows:

1. Fainting

Cause

This is often due to nervousness delicate constitution, hunger, fatigue, improper position or manipulation, such as too forceful manipulation.

Manifestations

During acupuncture treatment, there may appear palpitation, dizziness, vertigo, nausea, cold sweating, pallor, and weak pulse. In severe cases, there may be cold extremities, drop of blood pressure, incontinence of urine and stool, and loss of consciousness.

Management

Stop needling immediately and withdraw all the needles, then help the patient to lie down, and offer some warm or hot water to the patient. The symptoms will disappear after a short rest. In severe cases, press hard with the fingernail or needle Renzhong(GV 26), Hegu(LI 4), Neiguan(PC 6)and Zusanli(ST 36), or apply moxibustion to Baihui(GV 20), Qihai(CV 6), Guanyuan (CV 4) and Yongquan(KI 1). Generally, the patient will recover, but if not, other emergency measures should be taken.

Prevention

For patients being treated by acupuncture for the first time, or those of sensitive individuals, a brief account of needling should be given to them prior to the treatment to relieve their nervousness, and supine posture is adopted. The manipulation should not be too forceful. Needles are not retained for long time. During the treatment, if there appear some prodromal symptoms such as pallor, sweating or dizziness, management should be taken promptly.

2. Stuck needle

Cause

This may result from nervousness, strong spasm of the local muscle after the insertion of the needle, twirling the needle with too large amplitude or in one direction only causing muscle fibers to bind, or from a change of the position of the patient after the insertion of the needles.

Manifestations

After the needle is inserted, it is found difficult or impossible to rotate, lift and thrust the needles.

Management

Ask the patient to relax. If the needle is stuck due to excessive rotation in one direction, the condition will release when the needle is twirled in the opposite direction. If stuck needle is caused by temporary muscle spasm, leave the needle in place for a while, then withdraw it by rotating, or by inserting another needle nearby to disperse the Qi and blood, and to relieve the spasm. If the stuck needle is caused by the changing of the position of the patient, the original posture should be resumed and then withdraw the needle.

Prevention

Nervous patients should be encouraged to relax their tension. Manipulation should not be too forceful. Avoid puncturing the muscular tendon during insertion. Twirling the needle in only one direction shall not be allowed. During retention of the needles, the posture of the patient should remain unchanged.

3. Bent needle
Cause

This may arise from unskillful manipulation or too forceful manipulation, or the needle striking on the hard tissue, or a sudden change of the patient's posture, or the handle of needle being touched or pressed by something, or from an improper management of the stuck needle.

Manifestations

It is difficult to lift, thrust, rotate and withdraw the needle, and the patient feels painfull.

Management

When the needle is bent, lifting, thrusting and rotating shall be no longer conducted. The needle may be removed slowly and withdrawn by following the course of bend. If the bent needle is caused by the change of the patient's posture, help him to resume the original position, relax the local muscle and remove the needle. Never try to withdraw the needle with force so as not to break the needle inside the body.

Prevention

Skillful insertion and even manipulation are required. Prior to treatment, the patient should have a comfortable position. During the retention of the needle, a patient is not allowed to change the position as he pleases. The needling place shall in no case be impacted or pressed by an external force.

4. Broken needle
Cause

This may result from the poor quality of the needle or eroded base of the needle, from too strong manipulation of the needle, from strong muscle spasm, or a sudden movement of the patient when the needle is in place, or from withdrawing a stuck needle.

Manifestations

The needle body is broken during manipulation and the broken part is below the skin surface or a little bit out of the skin surface.

Management

When it happens, the patient should be told to keep calm to prevent the broken needle from going deeper into the body. If the broken part protrudes from the skin, remove it with forceps or fingers. If the broken part is at the same level of the skin, press the tissue around the site until the broken end is exposed, then remove it with forceps. If it is completely under the skin, surgery should be resorted with the help of x-ray to find out the exact location of the broken needle.

Prevention

To prevent accidents, careful inspection of the quality of the needle should be made. Prior to the treatment, reject the needles which are not in conformity with the requirements specified. The needle body should not be inserted into the body completely, and a little part should be exposed outside the skin. On needle insertion, if it is bent, the needle should be withdrawn immediately. Never try to insert a needle violently.

5. Hematoma
Cause

This may arise from injury of the blood vessels during insertion, or from no pressing of the point after withdrawing the needle.

Manifestations

Local swelling, distension and pain after the withdrawal of the needle. The skin of the local place is blue and purplish.

Management

Generally, a slight hematoma may disappear by itself. If the local swelling, distension and pain are serious, first press it or apply cold compression locally to stop bleeding, hot compression can be applied to promote resolution of the blood stasis after bleeding completely ceased.

Prevention

Avoid injuring the blood vessels and points are pressed with sterilized cotton ball as soon as the needle is withdrawn.

Section 6 Precautions in Acupuncture Treatment

1. It is advisable not to give acupuncture treatment to the patients who are either hungry or overeaten, drunk and overfatigued. For the very weak patient, the manipulation of needle should not be too strong, and supine posture of the patient is preferable.

2. It is contraindicated to puncture points on the abdomen and lumbosacral place for pregnant women, or the points that may cause contraction of the uterus, such as Hegu (LI 4), Sanyinjiao (SP 6), Kunlun (BL 60), and Zhiyin (BL 67). In the period of menstruation, if it is not for the regulation of menstruation, acupuncture treatment is not suggested to the woman.

3. Points on the vertex of infants should not be needled when the fontanel is not closed. In addition, retention of needles is forbidden since the infants are unable to cooperate with the practitioner.

4. To avoid puncturing the blood vessels so as to prevent bleeding, for patients with a tendency of spontaneous bleeding or unceased bleeding after injury, acupuncture should not be applied.

5. Acupuncture is forbidden on the places with infection, ulcer and soars.

6. To avoid an accident, the practitioner should be careful on the angle, direction and depth of needling where the points located around the eye, at the neck, the chest, the back and the hypochondriac places are punctured.

Chapter 2 Moxibustion

Moxibustion is a therapy which treats and prevents diseases by means of moxa wool, the main material in the therapy in the forms of moxa cones or sticks. The combustion of moxa wool permits transmission of heat to points or certain locations of human body. With the heat, the points and meridians would be simulated so that the purpose of warming the meridians and collaterals, invigorating the flow of Qi and blood, strengthening the body resistance and eliminating pathogens from the body is achieved.

The moxa wool comes from the moxa leaf which is warm in property and smells fragrant. Being easy to ignite and with mild heat that penetrates deep into the affected location of the body, "it regulates Qi and blood, expels cold and dampness, warms meridians, stops bleeding and calm the fetus," this exposition of moxibustion is recorded in *A New Edition of Materia Medica*. It is therefore indicated for wind, cold, damp Bi syndromes, weakness of Qi and blood, collapse of Yang Qi, carbuncles, furuncles and boils. Applying moxibustion frequently at Guanyuan(CV 4), Qihai(CV 6), Zusanli(ST 36)etc., may prevent and treat diseases as the body resistance invigorated and the immunity strengthened.

Section 1 Classification of Moxibustion

1. Moxibustion with Moxa Cone

Put the pure moxa wool on a plate, twrist and knead the wool into cones of different sizes, the commonly used ones are as big as a grain of wheat, a lotus seed, a cocklebur fruit, or half an olive. (Fig. 2-161)

Moxibustion with moxa cones is classified into direct, and indirect moxibus-

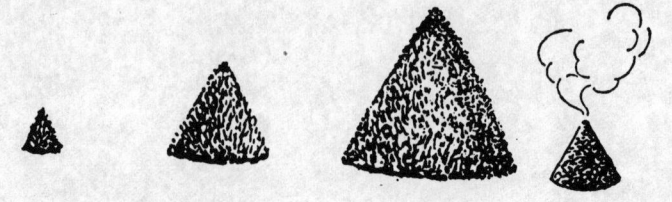

Fig. 2-161 A Moxa Cone

tions.

(1) Direct Moxibustion

A moxa cone placed directly on the point and ignited is called direct moxibustion. It is subdivided into scarring moxibustion, and no scarring moxibustion, in the former, the local place is desired to be burnt, blistered and left with a scar when healed, and in the latter, moxibustion conducted on the points will not cause burning, blistering and scarring. (Fig. 2-162)

Scarring Moxibustion (also known as "blistering moxibustion")

Prior to moxibustion, apply some garlic juice to the site in order to increase the adhesion and stimulation of the moxa cone to the skin, then put the moxa cone of the required size on the point and ignite it until it completely burns out, remove the ash. Repeat this procedure till all the cones burn out. Generally, for one session of treatment, five to seven cones are burnt. During the combustion when a patient feels painful, the surrounding place of the moxibustion site can be gently tapped with hand so as to reduce pain. Normally, one week after the moxibustion, the treatment site would blister and post-moxibustion sore appears. Five to six weeks later, the sore heals and a scar forms when the crust falls away. This method is indicated for certain chronic diseases, such as asthma, the impairment of the lung due to overstrain and intractable pain. It is advisable that the post-moxibustion sore should be kept clean and avoid secondary infection.

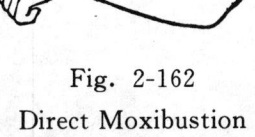

Fig. 2-162
Direct Moxibustion

No Scarring Moxibustion

A moxa cone is placed on a point and ignited. When about two thirds of it is burnt or the patient feels a burning discomfort, remove the cone and place another one. Three to seventeen cones are continuously burnt to cause flush in the local site, but no blister should be formed. This method is used widely, often for cold and deficient disorders such as asthma, chronic diarrhea, indigestion etc.

(2) Indirect Moxibustion (also known as moxibustion with material insulation)

The ignited moxa cone does not contact on the skin directly, but is insulated from the skin by the materials of ginger, salt, garlic, and monkshood cake.

Moxibustion with Ginger

Cut a slice of ginger about 2-3 cm wide and 0.2-0.3 cm thick, punch numerous holes on it and place it on the point selected. On top of this piece of ginger, a moxa cone is placed and ignited. (Fig. 2-163)

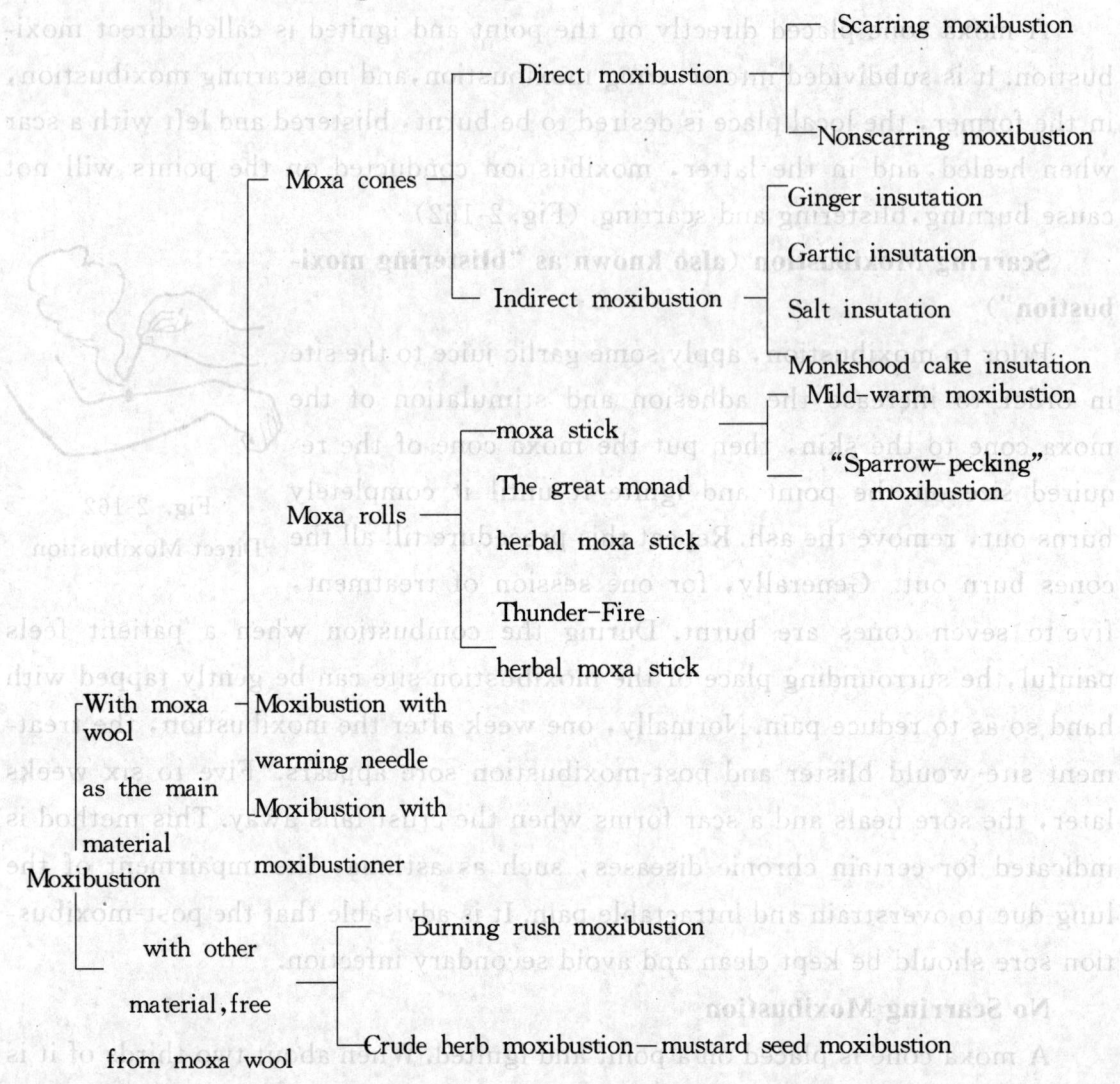

```
Moxibustion
├─ With moxa wool as the main material
│   ├─ Moxa cones
│   │   ├─ Direct moxibustion
│   │   │   ├─ Scarring moxibustion
│   │   │   └─ Nonscarring moxibustion
│   │   └─ Indirect moxibustion
│   │       ├─ Ginger insutation
│   │       ├─ Gartic insutation
│   │       ├─ Salt insutation
│   │       └─ Monkshood cake insutation
│   ├─ Moxa rolls
│   │   ├─ moxa stick         ┐ Mild-warm moxibustion
│   │   ├─ The great monad    │
│   │   ├─ herbal moxa stick  │ "Sparrow-pecking" moxibustion
│   │   └─ Thunder-Fire herbal moxa stick
│   ├─ Moxibustion with warming needle
│   └─ Moxibustion with moxibustioner
└─ with other material, free from moxa wool
    ├─ Burning rush moxibustion
    └─ Crude herb moxibustion — mustard seed moxibustion
```

When the patient feels scorching, remove it and ignite another. Repeat this till all the cones burn and the skin becomes reddish. This method has the effects of warming the spleen and stomach and dispersing the cold. It is therefore indicated for symptoms caused by weakness and cold of spleen and stomach, such as abdominal pain, diarrhea, painful joints and other symptoms due to Yang deficiency.

Moxibustion with Garlic

Cut a slice of garlic some 0.2 to 0.3 cm thick (a large single clove of garlic is desirable), punch holes on it, put it on the point with the ignited moxa cone above. Renew the cone when the patient feels scorching. This method has the effect of relieving swelling and pain, is often used for the early stage of skin ulcer with boils, scrofula, etc.

(3) Moxibustion with Salt

This method is usually applied at the umbilicus. Fill the umbilicus with salt to the level of the skin, place a moxa cone on the top of the salt and then ignite it. (Fig. 2-164) When it burns out, renew another until all the cones have combusted. As this method has the action of restoring Yang from collapse and warming the spleen and stomach, it is effective for the symptoms of sweating, cold limbs and undetectable pulse resulted from acute vomiting and diarrhea, or flaccid type of wind stroke and postpartum fainting.

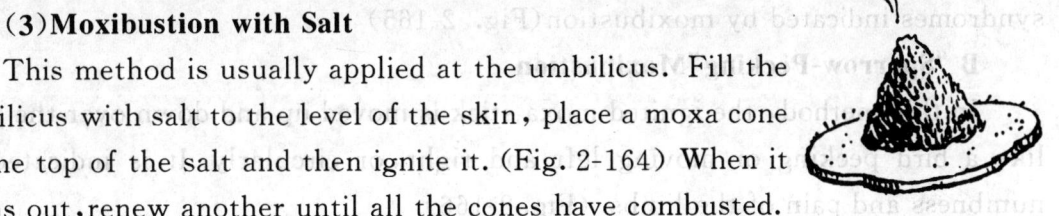

Fig. 2-163 Moxibustion with Ginger

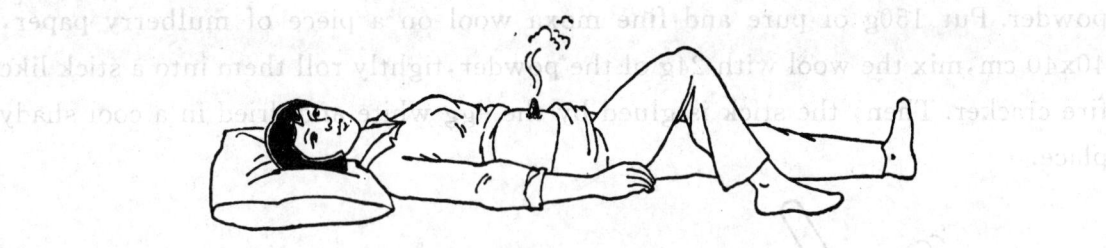

Fig. 2-164 Moxibustion with Salt

(4) Moxibustion with Monkshood Cake

A cake 3 cm in diameter and 0.3 cm in thickness, made of monkhood powder mixed with alcohol, is punched with holes in it, and placed on the site for moxibustion with the moxa cone, which is ignited and burnt on the top of it. This method is good for warming and strengthening kidney-Yang and thus adopted to treat impotence, spermatorrhea, ejaculate precox, infertility and ruptured abscess resistant to healing.

2. Moxibustion with Moxa Roll

This method includes moxibustion with moxa stick, with the great monad herbal moxa stick and with thunder fire herbal moxa stick.

(1) Moxibustion with Moxa Stick

Roll the moxa wool with a sheet of paper into a moxa stick, apply a burning moxa stick with a certain distance apart over the selected point. There are two kinds of method: mild-warm moxibustion and sparrow-pecking moxibustion.

A Mild-Warm Moxibustion

Ignite a moxa stick at its one end and place it two to three centimeters away over the site to bring a mild warmth to the local place, but not burning, for some fifteen minutes until the skin becomes slightly red. It is suitable for all the syndromes indicated by moxibustion (Fig. 2-165)

B "Sparrow-Pecking" Moxibustion

In this method, the ignited moxa stick is moved up and down over the point like a bird pecking or moving left and right, or circularly. It is indicated for numbness and pain of the limbs. (Fig. 2-166)

(2) Great Monad Herbal Moxibustion

Mix together the herbs of Radix Giseng 125g, Squama Manitis 250g, the blood of goat 90g, Rhizoma Homalomenae 500g, Zuan Di Feng 300g, Cortex Cinnamomi 500g, Fructus Foenicuii 500g, Rhizoma Atractylodis 500g, Radix Glycyrrhizae 1000g, Radix ledebouriellae 2000g, musk a little, ground them into fine powder. Put 150g of pure and fine moxa wool on a piece of mulberry paper, 40×40 cm, mix the wool with 24g of the powder, tightly roll them into a stick like fire cracker. Then, the stick is glued by the egg white and dried in a cool shady place.

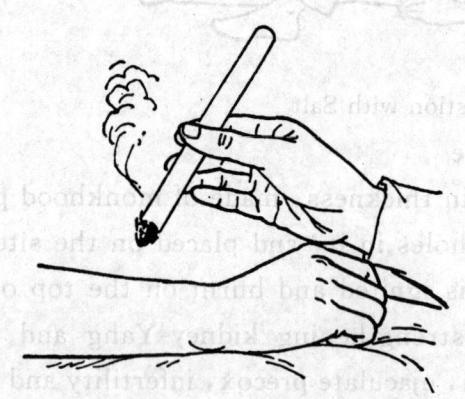

Fig. 2-165
Mild-warm Moxibustion

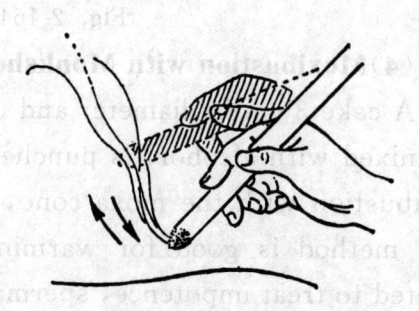

Fig. 2-166 Sparrow
-Pecking Moxibustion

In the operation, ignite the one end of the stick and wrap it into a piece of cloth of seven layers, then immediately press it on the point or the affected place to iron the place. When it becomes cool, reignite it and do the process again. Repeat it for seven to ten times. It is effective for wind, cold and damp Bi syndromes, intractable numbness, leanness with weakness and hemiplegia.

(3) Thunder-Fire Moxibustion

The way of making this sort of moxa stick is the same as that of the great monad herbal moxa stick, except that the ingredients in this moxa stick are different. It consists of pure fine moxa wool 125g and the powders of Lignum Aquilariae Resinatum 9g, Radix Aucklandiae 9g, Resina Olibani 9g, Rhizoma Seu Radix Notopterygii 9g, Rhizoma Zingiberis 9g, Squama Manitis 9g and a little musk.

The method of application and its indications are basically the same as that of the great monad herbal moxibustion with.

3. Warming Needle Moxibustion

Moxibustion with warming needle is an integration of acupuncture and moxibustion, and is used for conditions in which both retaining of the needle and moxibustion are needed. It is applied as follows:

After the arrival of Qi and with the needle retained in the point, get a small section of a moxa stick (about 2 cm long) and cuff on the handle of the needle, ignite the moxa stick from its bottom till it burns out. This method has the function of warming the meridians and promoting the flow of Qi and blood so as to treat Bi syndrome caused by cold-damp and paralysis. (Fig. 2-167)

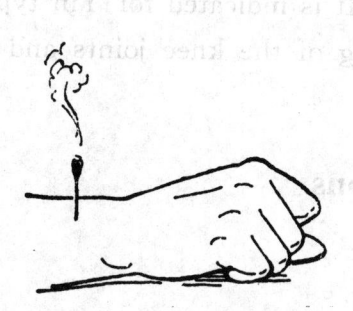

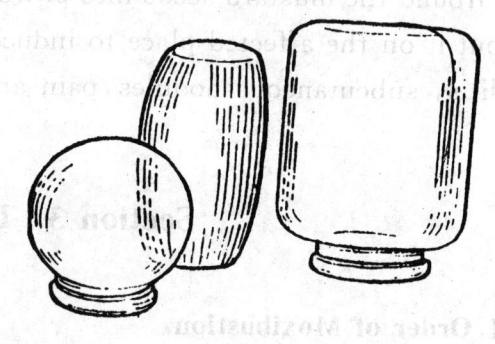

Fig. 2-167 Moxibustion with Warming Needle

Fig. 2-168 Glass Cup, Bamboo Jar

4. Moxibustion with Mild Moxibustioner

Mild moxibustioner, also known as container for moxibustion, is a metal cylindrical container made of 2 shells. The inside one being a small cylinder with cross-openings on its wall to hold the moxa floss, the outside one is cylindrical or circular cone in shape, also with cross-openings on its wall, it is attached with handle and support. Clinically, there may be other types of mild moxibustioner, however, the basic structure is similar.

Method of application: Ignite the moxa floss placed inside the container, and move the container forward and backward over the point or the affected place to let heat radiate from the bottom, or keep the container on certain distance away from the point until the local place becomes red. It is suitable for the disorders over large area, particularly, for women and children, and those who fear to be treated by other ways of moxibustion.

Section 2 Moxibustion with Other Materials

1. Burning Rush Moxibustion

Use a thread of medulla Junci, dip it into the sesame oil and ignite it, touch the point immediately with it. This method can eliminate the pathogenic wind and relieve the symptoms of the exterior syndrome, promote Qi flow and represhment, resolve phlegm and stop convulsion. It is mainly applied for paediatric diseases, such as tetanus neonatorium, gastralgia, abdominal distension and parotitis.

2. White Mustard Seed (Semen Sinapis Albae) Moxibustion

Ground the mustard seeds into powder and mix it with water or ginger juice and put it on the affected place to induce blister. It is indicated for Yin type of cellulitis, subcutaneous nodules, pain and swelling of the knee joints and wry face.

Section 3 Precautions

1. Order of Moxibustion

Generally, it starts from the upper part of the body, then to the low part; first the back, second the abdomen; first the head, then the four limbs. Clinically, it may be applied freely in accordance with the pathological state.

2. Reinforcement and Reduction with Moxibustion

For reinforcement, do not assist combustion by blowing, let the moxa burn naturally till it burns out; for reduction, while the moxa is burning, blow air to it time after time to make the combustion vigorous. This method is recorded in the book *Miraculous Pivot*.

Section 4 Contraindications of Moxibustion

1. In principle, excess heat syndrome or the syndrome of Yin deficiency with heat signs are contraindicated to moxibustion.

2. Scarring moxibustion is prohibited on face and head, and the place close to the large blood vessels.

3. The abdomen and lumbosacral region are not allowed to use moxibustion in pregnancy.

Section 5 Management After Moxibustion

After moxibustion, it is normal to have a slight redness of skin due to burning on the local place, sometimes, heavier or long-time moxibustion may cause a few blisters locally. Take care not to let small blisters break, they will heal by themselves. Large blisters should be punctured with sterilized needle and drained. Then applied with gentian violet and covered with gauze pad. If the patient receives scarring moxibustion and pus is formed during the period of festering, the patient should be advised to take proper rest and nutrious diet to keep the local area clean to prevent further infection. In case the wound is infected and the pus becomes yellow or green, and bloody, ointment of anti-infection or Yuhong ointment is necessary.

(Appendix: Cupping Therapy)

Cupping, also termed as "horn method" in the ancient China, is a therapy in which a jar is attached to the skin to induce local congestion and blood stasis through the negative pressure created by introducing heat by an ignited material inside the jar. It is commonly applied for Bi syndrome.

Cupping in conjunction with blood letting is indicated for treatment of acute sprains with blood stasis, carbuncles and ulcers, some skin diseases, such as erysipelas, neurodermatitic, etc.

(1) **Types of Jars**

There are three types commonly used in the clinic: glass cup, bamboo jar and ceramic cup. (Fig. 2-168)

(2) **Manipulations**

Cupping with glass cup and ceramic cup

A cup is attached to the skin surface through the negative pressure created by a fire inside the cup. Following are the four methods:

(a) Fire Twinkling Method

Clamp a cotton ball soaked with 95% alcohol with a forceps or nipper, ignite it and insert it into the cup, turn the ignited cotton for one circle inside the cup and immediately take it out and press the cup on the selected location. This method being simple and safe, not restricted by the body postures, is commonly applied in the clinic. (Fig. 2-169)

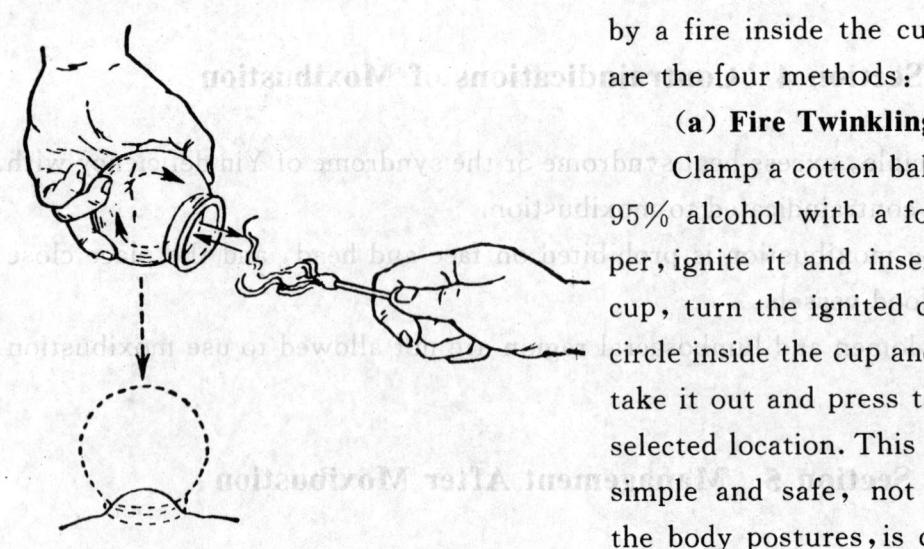

Fig. 2-169 Fire Twinkling Method

(b) Fire Throwing Method

Throw a piece of ignited paper or an alcohol cotton ball into the cup, then rapidly put the mouth of the cup firmly against the skin on the desired position. This method is applied to the lateral side of the body. (Fig. 2-170)

(c) Alcohol Firing Method

Place one to three drops of alcohol into a cup (not much so as to prevent it from dripping out of the cup to burn the skin), distribute evenly the alcohol on the wall by turning the cup. Then the alcohol is ignited and the cup is immediately pressed on to the place to be treated.

(d) Cotton Firing Method

Stick a piece of proper sized alcohol cotton on the lower one third of the inner wall of the cup, ignite the cotton and the cup is then placed on the selected location.

(e) Firing Method for Cup Laid on Treatment Location

Prior to firing, place a few drops of 95% alcohol or a piece of alcohol cotton into a non-combustive and slow heat conducting container, such as bottle cover, or small wine cup which previously

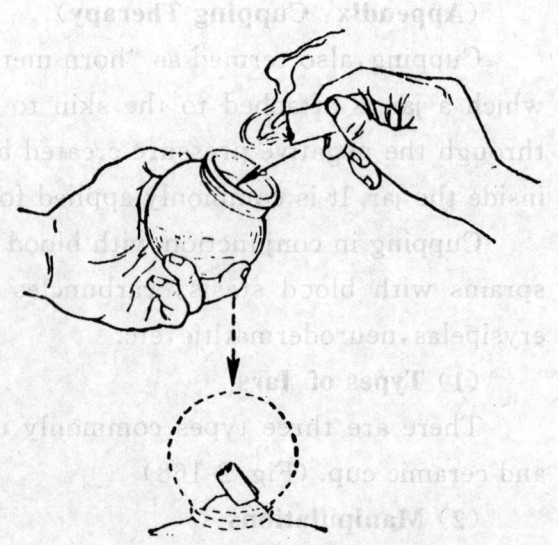

Fig. 2-170 Fire Throwing Method

laid on the treatment location, ignite the alcohol or cotton, press the cup rapidly on the position.

(f) Boiling Method

Fasten herbs in a cloth pouch, boil the herbal pouch in plain water to make into liquid of proper density, put the bamboo jar into the liquid, boiling about 15 minutes, take out the jar form the liquid and pour out the liquid inside the jar, the mouth of the jar is firmly pressed against a cold towel, the jar is then immediately placed on the selected location on the skin surface. The herbs in this method serve to enhance the effect of dispelling wind and relieving pain, often applied for wind-damp Bi syndrome and some soft tissue disorders. The herbs used possess the properties of dispelling wind, clearing obstruction in the meridians and promoting blood circulation.

(3) Removal of the Cup

Generally, the cup is retained in the location for 10 to 15 minutes, in this period, the local place would become hyperemic. The cup is then removed. On removal, hold the cup with the left hand and press the skin beside the edge of the cup with the right hand to let the air come into the cup, and release cup. It is not allowed to remove the cup by pulling or turning it hard, which may injure the skin. If cupping is conducted by a big cup and the suction is very strong, the cup should be retained for shorter time so as to avoid causing blister. (Fig. 2-171)

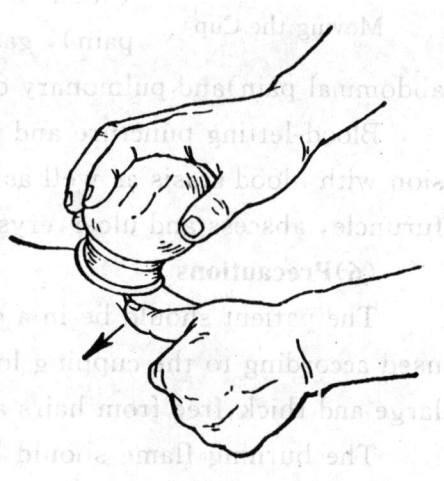

Fig. 2-171 Withdrawing the Cup

(4) Special Methods

Clinically in different pathological conditions, following options of cupping may be applied.

Movable Cupping

Prior to the treatment, apply lubricant oil, such as vaseline, on the skin, the cup then is sucked to the skin in the way as explained in the previous methods. Hold the cup with the right hand and slide it around and back to the affected area until the skin becomes congested. It is suitable for treatment of a large area, such as the back, the lumbus, the buttocks and the thigh. (Fig. 2-172)

Successive Flash Cupping

In this method, apply repeatedly and swiftly the cup over the same place until the skin becomes hyperaemic.

After the disinfection of the local place, puncture it with three-edged needle to let blood or tap with plum-blossom needle, then apply cupping. It enhances blood circulation and relieves swelling and pain by removing the blood stasis.

(5) Indications

The cupping method has the actions of warming meridians, invigorating Qi and blood circulation, dispelling damp and cold, relieving blood stagnation, swelling and pain. It is commonly applied in Bi syndromes (such as lumbago, low limb pain, shoulder and back pain), gastrointestinal tract disorders (such as gastralgia, abdominal pain) and pulmonary diseases (such as cough and asthma).

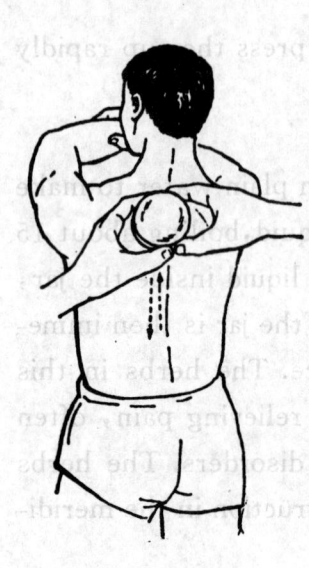

Fig. 2-172 Moving the Cup

Blood-letting puncture and cupping are suitable for acute sprain and contusion with blood stasis as well as skin and external diseases, including carbuncle, furuncle, abscess and ulcer, erysipelas, neurodermatitis, psoriasis, etc.

(6) Precautions

The patient should be in a comfortable position. Cups in different sizes are used according to the cupping location. Generally, the place where the muscle is large and thick, free from hairs and bone ridges are selected.

The burning flame should be strong enough to create a vacuum. Hold the cup with the rim close to the local place and cup it to the skin rapidly and deftly, otherwise the therapeutic effect will be attenuated.

It is not advisable to apply cupping to the patient with skin ulcer, edema, or on a place supplied with large blood vessels, to the patient with high fever and convulsion; or to the abdominal and sacral locations of the pregnant women.

It is not suitable to apply cupping to the patient with bleeding tendency. Caution for burning or scalding the skin. If blisters appear due to scalding or long retaining of cup, no treatment is needed. Blister for the small blister or the big one, drainage of liquid with a sterile syringe, application of gentian violet and gauze to prevent infection are indicated.

Chapter 3
Other Acupuncture Therapies

Section 1 The Three-Edged Needle

The three-edged needle, a needle for bloodletting, presently made of stainless steel, being 2 cun long, is shaped in a round handle, a triangular head and a sharp tip. (Fig. 2-173)

Fig. 2-173 The Three-Edged Needle

1. Manipulations

Hold the handle of the three-edged needle with the thumb and the index finger of the right hand, the middle finger supporting against the lower shaft of the needle with 0.1-0.2 cun of the tip exposed. (Fig. 2-174)

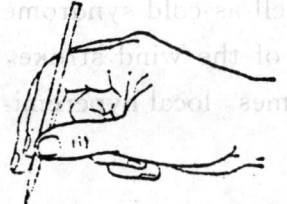

On pricking, the left hand holds the finger, the toe, or pinches, stretches the skin of the selected point. There are four commonly applied methods.

(1) Point Pricking

First, push and press the skin around the point to gather the blood, hold the handle of the three-edged needle with the right hand, prick the disinfected point swiftly about 0.1-0.2 cun deep for bloodletting and withdraw the needle immediately, gently squeeze the skin around the pricked spot to let a few drops of blood, afterwards, press the punctured point with a sterilized cotton ball to stop bleeding, for instance, pricking Shaoshang(LU 11) to treat sore throat, pricking the apex of the auricle for conjunctivitis.

Fig. 2-174 Holding the Three-Edged Needle

(2) Collateral Pricking

After disinfection of the skin, prick the selected superficial vein to let a little blood, afterwards, press the punctured hole with a sterilized dry cotton ball to stop bleeding, e.g. pricking the superficial vein at the popliteal space and the medial side of the elbow for sun stroke and pricking several spots on the red threads of the affected location for acute lymphangitis.

(3)**Clumpy Pricking**

Prink a number of spots at the affected location, or around a small place of a red swelling, then press the skin or apply cupping to let the stagnated blood escape to alleviate swelling and pain. In case of intractable tinea, carbuncles, erysipelas, sprain and contusion, the local place can be pricked by this method.

(4)**Prinking**

In the operation, the left hand presses or pinches up the disinfected skin, prick superficially the point or the reactionary spot with a three-edged needle to let blood or fluid, or further prick 0.5 cm deep to break the tissue fiber, afterwards, cover the punctured site with gauze. This method is applied for multiple folliculitis, neck scrofula which are treated by pricking the reactionary spots at the both sides of the vertebra. For hemorrhoids, prick the reactionary spots at the lumbar sacral place.

2. Indications

The three-edged needling has the function of dispelling blood stasis and heat and assisting resuscitation, promoting the flow of Qi and blood in meridians. It is advisable to treat excess syndrome and heat syndrome as well as cold syndrome of excess type, e.g. high fever, syncopy, tense syndrome of the wind stroke, sore throat, carbuncles, hemorrhoids, intractable Bi syndromes, local hyperemia, swelling, numbness, etc.

3. Precautions

(1) Puncturing the skin with three-edged needle is a strong stimulation, thus, fainting should be prevented.

(2) Aseptic manipulation should be observed to prevent infection.

(3) For spot pricking, the operation should be slightly superficial and rapid to avoid excessive bleeding, injuring the deep large arteries.

(4) Pricking shall in no case be applied for those with weak constitution, pregnancy and bleeding tendency.

(5) Bleeding is applied once daily or once every other day, three to five sessions constitute one course, for acute case, it may be given twice daily; if a large amount of bloodletting is made, it is advisable to apply the treatment once or twice a week; to apply the pricking method, it is performed once for 3-7 days and

one course consisting of 3-5 sessions of treatment, and 10—14 days break between two courses.

Section 2　The Cutaneous Needle

The cutaneous needle is also termed as the plum-blossom needle and seven-star needle, which is made of five to seven stainless needles inlaid onto the end of a handle. (Fig. 2-175)

1. Manipulation

After routine disinfection, hold the handle of the needle with the index finger against the handle and tap vertically on the skin with a gentle movement of the wrist. (Fig. 2-176)

The tapping may be light, moderate or heavy in accordance with the constitution, the age, the pathological state and the location of the patient. Light tapping is made by exerting a slight force until the skin becomes congested, it is applied for the kids, the women, the weak and the elderly, on the neck, face and five sense organs, also on the places with thin muscles; heavy tapping is conducted by exerting a relatively strong force until a slight bleeding appears with a little pain, suitable for the strong, the excess syndrome, or used on the places with thick muscles; the force exerted in the moderate tapping is between that of the light and heavy tappings. The moderate tapping is required to cause congestion and with slight pain, but no bleeding, suitable for the majority of the patients, ordinary diseases and general locations. The places to be tapped may be along the course of meridian, or on the points selected, or on the affected locations.

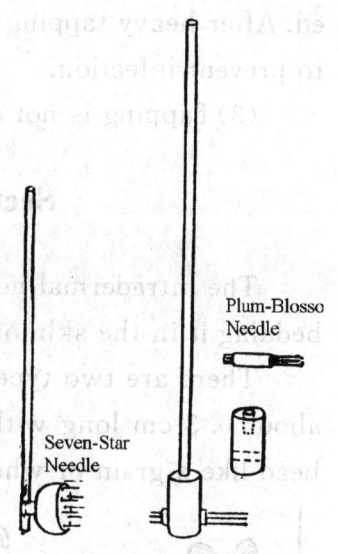

Fig. 2-175 Skin Needle

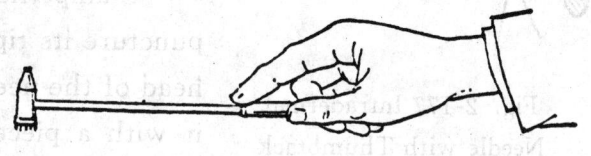

Fig. 2-176 Holding the Skin Needle

2. Indications

The cutaneous needling is used to treat disorders of the nervous system and dermatosis, e. g. headache, hypochondriac pain, dizziness and vertigo, insomnia, myopia, painful joints and paralysis, gastrointestinal disease, gynaecological disease and various kinds of skin disease.

3. Precautions

(1) The tips of the needles should be sharp, smooth and free from any hooks. On tapping, the tips of the needles should strike the skin at a right angle to the surface to reduce pain.

(2) Sterilize the needles, and the location of treatment should be disinfected. After heavy tapping, the local skin surface should be cleaned and disinfected to prevent infection.

(3) Tapping is not allowed to apply to the location of trauma and ulcers.

Section 3 The Intradermal Needle

The intradermal needle is a sort of specially made short needle used for embedding it in the skin or subcutaneously for relatively long time.

There are two types, the thumbtack type and grain-like type, the former is about 0.3 cm long with a circular head, and the latter some 1 cm long with a head like a grain or wheat. (Fig. 2-177)

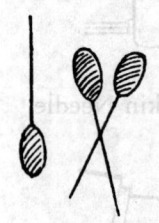

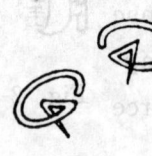

Fig. 2-177 Intradermal Needle with Thumbtack Type and Grain-like Type

1. Manipulations

(1) **The Thumbtack Needle**

Clamp the head of the needle with a forceps, puncture its tip into the disinfected point, leave the head of the needle on the surface of the skin and fix it with a piece of adhesive. It is suitable for the points on the face and the ear.

(2) **The Grain-like Needle**

Clamp the body of the needle with a forceps, insert the needle horizontally into the disinfected point some 0.5-1 cm deep, fix external part of the needle outside the skin with a piece of adhesive. It is used for points or trigger points at the various parts of the body.

2. Indications

It is mainly used for chronic, intractable or painful diseases which need long period retention of the needle, such as headache, stomachache, biliary colic, insomnia, hypertension, irregular menstruation, enurisis, cough, asthma, etc.

3. Precautions

(1) No intradermal needle are close to the joints so as to avoid pain by motion.

(2) Intradermal needle is not allowed at the inflammatory location or skin ulcers.

(3) During the embedding period, keep the place around the needle clean to prevent infection.

(4) The duration of implantation is varied with the pathological conditions as well as seasons, in summer when one tends to sweat, the needles are generally retained for 1-2 days to avoid infection. In autumn or winter, retention of the needle may last 3-7 days. During the retention, press the embedded site for 1-2 minutes at every 4 hours to enhance the stimulation and raise the therapeutic effect.

Section 4 Electro-Acupuncture

Electro-acupuncture is an approach of preventing and treating diseases, in which electrical stimulator is connected to the points after the needling sensation is obtained, and the sensation would be enhanced via the pulsative current to the points.

There are different types of electro-stimulator which vary in the mode of output, the pulsatory current is generated by an oscillator, the output voltage ranges from 40-80V, and the output current is less than 1mA with the advantage of being safe and providing strong stimulation, it may be adopted to replace the hand manipulation.

1. Manipulation

In general, 1 to 2 pair of points are selected from the same side of the body or limbs, puncture the point with the filiform needle after the needling sensation occurs and reinforcing or reducing needling manipulation is conducted, set the output potentionmeter of the stimulator to "0", connect the two wires of the output respectively to the handles of the two needles, switch on the power supply, select the desired wave pattern and frequency, gradually increase the output current until the patient gets a tolerable soreness and numbness sensation. The electro-stimulation may last 10-20 minutes. When used in the acupuncture analgesia, the stimulation may be longer. In case the stimulative sensation decreases, the current may be increased properly, or turn off the power supply for 1-2 minutes, then reswitch it on or adjust the output current to have a constant stimulative effect. When the treatment is over, turn the potential to "0" and switch off the stimulator, disconnect the wires from the needles and withdraw the needles.

2. The Actions of the Electro-Pulsation and the Indications of Electro-Acupuncture

(1) The Actions of Electro-Pulse

The low frequency pulsation of the stimulator would stimulate the point via the inserted filiform needle so as to affect the physiological function of the body, relieve the muscular spasm and pain, induce sedation and promote the blood circulation. As the pulsation varies in frequency and wave pattern, the actions of the pulses may be different. The high frequency pulse 50-100/sec. is known as dense wave, the low frequency pulse 2-5/sec. termed as rarefaction wave. A electro-stimulator may consist of a number of wave patterns, such as dense wave, rarefaction wave, dense-rarefaction wave and intermittent wave. The wave pattern is selected in accordance with the pathological condition.

Dense Wave: It may induce an inhibitory effect on the sensory nerve and motor nerve, commonly used for sedation and pain relief, relaxation of muscles and vessels spasm, acupuncture analgesia, etc.

Rarefaction Wave: It provides stronger stimulation to the points via the needles, thus causing contraction of muscle and the increment of the tension of muscles and ligaments. It induces a retarded inhibitory effect on the sensory and motor nerves. This kind of wave pattern is suitable for paralysis, injury of muscles, joints, ligaments, and muscular tendons, etc.

Rarefaction-Dense Wave: It provides an alternation of rarefaction wave and dense wave, each wave lasting for one and a half second. This pattern has the advantage of avoiding sensory adaptation to the electro-stimulation which may occur in the treatment with single wave pattern, being good for the promotion of metabolism and the flow of Qi and blood, improving the nutrition of tissues and relieving the inflammatory edema. It is commonly used for pain, sprain and contusion, peripheral arthritis, disturbance of Qi and blood circulation, sciatica, facial paralysis, myasthenia, local frozen bite.

Intermittent Wave: A regular intermittent rarefaction wave, it is an alternation of one and a half second stimulation in rarefaction wave and one and a half second on stimulation. This kind of wave may increase the excitability of muscular tissue and have a fine stimulative and contractive effect on the striated muscle. It is commonly used for muscular weakness and atrophy, paralysis, etc. (Fig. 2-178)

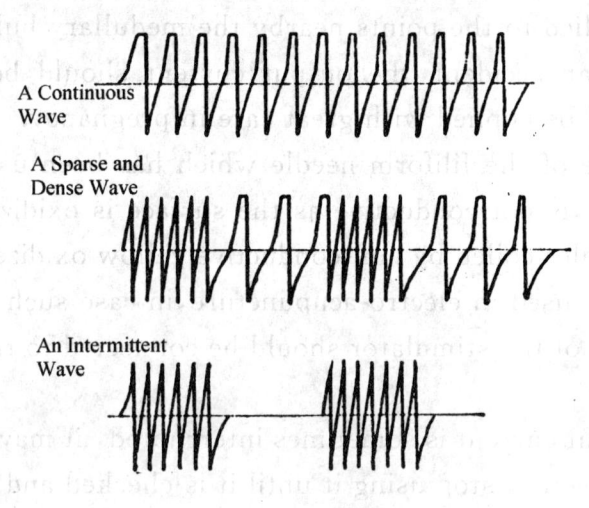

Fig. 2-178

Sawtooth Wave: It is a kind of fluctuation wave in sawtooth form, the frequency ranging from 16-25/min which is close to human's respiration, therefore also known as respiratory wave. It is used for stimulating the phrenic nerve, (Tianding LI 17) artificial electric breathing and respiratory failure. It also has the actions of raising the excitability of nerves and muscles, regulating the meridians and collaterals, improving the flow of Qi and blood.

(2) Indications

The electro-acupuncture is indicated for the diseases that can be treated by filiform needling, particularly for manic-depressive psychosis, neurasthenia, neuralgia, sequelae of cerebrovascular accident, sequelae of poliomyelitis, muscular flaccidity, gastrointestinal diseases, arthralgia syndrome, painful joints as well as acupuncture analgesia.

3. Precautions

(1) Prior to the treatment, inspect whether the output of the stimulator is normal, post to the treatment, turn all the buttons of the stimulator into "0", switch off the power supply and disconnect all the wires from the needles.

(2) Electro-acupuncture generally provides strong stimulation to the points, prevention of fainting should be kept in mind. On setting the output of the stim-

ulator, it is advisable to adjust it gradually, from small to large to avoid sudden and big increment, which may cause strong muscular contraction and bending or breaking needles.

(3) For patient with cardiac diseases, the electric stimulation is so connected that the current loop is not allowed to pass through the heart. When the electro-stimulation is supplied to the points nearby the medullary bulb and spinal cord, in order to avoid an accident, the output current should be smaller. Electro-acupuncture should be applied with great care in pregnancy.

(4) The handle of the filiform needle which has been used in the warming needle moxibustion, is not conductive as the surface is oxidized, and some needles with their handles coiled by non-conductive yellow oxidized alumina wire are not suggested to be used in electro-acupuncture, in case such needles have to be used, the connector of the stimulator should be connected to the body of the needle.

(5) If the output current is sometimes interrupted, it may be due to the poor contact of the connector, stop using it until it is checked and fixed.

Section 5   Hydro-Acupuncture

Hydro-acupuncture, also known as point injection, is a recently developed therapy, in which acupoint or relevant location is treated by drug injection. Exerting a stimulative and pharmaceutical effect on the point via puncture and drug injection, this therapy can improve physiological functions, correct the pathological state, and raise the therapeutic effects.

The sizes of the syringe needle and the syringe used in the treatment vary with drug dosage and the selected location. In general, 1ml, 2ml, 5ml, 10ml, 20ml syringes and No. 5, No. 6 ordinary syringe needles are adopted, or select No. 5 needle used by the dentists, or No. 9 long needle used in block therapy.

1. Commonly Used Drugs

The drugs for muscular injection can be adopted in hydro-acupuncture, such as the herbal injection: Chinese Angelica Root, Safflower, Compound Radix Angelicae Sinensis, Compound Radix Salviae Miltiorrhizae, Rhizome ligustici Chuangxiong, Radix Isatidis, Radix Bupleuri, Herba Houttuyniae, Radix Clematidis, Radix Lynanchi Paniculati; and western drug injection: Vitamin B, Vitamin B6, Vitamin C, Vitamin K3, 5-10% glucose, 0.25-2% procaine hydrochloride, 25% magnesium sulfate, normal saline, atropine, reserpine, adrenosem salicylate, ephedrine, antibiotics, placental extract etc.

2. Administration
(1) Selection of Points
Based on the differentiation of syndromes, select 2-4 relevant points or Ashi points, or reactionary masses as location for injection

(2) Dosage of Injection
The dosage in hydro-acupuncture depends on the location of injection, the property and density of the injection. For adults, with the herbal extract injection and vitamin injection, each point is injected 1-2ml in one session. With antibiotics, 1/10 to 1/2 of the original dosage is injected. With 5-10% glucose, in each session 5-20 ml is injected. The locations on the four limbs, waist and buttocks where the muscles are abundant can be injected with a little more dosage and those points at the head, face and auricle where the muscles are thin may be injected with 0.1-0.5 ml per point.

(3) Manipulation
In the treatment, select the right syringe and syringe needle, draw the injection into the syringe, disinfect the locations to be injected on the patient who is on an appropriate position for the injection. Puncture rapidly the syringe held with the right hand into the point (or the reactionary mass), then the needle is gradually inserted deeper, after the needling sensation occurs, withdraw the handle of the syringe a little bit to see whether blood is withdrawn into to the tube or not, if not inject the solution into the point. In general, moderate speed of injection is adopted. For acute and excessive heat syndromes, rapid injection is indicated and for chronic and deficient syndromes, the injection should be slow. In case a big amount of solution is injected, it should be injected into the point in a few steps, from the deep to the superficial, or the syringe needle can be inserted in a few directions from the punctured point to inject the solution.

(4) Course of Treatment
Hydro-acupuncture is applied once or twice daily for acute disease; and once daily or every other day for chronic disease, the points on both sides can be alternatively treated. One course consists of 6-10 sessions of treatment. Duration between two courses is one week.

Indications
The majority of the diseases indicated by acupuncture can be treated by hydro-acupuncture. It is suitable for cough, asthma, gastralgia, neuralgia, Bi syn-

drome, flaccid syndrome, lumbago and pain of the low limb, sprain and contusion, skin diseases, etc.

3. Precautions

(1) Great attention should be paid to the pharmacological property, action, dosage, quality, validity, contraindications, side effects and allergic reaction of the solution to be used. The solution may cause allergic reaction (e. g. Penicillin, etc) to some patients, skin test should be made before the treatment, the solution with relatively strong side effects should be used very cautiously.

(2) The solution in general should not be injected into the joint cavity, the spinal cord cavity and the vessels, the Misinjection of the solution into the joint cavity may lead to redness and swelling of the joint or fever and pain. Misinjection into the spinal cord cavity may impair the spinal cord.

(3) Deep injection is not allowed on the points at the neck, chest and back, and the dosage should be carefully controlled. In case the points are near the nerve trunk, avoid puncturing the nerve trunk. If the patient has electric shock sensation, withdraw the syringe a little bit to avoid injury the nerve, then inject the solution.

(4) To prevent abortion, in general, the low abdomen, the lumbar and sacral places as well as the points of Hegu (LI 4) and Sanyinjiao (SP 6), hydro-acupuncture is avoided in pregnancy.

(5) To avoid infection, aseptic manipulation in hydro-acupuncture is strictly required.

Chapter 4
The Nine Needles in the Ancient Times and the Methods Listed in Internal Classic

The record of nine needles first appeared in *Internal Classic*, in which the shapes, lengths and indications of the nine needles were mentioned in a number of chapters. The invention of the nine needles is of great significance in the development of needling techniques.

Section 1 Nine Needles

1. The Arrow-Headed Needle (Chan Zhen)

Shape: 1.6 inches long, with a sharp tip like an arrow, the cutaneous needle is developed from this needle.

Use: Superficial puncture of the skin for bloodletting, indicated for heat syndromes of the head and body.

2. Round Needle (Yuan Zhen)

Shape: 1.6 inches long with a oval-rounded tip and a cylindrical body.

Use: Rubbing the skin for Qi stasis in interstitial space and for massage

3. Blunt Needle (Di Zhen)

Shape: 3.5 inches long with a millet head, the tip is round and slightly sharp.

Use: For pressing the meridians not insertion, a tool for point pressing.

4. Sharp-Edged Needle (Feng Zhen)

Shape: 1.6 inches long with a triangular sharp three edged head and a cylindrical body, termed as "three-edged needle" by the later generations.

Use: Pricking to let blood for superficial carbuncles and painful swelling and febrile diseases.

5. Sword-Shaped Needle (Pi Zhen)

Shape: 4 inches long, 0.25 inches wide, shaped as a sword.

Use: For drainage of pus, a tool for external diseases.

6. Round-Sharp Needle (Yuan Li Zhen)

Shape: 1. 6 inches long with a slightly large head and a thin body, being round and sharp. It can be punctured deep into the point.

Use: For carbuncles and painful swelling, Bi syndrome.

7. Filiform Needle (Hao Zhen)

Shape: 2. 6 inches long, with a very fine body like a hair, a needle, for common use.

Use: Regulating meridians for cold, heat and painful syndromes.

8. Long Needle (Chang Zhen)

Shape: 7 inches long, with a round and sharp tip and a long fine body. The elongated needle is developed by the later generations from this needle.

Use: Puncture the deep tissue attacked by pathogens or persistent Bi syndrome.

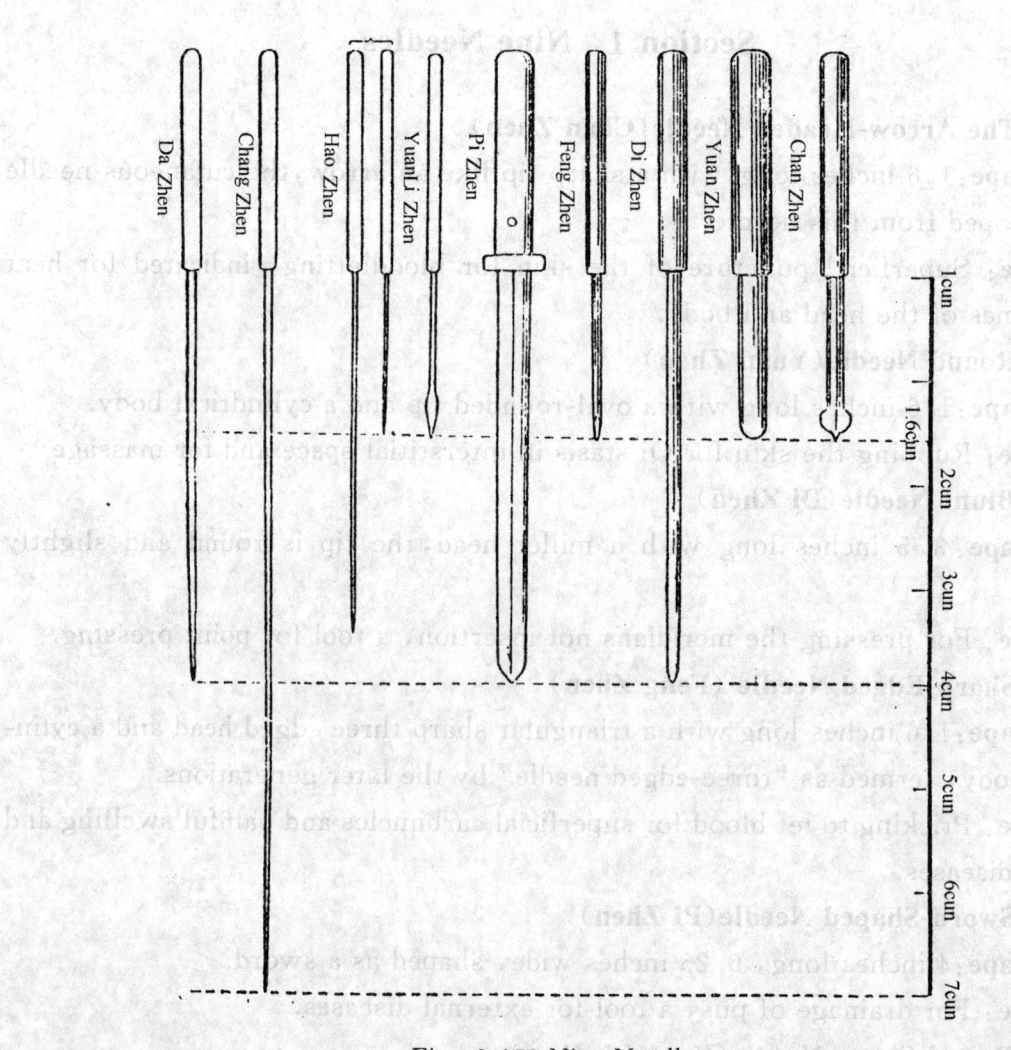

Fig. 2-179 Nine Needles

9. Large Needle (Da Zhen)

Shape: 4 inches long with a round and thick body.

Use: Removing water for joint disease with retention of water. The later generations use it as firing needle. (Fig. 2-179)

Many needling methods are described in *Internal Classic*, in which the seventh chapter of *Miraculous Pivot* has collected a lot of needling methods. Following are the brief description of the methods.

Section 2 The Nine Needling Methods

In Chapter Seven of *Miraculous Pivot*, it says: "there are nine ways of needling applied to deal with nine different diseases."

1. Shu-Point Needling

For disorders of the Five Zang-organs, by which the Ying-Spring point, Shu-stream point and the Back-Shu point of the relevant meridian are needled.

2. Distant Needling

Needling distal points on the affected meridians, by which the points in the lower part of the body are needled for diseases at the upper part, is used to treat diseases of the Six Fu-organs by selecting the lower He-(Sea) points of the Six Fu-organs from the three Yang Meridians of Foot.

3. Meridian Needling

Used to treat an affected meridian by needling along that meridian or the meridian related to the affected part, for meridian disorders.

4. Collateral Needling

Used to let blood of the subcutaneous small vessels to eliminate blood stasis and treat the collateral diseases.

5. Crack Needling

A method of needling the interstitial space to treat muscular pain, flaccidity and old injury.

6. Evacuation Needling

Use a sword-shaped needle to remove pus, purulent blood and fluid, often for external diseases.

7. Shallow Needling

A method to treat superficial disorders. The cutaneous needle used currently is developed from this method.

8. Contralateral Needling

Needling the point on the right side when the affected place is on the left or vice versa.

9. Heat Needling

A method with a red-hot fired needle to treat rheumatism, scrofula, ulcers of Yin nature, etc.

Section 3　The Twelve Needlings

In Chapter Seven of *Miraculous Pivot*, it says: "there are twelve needlings in response to various diseases of the twelve regular meridians."

1. A Coupled Puncture

A method in which two corresponding points in the anterior (the chest) and posterior (the back) aspects of the body are needled respectively known as coupling points from Yin side and Yang side in order to treat cardialgia, etc.

2. Trigger Puncture

For wandering pains, when pains are not localized in one definite spot, perpendicularly insert the needle into a trigger point with no immediate withdraw, the needle is then removed to puncture another trigger point which is later on found out by pressing with the left hand.

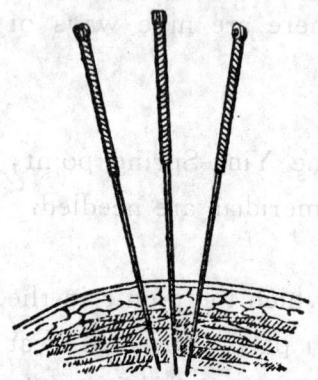

Fig. 2-180
Triple Puncture

3. Lateral Puncture

Perpendicular insertion needle at one side of the painful muscle, after needling sensation appears, ask the patient to move the affected part gently to promote the Qi flow in the meridians and relieve the spasm of the muscle. This method is used to treat rheumatic pain.

4. Triple Puncture

The needles are inserted at three spots with one in the center and two on both sides to treat rheumatism caused by pathogenic cold that attacks the body on a small scale but with a deep invasion. (Fig. 2-180)

5. Quintuple Puncture

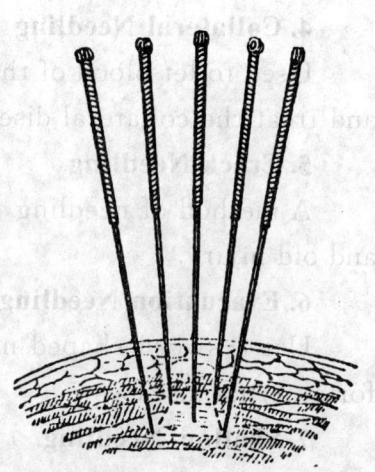

Fig. 2-181
Quintuple Puncture

A method in which the needles are inserted at five spots with one in the center and the four scattered around. This method is for the disorders involving relatively a large area by pathogenic cold. (Fig. 2-181)

6. Horizontal Puncture

A method in which the skin at the point is pinched up with a transversal insertion towards the affected place. This method is for superficial pathogenic cold invasion.

7. Shu-Point Puncture

A method in which the needles are perpendicularly inserted into a few points deeply and withdrawn rapidly to promote Qi flow and clear heat to treat heat syndrome of Qi excess.

8. Short-Puncture

A method in which the needle is inserted with slightly shaking down to the bone, then gently lifting, thrusting and twirling. This method is for deep diseases e.g. rheumatism involving the bone.

9. Superficial Puncture

A method in which an oblique or shallow insertion is applied to treat muscular spasms caused by cold. The intradermal needling is developed from this method.

10. Yin Puncture

A method in which the needling is applied to Taixi(KI 3), a point of Kindey Meridian on both feet behind the medial malleolus to treat cold limbs and cold syndrome.

11. Adjacent Puncture

A method in which the needles are inserted to the affected part perpendicularly and obliquely with one needle each to treat chronic rheumatism. (Fig. 2-182)

12. Repeated Shallow Puncture

A method in which the needle is repeatedly inserted vertically and superficially and withdrawn rapidly to cause bleeding of the affected part to treat carbuncles and erysipelas.

Section 4 The Five Needling Techniques

In the seventh Chapter of *Miraculous Pivot*, it says: "there are five needling techniques developed to treat various diseases associated with the Five Zang-organs."

1. Extreme Shallow Puncture

A technique of shallow insertion and immediate withdrawal without injury of the muscles. This technique is developed in response to the diseases associated with the lung which functionally dominates the superficial portion of the body. The technique with the action of relieving the pathogens retained in the superficies is used in the treatment for fever, cough, gasp due to pathogenic wind and superficial cold attacking and skin diseases.

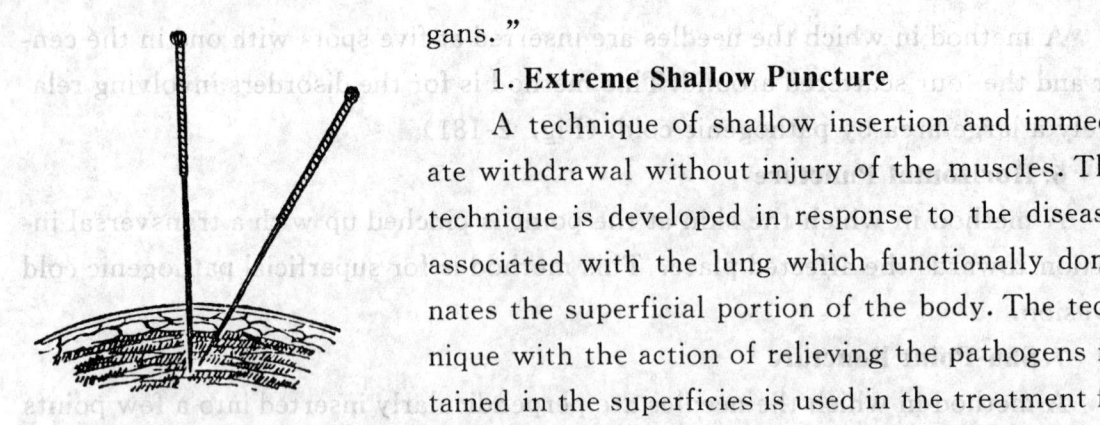

Fig. 2-182 Adjacent Puncture

2. Leopard-Spot Puncture

A technique of needling the small blood vessels superior, inferior, left and right to the diseased area to make bleeding. As the heart controls blood circulation and blood vessels, this technique is aimed at Qi and blood. This technique is used to treat swelling, redness, heat and pain.

3. Joint puncture

A technique of needling the muscles around the joints of the extremities, but to avoid bleeding, to treat rheumatism. This technique is aimed at the disease linked with the liver as the liver control tendons.

4. Hegu Puncture

A technique in which the needle is inserted obliquely and deeply between the muscles of the diseased area, then it is withdrawn to the superficial level, afterwards inserted obliquely right and left like the claws of the chicken to treat muscular rheumatism. This technique is aimed at the diseases linked with the spleen which controls muscles. (Fig. 2-183)

5. Shu-Point Puncture

A technique in which the needle is thrusted deeply to the bone to treat osteal pain. This technique is aimed at the diseases linked with the kidney which dominates bones.

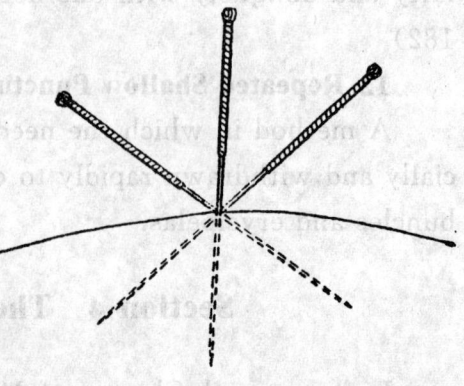

Fig. 2-183 Hegu Puncture

Chapter 5 Scalp Acupuncture

Scalp acupuncture refers to the therapeutic approach of needling the specific areas on the scalp. It is often applied for cerebral diseases. The needling points are scalp areas corresponding to the functional areas of the cerebral cortex, the nomenclature of the areas (lines) are in accordance with the functional area of the cerebral cortex.

Section 1 The Locations and Indications of the Stimulating Areas

In order to locate the stimulating areas more conveniently, two nominal lines, i. g. the anterior-posterior midline of the head and the eyebrow occipital line can be used as the landmarks.

The anterior-posterior midline: a midline of the head connecting the glabella with the lower border of external occipital protuberance.

The eyebrow-occipital line: a line from the mid-point of the upper border of the eyebrow diagonally to the tip of the external occipital protuberance (Fig. 2-184)

There are 13 common stimulating areas in scalp acupuncture.

Motor Area

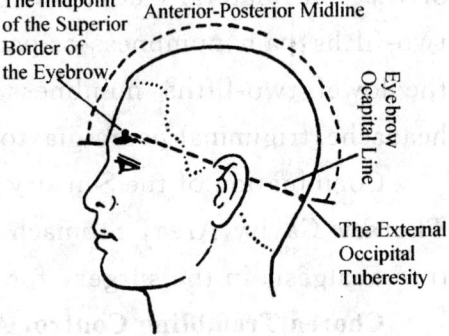

Fig. 2-184 Standard Lines

Location: It is located over the anterior central convolution of the cerebral cortex, being a line starting from a point (Know as the upper point of the Motor Area) 0.5 cm posterior to the midpoint of the anterior-posterior midline of the head and stretching diagonally to the juncture between the eyebrow-occipital line and the anterior border of the corner of temporal hairline. It is the projection of the Motor Area. In case the anterior corner of the temporal hairline is indistinct, draw a vertical line upward from the middle point of the zygomatic arch to the eyebrow-occipital line, the intersection of the two lines is the projection of the Motor Area. Motor Area is divided into five equal parts: the upper one-fifth be-

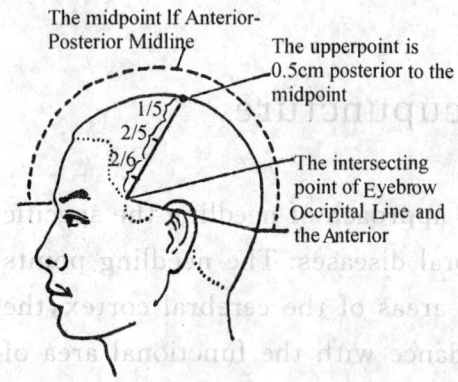

Fig. 2-185 Locating the Motor Area

ing the Motor Area of the lower limb and the trunk, the middle two-fifths being the Motor Area of the upper limb, the lower two-fifths, the Motor Area of the face. (Fig. 2-185)

Indications: The upper one-fifth: paralysis of the lower limb of the contralateral side; the middle two-fifths: paralysis of upper limb of the contralateral side; the lower two-fifths: central facial paralysis of the contralateral side, moter aphasia, dropping saliva, impaired speech.

Sensory Area

Location: Over the posterior central convolution of cerebral cortex, a line parallel and 1.5 cm posterior to the Motor Area, the upper one-fifth is the Sensory Area of the lower limb, the head and the trunk, the middle two-fifths is the Sensory Area of the upper limb, the lower two-fifths, the Sensory Area of the face. (Fig. 2-186)

Indications: The upper one-fifth of Sensory Area line: low back and leg pain of the contralateral side, paresthesia, numbness, neck pain, tinnitus; the middle two-fifths: pain, numbness or paresthesia of upper limb of the contralateral side; the lower two-fifths: numbness of the face of the contralateral side, one side headache, trigiminal neuralgia, toothache and mandibular joint arthritis.

Combination of the Sensory Area with the relevant areas of the viscera (e.g. Thoracic Cavity Area, Stomach Area, Genital Area) may be used for acupuncture analgesia in the surgery for certain areas.

Chorea Trembling Control Area

Location: Parallel with and 1.5 cm anterior to Motor Area Line. (Fig. 2-186)

Indications: Chorea, parkinsonian syndrome. If the disease involving only one side, treat the contralateral side of the Chorea Trembling Control Area, in case both sides are involved, treat both sides.

Vertigo and Auditory Area

Location: With a point 1.5 cm directly above the apex of ear as the midpoint, draw a 4 cm horizontal line. (Fig. 2-186)

Indications: Dizziness and vertigo, tinnitus, hearing impairment, etc.

The Second Speech Area

Location: Over the angular gyrus of the cerebral parietal lobe, a vertical line 3 cm long, starting from the point 2 cm inferior to the parietal tubercle, extending downward, parallel with the anterior-posterior midline of the head. (Fig. 2-186)

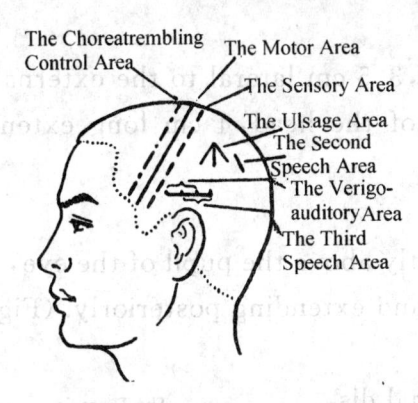

Fig. 2-186 Stimulation Areas of the Lateral Side of the Head

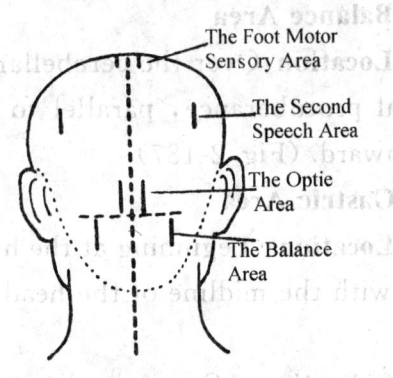

Fig. 2-187 Stimulation Areas of the Posterior Side of the Head

Indication: Nominal aphasia.

The Third Speech Area

Location: A parallel line overlaps half of the Vertigo and Hearing Area, starting from the midpoint of the Vertigo and Hearing Area and continues 4 cm posteriorly. (Fig. 2-186)

Indication: Sensory aphasia.

Praxis Area

Location: From the parietal tubercle, draw a line to the middle of mastoid process, and the other two lines anteriorly and posteriorly, forming a 40 angle respectively with it, all three lines 3 cm in length. (Fig. 2-186)

Indication: Apraxia.

Foot Motor Sensory Area

Location: Starting from the point 1cm lateral to the midpoint of the anterior and posterior midline of the head with which it paralles and continues for 3 cm long. (Fig. 2-187, 2-189)

Indications: Pain, numbness or paralysis of lower limb of the contralateral side, acute lumbar sprain, cortical polyuria, nycturia, prolapse of uterus, etc.

Optic Area

Location: A line 1 cm lateral and parallel to the anterior-posterior midline of the head, intersecting the horizontal line of the external occipital protuberance, draw a line 4 cm long from the intersecting point of these two lines, extending upward. (Fig. 2-187)

Indication: Cortical vision problems.

Balance Area

Location: Over the cerebellar hemisphere, 3.5 cm lateral to the external occipital protuberance, parallel to the midline of the head, 4 cm long extending downward. (Fig. 2-187)

Gastric Area

Location: Beginning at the hairline, directly above the pupil of the eye, parallel with the midline of the head, 2 cm long and extending posteriorly. (Fig. 2-188)

Indications: Stomachache, upper abdominal discomfort, etc.

Thoracic Cavity Area

Location: Midway between the Stomach Area and the midline of the head, draw 2 cm line respectively upward and downward from the hairline, parallel with the midline of the head. (Fig. 2-188)

Indications: Chest pain and stuffiness, palpitation, ischemia of coronary artery, asthma, hiccup, etc.

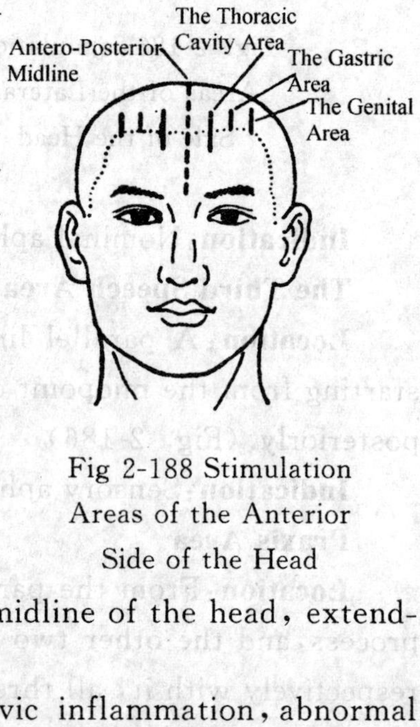

Fig 2-188 Stimulation Areas of the Anterior Side of the Head

Genital Area

Location: From the corner of the head, draw a line 2 cm long, parallel with the anterior-posterior midline of the head, extending upward. (Fig. 2-188)

Indications: Disfunctional uterine bleeding, pelvic inflammation, abnormal leukorrhea. It combines with Foot Motor Sensory Area for prolapse of uterus.

Section 2   Operations

Patient may be treated with a sitting position or lying position. After the stimulating area is selected, which is based on the pathological state of the patient, disinfect the local place routinely.

1. Insertion of the Needle

Select a 1.5 cun or 2 cun long filiform needle No. 28-30, swiftly insert the needle subcutaneously, in 30 angle to the scalp, when the needle reaches the subgaleal layer and the practitioner feels the insertion resistance becomes weak, further insert the needle by twirling method, which parallels with the scalp until it goes to the periosteum, the depth of insertion varies with the areas, generally 0.5-1.5 cun. After the needle being inserted to the required depth, conduct manipulation. (Fig. 2-190)

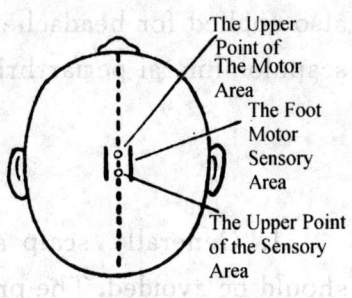

Fig. 2-189 Stimulation Areas of the Top of the Head

2. Manipulation

In scalp acupuncture, the needle is manipulated only by twirling method, no lifting or thrusting of the needle. The depth of insertion keeps constant, and the needle is twirled in a frequency of 130-200 times per minute, it is first manipulated for 2 to 3 minutes and the needle is retained for 5 to 10 minutes, afterwards, repeat this process twice or three times, then the needle is withdrawn. For hemiplegia, during the manipulation and retention of the needle, the patient is encouraged to exercise the affected limbs so as to raise the therapeutic effect. (In severe case, passive movement of the limbs of the patient is conducted). (Fig. 2-191)

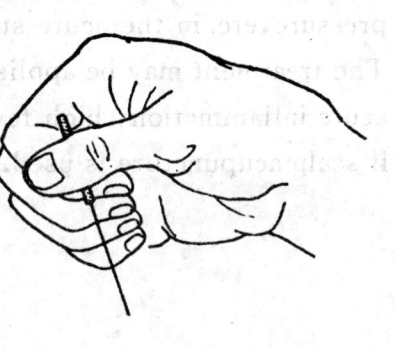

Fig. 2-190 Holding the Needle of Scalp Acupuncture

3. Electro-Stimulation

Electro-stimulator can be connected to the needles in the main areas to replace the hand manipulation. It is in a mode of high frequency and weak stimulation.

4. Course of Treatment

Scalp acupuncture is applied once daily or once every other day, one course consisting of ten sessions of treatment. Between two courses, there is five to seven days break.

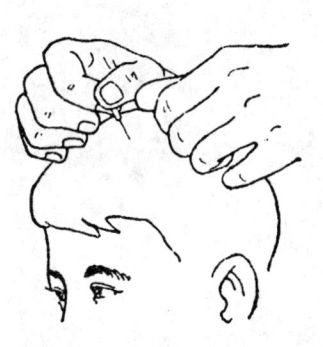

Fig. 2-191 Twirling Manner of Scalp Acupuncture

Section 3 Indications

It is mainly indicated for cerebral disorders, such as hemiplegia, numbness, aphasia, dizziness and vertigo, tinnitus, chorea, etc. It is also applied for headache, low back and leg pain, nocturia, trigiminal neuralgia, scapulohumeral periarthritis and other diseases of nervous system.

Section 4 Precautions

1. Generally, scalp acupuncture is a strong stimulation, fainting therefore should be avoided. The practitioner should keep a close eye on the complexion of the patient and the intensity of the stimulation should be appropriately controlled.

2. Wind stroke due to cerebral hemorrhage with coma, fever, high blood pressure, etc. in the acute stage is not suggested to treat by scalp acupuncture. The treatment may be applied until the pathological state is stable. Patients with acute inflammation, high fever and heart failure should be dealt with great care if scalp acupuncture is used.

Chapter 6 Ear Acupuncture

Ear acupuncture treats and prevents diseases by stimulating certain points on the auricle with needles or other tools. Diagnosis can be made by observing, pressing and measuring the electrical resistance on the auricular points.

In China, diagnosis and treatment on ear point have developed in a long history. As early as in the book *the Yellow Emperor's Canon of Internal Medicine*, it was recorded. For instance, *Miraculous Pivot* Syncope says: "Point Middle Ear is selected for deafness."Afterwards, it has been developed in the past dynasties. For instance, in Ming dynasty, Yang Jizhou pointed out in *Compendium of Acupuncture and Moxibustion*: "There are two points on the tip of ear, which can be got by folding the ear. These points can be used to treat nebula."There were some reports about using auricular points to make diagnosis in *Standard for Diagnosis and Treatment*: "If the ear is big this, this indicates the kidney is big, the ear is black, the kidney failure."In recent decades, it has a new breakthrough about ear points diagnosis and treatment, which became a special kind of acupuncture and moxibustion widely used.

Section 1 Relations between the Auricle and Zang-Fu Organs and Meridians

Relations between the Auricle and Zang-fu Organs: It is held in TCM that although the body can be divided into Zang-fu Organs, meridians and collaterals, five sense organs and nine orifices, four extremities and joints, etc., they are all parts of an organic whole.

The ear is not a separate sense organ but closely connected with Zang-Fu organs. As it is pointed out in *Miraculous Pivot Measurement of Meridians and Vessels*: "The Qi of the kidney reaches the ear to make auditory function normal." *Standard for Diagnosis and Treatment* pointed out: " The kidney is the governor of the ear while the heart is a visitor." *Revised Synopsis of Massage* further divided the ear into five aspects of heart, liver, spleen, lung and kidney. e. g. "Tragus belongs to the kidney; helix, the spleen; the superior helix, the heart; the surface intracutaneous and subcutaneous of the auricle, the lung; the back auricle, the liver." In addition, the doctors in the past and today make a determination about the development of the diseases in the Zang-Fu organs and explain the close relationship between the ear and Zang-Fu organs by observing the changes of the shape and colour, the tender and sensitive point of the auricle and the electrical resistance of the skin.

Relations between the Auricle and Meridians: The auricle meridians were recorded as early as in the book *Classic Moxibustion of Yin-Yang Eleven Meridian*, till the book of *Canon of Internal Medicine*, the auricle meridians were developed to Triple Energizer Meridian, and the relation between the auricle and meridians, divergent meridians, muscle regions were recorded systematically.

The Meridians of Small Intestine, Triple Energizer, Gallbladder and Large Intestine go or have branches to the ear separately. The Stomach Meridian passes the front of ear; the Bladder Meridian up to the superior angle of the ear. Although the six Yin Meridians don't go to the ear, they combine the Yang Meridians with the divergent meridians. Hence, all the twelve regular meridians go up to the ear directly or indirectly. As pointed out in *Miraculous Pivot the Evil-Qi and Diseases in the Zang-Fu Organs*, "The Qi, blood of all twelve meridians and their 365 collaterals ascend to the face and brain, the essential Yang-Qi ascend to the eyes to make vigorous eyes, their branches-Qi reaching the ear to make auditory function normal." This generalizes the relation between the auricle and meridians.

Section 2 Anatomical Names of the Auricles Surface (Fig. 2-192)

1. Helix: The curling rim of the most lateral border of the auricle.

2. Helix Tubercle: A small tubercle at the posterior-superior aspect of the helix.

3. Helix Crus: A transverse ridge of the helix continuing backward into the ear cavity.

4. Antihelix: An elevated ridge parallel to the helix. Its upper part tubercle out into the superior antihelix crus and the inferior antihelix crus.

5. Triangular Fossa: The triangular depression between the superior and inferior antihelix crura.

6. Scapha: The narrow curved depression between the antihelix and the helix.

7. Tragus: A curved flap in front of the auricle. It is also known as "the ear ball".

8. Supratragic Notch: The depression between the upper border of the tragus and the helix crus.

9. Antitragus: A small tubercle opposite to the tragus and superior to the ear lobe.

10. Intertragic Notch: The depression between the tragus and antitragus.

11. Helix Notch: The depression between the antihelix and antitragus.

12. Cymba Conchae: The depression between the helix crus and the antihelix.

13. Cavum Conchae: The cavum inferior to the helix crus.

14. Orifice of the External Anditory Meatus: The opening in the cavum concha.

15. The Root of the Upper Auricle: At the junction of the upper border of the auricle and the scalp.

16. The Root of the Lower Auricle: At the lower border of the root of the auricle.

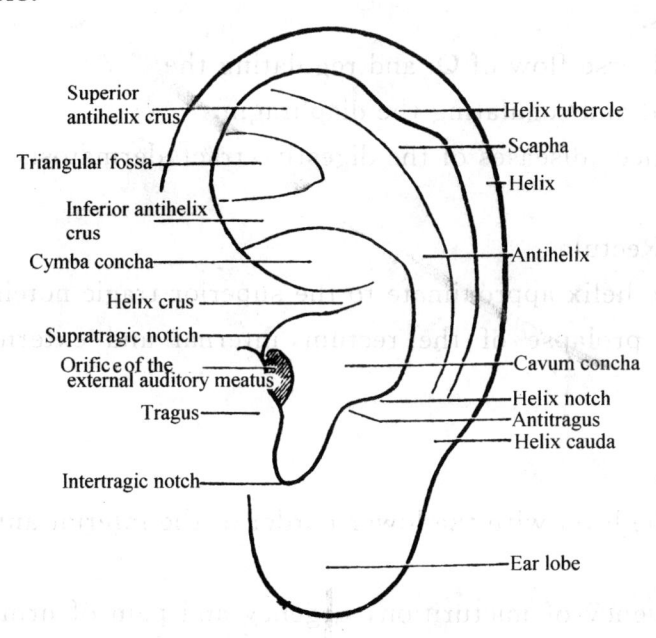

Fig. 2-192
Anatomical Structure of
the Auricular Surface

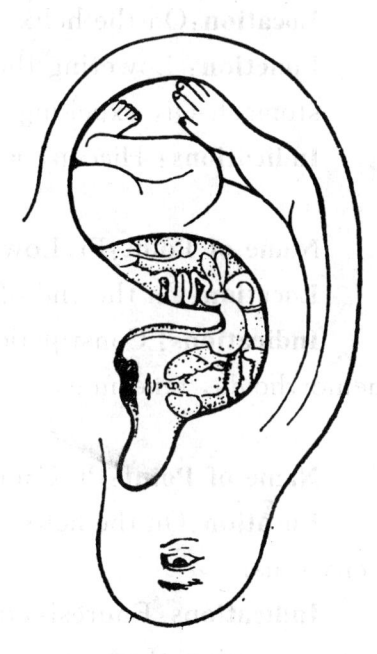

Fig. 2-193
Distribution of the
Imagery Auricular Points

Section 3 Auricular Points

Auricular points are some certain stimulating spots or areas on the auricle. The distribution of auricular points on the auricle is just like a fetus with the head downwards and the buttocks upwards (Fig. 2-193).

The distribution of auricular points is as follows: Points located on the lobule and around it are related to the head and facial region, those on the scapha to the upper limbs, those on the antihelix and its two crura to the trunk and lower limbs, those in the cavum and cymba conchae to the internal organs, and those arranged as a ring around helix crus to the digestive tract.

Locations and Indications of Auricular Points Commonly Used (Fig. 2-194). (Table. 2-14)

Locations, Functions and Indications of Auricular Points

Anatomical Region: The Helix Crus and Helix

Name of Point: Pt. Middle Ear

Original Name: Diaphragm

Location: On the helix crus.

Function: Lowering the adverse flow of Qi and regulating the stomach-Qi, expelling wind and regulating the diaphragm.

Indications: Hiccup, jaundice, diseases of the digestive tract, dermatosis.

Name of Point: Pt. Lower Rectum

Location: On the end of the helix approximate to the superior tragic notch.

Indications: Constipation. prolapse of the rectum, internal and external hemorrhoids, tenesmus.

Name of Point: Pt. Urethra

Location: On the helix at the level with the lower border of the inferior antihelix crus.

Indications: Enuresis, frequency of micturition, urgency and pain of urination, retention of urine.

Name of Point: Pt. External Genitalia

Location: On the helix at the level with the upper border of the inferior antihelix crus.

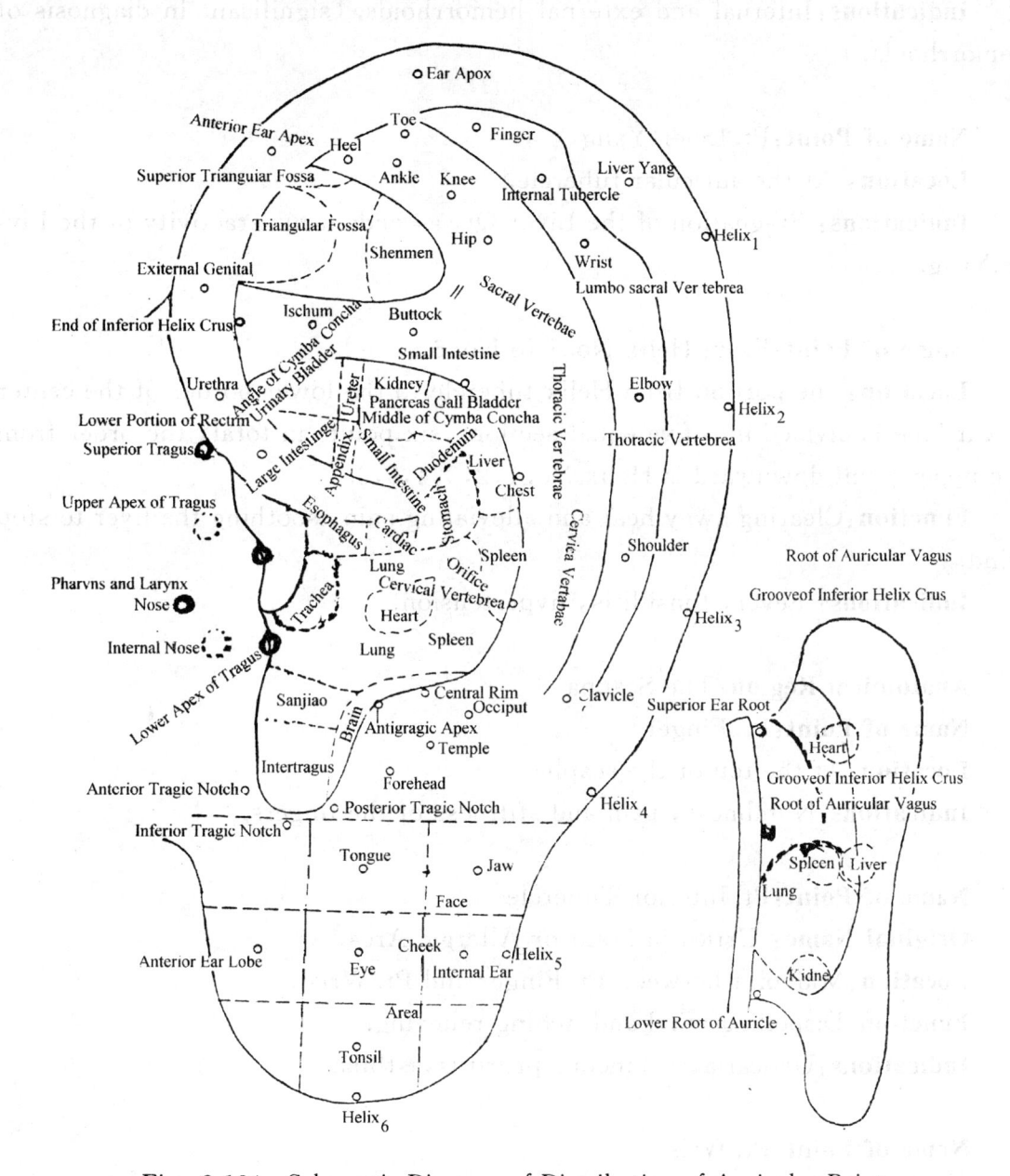

Fig. 2-194 Schematic Diagram of Distribution of Auricular Points

Indications: Inflammation and skin diseases of external genital organs, impotence.

Name of Point: Pt. Front Ear Apex
Original Name: Hemorrhoidal Nucleus
Location: At the point between Pt. Ear Apex and Pt. Root of the Upper Au-

277

ricle.

Indications: Internal and external hemorrhoids. (significant in diagnosis of hemorrhoids.)

Name of Point: Pt. Liver-Yang
Location: At the auricular tubercle.
Indications: Stagnation of the Liver-Qi, ascendent hyperactivity of the Liver-Yang.

Name of Point: From Helix No. 1 to No. 6
Location: The portion from Helix tubercle to the lower border of the center of ear lobe is divided into five equal sections, six points in total, the order from the upper point downward is Helix No. 1,2,3,4,5,6.
Function: Clearing away heat and alleviating pain, soothing the liver to stop wind.
Indications: Fever, tonsillitis, hypertension.

Anatomical Region: The Scapha
Name of Point: Pt. Finger
Location: At the top of the scapha.
Indications: Numbness, pain and stiffness of the fingers.

Name of Point: Pt. Interior Tubercle
Original Name: Urticaria Point or Allergic Area.
Location: Midpoint between Pt. Finger and Pt. Wrist.
Function: Dispelling wind and itching relieving.
Indications: Urticaria, cutaneous pruritus, asthma.

Name of Point: Pt. Wrist
Location: Midpoint between Pt. Elbow and Pt. Finger.
Indications: Wrist sprain, swelling and pain and dysfunction.

Name of Point: Pt. Elbow
Location: Midpoint between Pt. Finger and Pt. Clavicle.
Indications: Pain and dysfunction at corresponding areas of the body.

Name of Point: Pt. Shoulder
Location: Midpoint between Pt. Elbow and Pt. Clavicle.
Indications: Pain and dysfunction at corresponding areas of the body.

Name of Point: Pt. Clavicle
Location: On the scapha at level with the helix-tragic notch.
Indications: Pain at corresponding areas of the body, peripheral arthritis of the shoulder, pulseless disease.

Anatomical Region: The Superior Antihelix Crus
Name of Point: Pt. Toe
Location: Lateral and superior angle of the superior antihelix crus
Indications: Numbness, pain and dysfunction of the toe.

Name of Point: Pt. Heel
Location: Medial and superior angle of the superior antihelix crus.
Indications: Heel pain.

Name of Point: Pt. Ankle
Location: Midpoint between Pt. Heel and Pt. Knee.
Indications: Ankle sprain, pain and dysfunction at the corresponding part of the body.

Name of Point: Pt. Knee
Location: Middle portion of the superior antihelix crus.
Indications: Pain and dysfunction at the corresponding part of the body. (such as the knee joint sprain and arthritis, etc.)

Name of Point: Pt. Hip
Location: At inferior 1/3 of the superior antihelix crus.
Indications: Pain at the corresponding part of the body.

Anatomical Region: The Inferior Antihelix Crus
Name of Point: Pt. Buttocks
Location: At lateral 1/3 of the inferior antihelix curs.

Indications: Pain at the corresponding area, sciatica.

Name of Point: Pt. Sciatic
Original Name: Pt. Sciatic Nerve
Location: At internal 2/3 of the inferior antihelix crus.
Indication: Sciatica.

Name of Point: Pt. End of Inferior Antihelix Grus
Original Name: Pt. Sympathetic Never
Location: The terminal of the inferior antihelix crus.
Function: Relieving spasm and pain, nourishing Yin and strengthening Yang.
Indications: Pain in the internal organs, palpitation, spontsneous sweating, night sweating, functional disorders of autonomous nerve.

Anatomical Region: The Antihelix
Name of Point: Pt. Cervical Vertebrae, Pt. Thoracic Vertebrae, Pt. Lumbosacral Vertebrae
Location: A curved line from the helix-tragic notch to the bifurcation of the superior and inferior antihelix crura can be divided into three equal segments. The lower 1/3 of it is Pt. Cervical Vertebrae, the middle 1/3 is Pt. Thoracic Vertebrae and the upper 1/3 is Pt. Lumbosacral Vertebrae.
Function: Strengthening the spine and replenishing the marrow.
Indications: Pain at the corresponding region.

Name of Point: Pt. Neck
Location: On the border of cavum conchae level to Pt. Cervical Vertebrae.
Indications: Stiff neck, wry neck, and other diseases at the corresponding areas.

Name of Point: Pt. Chest
Location: On the border of the cavum conchae level to Pt. Thoracic vertebrae.
Indications: Stuffiness and pain of the chest, mastitis, and other diseases at

the corresponding regions.

Name of Point: Pt. Abdomem
Location: On the border of the cavum conchae level to Pt. Lumbrosacral Vertebrae.
Indications: Abdominal diseases and gynecopathy, pain of the lowback.

Anatomical Region: The Triangular Fossa
Name of Point: Pt. Shenmen
Location: At the bifurcating point between superior and inferior antihelix crus, and the lateral 1/3 of the triangular fossa.
Function: Tranquilizing, alleviating pain, anti-inflammation, clearing away heat.

Name of Point: Pt. Depression of the Triangular
Original Name: Pt. Tiangui, Pt. Uterus, or Pt. Seminal Palace.
Location: In the triangular fossa, depression in the midpoint of the helix.
Function: Strengthening Yang and replenishing the essence, regulating menstruation.
Indications: Diseases of woman, impotence, prostatitis.

Name of Point: Pt. Superior of the Triangular
Original Name: Pt. Lowering Blood Pressure Point
Location: At the lateral superior of the triangular fossa.
Function: Soothing the liver to stop wind.
Indications: Hypertension.

Anatomical Region: The Tragus
Name of Point: Pt. External Ear
Original Name: Pt. Supratragic
Location: On the supratragic notch close to the helix.
Function: Nourishing the kidney-water, settling the liver-Yang.
Indications: Dizziness, deafness, tinnitus.

Name of Point: Pt. Nose

Original Name: Pt. External Nose
Location: In the center of the lateral aspect of the tragus.
Function: Dredging meridians of the nasal region.
Indications: Rhinitis, nasal furuncle, nasal obstruction, etc. and other diseases of the nasal region.

Name of Point: Pt. Upper Tragic Apex
Original Name: Pt. Tragic Apex
Location: At the tip of the upper protuberance on the border of the tragus.
Function: Clearing away heat and alleviating pain.

Name of Point: Pt. Infratragic Apex
Original Name: Pt. Adrenal
Location: At the tip of the lower protubercle on the border of the tragus.
Function: Clearing away heat and alleviating pain, relieving spasm and dispelling wind.
Indications: Hypotension, syncope, pulseless disease, cough and asthma, cold, sunstroke, malaria, mastitis.

Name of Point: Pt. Pharynx-Larynx
Location: Upper half of the medial aspect of the tragus.
Function: Clearing and comforting the throat.
Indications: Acute and chronic pharyngitis, tonsillitis, etc.

Name of Point: Pt. Internal Nose
Location: Lower half of the medial aspect of the tragus.
Function: Dredging the nasal cavity.
Indications: Allergic rhinitis and other nasal disease.

Anatomical Region: The Antitragus
Name of Point: Pt. Antitragus
Original Name: Pt. Soothing Asthma, Pt. Parotid Gland
Location: At the tip of the antitragus.
Function: Soothing the lung and relieving asthma, clearing away heat and poison, expelling wind pathogenic factor.

Indications: Asthma, bronchitis, mumps, pruritus.

Name of Point: Pt. Middle Border
Original Name: Pt. Brain
Location: Midpoint between the antitragic apex and helix-tragic notch.
Function: Tonifying the brain and tranquilizing.
Indications: Oligophrenia, enuresis, etc.

Name of Point: Pt. Occiput
Location: At the posterior superior corner of the lateral aspect of the antitragus.
Function: Alleviating pain, tranquilizing and stopping wind.
Indications: Dizziness, headache, insomnia, etc.

Name of Point: Pt. Temple
Original Name: Pt. Taiyang
Location: At the midpoint between Pt. Occiput and Pt. Forehead.
Function: Alleviating pain.
Indication: Shaoyang type headache.

Name of Point: Pt. Forehead
Location: At anterior inferior corner of the lateral aspect of the antitragus.
Function: Alleviating pain.
Indications: Yangming type headache.

Name of Point: Pt. Brain
Original Name: Pt. Subcortex
Location: On the medial aspect of the antitragus.
Function: Replenishing the marrow and tonifying the brain, alleviating pain and tranquilizing.
Indications: Oligophrenia, insomnia, dreamy, tinnitus due to kidney deficiency. etc.

Anatomical Region: Periphery Helix Grus
Name of Point: Pt. Mouth

Location: Close to the posterior and superior border of the orifice of the external auditory meatus.
Function: Clearing away heart-fire and expelling wind.
Indications: Facial paralysis, stomatitis.

Name of Point: Pt. Esophagus
Location: At middle 2/3 of the inferior aspect of the helix crus.
Function: Soothing the diaphragm and harmonizing the stomach.
Indications: Difficulty in swallowing, esophagitis, etc.

Name of Point: Pt. Cardiac Orifice
Location: At lateral 1/3 of the inferior aspect of the helix crus.
Function: Soothing diaphragm and lowering the adverse flow of Qi.
Indications: Cardiospasm, nervous vomiting, etc.

Name of Point: Pt. Stomach
Location: The area where the helix crus terminates.
Function: Harmonizing the stomach and nourishing the spleen, reinforcing the middle and tranquilizing the mind.
Indications: Gastritis, gastric ulcer and other diseases of stomach, insomnia, etc.

Name of Point: Pt. Duodenum
Location: At lateral 1/3 of the superior aspect of the helix crus.
Function: Warming the middle and harmonizing the stomach.
Indications: Duodenal ulcer, pylorospasm, etc.

Name of Point: Pt. Small Intestine
Location: At middle 1/3 of the superior aspect of the helix crus.
Function: Tonifying the spleen and harmonizing the middle.
nourishing the heart and promoting the generation of blood.
Indications: Indigestion, palpitation, etc.

Name of Point: Pt. Appendix
Location: Between Pt. Small Intestine and Pt. Large Intestine.

Function: Clearing away the damp-heat from the Lower-Energizer. activating the lung-Qi.
Indications: Appendicitis, diarrhea.

Name of Point: Pt. Large Intestine
Location: At medial 1/3 of the superior aspect of the helix crus.
Function: Clearing the Lower-Energizer, soothing the lung-Qi.
Indications: Diarrhea, constipation.

Anatomical Region: Cymba Conchae
Name of Point: Pt. Liver
Location: On the lateral of Pt. Stomach and Pt. Duodenum.
Function: Clearing the liver to improve vision, relaxing tendons and promoting blood circulation.
Indications: Stagnation of Qi due to stagnation of the liver-Qi, diseases of the eye, diseases of lower abdomen, etc.

Name of Point: Pt. Pancrease and Biliary Tract
Location: Between Pt. Liver and Pt. Kidney.
Function: Soothing the gallbladder and harmonizing the stomach, soothing the liver and expelling wind.
Indications: Diseases of the biliary tract, pancreasitis, migraine.

Name of Point: Pt. Kindey
Location: On the lower border of the inferior antihelix crus, directly above Pt. Small Intestine.
Function: Tonifying the kidney and clearing hearing, strenthening the bone and replenishing marrow.
Indications: Lumbar pain, tinnitus, deafness, spermatorrhea, impotence.

Name of Point: Pt. Ureter
Location: Between Pt. Kidney and Pt. Bladder.
Indication: Colic pain of the ureter calculus.

Name of Point: Pt. Bladder

Location: On the inferior border of the inferior antihelix crus, directly above Pt. Large Intestine.
Function: Clearing the Lower-Energizer, invigorating the lower premordial Qi.
Indications: Lower back pain, sciatica, cystitis, enuresis, retention of urine.

Name of Point: Pt. Angle of Cymba Conchae
Location: At the medial superior angle of cymba conchae.
Function: Clearing heat from the Lower-Energizer and promoting urination.
Indications: Prostatitis.

Name of Point: Pt. Center of Cymba Conchae
Original Name: Pt. Around Umbilicus
Location: On the center of the cymba conchae.
Function: Regulating the stomach and spleen.
Indications: Lower fever, abdominal distension, ascariasis of biliary tract, hypoacusis, mumps, etc.

Anatomical Region: The Cavum Conchae
Name of Point: Pt. Heart
Location: In the central depression of the cavum conchae.
Function: Tranquilizing the heart and the mind, harmonizing nutrient-Qi and blood, alleviating pain and relieving itching.
Indications: Insomnia, palpitation, hysteria, night sweat, angina pectoris, etc.

Name of Point: Pt. Lung
Location: Around Pt. Heart
Function: Promoting the activating of the Qi and blood, promoting urination, reinforcing the deficiency to clearing away heat, treating skin and hair diseases.
Indications: Cough and asthma, dermatosis, hoarseness. It is a common point for acupuncture anesthesia.

Name of Point: Pt. Trachea
Location: Between the orifice of the external auditory meatus and Pt. Heart.
Function: Relieving cough and resolving phlegm.
Indications: Cough and asthma.

Name of Point: Pt. Spleen
Location: Inferior to Pt. Liver, at the lateral and superior of the cavum conchae.
Function: Relieving food retention, promoting the generation of blood, nourishing muscle, invigorating the spleen and Qi.
Indications: Abdominal distention, chronic diarrhea, indigestion, anorexia, dysfunctional uterine bleeding.

Name of point: Pt. Triple Energizer
Location: Superior to the intertragic notch.
Function: Dredging and regulating water passage, clearing away heat and alleviating pain..
Indications: Constipation, edema, abdominal distention, pain of the lateral aspect of hand and arm.

Name of point: Pt. Intertragus
Original Name: Pt. Endocrine
Location: At the base of the cavum conchae in the intertragic notch.
Function: Soothing the liver and regulating Qi, promoting menstral flow and blood, expelling wind, invigorating the lower premordial Qi.
Indications: Dysmenorrhea, impotence, irreguler menstruation, climacteric syndrome, dysfunction of endocrine, etc.

Anatomical Region: The Ear Lobule
Name of Point: Pt. Anterior Tragic Notch.
Original Name: Pt. Eye 1
Location: On the lateral, anterior and inferior aspect of the intertragic notch.
Function: Clearing the liver to improve vision.

Indications: Glaucoma, pseudomyopia, and other diseases of the eyes.

Name of Point: Pt Lower Tragic Notch.
Original Name: Elevating Blood Pressure Point.
Location: On the inferior aspect of the intertragic notch.
Function: Invigorating Qi to support yang.
Indications: Hypotension.

Name of point: Pt. Positerior Tragic Notch
Original Name: Pt. Eye 2
Location: On the posterior and inferior aspect of the intertragic notch.
Function: Clearing liver-fire to improve vision.
Indications: Ametropia, inflammation of external eye.

Name of Point: Pt. Facial Area
Location: At the ear lobule area, on the posterior and superior aspect of the eye point
Function: Clearing facial meridians.
Indications: Facial paralysis, acne and other diseases on the face.

Name of point: Pt. Tongue
Location: At the 2nd section.
Function: Clearing away the heart-fire.
Indications: Glossitis, etc.

Name of Point: Pt. Jaw
Location: At the 3rd section.
Indications: Toothache, mandibular arthritis etc.

Name of Point: Pt. No 4 of Ear Lobe
Original Name: Neurasthenic Point
Location: At the 4th section.
Function: Harmonizng the water (kidney) and fire (heart), tranquilizing the heart and mind.
Indications: Toothache, neuro-asthenia.

Name of Point: Pt. Eye
Location: At the 5th section.
Function: Improving vision.
Indications: Acute conjunctivitis, electric ophthalmitis, myopia, and other diseases of the eyes.

Name of Point: Pt. Internal Ear
Location: At the 6th section.
Function: Relieving dizziness and improving hearing.
Indications: Tinnitus, hypoacusis, aural vertigo.

Name of Point: Pt. Tonsil
Location: At the 8th section.
Function: Clearing and soothing the throat.
Indications: Acute tonsillitis, etc.

Anatomical Region: The Back Auricle
Name of Point: Pt. The Root of the Upper Auricle
Original Name: Pt. Yuzhong, Pt. Spinal Cord
Location: At the upper border of the root of the auricle.
Function: Alleviating pain and relieving asthma.
Indications: Headache, abdominal pain, asthma.

Name of Point: Pt. The Root of the Lower Auricle
Original Name: Pt. Yuzhong, Pt. Spinal Cord
Location: At the lower border of the junction of the ear lobule and facial region.
Function: Alleviating pain and relieving asthma.
Indications: Headache, abdominal pain, asthma.

Name of Point: Pt. Ermigen
Location: At the root of the junction of the back auricle and mastoid process, at the level with the helix crus.
Function: Clearing orifice and alleviating pain, regulating Zang-Fu organs.
Indications: Headache, nasal stuffiness, ascariasis of biliary tract, etc.

Name of Point: Pt. Groove of Inferior Antihelix Crus
Original Name: Pt. Groove of Lowering Blood Pressure
Location: Through the backside of the superior antihelix crus and inferior antihelix crus, in the depression as a "Y" form.
Function: Soothing the liver and lowering the adverse flow of Qi, treating the skin diseases.
Indications: Hypertension, skin diseases.

Name of Point: Pt. Heart
Location: On the upper part of the back auricle.
Function: Clearing away the heart-fire, tranquilizing, alleviating pain and itching.
Indications: Furuncle, insomnia, dreamy, hypertension, headache, etc.

Name of Point: Pt. Spleen
Location: On the middle part of the back auricle.
Function: Invigorating the spleen and harmonizing the stomach, promoting the generation of blood, nourishing the muscle.
Indications: Abdominal distention, diarrhea, indigestion, etc.

Name of Point: Pt. Liver
Location: At the lateral aspect of spleen area on the back auricle.
Function: Soothing the liver and harmonizing the stomach, relaxing tendons and promoting blood circulation.
Indications: Chest and hypochondriac congestion, acute appendicitis, lumbar and back pain, etc.

Name of Point: Pt. Lung
Location: The medial aspect of the spleen area on the back auricle.
Function: Invigorating the lung to stop asthma, clearing away heat, treating skin and hair diseases.
Indications: Asthma, fever, diseases and symptom of digestive system, etc.

Name of Point: Pt. Kidney
Location: On the lower part of the back auricle.

Function: Enriching the kidney-water, clearing the hearing, strengthening the bone and replenishing essence.

Indications: Headache, insomnia, dizziness, irregular menstruation.

Section 4 Application of Ear Acupuncture

1. Diagnosis by Auricular Points

When Zang and Fu organs disorder or abnormal of certain part of the body are present, reactions can be detected at the corresponding areas on the auricle, manifested by changes of the shape and skin colour, scales, papules, tenderness, low electrical resistance on the skin, etc. Diagnosis can be made according to these manifestations. Generally speaking, there are three methods:

(1) **Direct Observation**: Inspection is made from upper to lower, under internal to external ear with eyes or magnifying glass under the natural light, while special attention is paid to the changes of the shape and colour, e.g. scales, blisters, papules, hyperemia, knots, verrucous, chondral hyperplasia, pigmentation and the shape of blood vessel, changes of colour, etc.

(2) **Ashi-Point Pressure**: Detect the tender spot by pressing. After preliminary diagnosis, press on certain area or the whole ear gently, slowly, evenly. When a doctor's hand gets the tender spot, a patient will appear frown, blink, yelling or dodge, etc. Make a diagnosis and give the treatment according to them.

(3) **Electric Measure**: It is a method to measure the changes of the electrical resistance and electric potential of acurical point with special electronic instrument in order to help make a diagnosis. The patient holds the electrode stick with one hand, a doctor holds the probe to press on the acuricle to detect the tender spots. When the head of probe touches the sensitive spot, indicative signal, sound or hand of meter will show.

2. Selection of Points and Manipulation of Ear Acupuncture

There are four methods for selection of ear points:

(1) **Selection of Points Base on Differentiation of Syndromes and Signs**: Selection of points according to the theories of Zang-Fu and meridians, e.g. Pt. Lung can be selected for skin diseases for the reason that lung dominates the skin and body hair.

(2) **Selection of Points according to Experience**: Point Middle Ear for blood

and skin diseases; not only can Pt. Stomach be used to treat the gastrointestinal diseases but also the diseases of nervous system; Pt. Shenmen for pain and tranquilizing; Pt. Ear Apex for inflammation, fever and muscular spasm.

(3) **Selection of Points according to Physiology and Pathology of Modern Medicine:** For instance, Pt. Endocrine is selected for irregular menstruation; Pt. Brain(Subcortex) for neuro-asthenia.

(4) **Selection of Points according to Auricular Points Corresponding to the Diseased Areas:** For example, Pt. Eye, Pt. Eye 1, Pt. Eye 2 for diseases of the eyes; Pt. Stomach for gastric diseases; Pt. Uterus for diseases of woman, etc.

Manipulation of Ear Acupuncture:

After diagnosis and point prescription are made, detect the tender spots on the area where the ear points are selected. If marked tenderness is not located, give the treatment with auricular points therapy. After the selected points are located, strict skin disinfection is necessary. Auricular points selected for needling should be swabbed with 2% tincture iodine first and then it is removed by a 75% alcohol cotton ball as routine disinfection. If disinfection is not strict, it is easy to lead to auricular perichondritis due to infection. The manipulation techniques are as follows:

(1) **The Filiform Needle Methods:**

Insertion of Needle: The thumb, the index finger of the left hand hold the auricle, the middle finger supports the back of the ear. Hold a filiform needle with the right hand and insert it into the point, with the pain limited in the patient's maximal tolerance. If no reaction appears, the direction of the insertion should be changed. The required depth is flexible according to the thickness or thinness of the auricular. The needles are retained for 20-30 minutes. The needles should be retained longer for chronic diseases, painful diseases, shorter and mild stimulation in children and elders.

Removal of Needle: Hold the back of ear with the left hand, withdraw the needle with the right hand. After the needle is removed, press the puncture hole with a dry sterilized cotton ball for a while to prevent bleeding. If necessary, swab with alcohol cotton ball again.

(2) **Electrotherapy:** This method is used to treat diseases of the nervous system, spasm and pain in Zang and Fu organs, asthma, etc.

(3) **Needle-Embedding Therapy:** After the thumb-tack needle is embedded, ask the patient to press it 3 times a day by himself; retain the needle on the point

for 3-5 days.

(4) **Auricular-Seed-Pressing Therapy**: It is a simple stimulating method by tapping small seed-shape herb on the auricular point. This method is safe, painless and fewer side-effects. It will not cause auricular perichondritis. It is suitable for the elderly people and children or the patient who is afraid of acupuncture. The material, such as rape seed, a mung bean, radish seed, a seed of Vaccaria segetalis, magnetic bead, etc. can be used.

Section 5 Precautions

1. Strict disinfection is necessary to prevent infection. If redness and swelling occur on the puncture point, swab 2% tincture of iodine, or apply an ignited moxa stick to the area.

2. Filiform needles are usually selected. Give the electrotherapy every other day; give the irradiate with laser treatment once every day; give the auricular-seed(or magnetic bead)-pressing therapy treatment, retain the seed on the sensitive spot or the acupuncture point for 5-7 days, the points can be used alternately. 5-10 treatments make up a course.

3. Needling is contraindicated in pregnancy with history of habitual abortion. It is necessary for elderly or weak patients to take proper rest before and after needling, also gentle manipulation to guarantee safety is needed.

4. In a patient with motor impairment of the extremities or sprain, it is necessary after the needle are retained to ask the patient to move the affected limb in order to enhance the therapeutic effect.

Section 6 Examples of Point Prescriptions for Some Common Diseases

1. **Headache**: Pt. Forehead, Pt. Occiput, Pt. Brain, Pt. Middle Border, Pt. Ear Apex.
2. **Stiff Neck**: Pt. Forehead, the tender sensitive spots on Pt. Cervical Vertebrae.
3. **Common Cold**: Pt. Lung, Pt. Internal Nose, Pt. Infratragic Apex.
4. **Sunstroke**: Pt. Heart, Pt. Occiput, Pt. Brain.
5. **Cough**: Pt. Trachea, Pt. Lung, Pt. Shenmen.
6. **Asthma**: Pt. Soothing Asthma, Pt. Lung, Pt. End of Inferior Antihelix

Crus, Pt. Infratragic Apex.

7. Dizziness: Pt. Kidney, Pt. Shenmen, Pt. Internal Ear.

8. Gastric pain: Pt. Stomach, Pt. Shenmen, Pt. Brain, Pt. End of Inferior Antihelix Crus.

9. Enuresis: Pt. Kidney, Pt. Urinary Bladder, Pt. Middle Border, Pt. Brain.

10. Post-Operative Wound Pain: Auricular points corresponding to incised area, Pt. Shenmen, Pt. Lung.

11. Abdominal Distension after Surgical Operation: The tender spots of Large Intestine, and Small Intestine, Pt. Stomach, Pt. End of Inferior Antihelix Crus, Pt. Spleen.

12. Cancer Pain: Pt. Brain, Pt. Heart, Pt. Ear Apex, auricular points corresponding to the affected area, Pt. End of Inferior Antihelix Crus, Pt. Liver, Pt. Shenmen.

13. Ureter Colic due to Stones: Pt. Kidney, Pt. Abdomen, Pt. End of Inferior Antihelix Crus, Pt. Brain.

14. Dysentery: Pt. Large Intestine, Pt. Small Intestine, Pt. Lower Rectum.

15. Malaria: Pt. Infratragic Apex. Pt. Brain, Pt. Intertragus.

16. Hypertension: Pt. Infratragic Apex, Pt. End of Inferior Antihelix Crus, Pt. Heart, Pt. Shenmen.

17. Hiccup: Puncture the tender spots on the Point Middle Ear.

18. Vomiting: Pt. Stomach, Pt. Liver, Pt. Spleen, Pt. Shenmen.

19. Diarrhea: Pt. Large Intestine, Pt. Stomach.

20. Hysteria: Pt. Heart, Pt. Brain, Pt. Occiput, Pt. Middle Border, Pt. Shenmen.

Part III Acupuncture and Moxibustion Treatment

Chapter 1 Introduction

Acupuncture and moxibustion therapy takes the theories of differentiation of syndromes as guidance in treatment, that is, it is based on the theories of Zang and Fu organs and the meridians, the four diagnostic methods, and the eight principal syndromes, to analyze clinical data collected on a wide scale so as to determine the location of pathologic changes (in meridians and collaterals, Zang and Fu organs, and the exterior and the interior), the nature of pathology (Yin and Yang, heat and cold, and excessive and deficient), to weigh the severity of the disease and the state of the Qi and to get hold of the nature of the disease and its internal relations between manifestation and root. Then according to differentiation of syndromes, doctors work out principles and prescriptions to select the points and apply the therapy in order to invigorate meridians, regulate Qi and blood, and keep Yin and Yang in balance, Zang and Fu organs in harmony to guarantee Yin flourishing smoothly and Yang vivified steadily, hence a relative equilibrium and health are maintained. This is a process of proper therapeutic program.

Section 1 Differentiation according to the Principles of Acupuncture and Moxibustion Therapy

Acupuncture is a precious jewel in the treasure house of Traditional Chinese Medicine. Base on different theories or principles such as: eight principles, the theory of Zang and Fu organs, the theory of meridians, the theory of Qi and blood, the theory of six meridians, the development of an epidemic febrile disease by analyzing the four syndromes (Wei, Qi, Ying and Xue Systems), the pathology of the Triple Energizer, analysis of the pathogenic factors, there are a number of methods in Traditional Chinese Medicine for differentiating syndromes. Each method has its own strongness and weakness and stresses on a particular aspect, while differentiation according to the theory of meridians is widely adopted in acupuncture practice. Because meridians and collaterals pertain to Zang-Fu organs interiorly and link with limbs and joints exteriorly. When it is abnormal in the circulation of meridians, it reflects on Zang-Fu organs, meridians, five sense organs, nine orificies, skin, muscle, tendon and bone where the affected meridian passes by. They are the symptoms of the twelve meridians (See the chapter concerned with the meridians and collaterals); the symptoms of the Eight Extra Meridians and symptoms of the Fifteen Collaterals. This is the basis of diagnosis and treatment.

Section 2 Principles of Acupuncture and Moxibustion

There are two methods to establish principles. One is to select points according to the location of disease, the other is to work out treatment method according to the nature of disease. That is "Strengthening Deficiency" refers to the deficiency syndrome that should be treated with tonification and support of the Primordial Qi in acupuncture. "The excess should be relieved" refers to treating excess syndrome by dispelling the pathogenic factors "Wan Chen Ze Chu Zhi" means treating stasis symptom of meridians with blood-letting method to remove stasis " Re Zhe Ji Zhi" means treating febrile disease with swift-needling method to relieve pathogenic heat. "Retaining the needle for symptom of pathogenic cold" means treating cold symptoms by retaining the needle. "Xian Xia Ze Jia Zhi" means treating continuous sweating, prostration of Yang exhaustion, prolapse of uterus and rectum by moxibustion to invigorate the spleen function and send vital energy and nutrients upward for prolapse of rectum and uterus. "If symptom appears neither excessive nor deficient, the method of even reinforcing and reducing can be used" refers when the symptoms of deficiency syndrome and the excess syndrome are not obvious, the method of even reinforcing and reducing can be used on selected points of the affected meridian.

With the development of acupuncture, there appear more and more methods such as intradermal needling therapy, acupoint injection therapy, electric needling therapy, laser therapy, and microwave therapy.

Section 3 Acupuncture and Moxibustion Prescription

Acupuncture and moxibustion prescription refers to the realization of acupoints according to the decided principle. That is, principal points for main pathology, accessory points for symptomatic treatment, which make principal and supplementary points functionize together. Because diseases vary in their occurrence and development, the meridians which they affect are different. Thus, there are complicated prescription and simple prescription according to the number of points selected. Sometimes, only one point is used for main disease without accessory points, that is, a simple prescription. But, when disease affects several meridians complicated prescription is necessary which refers to the selection of a great number of points to get effective in treatment. It is stated in Chapter 74 of *Plain Question* that "diseases may appear severe or mild, treatment should be given according to individual conditions and prescriptions may be complicated or simple." In Chapter 59 of *Miraculous Pivot*, it says: "diseases are changeable, thus there are countless methods of treatment to be considered by the condition. A mild case should be treated by a few points, while a severe case treated by many points".

In the prescription, the following symbols are commonly used for manipulation:

T or $+$: reinforcing
⊥ or $-$: reducing
| or $\pm$: even movement
※: cutaneous needle
↓: bleeding with a three-edged needle
◯₋ : imbedding needle
/⁴ : electric needle
△: moxibustion
◯: cupping

Point prescription includes selection of nearby points, distant points, symptomatic points, corresponding points, and specific points. However, no matter which selection is applied, it must depend on the theory of meridians, that is, diseases can be treated or treatment can reach where the meridians pass through.

1. Selection of Nearby Points

Selection of nearby points refers to selecting points in the local area and the adjacent area of the disease. All the points selected can treat the diseases of the local area and the adjacent area. For instance, Jingming (BL 1) is selected for eye disease, Yingxiang (LI 20) for nose disease, Tinggong (SI 19) for ear disease, and Zhongwan (CV 12) for epigastric disease. This is called the selection of local points, it is mainly used for chronic diseases. When there are ulcer, injury and scar in the local area of disease, acupuncture may not be applied; points of the adjacent area can be selected. Selection of adjacent points refers to selecting points in the adjacent area of disease, for example, Yintang (EX-HN3) and Shangxing (DU 23) are selected for nose disease; Qihai (CV 6) and Tianshu (ST 25) for gastric disorder. This is chiefly employed for diseases of Zang-Fu organs and five sense organs.

2. Selection of Distant Points

Selection of distant points refers to selecting points located far from the diseased area. Generally, these points are located below the elbows and knees. It is said in Chapter 70 of *Plain Questions*, "Points on the lower portion should be selected for the diseases of upper part, points on the upper should be selected for the diseases of the lower part and points on the side of the body should be selected for the diseases of the middle part". For instance, Zusanli (ST 36) is selected for epigastric and abdominal disorders. Weizhong (BL 40) is selected for the disorders of back and lumbar region. Hegu (LI 4) is selected for facial disorders, and Neiguan (PC 6) is selected for hypocondriac diseases. In clinical practice, selection of nearby points can be combined with distant points to strengthen the therapeutic effect, the table as follows: (Table 2-15)

Table 2-15 Examples for Local, Nearby and distant Point Selection

Diseased Area	Local Points	Adjacent Points	Distant Points
Forehead	Yangbai (GB 14)	Baihui (GV 20)	Hegu (LI 4) Neiting (ST 44)
Temple	Taiyang (EX-HN 5) Shuaigu (GB 8)	Fengchi (GB 20)	Zulinqi (GB 41) Huantiao (GB 30) Zuqiaoyin (GB 44)

Diseased Area	Local Points	Adjacent Points	Distant Points
Nape	Yamen(GV 15)	Dazhui(GV 14)	Houxi(SI 3) Yaoyangguan(GV 3)
Eye	Jingming(BL 1)	Fengchi(GB 20)	Hegu(LI 4) Guangming(GB 37)
Nose	Yingxiang(LI 20)	Tongtian (BL 7) Juliao(ST 3)	Zusanli(ST 36)
Mouth	Dicang(ST 4)	Jiache(ST 6)	Hegu(LI 4) Taichong(LR 3)
Ear	Tinggong(SI 19)	Fengchi(GB 20)	Zhongzhu(TE 3) Fengshi(GB 31)
Throat	Renyin(ST 9)	Tianrong (SI 17) Dazhu(BL 11)	Shaoshang(LU 11) Zhaohai(KI 6) Lieque(LU 7)
Chest	Tanzhong(CV 17)	Feishu(BL 13)	Neiguan(PC 6) Qiuxu(GB 40)
Costal Region	Dabao(SP 21)	Ganshu(BL 18)	Zhigou(TE 6)
Upper Abdomen	Zhongwan(CV 12)	Liangmen(ST 21)	Zusanli(ST 36) Neiguan(PC 6)
Lower Abdomen	Guanyuan(CV 4)	Tianshu(ST 25)	Sanyinjiao(SP 6)
Lumbar Region	Shenshu(BL 23)	Juliao(GB 29)	Weizhong (BL 40) Yanglao(SI 6)
Rectum	Changqiang (GV 1)	Dachangshu (BL 25)	Chengshan(BL 57) Erbai(EX-UE 2)

3. Selection of Symptomatic Points

The effects of some points are relatively specific. In clinic, a group of points can be selected for corresponding symptoms. The application of sole point is its finest portion, the table as follows: (Table 2-16)

Table 2-16 Examples for Symptomatic Point

Symptoms	Points
Fever	Dazhui(GV 14), Quchi(LI 11), Waiguan(TE 5), Hegu(LI 4), Shixuan(EX-UE 11)

Symptoms	Points
Coma	Shuigou(GV 26), Shixuan(EX-UE 11), Shenque(CV 8)
Nigth Sweating	Yinxi(HT 6), Houxi(SI 3)
Lock Jaw	Jiache(ST 6), Xiaguan(ST 7), Hegu(LI 4)
Cough, Asthma	Dingchuan(EX-B 1), Yuji(LU 10), Tiantu(CV 22), Lieque(LU 7)
Chest Congestion	Tanzhong(CV 17), Neiguan(PC 6), Jiquan(HT 1)
Cardiac Pain	Tanzhong(CV 17), Neiguan(PC 6), Xinshu(BL 15), Ximen(PC 4)
Gastric Pain	Zusanli(ST 36), Liangqiu(ST 34), Neiguan(PC 6)
Constipation	Zhigou(TE 6), Zhaohai(KI 6)
Malposition of Fetus	Zhiyin(BL 67)
Debility	Zusanli(ST 36), Guanyuan(CV 4), Dazhui(GV 14)
Infantile Malnutrition	Sifeng(EX-UE 10)
Pile Bleeding	Erbai(EX-UE 2)

Selection of corresponding points: The meridian system is a crisscross network running up and down, connecting the exterior and the interior and the same named meridians are corresponding each other. When the location of disease is limited or acute pain appears, the corresponding points of related meridians of health side can be selected. For instance. Quchi(LI 11) in the right elbow is selected for the pain on the left arm; Yanglao(SI 6) is selected for sprain of external malleolus, Daling (PC 7) is selected for pain in heel.

4. Selection of Points by Reinforcing the Mother and Reducing the Son:

It is based on the theory of reinforcing the mother for deficiency syndrome and reducing the son for excess syndrome of *Classic on Medical Problems*. It combines the therapeutic properties of the Five Shu Points with Five Elements Theory: wood, fire, earth, metal and water, the Five Shu Points can be selected according to the interpromotion, and counteraction relations of the Five Elements. For instance, Lung relates to metal, when the excess symptom of Lung Meridian appears, select the He-(Sea)point of Lung Meridian, Chize(LU 5) which attributes to water, because metal generates water, water is the son of metal, selecting Chize (LU 5) is so-called "Reduce the son for excess syndrome." When deficiency syndrome of the Lung Meridian appears, select Shu-(Stream) point of the Lung Meridian, Taiyuan (LU 9) which attributes to earth, because earth generates metal, earth is the mother of metal, selecting Taiyuan (LU 9) is so-called "Reinforce the mother for deficiency syndrome." Other points are on the analogues of this. See the details in the following table: (Table 2-17)

Table 2-17 The "Mother" and "Son" Points for Reinforcing and Reducing

Five Elements		Zang-Fu Organs	Mother Point	Son Point
Metal		Lung	Taiyuan (LU 9)	Chize (LU 5)
		Large Intestine	Quchi (LI 11)	Erjian (LI 2)
Water		Kidney	Fuliu (KI 7)	Yongquan (KI 1)
		Bladder	Zhiyin (BL 67)	Shugu (BL 65)
Wood		Liver	Quguan (LR 8)	Xingjian (LR 2)
		Gallbladder	Xiaxi (GB 43)	Yangfu (GB 38)
Fire	King	Heart	Shaochong (HT 9)	Shenmen (HT 7)
		Small Intestine	Houxi (SI 3)	Xiaohai (SI 8)
	Premier	Pericardium	Zhongchong (PC 9)	Daling (PC 7)
		Triple Energizer	Zhongzhu (TE 3)	Tianjing (TE 10)
Earth		Spleen	Dadu (SP 2)	Shangqiu (SP 5)
		Stomach	Jiexi (ST 41)	Lidui (ST 45)

5. Selecting Points by Earth Meridian Ebb-Flowing Rule

Considering the earth meridians is also called considering the earth branches. By this method, a day (24 hours) is divided into 12 hour period. Each is represented by a Chinese character called earth branch which, in turn, corresponds with Zang-Fu organ respectively. Then according to different hour periods, the Qi and blood flow ebbs or flows in considering the symptoms at the same time to choose the points to strengthen the mother and reduce the son. In application, when the affected Zang (or Fu) organ is in excess of Qi-blood flow, reduce the son point. When the organs are deficient, strengthen the mother point at the next hour-period when the Qi-blood flow begins to wane. If time for reinforcing or reducing has passed, the excess and deficiency syndromes don't appear obviously, select the Yuan-(primary)point of the affected meridian or the points of the affected meridian for treatment. Even reinforcing and reducing can be employed. (see the following table)

Table 2-18 Selecting Points by Earth Meridian Ebb-Flowing Rule

Zang-Fu Organs	Period of Ebb-Flow	Earthly Branches	Period for Reducing Excess and Points	Period for Reinforcing Deficiency and Points	Yuan Point Point of Affected Meridian
Lung	3-5	Yin the 3rd	3-5 Chize (LU 5)	5-7 Taiyuan (LU 9)	Taiyuan (LU 9) Jingqu (LU 8)
Large Intestine	5-7	Mou the 4th	5-7 Erjian (LI 2)	7-9 Quchi (LI 11)	Hegu (LI 4) Shangyang (LI 1)
Stomach	7-9	Chen the 5th	7-9 Lidui (ST 45)	9-11 Jiexi (ST 41)	Chongyang (ST 42) Zusanli (ST 36)
Spleen	9-11	Si the 6th	9-11 Shangqiu (SP 5)	11-13 Dadu (SP 2)	Taibai (SP 3) Taibai (SP 3)
Heart	11-13	Wu the 7th	11-13 Shenmen (HT 7)	13-15 Shaochong (HT 9)	Shenmen (HT 7) Shaofu (HT 8)
Small Intestine	13-15	Wei the 8th	13-15 Xiaohai (SI 8)	15-17 Houxi (ST 3)	Wangu (SI 4) Yanggu (SI 5)

302

Zang-Fu Organs	Period of Ebb-Flow	Earthly Branches	Period for Reducing Excess and Points	Period for Reinforcing Deficiency and Points	Yuan Point Point of Affected Meridian
Bladder	15-17	Shen the 9th	15-17 Shugu (BL 65)	17-19 Zhiyin (BL 67)	Jinggu (BL 64)
Kidney	17-19	You the 10th	17-19 Yongquan (KI 1)	19-21 Fuliu (KI 7)	Taixi (KI 3) Yingu (KI 10)
Peri-Candium	19-21	Xu the 11th	19-21 Daling (PC 7)	21-23 Zhongchong (PC 9)	Daling (PC 7) Laogong (PC 8)
Triple Energizer	21-23	Hai the last	21-23 Tianjing (TE 10)	23-1 Zhongzhu (TE 3)	Yangchi (TE 4) Zhigou (TE 6)
Liver	23-1	Zi the 1st	23-1 Yangfu (GB 38)	1-3 Xiaxi (GB 43)	Qiuxu (GB 40) Zulinqi (GB 41)
Gallbladder	1-3	Chou the 2nd	1-3 Xingjian (LR 2)	3-5 Ququan (LR 8)	Taichong (LR 3) Dadun (LR 1)

303

Chapter 2
Acupuncture Therapy

Section 1 Internal Diseases

1. Stroke

Stroke refers to a disease characterized by sudden loss of consciousness, wry face, slurred speech and hemiplegia, or with hemiplegia but without sudden coma. Stroke is an emergency case accompanied with many symptoms, the pathological changes vary quickly like the wind, therefore it is also called "wind stroke". In mild cases, there are only symptoms showing dysfunction of the meridians and collaterals, while in severe cases, dysfunction of Zang-Fu organs may be subdivided into obstructive type and collapse type.

This disease includes cerebral hemorrhage, cerebral thrombosis, subarachnoid hemorrhage, cerebral vasospasm, even viral encephalitis and cerebral facial paralysis in western medicine.

Etiology and Pathogenesis

Wind stroke often occurs in the middle-aged and the aged who are in poor health, with constitutional deficiency of Qi and blood which cause functional disorder of liver, kidney, heart and spleen, with deficiency of liver Yin which leads to the excess of liver Yang, the deficiency of heart Yin which results in the excess of heart fire, deficiency of the Spleen-Yang which leads to production of damp phlegm. Under this condition, if emotional upset or depression, alcoholic indulgence, improper diet, invasion of exogenous pathogenic factors can lead to a sharp rise of liver—Yang that forces excessive flow of Qi and blood to ascend with the turbid damp phlegm to obstruct the clear orifices and cause the obstructive wind stroke. If the genuine primary Qi is feeble, Yin and Yang will be separated, the patient will collapse. There may also appear the wind stroke that if damp phlegm obstructs the meridians, hemiplegia will occur.

Differentiation

(1) **Wind Stroke Attacking the Zang-Fu Organs**

Obstructive Type

Main Manifestations: Falling down with loss of consciousness, tightly clinched hands and clenched jaws, flushed face, coarse breathing, stridor, retention of urine, constipation, red tongue with thick yellow or dark grey coating, string-taut, rolling and forceful pulse.

Treatment

Principle: Resuscitation, quenching the wind and fire, clearing up phlegm by needling mainly on the Governor Vessel, the Liver Meridian plus the twelve Jing-well) points.

Either reducing method or pricking to cause little bleeding, is applied.

Prescription

Main Points: Shuigou (GV 26), twelve Jing-(well) points on both hands (LU 11, HT 9, PC 9, LI 1, TE1, SI 1), Laogong (PC 8), Fenglong (ST 40), Baihui (GV 20), Taichong (LR 3), and Yongquan (KI1).

Additional Points

Clenched Jaws: Xiaguan (ST 7), Jiache (ST 6) and Hegu (LI 14).

Aphasia and Stiff Tongue: Yamen (GV 15), Lianquan (CV 23) and Tongli (HT 5).

Explanation: Shuigou (GV 26) is for resuscitation. Pricking the twelve Jing (well) points helps to eliminate heat, resuscitation and promote Qi of the Twelve Meridians. Laogong (PC 8) is applied to eliminate heat from the heart. Fenglong (ST 40), the Luo-(connecting) point of Stomach Meridian, promotes the Qi mechanism of the spleen and stomach, resolves damp phlegm. Baihui (GV 20) and Taichong (LR 3) are selected to subdue the upsurging of Qi in the Liver Meridian and the Liver-Yang; Yongquan (KI 1) is selected to nourish the Kidney-Yin, pacify the Liver-Yang. All these points function to clear up obstruction, resuscitate, pacify the liver-Yang, and clear phlegm heat; Xiaguan (ST 7), Jiache (ST 6) and Hegu (LI 4) are chosen to promote the circulation of Qi and blood for relieving the clenched jaws; Yamen (GV 15) is chosen to clear up the obstruction and resuscitate. While being mixed with Lianquan (CV 23) and Tongli (HT 5), Yamen (GV 15) can relieve stiffness of tongue.

Collapsing Type

Main Manifestations: Sudden falling down with loss of consciousness, closed eyes, opening mouth, weak nasal breathing, incontinence of urine and stools, flaccid tongue, cold limbs, flushed face, fainting pulse or rootless superficial pulse.

Treatment

Principle: The points of Governor Vessel are mainly selected while heavy moxibustion is applied to these points to restore Yang from collapse.

Prescription: Shenque(CV 8), Guanyuan(CV 4), Qihai(CV 6) and Baihui (GV 20).

Explanation: Shenque(CV 8) is located in the center of the umbilicus, linking with the genuine Qi, as the root of life. Guanyuan(CV 4) and Qihai(CV 6) are located in the lower abdomen and intersect the Conception Vessel with the three Yin meridians of foot. Guanyuan(CV 4) is the place where Qi of Triple Energizer infuses. If connected with the real Yang of the vital gate, Qihai(CV 6) is the sea of the meridian Qi. The ways of applying indirect moxibustion with salt to Shenque(CV8), heavy moxibustoin to Guanyuan(CV 4) and Qihai(CV 6) can restore Yang from collapse and strengthen the primary Yang. Applying moxibustion to Baihui (GV 20) can invigorate the Governor Vessel, resuscitate and clear up obstruction.

(2) Wind Stroke of Meridians and Collaterals Type

The Wind-phlegm obstructs the meridians, but doesn't attack the Zang-Fu organs; or after wind stroke, the functions of the affected Zang-Fu organs have been restored, yet there exists stagnation of the wind-phlegm in the meridians and collaterals.

Main Manifestations: Hemiplegia, numbness of skin and limbs, wry mouth and eyes, stiff tongue with poor speech. It may also be accompanied by headache, dizziness, twitching of muscles, red eyes and flushed face, thirst, dryness of the throat, irritability and wiry or slippery slow pulse.

Treatment

Principle: Select mainly the points of Large Intestine, Stomach, Triple Energizer, Gallbladder, Small Intestine and Bladder Meridians. Needling with even reinforcing and reducing method, in order to regulate Qi and blood, remove obstruction from the meridians and collaterals, reduce the wind and keep Yin and Yang in balance.

Prescription

Upper limbs: Jianyu(LI 15), Quchi(LI 11), Shousanli(LI 10), Zhigou(TE 6), Hegu(LI 4) and Houxi(SI 3)

Lower limbs: Shenshu(BL 23), Huantiao(GB 30), Yanglingquan(GB 34), Zusanli(ST 36) and Taichong(LR 3)

Head and facial region: Baihui(GV 20), Jianche(ST 6), Yamen(GV 15), Liangquan(CV 23), Fengchi(GB 20) and Dicang(ST 4)

Explanation: The Yangming meridians are full of blood and Qi, where Qi and blood flourish, diseases are easy to occur. So Jianyu(LI 15), Quchi(LI 11), Shousanli(LI 10), Hegu(LI 4), Zusanli(ST 36), Dicang(ST 4) and Jiache(ST 6) are selected in order to regulate Qi and blood of upper limbs, lower limbs, hand and facial region, eliminate wind, remove phlegm. The Shaoyang meridians dominate the body movement. Zhigou(TE 6), Fengchi(GB 20), Huantiao(GB 30) and Yanglingquan(GB 34) are selected to clear the meridians and collaterals and promote the circulation in the upper and lower portions of the body. Baihui(GV 20), Fengchi(GB 20) and Taichong(LR 3) are selected to pacify the Liver-Yang and wind to treat accompanying symptoms; Dicang(ST 4) and Jiache(ST 6) are selected to treat wry mouth, Yamen(GV 15) and Lianquan(CV 23) are used to strengthen the root of the tongue. Needling Houxi(SI 3) can strongly remove the obstruction from the Governor Vessel and check spasm. It is an effective point for paralysis of upper limbs and chinched hands.

Alternative Treatment

(1) Scalp Acupuncture

Selection of Points: Contralateral motor area, sensory area, foot sensory area, chorea-trembling controlling area.

Method: The needling with routine disinfection is applied one after another in those areas. The needles are inserted as deeply as to the periostium, then are rotated 140-160 times per a minute, for 2 minutes. the patient is advised to perform exercises when the needles are rotated. Retain the needles for 5 minutes, then rotate them for another 2 minutes, then retain the needles for 30—40 minutes. Treatment should be given once a day or every other day, ten treatments for a course. This method has better therapeutic effect in the thrombosis of arteria cerebri media and branch of arteria cerebri anterior.

(2) Ear Acupuncture

Selection of Points: Pt. Brain 1, Pt. Central Rim, Pt. Liver, Pt. Triple Energizer and auricular points corresponding with the regions of paralysis. Add Pt. Heart, Pt. Spleen for aphona, add Pt. Mouth, Pt. Root of Ear Vagus, Pt. Pharynx and Larynx for difficulty in swallowing. The treatment should be given once every other day. Fifteen and twenty treatments make a course. Ear acupuncture is effective for sequela of cerebral accident (wind stroke attacking meridians and collaterals). It will be better to begin the treatment when the condition of the patient becomes stable, and the patient regains consciousness.

(3) Electric Stimulation

Select one or two points on upper limbs and lower limbs. After the insertion of the needle and arrival of Qi, the needles are connected with the electric stimulator, adjust the output current from small to large to make regular constractions appear in related muscle group until the patient feels comfortable and can tolerate it. The electric stimulation lasts 20 minutes for each treatment, treatment is given every other day. Ten treatments make a course. Electric stimulation is effective for wind stroke attack.

(4) Point Injection
Selection of Points:
Upper Limbs: Quchi(LI 11)
Lower Limbs: Yanglingquan(GB 34)

Select liquid medicine of 1ml 5% Danggui(Angelica sinesis) which may be injected into each point. The injection is advisable once every other day, ten treatments for a course, it is effective for wind stroke attacking meridians and collaterals.

(5) Cutaneous Acupuncture

Tap the skin lightly along the Governor Vessel and the Bladder Meridian on the head. Tap the skin heavily along the Gallbladder Meridian; tap the skin lightly in back and lumbar region; tap the skin heavily in the sacrum region; tap the skin lightly along the Meridians of Three Hand Yin of the medial side of upper limbs; tap the points of the finger tip and the skin along the meridians of Three Hand Yang; tap the skin lightly along the meridians of Three Foot Yin below knee; tap the points of the toe tip and skin heavily along the Meridians of Three Foot Yang. Treatment is given once a day. Ten treatments makes a course. This therapy is suitable for mild wind stroke attacking the meridians and collaterals.

Remarks
Prophylactic Measures for Wind Stroke

The aged with deficiency of Qi and excessive phlegm, or with manifestations of upsurging of Liver-Yang marked by dizziness and palpitations, may have prodromal symptoms such as stiff tongue, slurred speech, pain and weakness of limbs, irritation and numbness of the finger tips. Caution should be paid to diet and life style and avoid overstraining. Frequent moxibustion on Zusanli(ST 36) and Xuanzhong(GB 39) may prevent an attack of wind stroke.

2. Sunstroke

Sunstroke is an acute case occurring in summer, manifested by high fever, irritability, nausea, or even followed by collapse and loss of consciousness. The onset of this disease is due mostly to prolonged exposure to the sun, or to an environment with high temperature. This disease includes thermoplegia, heat cramp, heliosis, etc.

Etiology and Pathogenesis

Summer heat is prevalent in summer. When the weather is scorching, long exposure to the sun and to a heat environment, the high temperature will damage Qi. Invasion of summer heat in a condition of lower resistance brings about sunstroke. Clinically, sunstroke is mainly divided into mild and severe types with different severity.

Differentiation
(1) **Mild Type**

Main Manifestations: Headache, dizziness, profuse sweating, hot skin, coarse breathing, dry mouth and tongue, extreme thirst, superficial, large and rapid pulse.

Treatment

Principle: Reducing at the points of Governor Vessel, Pericardium and Large Intestine Meridians is applied to eliminate the summer heat.

Prescription: Dazhui(GV 14), Neiguan(PC 6), Quchi (LI 11) and Weizhong (BL 40)

Explanation: Dazhui (GV 14) is for eliminating general summer heat, Weizhong (BL 40) also named Xuexi is for eliminating pathological heat in the Xue (blood) system by applying blood-letting. Neiguan (PC6) is for eliminating heat from Triple Energizer. Quchi(LI 11) is the main point for eliminating heat.

(2) **Severe Type**

Main Manifestations: Headache, extreme thirst and shortness of breath at first, and then collapse, loss of consciousness, sweating, deep and faint pulse.

Treatment
Principle: Reducing manipulation is applied at the points of the Governor Vessel to resuscitate and eliminate heat.
Prescription: Shuigou(GV 26), Baihui (GV 20), Shixuan(EX-UE 11), Quze(PC 3)and Weizhong(BL 40)
Explanation: Shuigou(GV 26) and Baihui (GV 20) are selected to resuscitate. Quze(PC 3), the He-(Sea) point of Pericardium Meridian, Weizhong(BL 40)are pricked superficially to remove the heat from the blood. Blood-letting at Shixuan(EX-UE 11) can eliminate heat and resuscitate.

Alternative Treatment
Scrapping Method
It is indicated for mild type of sunstroke. A smooth spoon is used to scrap the skin with cooking oil or water. Scarp both sides of medical line of the Bladder Meridian, neck, space of the hypochondriac region, arm, shoulder, fossa cubitalis, and fossa malleolus, until local redness of the skin with red purplish blood stasis appear.

3. Syncope

Syncope is manifested by sudden fainting, cold limbs and loss of consciousness. A mild case of syncope only makes the patient faint for a short period of time, recover spontaneously without leaving any consequence while in severe cases it may lead to loss of consciousness for a long time, or even death. Syncope appears in simple fainting, postural hypotension, hypoglycemia, shock and the onset of hysteria.

Etiology and Pathogenesis
(1)Deficiency Syndrome
Syncope of deficiency type is often caused by general deficiency of the primary Qi and failure of clearing Yang in ascending due to over fatigue or grief and fight, or by exhaustion of Qi after profuse bleeding, which causes divorce of Yin and Yang, and syncope results.
(2)Excess Syndrome
It is mainly due to mental stress, such as anger, fear and fright, leading to rebellious flow of Qi, which rushes upwards to the heart and chest, blocking the air passage and orifices or due to upsurging of Liver-Yang, and upward flowing

of Qi followed by perversion of blood flow after a fit of anger, leading to blockage of orifices and resulting in loss of consciousness.

Differentiation
(1) **Deficiency Syndrome** Sudden fainting, feeble breathing with mouth agape, pale face, spontaneous sweating, cold limbs, deep and thready pulse.

Treatment
Principle: The points of Governor Vessel and Pericardium Meridian are selected as the main points to resuscitate, reinforce Qi and Yang. Moxibustion can be used together.

Prescription: Shuigou (VG 26), Baihuit (GV 20), Neiguan (PC 6), Guanyuan (CV 4) and Zusanli (ST 36)

Explanation: Shuigou (GV 26) is the point for resuscitation, Baihui (GV 20) ascends the primary Qi of Yang, Neiguan (PC 6) can relieve chest congestion, Guanyuan (CV 4) reinforces the primary Qi, Zusanli (ST 36) reinforces Qi and blood. These five points perform functions of resuscitating, clearing the orifices, reinforcing Qi and Yang.

(2) **Excess Syndrome** Sudden fainting, coarse breathing, rigid limbs, clenched jaws, deep and excessive pulse.

Treatment
Principle: The points of Governor Vessel and Pericardium Meridians are selected as main points to resuscite and regulate the flow of Qi. Reducing manipulation is applied at the points.

Prescription: Shuigou (GV 26), Zhongchong (PC 9), Laogong (PC 8), Hegu (LI 4), Taichong (LR 3) and Yongquan (KI 1).

Explanation: Shuigor (GV 26) and Zhongchong (PC 9) are used to resuscitate; Hegu (LI 4) and Taichong (LR 3) are used to regulate the circulation of Qi and blood; Laogong (PC 8) and Yongquan (KI 1) are to clear heart orifice and smooth flow of Qi and blood.

Alternative Treatment
Ear Acupuncture

Selection of Points: Pt. Heart, Pt. Subcortex, Pt. Shenmen, Pt. Central Rim, and Pt. Sympathetic.

Method: Select two or three points, retain the filiform needles for 30 minutes. Apply strong stimulation to excess syndrome, mild stimulation to deficiency syndrome, rotate the needles every five minutes.

4. Common Cold

Common cold is an exogenous ailment with headache, stuffy and running nose, aversion to wind and fever. It may occur around the year, but more often in spring and winter. According to the difference in pathogens and clinical manifestations, this condition can be classified into two types: wind cold and wind heat. Mild case is known as catching cold, the upper respiratory infection and influenza are included in this disease.

Etiology and Pathogenesis

This disease is often due to weak constitution and resistance which makes the body inadaptable to intense changes of the weather, then the exogenous pathogenic wind invades the body through the pores of skin, mouth and nose, leading to manifestation related to the Lung Meridian.

(1) Exogenous pathogenic wind-cold attacks the body superficies, leading to closed pores and dysfunction of lung in dispersing, this is called wind cold syndrome.

(2) Exogenous pathogenic wind-heat attacks the lung, leading to dysfunction of lung in descending and abnormal opening and closing of pores. This is called wind-heat syndrome.

Differentiation
(1) Wind—Cold
Main Manifestations: Chills, fever, headache, cough, anhidrosis, pain of the limbs, stuffy and running nose, itching of the throat, hoarse voice, profuse thin sputum, white tongue coating, floating and tense pulse.
Treatment
Principle: Eliminate wind, disperse cold from the body surface and promote the function of the lung in dispersing by puncturing points mainly from Lung Meridian, Large Intestine Meridian and Bladder Meridian with reducing manipulation.
Prescription: Lieque (LU 7), Hegu (LI 4), Fengchi (GB 20), Fengmen (BL 12).
Additional Points

Add Zhongwan (CV 12), Neiguan (PC 6) and Zusanli (ST 36) for excessive dampness.

Explanations: Lieque (LU 7), the Luo—(Connecting) point of the Lung Meridian, has the effect of promoting the lung to disperse, and treat nasal obstruction, itching of throat and cough, Fengmen (BL 12), a point of Bladder Meridian, which dominates the surface of the whole body is selected to regulate the circulation of Qi, to eliminate wind-cold and relieve aversion to cold, fever, and headache. Hegu (LI 4), the Yuan-(Primary) point of Large Intestine Meridian is used to promote the lung to disperse, and relieve the exterior symptoms. Fengchi (GB 20), a point at the intersection of the Gallbladder Meridian and the Yang Link Vessel is used to eliminate wind cold and relieve the exterior symptoms. These four points combined with each other perform the function of eliminating wind cold, promoting the lung to disperse and relieving the exterior symptoms. Zhongwan (CV 12), Neiguan (PC 6) and Zusanli (ST 36) are added for excessive dampness to strengthen the function of spleen and stomach, to remove dampness and regulate Qi and descend perversive flow of Qi.

(2) Wind—Heat

Main Manifestations: Fever, sweating, slight aversion to wind, pain and distending sensation of the head, cough with yellow thick sputum, congested and sore throat, extreme thirst, thin white or yellowish tongue coating, floating and rapid pulse.

Common cold in summer accompanying with damp heat, the chief manifestations include high fever, sweating can't reduce heat, general tiredness, thirst, yellow and red urinary, red and yellow tongue coating and soft, rapid pulse.

Treatment

Principle: Eliminate wind, disperse heat and promote the circulation of lung Qi by needling the points mainly from Governor Vessel, Lung Meridian, Large Intestine Meridian and Triple Energizer Meridian with reducing manipulation.

Prescription: Dazhui (GV 14), Chize (LU 5), Waiguan (TE 5), Hegu (LI 4), Yuji (LU 10) and Shaoshang (LU 11)

Additional Points

Add Zhongwan (CV 12) and Zusanli (ST 36) for excessive dampness.

Explanation: Dazhui (GV 14), a point where all the Yang meridians meet, is used to eliminate heat and other pathogens of Yang nature, Chize (LU 5), the He-(Sea) point of Lung Meridian, Yuji (LU 10), the Ying-(Spring) point of

Lung Meridian, and Shaoshang (LU 11), the Jing-(Well) point combined with each other can eliminate heat from the lung, clear throat, Waiguan (TE 5) the Luo-(Connecting) point of the Triple Energizer Meridian connecting with Yang Link Vessel can dispel pathogens of Yand nature in the exterior of the body and eliminate heat. Zhongwan (CV 12) and Zusanli (ST 36) are added for damp-heat to strengthen the function of spleen and stomach, and remove the pathogenic dampness.

Alternative Treatment
(1) Ear Acupuncture
Selection of Points: Pt. Lung, Pt. Trachea, and Pt. Ear Apex.
Method: Filiform needles are used to pierce both ears with strong stimulation and retain the needles for 10—12 minutes.
(2) Cutaneous Acupuncture
The plum-blossom needle is used to tap the skin along the Governor Vessel and Bladder Meridian of the back for the pain in neck and back, and fever without sweating, Then cupping therapy is applied.

Remarks
Prophylactic Measure: Moxibustion is applied to Fengmen (BL 12) or Zusanli (ST 36) to prevent common cold during its prevalence.

5. Malaria

Malaria is an epidemic disease characterized by shivering chills, strong fever and sweating at regular intervals, mostly found in late summer and early autumn, but also sporadically occurring in other seasons. The causative factor is the malarial pestilential air. The recurrence of chills and fever may be once every day, every second day, or every third day, known respectively as quotidian malaria according to the interval between attacks. In chronic cases, there may be a mass in the hypochondriac region, termed "malaria with splenomegaly."

Etiology and Pathogenesis
Malaria is mainly caused by the invasion of pestilential factor and that of exogenous pathogenic heat, wind, cold, summer heat and dampness dormant in the semi-exterior and semi-interior and wandering between the nutrient and defensive systems. Chills appears if such factors run into the nutrient system, and

heat appears if they outwardly disturb the defensive system, the imbalance between nutrient and defensive systems and the struggle between the genuine Qi and pathogenic Qi develops malaria. If the pathogenic factors and the antipathogenic factors are separated from each other, or if the pathogenic factors avoid fighting with the nutrient and defensive systems, there appears an interval between the paroxysms.

Only when the body resistance is weak, the pestilential factor invades the body. Weakened body resistance may be due to abnormal daily life, overfatigue, or deficiency of Qi and blood caused by disorder in transportation and transformation function of the spleen and stomach as a result of irregular food intake. Zhang Jingyue said: "Malaria is an exogenous disease... only in the condition of delicate health, or overfatigue and stress, one is apt to be attacked by malarial pathogenic factor."

Differentiation

Main Manifestations: Shivering chills and fever appear at regular intervals. Shivering chills occurs at first, then fever appears. Sweating makes the symptoms release.

This disease starts with yawning and forcelessness, and then with shivering chills. When the chills retreat, general fever takes place. There appear intolerable headache, flushed face and red lips, extreme thirst, bitter taste and dry mouth, congestion in the hypochondriac region.

At the end of the paroxysm, the patient breaks out in profuse perspiration and fever subsides with the body feel cool, thin, sticky and yellow tongue coating, the pulse is wiry and rapid. In chronic cases, a mass in the hypochondronic region-splenomegaly is usually found.

Treatment

Principle: Reducing manipulation is applied at the points of Governor Vessel and Shaoyang Meridians to regulate the Governor Vessel and to harmonize the Shaoyang Meridians. Treatment is given two hours prior to the paroxysm, if chill is predominant during the paroxysm, acupuncture is advised to combine with moxibustion, if fever is the dominant symptom, acupuncture alone is employed.

Prescription: Dazhui (GV 14), Taodao (GV 13) Houxi (SI 3), Jianshi (PC 5), Yemen (TE 2), and Zulinqi (GB 41)

Additional Points

Quchi (LI 11) is used with reducing manipulation for high fever. Zhangmen (LR 13) is added for malaria with splenomegaly, moxibustion is applied to Pigen (EX-B 4), prick the twelve Jing-(Well) points for high fever with delirium.

Explanation: Dazhui (GV 14), the meeting point of the three Yang Meridians and the Governor Vessel can promote the circulation of Qi in the Yang Meridians and help to eliminate pathogenic factors, in combination with Taodao (GV 13), which can eliminate pathogenic heat, and regulate Yin and Yang. They are the chief points for malaria. Yemen (TE 2) and Zulinqi (GB 41) can harmonize Qi of the Shaoyang Meridian, Houxi (SI 3), the Shu-(Stream) point of Small Intestine Meridian can activate the circulation of Qi in the Taiyang Meridian and Governor Vessel, and drive pathogenic factors out. Jianshi (PC 5), is the He-(Sea) point of Pericardium Meridian, because the Jueyin Meridian links with the Shaoyang Meridian exteriorly-interiorly, Jianshi (PC 5) can regulate the circulation of Qi and drive pathogenic factors out, combination of all the abovementioned points can promote the circulation of Qi in the Yang Meridians and help to eliminate pathogenic factors, harmonize the interior and exterior, Yin and Wei, and control malaria. Quchi (LI 11) combined with Dazhui (GV 14) can dispel heat. Zhangmen (LR 13), the influential point dominating Zang-organs can regulate Qi in the Zang-organs. Pigen (EX-B4), an extra point, is selected to treat the mass in the hypochondriac region.

Alternative Treatment

(1) **Ear Acupuncture**

Selection of Points: Pt. Adrenal Gland, Pt. Subcortex, Pt. Endocrrine, Pt. Liver and Pt. Spleen.

Method: Apply filiform needles with strong stimulation at points.

Treatment is given one or two hours in advance of the next attack. Retain the needles for 1 hour, the therapy is applied to the patient for 3 days.

(2) **Topical Application of Drugs**

Dazhui (GV 14) is selected and fine powders of pepper of smashed chilli (one or two chillis) are applied topically for 3—4 hours. This application should be used two hours in advance of the next attack.

Neiguan (PC 6) is selected and tobacco (two portions) and ginger (one portion) smashed are applied in size of a coin.

Neiguan (PC 6) is selected and a certain amount of smashed wild herba menthae and garlic is applied. Paste should be fixed with paster for 3—4 hours. This therapy should be employed one or two hours in advance of the next attack.

Remark
Acupuncture treatment of tertian malaria has better effects.

6. Cough

Cough, a main symptom of the lung problems, may result either from attack by exogenous factors disturbing the dispersion of Qi of the lung, or from disorders of the lung itself or other diseased Zang-Fu organs affecting the lung. In modern medicine, cough is commonly seen in upper respiratory tract infection, acute and chronic bronchitis bronchicetasis, and tuberculosis.

Etiology and Pathogenesis
(1) Invasion by the Exogenous Pathogenic Factors

The lung dominates Qi and is regarded as an umbrella protecting the five Zang-organs. Upward it connects the throat and has its opening in the nose, governing respiration. Externally it associates with the skin and hair. Once the lung is attacked by the exogenous pathogenic factors, the defensive system of lung is invaded by pathogenic factors, the Qi of the lung is blocked and fails to descend, thus resulting in cough. Since the weather changes in different seasons, the exogenous pathogenic factors attacking the human body are various, cough is therefore divided into two types: wind-cold and wind-heat.

(2) Internal Injury

Cough resulted from functional impairment in the Zang-Fu organs, falls into the category of cough due to internal injury such as cough caused by dryness of the lung with deficiency of Yin leading to failure of the Qi of the lung to descend; cough caused by the deficiency of the spleen which gives rise to internal dampness whose excessive accumulation produces phlegm. Phlegm damp in return may go up into the lung, causing the dysfunction in descending, cough resulting from stagnation of liver-Qi may be turned into fire, flares up and injures the lung fluid, and cough is due to deficiency of liver and kidney-Yin, and the dysfunction of the lung in descending and dispersing.

Differentiation
Invasion by the Exogenous Pathogenic Factors
(1) Wind-Cold

Main Manifestations: Cough, itching of the throat, thin and white sputum, aversion to cold, fever, anhidrosis, headache, stuffy and running nose, thin, white tongue coating and superficial pulse.

(2) Wind-Heat

Main Manifestations: Cough with yellow and thick sputum, choking cough, thirst, sore throat, fever, or headache, aversion to wind, sweating, thin, yellow tongue coating, floating and rapid pulse.

Treatment
Principle: Points mainly from the Lung Meridian and Large Intestine Meridian are selected. Both acupuncture and moxibustion are applied in case of wind cold. While only acupuncture is used in case of wind heat to activate the dispersing function of the lung and to relieve the symptoms.

Prescription: Lieque (LU 7), Hegu (LI 4), Feishu (BL 13)

Additional Points

Add Shaoshang (LU 11) for pain and swelling of the throat. Dazhui (GV 14) and Waiguan (TE 5) for fever and aversion to cold.

Explanation: The lung dominants skin and hair, it links with the large intestine exteriorly-interiorly. Lieque (LU 7), the Lou-(Connecting) point of the Lung Meridian and Hegu (LI 4), the Yuan-(Primary) point are selected to eliminate wind and remove pathogenic factors, and activate the dispersing function of the lung and relieve the symptoms. Feishu (BL 13), the Back-Shu point can strengthen the functional activities of the lung, to relieve symptoms and to eliminate the exogenous pathogenic factors. Shaoshang (LU 11) is selected to disperse heat of lung, Dazhui (GV 14) is used for fever and aversion to cold. Waiguan (TE 5) is applied to eliminate heat and relieve symptoms.

Internal injury
(1) Blockage of the Lung by Phlegm

Main Manifestations: Cough with profuse, white and sticky sputum, stuffiness and chest congestion, loss of appetite, white, sticky tongue coating and rolling pulse.

Treatment

Principle: The Back-Shu point and the points of the Stomach Meridian are selected as the principal points. Both reinforcing and reducing manipulations should be considered in acupuncture treatment, or combined with moxibustion to strengthen the function of the spleen and to resolve phlegm.

Prescription: Feishu (BL 13), Pishu (BL 20), Zhongwan (CV 12), Zusanli (ST 36), Chize (LU 5), Fenglong (ST 40).

Explanation: Feishu (BL 13) and Pishu (BL 20) are selected to reinforce the Qi of lung and spleen, and activate the dispersing function of the lung, and strengthen the function of the spleen. Zhongwan (CV 12) and Zusanli (ST 36) are selected to remove dampness and resolve phlegm. Chize (LU 5) is able to reduce the pathogenic factors from the lung and relieve cough. Fenglong (ST 40) is selected to strengthen smooth transportation of Qi in the spleen and stomach, and resolve phlegm.

(2) **Deficiency of Yin with Dryness of the Lung**

Main Manifestations: Dry cough without sputum or with scanty sputum, dryness of the nose and throat, sore throat, spotting blood or even coughing blood, afternoon fever, malar flush, red tongue, thin coating, threadly and rapid pulse.

Treatment

Principle: The Back-(Shu) point and the Front-(Mu) point of Lung Meridian are selected as the principal points. Even reinforcing and reducing is applied in acupuncture treatment to nourish Yin, eliminate dryness and descend lung-Qi.

Prescription: Feishu (BL 13), Zhongfu (LU 1), Lieque (LU 7), Zhaohai (KI 6)

Additional Points

Add Kongzui (LU 6) and Geshu (BL 17) for hemoptysis

Explanation: The selection of Feishu (BL 13) and Zhongfu (LU 1) is a method of combining Back-(Shu) point and Front-(Mu) point. It is used to nourish lung-Yin and regulate Qi of lung. Lieque (LU 7), the Luo-(Connecting) point of the Lung Meridian is connected with the Conception Vessel to descend the lung-Qi and relieve cough. Lieque (LU 7) combining with Zhaohai (KI 6) can nourish Yin, clear the throat; Kongzui (LU 6), the Xi-(Cleft) point of the lung. Geshu (BL 17) is a blood point of the Eight Influential Points which specializes in stopping blood. Geshu (BL 17) combining with Kongzui (LU 6) can stop coughing blood. All the points above-mentioned can perform function of nourishing Yin, eliminating dryness, descending the lung-Qi, relieving cough and stopping bleeding.

Alternative Treatment
(1) Ear Acupuncture

Selection of points: Pt. Lung, Pt. Bronchea, Pt. Shenmen, Pt. Spleen

Method: Points of both ears are selected with moderate stimulation and retain the needles for 10—20 minutes. Treatment is given once every other day. Ten treatments constitute a course. Embedding seeds in ear is also applicable.

(2) Cutaneous Acupuncture

Tap lightly the skin of the neck and back along the Governor Vessel and the Bladder Meridian and both sides of the throat. Once a day, ten treatments make a course.

7. Asthma

Asthma is a common illness characterized by repeated attacks of paroxysmal dyspnea with wheezing. Dyspnea refers to difficulty in breathing, wheezing is marked by the noise when breathing. Since both of them appear at the same time and their causes and mechanisms are quite similar, they are combined together and termed asthma. This disease results from disturbance of Qi activities and can be divided into two types: deficiency and excess. It includes bronchial asthma, asthmatic bronchitis and obstructive pulmonary emphysema in modern medicine.

Etiology and Pathogenesis

Numerous factors may lead to asthma, they are categorized to exogenous and endogenous injuries. Zhang Jingyue, doctor of the Ming Dynasty, said: "Excess asthma is due to pathogenic factors, which manifest excess symptom, deficiency asthma has no pathogenic factors, involved and manifests constitutional asthenia only." Exogenous pathogenic factors show excess symptom, while endogenous injuries show deficiency symptom.

Excess type
(1) Wind-Cold Type

It denotes asthma due to invasion of wind cold, which impairs the smooth flow of the lung-Qi and makes the pore closed, since the lung and the superficial defensive system are weakened, the lung-Qi is accumulated and fails to disperse and descend, which leads to asthma.

(2) Phlegm-Heat Type

It refers to asthma due to improper food intake, failure of the spleen in transformation and transportation resulting in production of phlegm from the accumulated dampness or long-standing retention of phlegm turns into heat, or excessive fire of the lung evaporates the fluids to phlegm, when the phlegm fire stays in the lung, the lung-Qi is stagnated and the normal activity of the lung is impaired. Failure of the lung-Qi in descending function results in asthma.

Deficiency type
(1) Lung Deficiency

A prolonged and protracted cough can weaken and injure the lung-Qi. Overstrain and endogenous injuries can also bring about deficiency of the lung-Qi, then shortness of breath and dyspnea may occur.

(2) Kidney Deficiency

Oversex can injure the kidney. A severe or chronic disease weakens the body resistance and the essential Qi. Long-standing asthma also affects the kidney. In any of the above-mentioned cases, impairment of the kidney in receiving Qi may give rise to asthma.

Differentiation
Excess Type
(1) Wind-Cold Type

Main Manifestations: Cough with thin sputum, accompanied by aversion to cold and fever, headache, without sweat, absence of thirst, white tongue coating, floating and tense pulse.

Treatment

Principle: The points of Governor Vessel, Lung Meridian and Large Intestine Meridian are selected as the principal points. Filiform needles are applied with reducing manipulation in combination with moxibustion to eliminate wind cold, relieve symptom, disperse the lung-Qi and soothe asthma.

Prescription: Dazhui (GV 14), Hegu (LI 14), Lieque (LU 7), Feishu (BL 13), Fengmen (BL 12).

Explanation: Dazhui (GV 14) affects to promote Yang and relieve superficial cold from the body. Hegu (LI 4) is to regulate Qi and relieve the superficial cold Lieque (LU 7) affects to disperse lung-Qi and relieve the superficial cold, Feishu (BL 13) is to regulate the lung-Qi, Fengmen (BL 12) is to dominate wind and relieve the superficial cold. All these points are able to relieve the superficial cold, disperse the lung-Qi and soothe asthma.

(2) Phlegm-Heat Type

Main Manifestations: Rapid and short breathing, coarse voice, chest stuffiness, dry mouth, cough with thick yellow sputum, thick yellow or sticky coating, rolling and rapid pulse.

Treatment

Principle: The points of Lung and Stomach Meridians are selected as the principal points with reducing manipulation to resolve phlegm, reduce heat, disperse the lung-Qi and soothe asthma.

Prescription: Yuji (LU 10), Chize (LU 5), Dingchuan (EX-B 1), Fenglong (ST 40).

Explanation: Yuji (LU 10), the Ying-(Spring) point of Lung Meridian pertaining to fire, affects to reduce the heat of lung and relieve asthma. Chize (LU 5), the He-(Sea) point of Lung Meridian pertaining to water, is in charge of calming rebellious Qi, since water can control fire, so Chize (LU 5) can reduce lung heat to soothe asthma.

Dingchuan (EX-B 1) is an empirical point to pacify breathing, Fenglong (ST 40), the Luo-(Connecting) point of the Stomach Meridian, is able to strengthen the spleen function, reduce phlegm heat, disperse the lung-heat and soothe asthma.

Deficiency Type

(1) Lung Deficiency

Main Manifestations: Short and rapid breathing, feeble voice, weak and low sound of coughing, sweating on exertion, pale tongue, pulse of deficiency type.

Treatment

Principle: The points of Lung and Stomach Meridians are selected as the principal points with reinforcing method applied to strengthen the lung-Qi, and soothe asthma, moxibustion is also advisable.

Prescription: Feishu (BL 13), Zhongfu (LU 1), Taiyuan (LU 9), Taibai (SP 3), Zusanli (ST 36).

Explanation: Feishu (BL 13) and Zhongfu (LU 1) the combination of the Back-(Shu) and Front-(Mu) points, and Taiyuan (LU 9), the Yuan-Primary point of Lung Meridian, all these three points combined can strengthen the lung-Qi and soothe asthma. Zusanli (ST 36), the He-(sea) point of Stomach Meridian, and Taibai (SP 3), the Yuan-(Primary) point of Spleen Meridian, are combined to reinforce earth and promote metal, which refers to "Reinforce the mother when deficiency is found in the son", thus they are able to strengthen the lung through invigorating the spleen and stomach, and soothe asthma.

(2) **Kidney Deficiency**

Main Manifestations: Dyspnea on exertion after long-standing asthma, severe wheezing, short breath, lassitude and weakness, sweating, cold limbs, pale tongue, deep and thready pulse.

Treatment

Principle: The points of Kidney Meridian and Conception Vessel are selected as the principal points with reinforcing manipulation to strengthen the kidney function in receiving Qi and soothe asthma. Moxibustion is also advisable.

Prescription: Shenshu (BL 23), Taixi (KI 3), Feishu (BL 13), Gaohuang (BL 43), Tanzhong (CV 17), Pishu (BL 20), Zhongwan (CV 12), Guanyuan (CV 4).

Explanation: Long-standing asthma impairs the kidney-Qi, Taixi (KI 3) and Shenshu (BL 23) can strengthen the kidney function in receiving Qi and soothe asthma. Feishu (BL 13) and Tanzhong (CV 17) are able to regulate Qi, Pishu (BL 20) and Zhongwan (CV 12) strengthen the function of spleen and stomach, and invigorate the kidney-Qi, Guanyuan (CV 4) can reinforce the function of the spleen and strengthen the function of kidney. Gaohuang (BL 43) is an important point to reinforce Qi in general. All these points can strengthen kidney function in receiving Qi and reinforce the function of the spleen and pacify breathing.

Alternative Treatment

(1) **Ear Acupuncture**

Selection of Points: Pt. Relieving Asthma, Pt. Lung, Pt. Apex of Lower Tragus, Pt. Crus of Hexilx.

Method: Mild stimulation is applied, retain needles for 20 minutes.

(2) **Moxibustion Therapy**

Selection of Points: Feishu (BL 13), Gaohuang (BL 43), Pishu (BL 20), Shenshu (BL 23).

Method: Apply ignited moxa cones similar to the size of date nuts on slices of ginger at points proposed. Each point is heated with three to five moxa cones to make the local skin red without causing any blisters. Ten treatments are given once daily, commencing from the midsummer dog-days to the arrival of autumn season.

(3) **Cutaneous Acupuncture**

Selection of Points: The region along the Lung Meridian and musculus sternocleidomastideus of both sides.

Method: Tap the surface skin slightly in order for 15 minutes, to make the skin slightly red. The therapy is applied during the attack of asthma to relieve symptom.

(4) **Point Injection**

Selection of Points: Jiaji (EX-B 2) from the first thoracic vertebra to the sixth thoracic vertebra.

Method: Select a pair of points into which 0.5 ml placenta tissue extract is injected from upper parts to lower parts, change another pair the next day. This therapy is applied during the remission period of asthma.

(5) **Topical Application of Drugs**

Selection of Points: Feishu (BL 13), Dingchuan (EX-B 1), Tanzhong (CV 17), Chize (LU 5), Zusanli (ST 36).

Method: Select 3 or 4 points on which a bit of Xiao Chuan Gao (Paste for eliminating asthma) is applied by fixing the paste with the paster for 30-60 minutes, then eliminate this medical paste. This therapy is applied every ten days.

Remarks

Xiao Chuan Gao, the medical paste for eliminating asthma is made as follows: dried drugs such as White Mustard Seed (12g), Rhizome Corydalis (21g), Merba Asari (15g) and Radix Eaphorbiae Kansui (12g) are ground into fine powers and made into paste with ginger juice.

8. Epigastric Pain

Epigastric pain, refers to a syndrome manifested by frequent pain over the epigastric region and close to the cardia, so in ancient times, it was also named "cardiac pain" or "cardioabdominal pain". It is commonly seen in acute and chronic gastritis, stomach or duodental ulcer, functional stomach pain in modern medicine.

Etiology and Pathogenesis

(1) Irregular food intake, raw and cold food and hunger injure the spleen and stomach, causing failure of the spleen in transportation and transformation and failure of the stomach-Qi in descending, then pain appears.

(2) Anxiety, anger and mental depression damage the liver, causing failure of the liver in dominating free flow of Qi, adversely attacking the stomach, impeding its activity and hindering its Qi descending, then pain appears.

(3) Generally, lowered functioning of the spleen and stomach, due to invasion of pathogenic cold, which is stagnated in the stomach, causes failure of the stomach-Qi in descending, then pain occurs.

Differentiation
(1) Retention of Food

Main Manifestations: Distending pain in the epigastrium, aggravated on pressure, belching with fetid odour, anorexia, pain aggravated after meals, thick, sticky tongue coating, deep, forceful or rolling pulse.

Treatment

Principle: The Front-(Mu) point of the Stomach and the points of Stomach Meridian are selected with reducing manipulation to remove retention, pacify the stomach and relieve pain.

Prescription: Zhongwan (CV 12), Neiguan (PC 6), Zusanli (ST 36), Inner-Neiting (EX) and Tianshu (ST 25).

Explanation: Zhongwan (GV 12) is the Front-(Mu) point of stomach, and also one of Eight Influential Points, the influential point of Fu-organs, the principle point for diseases of Six Fu-organs, Zusanli (ST 36), the lower He-(Sea) point of the stomach and the principal point for diseases of stomach because of "the lower He-(Sea) point can treat diseases of Fu-organs". Neiguan (PC 6) is used to regulate Qi, pacify the stomach and relieve pain, and is also the principal point for relieving chest pain due to disorder of stomach. The joint use of the above-mentioned three points may relieve food retention, pacify stomach, and relieve pain. Inner-Neiting (EX) is an empirical point to treat retention of food. Tianshu (ST 25), the Front-(Mu) point of the large intestine may promote the Qi circulation in the large intestine to help to relieve food retention.

(2) **Attack of the Stomach by the Liver-Qi**

Main Manifestations: Paroxysmal pain in the epigastrium, radiating to the hypochondriae regions, frequent belching, nausea, acid regurgitation, abdominal distension, anorexia, thin, white tongue coating, deep, string-start pulse.

Treatment

Principle: The points of Liver and Stomach Meridians are selected as the principal points with the reducing manipulation to remove the stagnation of liver-Qi, to pacify the stomach and to relieve pain.

Prescription: Neiguan (PC 6), Qimen (LR 14), Taichong (LR 3), Zhongwan (CV 12), Zusanli (ST 36)

Explanation: Qimen (LR 14) is the Front-(Mu) point of the liver and Taichong (LR 3) is the Yuan-(Primary) point of Liver Meridian. The two are used in combination to remove the stagnation of liver-Qi, regulate the flow of Qi and relieve pain. Zusanli (ST 36), Neiguan (PC 6) and Zhongwan (CV 12) are applied to pacify the stomach, relieve pain, descend perversive flow of Qi and check vomiting.

(3) **Deficiency of the Stomach with Stagnation of Cold**

Main Manifestations: Dull pain in the epigastrium, which may be relieved by pressure and warmth, regurgitation of thin fluid, general lassitude, thin, white tongue coating, deep, slow pulse.

Treatment

Principle: The Back-(Shu) points and points of the Conception Vessel are selected as the principal points with both acupuncture and moxibustion to warm up the Middle Energizer and dispel cold and regulate the flow of Qi and relieve pain.

Prescription: Zhongwan (CV 12), Qihai (CV 6), Pishu (BL 20), Neiguan (PC 6), Gongsun (SP 4), Zusanli (ST 36).

Explanation: Moxibustion is applied for cold sympton, while reinforcing method for deficiency symptom. Acupuncture and moxibustion at Zhongwan (CV 12) and Zusanli (ST 36) warm the Middle Energizer, dispel cold, regulate the flow of Qi and relieve pain. Neiguan (PC 6) and Gongsun (SP 4), the Confluent Points can not only strengthen the function of spleen, and pacify the stomach, but also regulate the flow of Qi and relieve pain. Indirect moxibustion with ginger on Qihai (CV 6) is most desirable in treatment of chronic gastric disorder due to cold of deficiency, as ginger has the function of dispelling cold, and moxa has the function of removing stasis in meridians and collaterals and relieving pain.

Alternative Treatment
(1) Cupping
Points of back and upper abdomen are selected for this therapy. Cups of large size or middle size can be used, The treatment lasts for 10—15 minutes. The therapy is desirable in treating gastric pain due to cold of deficiency.
(2) Ear Acupuncture
Selection of points: Pt. Stomach, Pt. Shemen, Pt. Brain, Pt. Crus of Helix.
Method: Apply mild stimulation and retain needles for 20 minutes.
(3) Point Injection
Selection of Point: Zusanli (ST 36), Zhongwan (CV 12), Neiguan (PC 6).
Method: 1—2 ml of 1% procaine or 0.5 ml of 1 : 1000 atropine, or liquid of Radix Angelicae Sinensis of flos carthami can be used to inject into the above-mentioned points. Select one or two points for a treatment, 1—2ml for liquid herbal medicine for each point.

9. Vomiting

Vomiting is a common symptom, resulting from the failure of the stomach-Qi to descend, and regurgitation of Qi. Vomiting is divided into vomiting with vomitus and yelling sound, silent vomiting with vomitus and vomiting without vomitus, but yelling sound. Vomiting can be seen in nervous vomiting, acute and chronic gastritis, gastrectasia, cardiopasm, pylorospasm, pylorchesis, and choleystitis in modern medicine.

Etiology and Pathogenesis
(1) Exogenous Invasion into the Stomach
Invasion of exogenous pathogens such as wind, cold, summer-heat, and dampness into the stomach, or the stomach Meridian leads to derangement of stomach-Qi, resulting in vomiting.
(2) Food Retention in the Stomach

Over in take of cold, raw and greasy food and taking putrid and undean food by mistake, the stomach is injured the stomach-Qi can't descend, impairing the down ward movement of stomach-Qi, causing vomiting.

(3) Deficiency of the Spleen and Stomach

Door transformation and transportation, the aetention of food and gastric fluid, phlegm produced in accumulated in the stomach, impairing the dounward movement of stomach-Qi, causing vomiting.

(4) Liver-Qi Attacking the Stomach

Emotional disturbance and stagnation and depression of the liver-Qi harm the stomach, impairing the downward movement of the stomach-Qi, causing vomiting.

Differentiation

(1) Exogenous Invasion into the Stomach

Main Manifestations: Watery regurgitation, or thin fluid, aversion to cold, preference for warmth, loose stool, frequent vomiting, vomiting after intake of food, thirst, preference for cold drinking, constipation, slow or rapid pulse.

(2) Food Retention in the Stomach

Main Manifestations: Acid fermented vomitus, epigastric and abdominal distension, belching, anorexia, thick, greasy tongue coating, slippery and full pulse.

(3) Deficiency of the Spleen and Stomach

Main Manifestations: Discomfort in the stomach, after a big meal or vomiting in severe case, dizziness and nausea after overworking, poor appetite, lassitude, loose stools, pale tongue proper, thin, white tongue coating, thready and forceless pulse.

(4) Liver-Qi Attacking the Stomach

Main Manifestations: Vomiting, acid regurgitation, frequent belching, distending pain in the chest and hypochondriac regions, irritability with an oppressed feeling, thin, sticky tongue coating, string-taut pulse.

Generally speaking, the cause of vomiting comes from stomach, the failure in descending stomach-Qi which leads to abnormal ascending of stomach-Qi results in vomiting.

Treatment

Principle: The Front-(Mu) point and the lower He-(Sea) point of Stomach

Meridian are selected as principal points. Reducing manipulation is used for excess syndrome, while reinforcing manipulation for deficiency syndrome to pacify the stomach, activate the descent of Qi and check vomiting.

Prescription: Zhongwan (CV 12), Neiguan (PC 6), Zusanli (ST 36), Yongquan (KI 1)

Additional Points

Add Dazhui (GV 14) and Zhiyang (GV 9) for exogenous invasion into the stomach. Add Jianli (CV 11) and Tianshu (ST 25) for food retention in the stomach. Add Pishu (BL 20) and Sanyinjiao (SP 6) for deficiency of the spleen and stomach. Add Taichong (LR 3) and Yanglingquan (GB 34) for liver-Qi attacking the stomach.

Explanation: Zhongwan (CV 12), the Front-(Mu) point of the Stomach Meridian, and the converging point of Fu-organs is used to pacify the stomach and regulate the flow of Qi. Zusanli (ST 36), the lower He-(Sea) point of Stomach Meridian is applied to descend the Qi and check vomiting. Neiguan (PC 6), the Luo-(Connecting) point of Pericardium Meridian linking with Triple Energizer Meridian can regulate Triple Energizer, and is an effective point for descending the Qi and checking vomiting, the kidney is regarded as the pass for stomach, Yongquan (KI 1) can cause the stomach-Qi to descend, and is an empirical point for checking vomiting.

Since exogenous pathogenic cold invades the stomach, moxibustion is applied at Zhiyin (BL 67) to warm stomach, dispel cold and check vomiting. Warming the stomach and needling Dazhui (GV 14) with reducing manipulation can activate the descent of Qi and check vomiting. Jianli (CV 11) is used to reinforce the stomach and promote digestion, Tianshu (ST 25) is applied to remove stagnation from the intestine and descend the stomach-Qi. The joint use of these two points have the function of pacifying stomach and checking vomiting. It is a group of effective points for food retention in the stomach. Pishu (BL 20) and Sanyinjiao (SP 6) can invigorate the Qi of the spleen and stomach, and the function of Qi in ascending and descending. Taichong (LR 3) and Yanglingquan (GB 34) can pacify the liver to activate the descent of Qi.

Alternative Treatment

(1) **Ear Acupuncture**

Selection of Points: Pt. Stomach, Pt. Liver, Pt. Spleen, Pt. Shenmen.

Method: Apply mild stimulation, retain needles for 20 minutes.

(2) Topical Application of Drugs

Select Yongquan (KI 1) for vomiting due to the invasion of pathogenic cold. Fructus Euodiae is ground into fine powder and then made into the paste with vinegar or boiling water. Apply the paste on Yongquan (KI 1), this therapy is desirable for vomiting of children's indigestion. Generally, the paste does work after 1—4 hours, vomiting is checked.

10. Hiccup

Hiccup is a symptom referring to the adverse bursting of the Qi from the diaphragm manifested by an involunting short, quick sound in the throat, and the patient unable to stop it by himself. In severe case, it prevents patients from talking, eating, breathing and sleeping. Occasional attack of hiccup suggests a mild case and will stop itself. But if it persists, treatment is required.

In modern medicine, it is commonly seen in spasm of the diaphragm caused by functional disorder of gastroenteric tract, and spasm of the diaphragm due to disease of stomach, intestine, mediastinum and esophagus.

Etiology and Pathogenesis

Hiccup is mostly the result of adversely bursting up of stomach-Qi due to various causes.

(1) Irregular food intake makes Qi obstruction and retention of dryness and heat in the Middle Energizer, the failure of stomach-Qi to descend, and then adverse rise of stomach-Qi leads to hiccup.

(2) Emotional frustration stagnates the liver-Qi, leading to adverse rise of stomach-Qi, then hiccup occurs.

(3) The attack of the stomach by cold, overeating of cold and raw food, or taking medicine of cold nature gives rise to retaining of the stomach-Yang and adverse rise of Qi, leading to hiccup.

(4) The deficiency of the spleen and kidney caused by chronic diseases results in the decline of stomach-Qi, retaining of stomach-Qi and leads to hiccup.

Differentiation

(1) Retention of Food

Main Manifestations: Loud hiccup, epigastric and abdominal distention, anorexia, thick, sticky tongue coating, rolling and forceful pulse.

(2) Stagnation of Qi

Main Manifestations: Continual hiccups, the attack of hiccups is caused by emotional changes or in severe case. Distending pain and chest congestion and hypochondriac pain, thin tongue coating, string-taut and forceful pulse.

(3) Cold in Stomach

Main Manifestations: The Hiccup is alleviated by warmth and aggravated by cold, discomfort and pain in the epigastrium, preference for warmth, thin, white coating, slow pulse.

(4) Decline of Stomach-Qi

Main Manifestations: Hiccup is low and weak, lassitude, emaciation, light tongue proper, enlarged tongue with dental indentations, thready, weak and irregularly intermittent pulse.

Treatment

Principle: Select the points of the stomach meridian and some other related points as the principal points. Reducing manipulation is applied for retention of food and stagnation of Qi while both acupuncture and moxibustion are used for cold in the stomach. Heavy moxibustion is applied for the decline of stomach-Qi to pacify the stomach, facilitate the descent of Qi and check hiccup.

Additional Points

Add Liangmen (ST 21) and Tianshu (ST 25) for food retention. Add Tanzhong (CV 17) and Taichong (LR 3) for stagnation of Qi. Add Shangwan (CV 13) for cold in the stomach. Add Guanyuan (CV 4) for the decline of stomach-Qi.

Explanation: Zhongwan (CV 12), the Front-(Mu) point of stomach is combined with Zusanli (ST 36), the He-(Sea) point of Stomach Meridian to pacify the stomach, subdue the ascending Qi. Geshu (BL 17), the converging point of blood can tonify blood and Qi and check hiccup, Neiguan (PC 6) can regulate the flow of Qi and check hiccup. Taiyuan (LU 9) can descend stomach Qi and stop hiccup; Cuanzhu (BL 2) is an empirical point for hiccup.

Add Liangmen (ST 21) and Tianshu (ST 25) for retention of food to pacify the stomach, clear obstruction from intestine, invigorate the descent of Qi and check hiccup. Add Tanzhong (CV 17) and Taichong (LR 3) for stagnation of Qi to regulate the flow of Qi, pacify the liver and check hiccup.

Add Shangwan (CV 13) with moxibustion for cold in the stomach to warm stomach. Add Guanyuan (CV 4) with moxibustion for the decline of stomach-Qi to reinforce the Yang of the kidney.

Alternative Treatment
(1) Ear Acupuncture
Selection of Points: Ear center or tender points on the root of ear vagus.
Method: Apply mild stimulation, retain needles for 20 minutes.
(2) Cupping Therapy
Selection of Points: Geshu (BL 17), Geguan (BL 46), Ganshu (BL 18), Zhongwan (CV 12), Rugen (ST 18).
Method: Retain the needles for 5-10 minutes, until the skin turns red and blood stasis appears underneath the skin.

11. Diarrhea

Diarrhea refers to increased times of loose stools, and in severe case, watery feces. It is usually due to disorders of the spleen, stomach, large and small intestine. According to the clinical manifestations and duration, it is divided into the acute and chronic diarrhea. The acute type is mostly caused by indigestion, invasion of external cold dampness, which lead to dysfunction in transmission of intestinal contents, or by the attack of damp-heat in summer or autumn. The chronic diarrhea is caused by deficiency of spleen and kidney which leads to failure in transportation and transformation.

Diarrhea may be seen in acute and chronic enteritis, intestinal dysfunction, indigestion, allergic colitis, intestinal tuberculosis and neurogenic diarrhea.

Etiology and Pathogenesis
Acute Diarrhea
(1) **Cold-Dampness**: When the cold-dampness attacks the stomach and the intestines, it impairs the function of the spleen in sending food essence and water upward and that of the stomach in sending the contents downward. The food essence and the waste move downward unseparately to the large intestine, so watery diarrhea occurs.

(2) **Damp-Heat**: When the intestines and the stomach are attacked by damp heat in summer or autumn, the transmitting and transformation function are impaired, and diarrhea appears.

(3) **Retention of Food**: Excessive intake of food, or unclean food, or cold, raw, greasy food, leads to retention of food in Middle Energizer, injuries the stomach and spleen, impairs the stomach and spleen in transportation and transformation, then diarrhea occurs.

Chronic Diarrhea

(1) **Deficiency of Spleen**: When the spleen-Yang is deficient, it leads to impairment of the stomach and spleen in transportation and transformation, the food essence and waste can not be separated, remaining in intestines and stomach, so diarrhea occurs.

(2) **Deficiency of Kidney**: When the kidney-Yang is deficient, it leads to inadequate warming on the spleen and stomach to do digestion, therefore diarrhea is the consequence of dysfunction of the spleen and stomach.

Differentiation
Acute Diarrhea
(1) **Cold—Dampness**
Main Manifestations: Watery diarrhea, or remaining food, abdominal pain and borborygmi, chilliness which responds to warmth, absence of thirst, pale tongue, white tongue coating, deep, slow pulse.

(2) **Damp-Heat**
Main Manifestations: Diarrhea with abdominal pain, yellow, hot and fetid stools, burning sensation in the anus, scanty urine or accompanied by general feeling of fever, thirst, yellow, sticky tongue coating, rolling and rapid pulse.

(3) **Retention of Food**
Main Manifestations: Fetid stools smells like rotten eggs, abdominal pain, borborygmi, abdominal pain relieved after bowel movements, epigastric and abdominal fullness and distention, belching, anorexia, thick, filthy tongue coating, rolling rapid or string-taut pulse.

Treatment
Principle: The points of Stomach Meridian are selected as the principal points. Both acupuncture and indirect moxibustion with ginger are applied for cold dampness to warm the stomach and resolve dampness. Reducing manipulation is used to eliminate heat and dampness. Reducing manipulation is applied for retention of food to regulate the function of the spleen and stomach and remove

333

stagnation.

Prescription: Tianshu (ST 25) Zusanli (ST 36)

Additional Points

Add Zhongwan (CV 12) and Guanyuan (CV 4) for cold-dampness. Add Quchi (LI 11) and Yinlingquan (SP 9) for damp-heat. Add Neiguan (PC 6) and Liangmen (ST 21) for retention of food.

Explanation: Tianshu (ST 25), the Front-(Mu) point of the Large Intestine is applied to regulate the transmitting function of the intestines, Zusanli (ST 36), the He-(Sea) points of Stomach Meridian are used to adjust the flow of the stomach-Qi. Moxibustion to Zhongwan (CV 12) and Guanyuan (CV 4) is to warm the spleen and stomach, dispel cold, resolve dampness and check diarrhea. Quchi (LI 11) is used to eliminate damp-heat from the large intestine, Yin lingquan (SP 9) is used to promote the excretion of urine and remove dampness. The joint use of the two points can eliminate heat from stomach and intestines and treat diarrhea due to damp-heat. Neiguan (PC 6) is needled for retention of food to regulate the function of Qi of Triple Energizer. Liangmen (ST 21) is used to remove stagnation and retention of food. The joint use of the two points can regulate the function of spleen and stomach and remove the stagnation.

Chronic Diarrhea

(1) **Deficiency of the Spleen**

Main Manifestations: Loose stool, undigested food due to severe case, anorexia, epigastric distress after eating, sallow complexion, lassitude, pale tongue, white tongue coating, thready, forceless pulse.

(2) **Deficiency of Kidney**

Main Manifestations: Diarrhea usually occurs at dawn, abdominal pain and borborygmi may be relieved after bowel movement, symptoms aggravated by cold, abdominal distension sometimes, cold lower limbs, pale tongue, white tongue coating, deep, forceless pulse.

Treatment

Principle: The points of Stomach, Spleen Meridians, Conception and Governor Vessels are selected as principal points with the reinforcing manipulation and moxibustion to warm and reinforce the kidney-Yang, the function of intestines and stop diarrhea.

Prescription: Zhongwan (CV 12), Tianshu (ST 25), Guanyuan (CV 4), Zusanli (ST 36), Diji (SP 8).

Additional Points

Pishu (BL 20) and Taibai (SP 3) are applied for deficiency of spleen, Shenshu (BL 23) and Taixi (KI 3) for deficiency of spleen, Shenshu (BL 23) and Taixi (KI 3) for deficiency of kidney.

Explanation: Zhongwan (CV 12), the converging point of Fu-organs and the Front-(Mu)point of stomach can invigorate the stomach, regulate the function of intestines and check diarrhea. Tianshu (St 25), the Front-(Mu) point of large intestine can regulate the functions of intestines and check diarrhea. Guanyuan (CV 4) can warm kidney, Zusanli (St 36) invigorates the stomach. Diji (SP 8) can invigorate the spleen. The joint use of these three points can warm the stomach and spleen, dispel cold and check diarrhea. Moxibustion to Pishu (BL 20) and Taibai (SP 3) is applied for deficiency of spleen-Yang to invigorate the spleen and Yang. Add Shenshu (BL 23) and Taixi (KI 3) for deficiency of kidney to warm the kidney and check diarrhea.

Alternative Treatment

(1). Ear Acupuncture

Selection of Points: Pt. Large Intestine, Pt. Stomach.

Method: Needling with mild stimulation, retain needles for 20 minutes.

(2) Cupping Therapy

Selection of Points: Tianshu (St 25), Guanyuan (CV 4), Dachangshu (BL 25), Xiaochangshu (BL 27).

Method: Retain cups for 10 minutes, treatment is given twice a day.

12. Constipation

Constipation is a condition of dry compacted feces in the large intestine, difficulty and failure in defecating for more than two days. It is mainly caused by the impaired transmitting function of the large intestine and also related to the function of the spleen, stomach and kidney. Constipation can be divided into two types: deficiency and excess. Habitual constipation in modern medicine can be treated according to deficiency or excess.

Etiology and Pathogenesis

1. Execss Condition

(1) **Constitutional Excess of Yang and Food Exaggeration**: Constitutional Yang preponderance, and indulgence in spicy and greasy food may lead to accumulation of heat in the stomach and intestines, consumption of the body fluid which leads to dryness in intestines as well as dry stools.

(2) **Emotional Factors**: Anxiety and depression may cause stagnation of Qi, impairing the function of the large intestine in transmitting. As a result, the wastes are retained inside and unable to move downward, causing the constipation.

2. Deficiency Condition

(1) **Deficiency of Qi and Blood**: It may happen after an illness, or delivery, or in the aged people, which may lead to deficiency of Qi and blood. Qi deficiency results in weakness of the large intestine in transmission. While blood deficiency gives rise to shortage of body fluid, then the large intestine can no longer be moistened, which causes constipation.

(2) **Cold Deficiency of the Lower Energizer**

Deficiency of Yang Qi in the Lower Energizer leads to congealment of interiorying cold which obstructs the Qi flow of large intestine, resulting in constipation.

Differentiation

(1) **Excess Condition**

Main Manifestations: Difficult passage of dry, hard stool, defecation every three to five days, or even longer. General fever, thirst, foul breath, rapid pulse, yellow dry tongue coating or fullness and distending pain in the abdomen and hypochondria regions, frequent belching, loss of appetite, thin, sticky tongue coating, string-taut pulse.

(2) **Deficiency Condition**

Main Manifestations: Difficult passage of dry stools, pale complexion and lips, dizziness and palpitation, lassitude, shortness of breath, pale tongue, thin tongue coating, thready and weak pulse, or abdominal pain, preference for warmth and aversion to cold, pale tongue, white and moist tongue coating, deep, slow pulse.

Treatment

Principle: Select the Back-(Shu) and Front-(Mu) points of Large Intestine Meridian and the points of Triple Energizer and Kidney Meridians as principal points. For excess condition, the reducing manipulation is applied to remove the heat and Qi stagnancy and moisten the intestine, while for deficiency condition, the reinforcing manipulation is used to reinforce Qi and blood and moisten the intestines. Constipation due to cold can be relieved by moxibustion to warm the Lower Energizer for defecation.

Prescription: Dachangshu (BL 25), Tianshu (ST 25), Zhigou (TE 6), Zhaohai (KI 6), Shuidao (ST 28).

Additional Points

Add Quchi (LI 11), Hegu (LI 4) for accumulation of heat; Zhongwan (CV 12), Taichong (LR 3) for stagnation of Qi, Pishu (BL 20), Weishu (BL 21), Zusanli (ST 36) for deficiency of Qi and blood, Moxibustion to Shenque (CV 8) and Qihai (CV 6) is applied for congealment of cold.

Explanation: The causes of constipation are various, but they are common in impairing the transportation of the large intestine, because of the failure of body liquid to moisten the large intestine. Therefore, Dachangshu (BL 25), the back-(Shu) point of the large intestine, Tianshu (ST 25), the Front-(Mu) point of large intestine are used to promote the flow of Qi in the large intestine, the transportation can be regained when the Qi of the Fu-organ flows smoothly, then constipation can be relieved, Zhigou (TE 6), the fire point of Triple Energizer can eliminate fire from Triple Energizer to promote bowel motions. Zhaohai (KI 6) can nourish kidney to moisten the intestines. Quchi (KI 11) and Hegu (LI 4) can reduce the heat from the large intestine to promote bowel motions. Zhongwan (CV 12) can remove stagnation of Triple Energizer. Taichong (LR 3) is to soothe the liver-Qi in order to remove the stagnation of intestine. Reinforcing to Pishu (BL 20), Weishu (BL 21) and Zusanli (ST 36) is able to reinforce Qi in the spleen and stomach. Once the spleen and stomach-Qi is vigorous, Qi and blood can be produced as a natural consequence, so this is the approach of treating the main cause of constipation in deficiency conditions. Moxibustion to Shenque (CV 8) and Qihai (CV 6) is offered to regulate the flow of Qi and loosen the bowels. Zushuidao (EX) is an empirical point for constipation.

Alternative Treatment

Ear Acupuncture

Selection of Points: Pt. Lower Portion of Rectum, Pt. Large Intestine, Pt. Brain.

Method: Rotate the needles with moderate or strong stimulation. Retain the needles for 20—30 minutes.

Remarks

Acupuncture has good effect in treating constipation. If no effect after several treatments, other therapies should be employed. Meanwhile, further examination should be taken to find out the cause of disease and avoid missing treatment. In daily life, the patient should keep on physical exercise, take more vegetables, develop a habit of regular bowel movement.

13. Abdominal Distention

Abdominal distention refers to distention and fullness which occur in both the upper and lower abdomen. The stomach and spleen are located in the upper abdomen, while the small and large intestines are in the lower. Dysfunctions of these four organs may lead to abdominal distention. It may be seen in gastroptosis, acute gastrectasis, enteroparalysis, intestinal obstruction, and functional disorder of gastrointestinal tract in modern medicine.

Etiology and Pathogenesis

(1) Irregular or excessive food intake impairs the stomach and intestines, causing dysfunction of transportation and transformation, thus the retained food is stagnated and blocks the flow of Qi, causing abdominal distention.

(2) Because of the weakened function of the spleen and stomach or ageing, long illness, and general debility, the spleen and stomach fail in their transporting functions, so the circulation of Qi in the stomach and intestines is impaired, resulting in abdominal distention.

(3) Abdominal operations may disturb the circulation of Qi in stomach and intestines, leading to abdominal distention.

Differentiation

(1) **Excess Condition**

Main Manifestations: Distention and fullness in the abdomen which are aggravated by pressing, abdominal pain in severe case, belching, foul breath, dark yellow urine, constipation, occasional fever, vomiting, yellow, thick tongue coating, rolling, rapid and forceful pulse.

(2)Deficiency Condition

Main Manifestations: Abdominal distention, relieved by pressing, worsens and lessens from time to time, borborygmi, loose stools, lose of appetite, lassitude, listlessness, clear urine, pale tongue, white tongue coating, weak pulse.

Treatment

Principle: The points of Spleen, Stomach Meridians and Conception Vessel are selected as principal points. The excess condition is treated by the reducing manipulation to regulate the flow of Qi in Fu-organs while the deficiency condition is treated by the reinforcing or combined with moxibustion to invigorate the stomach and spleen and the circulation of Qi to relieve the distention.

Prescription: Gongsun (SP 4), Zhongwan (CV 12), Tianshu (ST 25), Qihai (CV 6), Zusanli (ST 36).

Additional Points

Add Shangqiu (SP 5) and Lidui (ST 45) for excess condition, Guanyuan (CV 4), Dadu (SP 2) and Jiexi (ST 41) for deficiency condition.

Explanation: Gongsun (SP 4), the Lou-(Connecting) point of Spleen Meridian can invigorate the function of the spleen and stomach; Zhongwan (CV 12), the converging point of Fu-organs can pacify stomach-Qi; Tianshu (ST 25), the Front-(Mu) point of large intestine may regulate the function of large intestine and remove the stagnation. Qihai (CV 6) can regulate the flow of Qi and relieve the distention; Zusanli (ST 36) removes the stagnation in stomach and intestines to descend stomach-Qi. The joint use of the five points can reinforce the spleen and stomach, promote the Qi circulation of the gastrointestines, remove the stagnation, regulate the flow of Qi and pacify stomach. Add Shangqiu (SP 5) and Lidui (ST 45) for excess condition to reduce the Qi of spleen and stomach based on the principle of reducing the son due to excess symptom. Add Dadu (SP 2) and Jiexi (ST 41) for deficiency condition to invigorate the function of spleen and stomach based on the principle of reinforcing mother due to deficiency symptom.

14. Dysentery

Dysentery is characterized by abdominal pain, tenesmus and frequent bowel movement with blood and mucus in stool. It is a common epidemic disease in summer and autumn. It is called "damp heat dysentery" in *Internal Classic*: It is called "Chanpi" meaning dysentery in *Synopsis of Prescription of the Golden Chamber*; It is called "red-white dysentery", "bloody dysentery", "purulent and bloody dysentery", or "heat dysentery" in *General Treatise on the Etiology and Symptomology of Diseases*. And it is known as "persistent dysentery" if it lasts for a long time and "intermittent dysentery" if it comes on and off. Clinically, it is divided into damp-heat dysentery, damp-cold dysentery, fasting dysentery, and intermittent dysentery. This disease is often due to the invasion by the epidemic damp heat and internal injury by intake of raw, cold and unclean food, which obstructs and damages the stomach and intestines. It includes acute, chronic bacillary dysentery, and amebic dysentery in modern medicine.

Etiology and Pathogenesis

(1) Invasion of Summer Heat Dampness

The summer epidemic heat dampness invades the stomach and intestines, impeding the flow of their Qi and blood. Pus and blood are formed from the stagnated Qi and blood in struggling against heat dampness, and hence occurs dysentery. In case, dampness is preponderant to heat, white dysentery results, in case, heat preponderant to dampness, red dysentery appears, and in case both dampness and heat are excessive, red-white dysentery occurs.

(2) Preference for Fatty and Sweet Food

Internal accumulation of damp-heat plus irregular diet, or intake of unclean food, leads to stagnation of Qi and blood in the Fu-organs, which turns into pus and blood in the stools and results in dysentery.

(3) Excessive Intake of Raw, Cold Food

Internal accumulation of cold dampness plus excessive intakes of raw, cold, unclean food impedes the stomach and intestines. The stagnated Qi injures the blood and results in cold-damp dysentery.

Although the above-mentioned etiological factors can be classified into the exogenous pathogenic factors and food intake, the two are usually mutually affected.

The disease is in the intestine, but closely related to the stomach. If the epidemic toxic and damp heat attack the stomach, which fails to receive food, fasting dysentery occurs. If dysentery lasts longer, the body resistance is weaker, persistent or intermittent dysentery appears.

Differentiation

(1) Damp-Heat Dysentery

Main Manifestations: Abdominal pain, tenesmus and frequent passage with pus and blood in stool, burning sensation of the anus, scanty and yellow urine, chills, fever, restlessness, thirst, yellow, sticky tongue coating, rolling, rapid or soft, rapid pulse.

(2) Cold-Damp Dysentery

Main Manifestation: White mucus in stools, preference for warmth and aversion to cold, lingering abdominal pain, fullness in the chest and epigastrium, tastelessness in the mouth, absence of thirst, white, sticky tongue coating, deep, slow pulse.

(3) Fasting Dysentery

Main Manifestations: Frequent passage with blood and pus, loss of appetite, nausea, vomiting, yellow, sticky tongue coating, soft, rapid pulse.

(4) Intermittent Dysentery

Main Manifestations: Dysentery occurring on and off, difficult to cure, lassitude, somnolence, anorexia, pale tongue, sticky tongue coating, soft pulse.

Treatment

Principle: The points of Large Intestine Meridian as well as the Front-(Mu) point and Lower He-(Sea) point of the Large Intestine are selected as the principal points to remove the stagnation from the intestines. Reducing manipulation is used for the damp-heat dysentery, both acupuncture and moxibustion are used for the cold-damp dysentery, and acupuncture and moxibustion with both reinforcing and reducing manipulations are used for the persistent dysentery.

Prescription: Tianshu(ST 25), Shangjuxu (ST 37).

Add Quchi (LI 11) and Hegu (LI 4) for damp-heat dysentery. Add Zhongwan (CV 12), Yinlingquan (SP 9), moxibustion to Qihai (CV 6) for damp-cold dysentery. Add Zhongwan (CV 12) and Neiguan (PC 6) for lasting dysentery. Add Pishu (BL 20), Weishu (BL 21), Guanyuan (CV 4) and Zusanli (ST 36) for intermittent dysentery.

Additional Points

Add Dazhui (GV 14) for fever; add Baihui (GV 20) with moxibustion and Changqiang (GV 1) with needling for prolapse of rectum.

Explanation: It is recorded in Internal Classics that the He-(Sea) points are applied for the disease of the Fu-organs, dysentery is in the Large Intestine, therefore, Tianshu (ST 25), the Front-(Mu) point of the Large Intestine, and Shangjuxu (ST 37), the Lower He-(Sea) point of the large intestine are selected as the principal points to remove the stagnation of Qi in the large intestine, regulate the flow of Qi and dampness will be resolved. Quchi (LI 11) and Hegu (LI 4) may dispel the damp-heat from the stomach and intestines to check dysentery. Moxibustion to Zhongwan (CV 12) and Qihai (CV 6) is applied to warm the spleen and stomach, regulate the flow of Qi. Yinlingquan (SP 9) is needled to strengthen the spleen function to resolve dampness. The joint use of these three points can treat cold-damp dysentery. For fasting dysentery, Zhongwan (CV 12) is used to improve digestion and appetite. Neiguan (PC 6) is used to remove stagnation from Triple Energizer. The two points can pacify stomach-Qi to eliminate dampness. Moxibustion to Pishu (BL 20) and Weishu (BL 21), Zusanli (ST 36) with needling can warm the spleen and stomach, and eliminate the intestinal stagnation. Guanyuan (CV 4), the Front-(Mu) point of the small intestine is applied to separate the food essence from the waste, reinforce Qi and activate Yang.

Alternative Treatment
(1) **Ear Acupuncture**
Selection of Points: Pt. Large Intestine, Pt. Small Intestine, Pt. Lower Portion of Rectum.
Method: Needle points with mild stimulation, retain the needles for 20 minutes.
(2) **Point Injection**
Selection of Points: Tianshu (ST 25), Zusanli (ST 36)
Method: 0.5 ml of 10% glucose or Vitamin B1 is injected into each point. Injection is given once a day.

15. Prolapse Ani
Prolapse ani refers to the condition in which the lower portion of the rectum or rectum mucosa lapses out of the anus and is called rectum prolapse in modern medicine.

Etiology and Pathogenesis
This disease is mostly caused by long-standing diarrhea or dysentery, constitutional weakness after severe diseases, deficiency of the primary Qi, sinking of

the spleen and stomach Qi and disability of restraining; or by persistent constipation, leading to anus exstrophy and failure in controlling.

Differentiation
Main Manifestations: The onset is slow. It stars with distending and draggling sensation of rectum during defecation, returning to normal after the bowel movement. If it is sustained without proper treatment, recurrence may happen by overstrain and the prolapsed rectum fails to return spontaneously without the aid of the hand, or accompanying with lassitude, weakness of limbs, shortness of breath, palpitation, sallow complexion, the pale tongue with white coating, thready and feeble pulse.

Treatment
Principle: The points of Governor Vessel, Bladder and Stomach Meridians are selected as the principal points with the reinforcing manipulation and moxibustion.

Prescription: Baihui (GV 20), Changqiang (GV 1), Dachangshu (BL 25) and Chengshan (BL 57).

Explanation: Large Intestine connects with anus, reinforcing Dachangshu (BL 25) can replenish the Qi of the large intestine. Changqiang (GV 1), a point of the collateral of Governor Vessel, located near the anus, needle this point to strengthen the anus'ability of restraining. Chengshan (BL 57), the point of Bladder Meridian, its divergent meridian enters the anus and its muscle region connects with the buttock, combining with Changqiang (GV 1) to strengthen the rectum's ability of restraining. Baihui (GV 20) located on the top of head, moxibustion to Baihui (GV 20) can invigorate Yang Qi and improve the elevating and contracting function. Combination of these points can elevate when there is subsidence and make rectum restore to normal state.

Alternative Treatment
Ear Acupuncture
Selection of Points: Pt. the Lower Portion of Rectum, Pt. Subcortex. Pt. Shenmen.

Method: Needle the points of both ears with moderate stimulation, retain the needles for 30 minutes. Treatment is given once daily.

16. Jaundice

Jaundice is mainly manifested by yellow discoloration of the sclera, skin and urine. The yellow sclera is considered as the main sign in the clinic. Clinically, it is divided into Yang jaundice and Yin jaundice according to its nature. It results from the dampness in the spleen and heat in the stomach, which lead to abnormal flooding of the bile to the skin and eyes.

This disease may commonly be seen in acute icteric hepatitis, obstructive jaundice and hemolytic jaundice in modern medicine.

Etiology and Pathogenesis

(1) The seasonal and epidemic pathogenic factors accumulate in the spleen and stomach, leading to internal formation and collection of damp-heat. The liver and gallbladder are steamed by the heat in the spleen and stomach, leading to overflow of the bile to the skin, thus jaundice appears.

(2) Irregular diet injures the spleen and stomach, disturbs transportation and transformation which causes internal formation of dampness, stagnation of which generates heat. Damp heat stains the skin, then jaundice appears.

(3) Overstrain or general weakness of the spleen-Qi may give rise to hypoactivity of the Yang in the Middle Energizer, leading to failure in transportation and transformation and stagnation of cold dampness, thus Yin jaundice results. As said in *A Guide to the Clinic Treatment* For "the cause of Yin jaundice if the dampness is produced from cold water. If the spleen Yang fails to resolve the dampness, the normal distribution of bile is impaired, affecting the spleen, soaking into the muscles and spreading to the skin which turns yellow as if it were smoked."

(4) Yin Jaundice can result from an improperly treated Yang jaundice which leads to injury of the Yang Qi, hypoactivity of the spleen-Yang, and internal accumulation of cold dampness.

Differentiation

(1) **Yang Jaundice**

Main Manifestations: Lustrous yellow skin and sclera, fever, thirst, scanty dark yellow urine, heaviness of the body, abdominal distention, chest congestion, nausea, yellow, sticky tongue coating, string-taut, rapid pulse.

Treatment

Principle: The points of Gallbladder, Spleen Meridians and Governor Vessel are selected as principal points. Reducing manipulation is applied to regulate the flow of Qi in the liver and gallbladder and remove heat and dampness.

Prescription: Zhiyang (GV 9), Danshu (BL 19), Yanglingquan (GB 34), Yinlingquan (SP 9), Taichong (LR 3).

Additional Points

Add Dazhui (GV 14) and Quchi (LI 11) for severe heat, Zusanli (ST 36) and Sanyinjiao (SP 6) for severe dampness, Zhigou (TE 6) for constipation.

Explanation: Zhiyang (GV 9), the spot where the Qi of Governor Vessel infuses, may activate the Qi of Governor Vessel. Reducing manipulation applied to Zhiyang (GV 9) can reduce heat, and is an important point to treat jaundice. Danshu (BL 19), the Back-(Shu) point of gallbladder, Yanglingquan (GB 34), the lower He-(Sea) point of the gallbladder, Taichong (LR 3), the Yuan-(Primary) point of the liver. Reducing method applied to these three points can regulate the flow of Qi in the liver and gallbladder. Yinlingquan (SP 9), the He-(Sea) point of Spleen Meridian, reducing manipulation applied to Yinlingquan (SP 9) can eliminate heat and dampness. The joint use of the above points may eliminate heat, dispel dampness, restore the normal bile excretion, so that jaundice can be relieved. Add Dazhui (GV 14) and Quchi (LI 11) to reduce severe heat; Zusanli (ST 36), Sanyinjiao (SP 6) to invigorate the spleen and pacify stomach to dispel severe dampness; Zhigou (TE 6) for constipation to reduce heat from the Triple Energizer and promote bowel movement.

(2) Yin Jaundice

Main Manifestations: Sallow skin, heaviness of the body, weakness, lose of appetite, epigastric stuffiness, lassitude, aversion to cold, absence of thirst, pale tongue, thick white tongue coating, deep and slow pulse.

Treatment

Principle: The points of Spleen and Stomach Meridians are selected as the principal points. Reducing manipulation and moxibustion are applied to strengthen the spleen, soothe liver and regulate the flow of Qi in gallbladder, and warm out the cold dampness.

Prescription: Pishu (BL 20), Danshu (BL 19), Zusanli (ST 36), Sanyinjiao (SP 6), Yinlingquan (SP 9).

Additional Points

Add Guanyuan (CV 4) and Mingmen (GV 4) for general lassitude; Qihai (CV 6) for distention and stuffiness in epigastric and abdominal regions; Tianshu (ST 25) for loose stools; Pigen (Ex-B 4) for mass.

Explanation: Yin jaundice is caused by cold-dampness, mainly by cold deficiency of the spleen and stomach. Moxibustion to Pishu (BL 20), Zusanli (ST 36), Sanyinjiao (SP 6), can reinforce the spleen and stomach by warming out the cold-dampness. Needling Danshu (BL 19) and Yanglingquan (GB 34), the combination of the Back-(Shu) point and the He-(Sea) point may promote bile excretion and relieve jaundice. Moxibustion to Guanyuan (CV 4) and Mingmen (GV 4) for the patient with lassitude due to deficiency of primary Qi to reinforce the primary Qi. Needle Qihai (CV 6) for abdominal distention to regulate the flow of Qi and relieve distention. Moxibustion to Tianshu (ST 25) may check diarrhea. Moxibustion applied to Pigen (EX-B 4) for mass may soften and resolve hard lumps.

Alternative Treatment
(1) Ear Acupuncture
Selection of Points: Pt. Gallbladder. Pt. Liver. Pt. Spleen, Pt. Stomach, Pt. the Root of Ear Vagus, Pt. Diaphragm.
Method: Apply filiform needles to two or three points with moderate stimulation once daily. Ten treatments make a course.
(2) Point Injection
Selection of Points: Ganshu (BL 18), Danshu (BL 19), Qimen (LR 14), Riyue (GB 24), Zhongdu (LR 6).
Medication: Radix Isatidis injection, Vitamin B1 injection.
Method: Select two or three points 0.5—1 ml liquid medicine is injected into each point once daily. Ten treatments constitute a course.

17. Edema
Edema refers to retention of fluid in the body, resulting in the puffiness of the head, face, eyelids, limbs, abdomen, back and even the general body. Edema is the manifestation of the functional derangement of Qi in the whole body and related with lung, spleen, kidney, Triple Energizer. Clinically, edema is divided into Yang edema and Yin edema. It may be seen in nephritis. cor-pulmonale, liver cirrhosis malnutrition, endocrinal disorder in modern medicine.

Etiology and Pathogenesis

(1) Invasion of the wind upon the lung causes dysfunction of the lung in dispersion which fails to regulate the water passage and leads to the overflow of water to the superficial part of the body, and thus edema appears.

(2) Improper diet and overstrain injury the spleen, which fails to control transporting and transforming fluid, internal retention of damp-water appears, leading to the overflow of water to the superficial part of the body, thus edema results.

(3) Indulgent sexual intercourse damages the kidney-Qi which fails to control water metabolism. Retention of water follows and results in the overflow of water to the superficial part of the body and edema appears.

Differentiation
(1) Yang Edema

Main Manifestations: Abrupt onset of edema with puffy face and eyelids, anasarca, severe edema above the lumbus, swelling of the scrotum, depression and irritability, shortness of breath, cold body without sweating, white, greasy tongue coating, superficial, and string-taut pulse, or sore throat, yellow, thin tongue coating, superficial, rapid pulse.

Treatment

Principle: The points of Lung and Spleen Meridians are selected as the principal points. Even reinforcing and reducing manipulation are applied to clear the lung, relieve the exterior symptoms and remove the retained fluid. After the exterior symptoms are relieved, give treatment on basis of the method for Yin edema.

Prescription: Lieque (LU 7), Hegu (LI 4), Pianli (LI 6), Yinlingquan (SP 9), Weiyang (BL 39).

Explanation: Yang edema is caused by failure in the descent of lung Qi, retention of water. Edema above the lumbus should be treated by diaphoresis, therefore Lieque (LU 7) and Hegu (LI 4) are used to cause sweating, relieve the muscles and skin, disperse the lung, while edema below the lumbus should be treated by diuresis. Pianli (LI 6) and Yinlingquan (SP 9) are applied to promote diuresis to relieve edema, Weiyang (BL 39), the lower He-(Sea) point of Triple Energizer is able to regulate the Qi activity of the Triple Energizer and subdue edema.

(2) Yin Edema

Main Manifestations: Slow onset of edema, at first on the pedis dorsum and then over the whole body, especially remarkable below the lumbar region. Depressions appearing upon hand pressing rebound slowly, sallow complexion, short urine, accompanied with epigastric fullness, abdominal distention, loss of appetite, loose stools, lassitude, weak limbs, sticky tongue coating, thready, slow pulse, or accompanied with lumbar pain and weakness of legs, aversion to cold, cold limbs, lassitude, pale tongue with white coating, deep, thready pulse.

Treatment

Principle: The points of Spleen and Kidney Meridians are selected as the principal points. Reinforcing manipulation in combination with moxibustion is applied to warm the spleen and kidney, remove the retained fluid and edema.

Prescription: Pishu (BL 20), Shenshu (BL 23), Shuifen (CV 9), Fuliu (KI 7), Guanyuan (CV 4), Sanyinjiao (SP 6).

Explanation: Yin edema is caused by deficiency of kidney-Yang and spleen-Yang. Acupuncture and moxibustion to Pishu (BL 20), Shenshu (BL 23) and Fuliu (KI 7) may warm the primary Yang of the spleen and kidney and promote the Qi activity of Triple Energizer. Moxibustion to Shuifen (CV 9) may remove the retained fluid and edema. Moxibustion to Guanyuan (CV 4) may reinforce the primary Qi to warm the lower energizer. Reinforcing manipulation applied to Sanyinjiao (SP 6) can strengthen the spleen, remove dampness and be diuretic.

Alternative Treatment

Ear Acupuncture

Selection of Points: Pt. Lung, Pt. Spleen, Pt. Kidney, Pt. Triple Energizer, Pt. Bladder, Pt. Subcortex.

Method: Apply filiform needles with moderate stimulation at two or three points each time, once every other day. Embedding of ear seeds is also applicable.

18. Enuresis

Enuresis refers involuntary discharge of urine during sleep at night. It is mostly seen in children over the age of three years and occasionally in adults. It is mainly caused by deficiency of kidney-Qi with disability of the bladder to restrain the urine discharge.

Etiology and Pathogenesis

If the kidney-Qi is insufficient, it will be unable to maintain the function of the bladder in restraining the urination, and thus occurs enuresis.

Differentiation

Main Manifestations: Involuntary micturition during sleep with dreams, or the victim is not aware of it until enuresis occurs, once in several nights in mild cases, or several times at night in severe cases. If this condition prolongs for a long time, then there appear sallow complexion, loss of appetite, weakness of limbs, pale tongue, white coating, thready, weak, slow pulse.

Treatment

Principle: The Back-(Shu) and Front-(Mu) points of the Kidney and Bladder are selected as the principal points, with reinforcing or moxibustion to strengthen the kidney and Qi, then improve the function of bladder.

Prescription

Shenshu (BL 23), Pangguangshu (BL 28), Zhongji (CV 3), Sanyinjiao (SP 6), Dadun (LR 1).

Additional Points

Add Shenmen (HT 7) for enuresis with dreams, Pishu (BL 20) and Zusanli (ST 36) for loss of appetite.

Explanation: The kidney has relation to the bladder as interior to exterior. Select the Back-(Shu) points of the kidney and bladder and Zhongji (CV 3), the Front-(Mu) point of the bladder. Combined use of the above three points can strengthen the kidney and Qi. Sanyinjiao (SP 6) is added to adjust the Qi of the Liver, Spleen and Kidney Meridians to strengthen the spleen, the liver and the kidney. Moxibustion to Dadun (LR 1), the Jing-(Well) point of the Liver Meridian can warm meridians and strengthen the Yang-source energy.

Alternative Treatment

Ear Acupuncture

Selection of Points: Kidney, Urinary Bladder, Subcortes, Urethra.

Methad: Apply filiform needles at two to three points with mild stimulation and retain the needles for 20 minute.

Embedding of ear seeds in also applicable.

Remarks

Acupuncture provides satisfactory effect to enuresis due to delayed maturation of nervous system. As for enuresis caused by organic diseases, such as deformity of urinary tract, cryptorachischisis, organic cerebral diseases and oxyuriasis, the treatment should be aimed to the primary disease.

19. Hesitancy and Obstruction

Hesitancy and obstruction refer to difficult urination, distending pain in the lower abdomen and even blockage of urine in severe case. The mild case refers to difficulty in urination and dripping of urine; while the severe cause to failure in urination with distention and feeling of urgency. In both mild and severe cases the lesion is at the bladder, and their mechanisms can be transformed each other, so it is called "Long Bi" in Chinese as a combination of them.

This disease results from dysfunction of Qi in the bladder. As said in *Internal Classics* "Hindrance of bladder is called "Long" (Hesitancy)". It is seen in retention of urine of various causes.

Etiology and Pathogenesis

(1) **Heat Accumulation in the Bladder**: Heat accumulation in the Lower-Energizer and bladder or heat of the kidney shifts to the bladder which impedes the Qi flow and leads to retention of urine.

(2) **Decline of Mingmen Fire**: The kidney and bladder are related interiorly and exteriorly. The Qi function of the bladder depends on the warming function of the kidney-Yang. In case of weakness of the kidney-Yang and decline of Mingmen fire, the bladder may be too weak to discharge urine.

(3) **External Injury**: Traumatic injury or surgical operation, hindering the Qi of meridians or damaging the bladder, causes retention of urine.

Differentiation

(1) **Heat Accumulation in the Bladder**

Main Manifestations: Dripping urinary discharge, heat pain in the urinary track, scanty yellow urine, or retention of urine, distension and fullness of the lower abdomen, thirst but without desire to drink, red tongue with yellow coating, rapid pulse.

Treatment

Principle: The Back-(Shu) Points and Front-(Mu) points of Bladder Meridian are selected as the principal points. Reducing manipulation is applied to remove heat and promote diuresis.

Prescription: Pangguangshu (BL 28), Zhongji (CV3), Sanyinjiao (SP6), Weiyang (BL 39), Shugu (BL 65).

Explaination: Heat accumulation in the bladder leads to the retention of urine. Pangguangshu (BL 28) and Zhongji (CV 3) known as the combination of Back-(Shu) and Front-(Mu) Points are used to clear up the retention of heat in the bladder and adjust the Qi function of bladder. Sanyinjiao (SP 6) is used to strengthen the function of spleen and eliminate the dampness, clear up heat and promote diuresis, Weiyang (BL 39), the lower He-(Sea) point of Triple Energizer promotes the Qi function of Triple Energizer, eliminates the damp-heat in the Lower-Energizer, Shugu (BL 65), the Back-(Shu) point of Bladder Meridian, pertaining to wood, can inhibit the son when excess syndrome occurs.

(2) **Decline of Mingmen Fire**

Main Manifestations: Dribbling urination, attenuating in strength of the urine discharge, distension and fullness in the lower abdomen, pallor, cold limbs, pale tongue, deep, thready pulse weak at the Chi region.

Treatment

Principle: The points of Governor Vessel, Conception Vessels and Bladder Meridian are selected as the principal points. Reinforcing manipulation or moxibustion is applied to warm the kidney-Yang and promote the Qi function of the bladder.

Prescription: Mingmen (GV 4), Shenshu (BL 23), Guanyuan (CV 4), Yingu (KI 10), Sanyinjiao (SP 6).

Explanation: In case of the decline of Mingmen fire and deficiency of the kidney-Qi, needle Mingmen (GV 4), Shenshu (BL 23), and Yingu (KI 10) to warm kidney-Yang and reinforce Mingmen fire. Guanyuan (CV 4) is used to warm the Lower Energizer and invigorate the Qi function of bladder. Sanyinjiao (SP 6) is used to promote diuresis and remove retention of urine.

(3) **External Injury**

Main Manifestations: Retention of urine, distension and pain in the lower abdomen.

Treatment

Principle: The Front-(Mu) point of Bladder and points of Kidney and Spleen Meridians are selected as the principal points. Even reinforcing and reducing manipulation is applied to promote the circulation of the Qi in the meridian and restore the function of the bladder.

Prescription: Liniaoxue (EX-CA), point for promoting diuresis. Zhongji (CV 3), Sanyinjiao (SP 6), Zhaohai (KI 6).

Explanation: Linjaoxue (EX) is located in the bladder, press this point with finger to promote the function of bladder and diuresis Zhongji (CV 3), the Front-(Mu) point of the bladder in combination with Sanyinjiao (SP 6) is needled to improve the function of the bladder, Zhaohai (KI 6) is needled to promote the kidney-Qi and diruesis. The joint use of these above points can promote Qi circulation in the meridian, the function of the bladder and diuresis.

Alternative Treatment

(1) **Ear Acupuncture**

Selection of Points: Pt Bladder, Pt Kidney, Pt Urethra, Pt Triple Energizer.

Method: Apply filiform needles at one to two points each time with moderate stimulation and retain the needles for 40—60 minutes. Rotate the needles once every ten to fifteen minutes.

(2) **Point Injection**

Selection of Points: Zusanli (ST 36), Guangyuan (CV 4), Sanyinjiao (SP 6).

Method: 0.2—0.3ml Vitamin B1 injection is injected into each point.

(3) **Electric Stimulation**

Selection of Points: Shuidao (ST 28).

Method: Apply filiform needle at Shuidao (ST 28) horizontally towards Qugu (CV 2) for two to three cun distance, this is then followed by electric stimulation for 15—30 minutes.

(4) **Topical Application of Drugs**

1) Cut spring onion into small pieces, mash them into paste, then put the paste at Shenque (CV 8). In 24 to 48 hours, urinary discharge will become normal. At the beginning, dripping urine appears, then it is turning normal gradually.

2) Two garlics and two mole crickets are mashed and wrapped in gauze, then appliy them at Shenque (CV 8).

20. Urination Disturbance

Urination disturbance includes frequency of urination, painful urination, and incontinence of urination, resulting mainly from accumulation of heat in the bladder, and sometimes also from emotional factors and deficiency of the kidney.

According to the clinic manifestations, urination disturbance is divided into five kinds, i. e. dysuria caused by Qi dysfunction, dysuria caused by calculi, painful urination with blood, dysuria with milky urine, and dysuria caused by overstrain.

This disease is mainly seen in infection of urinary system, and stone in the urinary tract.

Etiology and Pathogenesis

(1)**Dysuria Caused by Calculi**: Eating too much fatty or sweet food or drinking too much alcohol, leads to accumulation of damp heat in the lower energizer, where the urine is precipitated into calculi, which may be either small as gravel or large as stones, staying in the kidney, or the bladder or the urethra, so it is called dysuria caused by calculi.

(2)**Painful Urination with Blood**: In case, the damp heat accumulates in the bladder, or the heat fire shifts to the bladder, the heat injures the blood vessels, and forces the blood to extravagate, then painful urination with blood results.

(3)**Dysuria with Milky Urine**: If the damp heat accumulates in the lower energizer causing failure in the Qi function, impairing the control of the flow of the chylous fluid, viscous urine like milky urine appears, known as dysuria with milky urine.

(4)**Dysuria Caused by Qi Dysfunction**: Damage of the liver by anger, production of fire from stagnated Qi or obstruction of Qi due to stagnation, leading to accumulation of Qi and fire in the Lower Energizer, impede the activity of the bladder, therefore, urination is difficult, painful, and incontinent, known as dysuria caused by Qi dysfunction.

(5)**Dysuria Caused by Overstrain**: Indulgent sexual intercourse leading to deficiency of the kidney Qi, or sinking of the spleen Qi due to deficiency causes difficult and painful urination which often recurs on overstrain, known as dysuria caused by overstrain.

Differentiation

(1)**Dysuria Caused by Calculi**

Main Manifestation: Occasional presence of calculi in the urine, difficult urination, dark yellow turbid urine, or interruption of urination due to sudden obstruction, unbearable pricking pain during urination, unbearable pain of the lumbus and abdomen, or presence of blood in the urine, normal tongue coating.

(2) **Dysuria Caused by Qi Dysfunction**

Main Manifestations: Difficult and hesitant urination, fullness and pain of the lower abdomen, thin, white tongue coating, deep, string-taut pulse.

(3) **Painful Urination with Blood.**

Main Manifestations: Hematuria with pain and urgency of micurition, burning sensation and pricking pain in urination, thin, yellow tongue coating, rapid, forceful pulse.

(4) **Dysuria with Milky Urine**

Main Manifestations: Cloudy urine with milky or creamy appearance, urethral burning pain in urination, red tongue proper, sticky coating, thready, rapid pulse.

(5) **Dysuria Caused by Overstrain**

Main Manifestation: Difficulty in urination with dribbling of urine, occurring off and on, exacerbated after overwork, and usually refractory to treatment, weak pulse.

Treatment

Principle: The Back-(Shu) and Front-(Mu) points of Bladder Meridian are selected as the principal points. Reducing manipulation along with combination of reinforcing and reducing is applied to promote the activity of the bladder.

Prescription: Pangguangshu (BL 28), Zhongji (CV 3), Yinlingquan (SP 9).

Additional Points

Add Weiyang (BL 39) for dysuria caused by calculi, Xingjian (LR 2) for dysuria caused by Qi dysfunction, Xuehai (SP 10) and Sanyinjiao (SP 6) for painful urination with blood, Shenshu (BL 23), and Zhaohai (KI 6) for dysuria with milky urine, Baihui (GV 20), Qihai (CV 6) and Zusanli (ST 36) for dysuria caused by overstrain.

Explanation: Urination disturbance is chiefly due to the affections of the bladder, so Pangguangshu (BL 28) and Zhongji (CV 3), the Front-(Mu) point of the bladder are needled to improve the function of the bladder; Yinlingquan (SP 9), the He-(Sea) point of Spleen Meridian is combined to promote diuresis, restoring the Qi function and free urination, referring to the theory "Pain will disappear when obstruction is removed." Dysuria caused by calculi is due to the accumulation of damp heat in the Lower energizer and precipitation of urine, therefore, Weiyang (BL 39), the point of Bladder Meridian, and also the Lower He-(Sea) point of Triple Energizer Meridian, is applied to reduce damp-heat, from the lower energizer and strengthen the function of the bladder, Xingjian (LR 2), the Ying-(Spring) point of the Liver Meridian is used to dispel the fire from the Liver Meridian, regulate the flow of Qi and relieve dysuria. Xuehai (SP 10) and Sanyinjiao (SP 6) are applied to remove the heat from the low energizer and stop bleeding. If dysuria with milky urine lasts longer, deficiency of the kidney fails to check the downward flow of fatty liquid, so Shenshu (BL 23) and Zhaohai (KI 6) are needled to reinforce the kidney-Qi. Dysuria caused by overstrain is due to weakness of both spleen and kidney, Baihui (GV 20), the meeting point of all the Yang meridians in combination with Qihai (CV 6) and Zusanli (ST 36) may reinforce the Qi of the spleen and kidney.

21. Impotence

Impotence refers to poor erection of penis during sexual intercourse. It is called "Yinwei" in *Internal Classics* Zhang Jingyue said: "Yinwei refers to weak erection of penis". It is due to looseness of penis of various causes. It may mostly be seen in sexual neurasthenia or some other chronic diseases.

Etiology and Pathogenesis

(1) **Decline of Mingmen-Fire**: Excessive sex or masturbation makes Mingmen-fire decline and exhausts the kidney essence. Impotence may also be due to fear, fright or worry, consumption of essence of the kidney, and of penis. Just as said in *Treatment of Internal Disorders*: "The inability of penis to erect is due to the injury of the internal organs, which is mainly caused by exhaustion of kidney essence from indulgent sexual intercourse, or by worry damaging the mind, or by fright leading to dysfunction of the kidney."

(2) **Downward Flowing of Damp-Heat**: Greasy food and wine may damage the function of the spleen and stomach in transportation and transformation, causing dampness to turn into heat. The damp-heat drives downward to make the penis unable to erect resulting in impotence, however, impotence of the damp heat type is not very common. Just as Zhang Jingyue said: "Seven to eight out of ten impotence are caused by the decline of fire. Only a few of them are due to excess of fire".

Differentiation
(1) Decline of Mingmen-Fire
Main Manifestations: Failure or weakness of the penis in erection, pallor, cold limbs, dizziness, listlessness, soreness and weakness of the loins and knees, pale tongue with white coating, deep, thready pulse. If the heart and spleen Qi is damaged, palpitations and insomnia may be present.

Treatment
Principle: The points of Conception Vessel and Kidney Meridians are selected as the principal points.
Reinforcing method with moxibustion is applied to invigorate the kidney-Yang.
Prescription: Mingmen (GV 4), Guanyuan (CV 4), Shenshu (BL 23), Taixi (KI 3).

Additional Points
Add Xinshu (BL 15), Shenmen (Ht 7) Sanyinjiao (SP 6) for damage of the Qi of the heart and spleen.

Explanation: Impotence is caused by decline of Mingmen fire and deficiency of kidney-Yang. Mingmen (GV 4), Shenshu (BL 23) and Taixi (KI 3) are used to strengthen the kidney-Yang, Guanyuan (CV 4) is the meeting point of Conception Vessel and the three Foot Yin Meridians. Reinforcing method is used to promote the primary-Qi and invigorate the kidney function. Xinshu (BL 15), Shenmen (HT 7) and Sanyinjiao (SP 6) are good for activating the Qi of the heart and spleen.

(2) Downward Flowing of Damp-Heat:
Main Manifestations: Inability of the penis to erect accompanied with bitter taste in the mouth, thirst, hot and dark red urine, soreness and weakness of the lower limbs, yellow, sticky tongue coating, soft, rapid pulse.

Treatment
Principle: The points of Conception Vessel and Spleen Meridians are selected as the principal points. Reducing manipulation is applied to eliminate the damp heat.
Prescription: Zhongji (CV 3), Sanyinjiao (SP 6), Yinlingquan (SP 9), Zusanli (ST 36).

Explanation: This condition is caused by the downward flow of damp heat from the spleen meridian, disturbed by dampness of spleen turning into heat due to long-standing accumulation. Sanyinjiao (SP 6) and Yinlingquan (SP 9) are selected to soothe and regulate the Qi of spleen meridian to eliminate the damp heat. Zhongji (CV 3) is used to dispel damp heat from the lower energizer, Zusanli (ST 36) is chosen to dispel dampness by improving the function of the spleen in transportation and transformation.

Alternative Treatment
Ear Acupuncture
Selection of Points: Pt. Uterus, Pt. External Genitalia, Pt. Testis, Pt. Endocrine.

Method: Apply filiform needles with moderate stimulation, rotate the needles once every ten minutes and retain the needles for 30 minutes.

22. Spermatorrhea

Spermatorrhea refers to nocturnal emission and spontaneous spermatorrhea. Nocturnal emission happens during dreams in sleep, while spontaneous spermatorrhea happens when the patient has no sexual fantasy or provocation by female. This condition is due to unfirmness of the spermal gate of various causes. It may be seen in sexual neurasthenia, seminal vesiculitis, orchitis and other chronic disease.

Etiology and Pathogenesis

(1) **The Disharmony between the Heart and Kidney:** Overcontemplation or excessive sexual activities leads to disharmony between the heart and kidney. If the heart fire fails to descend and control the kidney water, the kidney water cannot ascend and cool the heart fire, when water deficiency and fire excess disturb the essence, nocturnal emission happens in dreams.

(2) **Failure in Storing Sperms Due to Deficiency of Kidney Yang:** Indulgent sexual intercourse, or damage of the kidney after a long-standing illness makes the kidney unable to store sperms, the spermal gate is not firm, resulting in spermatorrhea.

(3) **Downward Flowing of Damp Heat:** Damp-heat accumulated flows downward in the Lower Energizer and disturbs the essence, the spermal gate is not firm, leading to nocturnal emission.

Differentiation:

(1) Disharmony between the Heart and Kidney

Main Manifestations: Nocturnal emission happens in dreams, dizziness, palpitation, listlessness, lumbar soreness, tinnitus, yellow urine, red tongue, and thready, rapid pulse.

Treatment

Principle: Acupuncture is given with reducing manipulation to the points of the Heart Meridian and with reinforcing manipulation to the points of the Kidney Meridian to regain harmony between the heart and kidney and promote the function of kidney in storing essence and sperms.

Prescription: Shenmen(HT 7), Xinshu(BL 15), Taixi(KI 3), Zhishi(BL 52)

Explanation: Shenmen (HT 7) and Xinshu (BL 15) are needled to lower the heart-fire and harmonize the heart and kidney. Taixi (KI 3) is used to activate the kidney-Qi and Zhishi (BL 52) to control the essence.

(2) Failure in Storing Essence due to Deficiency of Kidney-Yang

Main Manifestations: Frequent spermatorrhea at day or night, particularly there is emission on sexual fantasy in severe cases, emaciation, pallor complexion, pale tongue, deep, thready pulse.

Treatment

Principle: The points of Bladder, Spleen Meridians and Conception Vessel are selected as principal points with reinforcing method and moxibustion to strengthen the primary Yang and the sperms in combination with Sanyinjiao(SP 6) can strengthen the kidney and control the essence and semen.

Prescription: Shenshu (BL 23), Zhishi (BL 52), Mingmen (GV 4), Guanyuan (CV 4), Sanyinjiao (SP 6).

Explanation: Shenshu (BL 23) and Zhishi (BL 52) are needled to reinforce the kidney-Qi and control the essence. Mingmen (GV 4) is needled to warm the kidney and store essence. Guanyuan (CV 4) is applied to strengthen the primary Yang and sperms in combination with Sanyinjiao (SP 6) can strengthen the spleen, nourish the liver and reinforce the kidney.

(3) Downward Flow of Damp-Heat

Main Manifestations: Frequent spermatorrhea, semen in urine, restlessness, poor sleep, dry mouth with bitter taste, difficult urine with hot sensation, yellow, sticky, tongue coating, soft, rapid pulse.

Treatment

Principle: The points of Conception Vessel and Spleen Meridian are selected as principal points with reducing manipulation to clear up damp-heat and control essence.

Prescription: Zhongji (CV 3), Yinlingquan (SP 9), Sanyinjiao (SP 6).

Explanation: Zhongji (CV 3) is the Front-(Mu) point of the bladder. Reducing manipulation applied to Zhongji (CV 3) can dispel the Qi of kidney and remove damp-heat with discharge of urine, Yinlingquan (SP 9) and Sanyinjiao (SP 6) can strengthen the spleen and resolve dampness, clear up heat and promote diuresis. Zhongji (CV 3) and Sanyinjiao (SP 6) are the crossing points of Three Foot Yin Meridians. Zhongji (CV 3) located in the lower abdomen in combination with Sanyinjiao (SP 6) can control essence. The joint use of the above points can clear up heat, remove dampness and prevent spermatorrhea.

Alternative Treatment

(1) **Ear Acupuncture**

Selection of Points: Pt. Sperm Place, Pt. Endocrine, Pt. Shenmen, Pt. Heart, Pt. Kidney.

Method: Apply filiform needles to two or three points with mild stimulation. Retain the needles for 15—20 minutes. Embedding of ear seeds is also applicable.

(2) **Point Injection**

Selection of Points: Guanyuan (CV 4), Zhongji (CV 3), Zhishi (BL 52).

Method: 0.2—0.5 ml of Vitamin B1 or Radix Angelicae Sinensis injection is injected into each point slowly while needling sensation is going to external genitalia.

23. Insomnia

Appendix: Poor Memory

Insomnia is a condition that makes the patient unable to have normal hours of sleep. It has different patterns: difficulty in falling asleep after retiring, early awakening, inability to sleep again after awakening, intermittent waking through the period of attempted sleep and even inability to sleep all the night.

Insomnia is often accompanied by dizziness, headache, palpitation, poor memory and mental astheria.

Etiology and Pathogenesis

(1)**Deficiency of Both the Heart and Spleen-Qi**: Anxiety and overwork damage the heart and spleen. Blood is exhausted, the deficient heart can not hold the mind while Qi and blood production becomes poor in case of deficiency of the spleen Qi. Blood deficiency is unable to nourish the heart, leading to insomnia. Just as Zhang Jingyue described: "Overwork and anxiety cause the exhaustion of blood and damage the storage of the mind. As a result, insomnia follows."

(2)**Disharmony between the Heart and Kidney**: Congenital deficiency, indulgent sexual intercourse, or a chronic illness damages the kidney Yin. The kidney water fails to ascend to the heart to check the heart fire. A violent emotional fit can induce flaring of the heart fire which fails to descend to the kidney to control the kidney water, then the heart Yang is hyperactive and excess of the heart fire injures the mind and hence insomnia results.

(3)**Upward Disturbance of the Liver-Fire**: Emotional depression causes the stagnation of Qi in the liver. The stagnation Qi of long duration is transformed into fire, which flares up and disturbs the mind, and then insomnia occurs.

(4)**Dysfunction of the Stomach**: Irregular food intake damages the spleen and stomach. The accumulated undigested food causes dysfunction of the stomach and insomnia as stated in *Internal Classics* that sleep is disturbed if the function of the stomach is in disharmony.

Differentiation

(1)**Deficiency of Both the Heart and Spleen-Qi**.

Main Manifestations: Difficulty in falling asleep, dreamy, palpitation, poor memory, lassitude, anorexia, sallow complexion, pale tongue with thin coating, thready, weak pulse.

(2)**Disharmony between the Heart and Kidney**

Main Manifestations: Restlessness, poor sleep, dizziness, tinnitus, dry mouth with little saliva, burning sensation of the chest, palms and soles, red tongue, thready, rapid pulse, or nocturnal emission, poor memory, palpitation, lumber pain.

(3)**Upward Disturbance of the Liver-Fire**

Main Manifestations: Irritability due to insomnia, dreamy sleep, headache, bitter taste in the mouth, distension in the costal region, string-taut pulse.

(4) **Dysfunction of the Stomach**

Main Manifestations: Insomnia, suffocating feeling and distending pain in the epigastric region, poor appetite, difficult defecation, sticky tongue coating, rolling pulse.

Treatment

Principle: The points of Heart Meridian and Three Foot Yin Meridians are selected as principal points. Reinforcing is applied for deficiency syndrome, while reducing for excess syndrome to calm the heart and soothe the mind. Acupuncture is desirable in the afternoon or in the evening before sleep.

Prescription: Shenmen (HT 7), Sishencong (EX-HN 1), Sanyinjiao (SP 6), Anmian (EX).

Additional Points

Add Xinshu (BL 15), Pishu (BL 20) for deficiency of the heart and spleen, Xinshu (BL 15), Taixi (KI 3), Zhaohai (KI 6) for disharmony between the heart and kidney, Xingjian (LR 2) for upward disturbance of the liver-fire, Zhongwan (CV 12), Zusanli (ST 36) for dysfunction of the stomach.

Explanation: Shenmen (HT 7) nourishes the heart, Sishencong (EX-HN 1) calms the mind. Anmian (EX) soothes the mind, Sanyinjiao (SP 6) can strengthen the spleen, nourish liver and reinforce kidney. The joint use of these four points can calm the heart and soothe the mind, Xinshu (BL 15) and Pishu (BL 20) reinforce the spleen and nourish the heart, reinforce Qi and nourish blood. Taixi (KI 3) and Zhaohai (KI 6) reinforce kidney water and harmonize the heart and kidney, Xingjian (LR 2) calms liver fire and the mind, Zhongwan (CV 12) and Zusanli (ZT 36) remove the retention of food, strengthen the spleen, pacify the stomach and the mind.

Alternative Treatment

(1) **Ear Acupuncture**

Selection of Points: Pt. Shenmen, Pt. Heart, Pt. Liver, Pt. Spleen, Pt. Subcortex.

Method: Apply filiform needles at two to three points with mild stimulation and retain the needles for 20 minutes.

(2) Cutaneous Acupuncture

Tap the regions along the Governor Vessel and the Bladder Meridians from head to back with mild stimulation from above downward, with strong stimulation in lumbar sacrum until local redness appears. Treatment is given once daily or every other day. Ten treatments constitute a course.

(3) Point Injection

Selection of Points: Xinshu (BL 15), Ganshu (BL 18), Pishu (BL 20), Shenshu (BL 23), Zusanli (ST 36), Sanyinjiao (SP 6), Shenmen (HT 7).

Method: Select two to three points. 0.1—0.5 ml of mixed medicine liquid of Vitamin B1 and Vitamin B 12 is injected into each point. Treatment is given once daily or every other day. Ten treatments constitute a course.

Poor Memory

Poor memory refers to the functional decline of the brain, hypomnesia or forgetfulness. This condition is caused by deficiency of kidney essence and insufficiency of the heart and spleen.

Etiology and Pathogenesis

The kidney is in charge of storing essence, and producing marrow, the brain is the sea of marrow, regarded as "the residence of mind". Indulgent sexual intercourse consumes the essence and marrow, the brain is therefore poorly nourished, causing forgetfulness. The spleen dominates the recollection and thinking, and thinking also depends on the action of the heart. Overthinking injuring the heart and spleen consumes blood and leads to poor memory. The aged also tend to have poor memory due to the kidney decline.

Treatment

Treatment is mainly to replenish the blood of the heart and reinforce the spleen and kidney.

Prescription: Sishencong (EX-HN1), Xinshu (BL 15), Pishu (BL 20), Shenshu (BL 23), Zusanli (ST 36), Zhaohai (KI 6), Xuanzhong (GB 39), reinforcing manipulation is applied.

Explanation: Sishencong (EX-HN 1) is an empirical point for poor memory, can replenish the brain and promote intelligence. Xinshu (BL 15) and Pishu (BL

20) are applied to replenish the blood of heart, Zusanli (ST 36) reinforces the spleen and stomach in transportation and transformation, Xuanzhong (GB 39), the converging point of marrow, in combination with Shenshu (BL 23) and Zhaohai (KI 6) promotes the kidney essence, produces marrow to replenish the brain.

24. Palpitation and Severe Palpitation

Palpitation refers to unduly rapid action of the heart which is felt by the patient and accompanied by nervousness and restlessness. Mild palpitation is mostly due to sudden fright, severe palpitation is not due to sudden fright but prolonged internal injury. The long-standing palpitation may result in cardiac condition. It may be seen in neurosis, disturbance of vegetative nervous system, arrhythmia due to various cardiac conditions.

Etiology and Pathogenesis

(1) **Fright**: A timid person is likely to have palpitation when being frightened by sudden noises, surprising objects or dangerous environments. In Chapter 19 of *Plain Questions*, it says: "Fright makes Qi disturbed because the heart has nothing to rely on, the mind has no place to house and the thinking has nothing to focus on".

(2) **Insufficiency of Qi and Blood**: Chronic consumptive disease, loss of blood, or mental stress damage the heart and spleen, and impede the production of Qi and blood. Deficiency of Qi and blood fails to nourish the heart, causing palpitation.

(3) **Hyperactivity of the Fire Due to Yin-Deficiency**: Injury of kidney-Yin caused by indulgent sex renders the kidney water unable to check the heart fire. Disharmony between the heart and kidney causes palpitation.

(4) **Retention of Harmful Fluid**: Deficiency of the spleen and kidney-Yang or depression of the heart-Yang, causes the heart to be attacked by vaporized water resulting in palpitation.

Differentiation

(1) **Fright**

Main Manifestations: Palpitation, fear and fright, irritability, restlessness, dreamy, white, thin tongue coating, mild, rapid pulse.

(2) **Insufficiency of Qi and blood**

Main Manifestations: Palpitation, lustreless complexion, dizziness, blurring of vision, shortness of breath, lassitude, pale tongue with tooth prints, thready, weak or intermittent pulse.

(3) **Hyperactivity of the Fire Due to Yin Deficiency**

Main Manifestations: Palpitation, restlessness, dizziness, tinnitus, irritability, insomnia, red tongue with little coating, thready, rapid pulse.

(4) **Vaporized Water Attacking Heart**

Main Manifestations: Palpitation, expectoration of mucoid sputum, fullness in the chest and epigastric region, lassitude, weakness, cold extremities, white tongue coating, string-taut, rolling pulse. In case of deficiency of Yang in the spleen and kidney, scanty urine, thirst without desire to drink, white, slippery tongue coating, string-taut, rolling pulse.

Treatment

Principle: The Back-(Shu) and Front-(Mu) points of Heart Meridian and the points of Heart and Pericardium Meridians are selected as the principal points. Reinforcing is applied for fright to calm the heart. Reinforcing is used for insufficiency of Qi and blood to reinforce Qi and nourish blood. Reinforcing is applied for hyperactivities of fire due to Yin deficiency to nourish the kidney-Yin and harmonize the heart and kidney. For vaporized water attacking, reinforcing is applied in combination with moxibustion to warm Yang and dissolve the condensed water.

Prescription: Neiguan (PC 6), Shenmen (HT 7), Xinshu (BL 15), Juque (CV 14).

Additional Points

Add Tongli (HT 5), Zusanli (ST 36), Qiuxu (GB 40) for fright, Zusanli (ST 36), Sanyinjiao (SP 6), and Pishu (BL 20) for insufficiency of Qi and blood, Shaofu (HT 8), and Zhaohai (KI 6) for hyperactivities of fire due to Yin deficiency, Shuifen (CV 9), Guanyuan (CV 4), Yinlingquan (SP 9) for vaporized water attack of heart

Explanation: Palpitation attributes to the heart, so treatment should rely on calming heart and easing mind. Neiguan (PC 6), the Luo-(Connecting) point of the Pericardium Meridian, linking with Yin Link Vessel can regulate Qi and blood of the heart is the empirical point for palpitation and cardiac pain, Shenmen (HT 7), the Yuan-(Primary) point of Heart Meridian, Xinshu (BL 15), and

Juque (CV 14) are the Back-(Shu) and the Front-(Mu) points. The joint use of these three points can regulate Qi and blood of heart to calm heart and ease mind. Tongli (HT 5), the Luo-(Connecting) point of Heart Meridian and Qiuxu (GB 40), the Yuan-(Primary) point of Gallbladder Meridian, Zusanli (ST 36) is an important point to reinforce Qi and blood. The joint use of these three points can calm the heart and reinforce gallbladder and strengthen body resistance. Sanyinjiao (SP 6) and Pishu (BL 20) can regulate the spleen and stomach to promote Qi and blood production. Shaofu (HT 8), the Ying-(spring) point of the Heart Meridian can clear up the fire of heart. Zhaohai (KI 6) can nourish kidney water to descend heart fire. The joint use of these two points can nourish kidney-Yin and descend the fire to harmonize the heart and kidney. Shuifen (CV 9) can remove fluid. Guanyuan (CV 4) can warm the kidney and spleen to strengthen the kidney Yang. Yinlingquan (SP 9) removes dampness. These three points can invigorate the heart-Yang, strengthen the spleen and remove the condensed water.

Alternative Treatment
(1) Ear Acupuncture
Selection of Points: Pt. Sympathetic, Pt. Heart, Pt. Subcortex.
Method: Apply filiform needles with mild stimulation and retain the needles for 20 minutes. Rotate the needles twice or three times. Treatment is given once daily. Ten treatments constitute a course.

(2) Point Injection
Selection of Points: Xinshu (BL 15), Pishu (Bl 20), Ganshu (BL 18), Shenshu (BL 23), Neiguan (PC 6), Shenmen (HT 7), Zusanli (ST 36), Sanyinjiao (SP 6).
Method: Select two to three points and apply injection of Radix Angelicae, or injection of compound Radix Salviae Miltiorrhizae or injection of Vitamin B 12, 0.5−1 ml of liquid medicine is injected into each point, injection is given once every other day.

25. Depressive Madness

Depressive madness is one kind of mental disorders. Most of the patients are in the young and middle age. The depression is manifested by reticence or incoherent speech, while madness by shouting restlessness and violent behaviours.

As described in The 20th Problem, a Chapter of *Classic on Medical Problems*, depression is caused by abundant Yin; madness by abundant Yang. Wang Bing holds that depression is manifested by overjoy, while madness by over anger.

The most important etiological factor of depression and madness is emotional injury. Pathogenetically, phlegm plays the primary role, in addition, this disease is also related to the hereditary factors. Although depression and madness are different in symptomatology, they are related to each other. A prolonged depression, in which fire is produced by phlegm stagnation, may change into manic disorder, while a protracted madness, in which the stagnated fire is gradually dispersed, but the phlegm which is still existing, can change into depressive psychosis. Therefore, they are termed together as depressive madness.

This disease corresponds to schizophrenia, psychosis of manic or depressive type and meno-pause psychosis in modern medicine.

Etiology and Pathogenesis
(1) **Depression**

Depression is caused by worry and emotional depression, which may damage the liver and spleen, then lead to dysfunction of the liver in maintaining the free flow of Qi and spleen in transportation and transformation. As a result, the accumulated fluid due to impaired transportation, turns into phlegm, which goes upward to disturb the mind.

(2) **Madness**

In most cases, it is caused by frustration and anger that injure the liver function of dispersing. The stagnated Qi transforms into fire, which evaporates the body fluid to produce phlegm fire. The phlegm fire perverted by rushes upward and disturbs the mind. As a result, madness occurs.

Differentiation
(1) **Depression**

Main Manifestations: Gradual onset, emotional dejection and dullness at early stage, followed by soliloquy non-stopping laughing or silence, anorexia, somnolence, thin, sticky tongue coating, string-taut rolling pulse.

Treatment

Principle: Even movement is applied to the point of Stomach Meridian, Governor Vessel, Conception Vessel, Spleen Meridian, Pericardium Meridian and

Liver Meridian to soothe the liver, calm the heart and dissolve the phlegm by strengthening the spleen.

Prescription: (1) Xinshu (BL 15), Ganshu (BL 18), Pishu (BL 20), Shenman (HT 7), Fenglong (ST 40). (2) Shenmen (HT 7), Dazhong (KI 4), Daling (PC 7), Fenglong (ST 40).

Explaination: This syndrome is caused by the stagnation of phlegm and Qi, which injures the heart, liver and spleen. Xinshu (BL 15) is used to open the heart orifice and calm down the mind, Ganshu (BL 18) to remove the liver stagnation, Pishu (BL 20) to promote the spleen Qi circulation, so as to dissolve the phlegm, Shenmen (HT 7) to nourish the heart to treat mental dullness, Fenglong (ST 40) to dissolve the phlegm for calming the mind, Dazhong (KI 4) and Daling (PC 7) to regulate Qi in the chest.

(2) Madness

Main Manifestations: Irritability, headache, insomnia, red face, then violent behaviours, followed by excessive motor activity, loss of appetite in few days but with full of vigour. Yellow sticky tongue coating, string-taut, rolling and rapid pulse.

Treatment

Principle: Reducing manipulation is applied to the points on Governor Vessel, Pericardium Meridian, Stomach Meridian to calm the heart, reduce the heat and dissolve the phlegm.

Prescription: Dazhui (GV 14), Shuigou (GV 26), Fengfu (GV 16), Neiguan (PC 6), Fenglong (ST 40).

Additional Points

Madness with Extreme Heat: Prick the twelve Jing-(Well) points on hand to cause bleeding for reducing heat.

Explanation: Dazhui (GV 14) is used to reduce heat for calming the mind. Shuigou (GV 26) is used to clear the mind. Since the brain is regarded as the palace of the primary mind, Governor Vessel enters the brain from Fengfu (GV 16). Fengfu (GV 16) can clear and clam the heart. Neiguan (PC 6) is combined with Fenglong (ST 40) to clear the heart and dissolve the phlegm.

Alternative Treatment

(1) Scalp Acupuncture

Thoracic Region and Foot Motor and Sensory Region are applied to be punctured along the scalp to the periosteum. Then, the needle is rotated for two minutes. The treatment is given once a day.

(2) Ear Acupuncture

Pt. Shenmen, Pt. Heart, Pt. Liver, Pt. Spleen, Pt. Subcortex, Select 3 — 4 points each treatment, mild stimulation is used for depression, strong stimulation is used for madness, the needles are retained for thirty minutes, rotate needles once every five minutes.

26. Epilepsy

Epilepsy occurs in seizures, manifested by falling down in fit, loss of consciousness, foam on the lips, or screams with eyes starting upward, and convulsions, when the consciousness regains, the patient becomes normal.

Besides the typical seizures, the manifestations of the disease may be various. It can be a momentary loss of attention or consciousness. Epileptic fits may occur at any time, in various frequency and with different severity. It is often preceded by an "aura" of dizziness, chest congestion and listlessness. Epilepsy is an excess condition, but frequent recurrence can lower the body resistance.

The above description refers to many types of epileptic seizures including grand mal, petit mal, psychomotor and focal seizures. For secondary epilepsy, the primary disease should be treated actively.

Etiology and Pathogenesis

(1) Fright makes Qi disordered and fear makes Qi descend. Fear and fright may damage the kidney and disturb the Qi activity affecting the liver and kidney; then Yin can not control Yand and wind is transformed from heat. As a result, epilepsy occurs.

(2) Stagnation of the liver-Qi injures the spleen and the stomach which make the accumulated dampness turn into phlegm. The stagnated Qi and phlegm go upward to disturb the mind then cause epilepsy.

(3) Epilepsy may result from hereditary factors, but in most of the hereditary cases, it happens in the childhood.

Differentiation

(1) Excess Type

Main Manifestations: Sudden falling down with loss of consciousness, pallor, clenched jaws, upward staring of the eyes, convulsion, foam on the lips screaming as pigs or sheep, and even incontinence of urine and feces. Later consciousness is gradually regained and the symptoms subside. Apart from fatigue and weakness, the patient can lead a normal life. Tongue coating is white sticky, and pulse is string-taut, rolling.

Treatment

Principle: Points of the Governor Vessel, Conception Vessel and Liver Meridian are selected as the main points with reducing manipulation to dissolve the phlegm resuscitate, soothe the liver and dispel the wind.

Prescription: (1)Shuigou(GV 26), Jiuwei(CV 15), Jianshi (PC 5), Taichong (LR 3), Fenglong (ST 40).

(2)Dazhui(GV 14), Zhongwan (CV 12), Fenglong (ST 40).

Explanation: Shuigon (GV 26), Dazhui (GV 14) are used for resuscitation. Juiwei (CV 15), Zhongwan (CV 12), Fenglong (ST 40) are used to clear the heart and the phlegm. Jianshi (PC 5), Taichong (LR 3) are used to regulate Qi, to eliminate the stagnation of liver-Qi and to dispel the wind of liver. All of these points are used for resuscitation to dissolve the phlegm and dispel the wind.

(2)Deficiency Type:

Main Manifestations: The longer the disease lasts, the more severe the spasm is, listlessness, lustreless complexion, dizziness, palpitation, anorexia, profuse sputum, weakness and soreness of the lions and limbs, pale tongue proper with little coating, thready, rolling pulse.

Treatment

Principle: To select the main points from Heart, Spleen and Kidney Meridians with even movement to nourish the heart, ease the mind, strengthen the spleen and reinforce the kidney.

Prescription: Xinshu (BL 15), Shenmen (HT 7), Baihui (GV 20), Sanyinjiao (SP 6), Yaoqi(EX-B9)

Additional Points

Daytime seizure: Shenmai (BL 62). Night seizure: Zhaohai (KI 6), phlegm stagnation: Zhongwan (CV 12), Fenglong (ST 40), severe deficiency of Qi and blood: Zusanli (ST 36), Guanyuan (CV 4).

Explanation: Deficiency type is due to weak resistance, leading to deficiency of Qi and blood, and phlegm, damp stasis. Xinshu (BL 15), Shenmen (HT 7) are used for nourishing the heart and easing the mind, Baihui (GV 20) is used for lifting the Qi and clearing mind, Sanyinjiao (SP 6), for strengthening the liver and kidney, to nourish the spleen and dissolve the phlegm. Yaoqi (EX−B9) is an experience point for epilepsy. Daytime seizure due to deficiency of Yang, to puncture Shenmai (BL 62) is to warm Yang. Night seizure is due to deficiency of Yin, to puncture Zhaohai (KI 6) is to nourish Yin, Zhongwan (CV 12), Fenglong (ST 40), are used to nourish spleen and dissolve phlegm. Guanyuan (CV 4) and Zusanli (ST 36) are used to regulate and replenish Qi and blood.

Alternative Treatments

(1) **Ear Acupuncture**: Pt. Shenmen, Pt. Subcortex, Pt. Heart, Pt. Occiput, Pt. Brain point, Pt. Stomach, two to three points of them can be selected with strong stimulation, the needles are retained for thirty minutes, and rotated intermittently. The treatment is given once every other day, ten treatments are taken as one course.

(2) **Point Injection**: Dazui (GV 14), Zusanli (ST 36) are injected by Vitamin B_1 or B_{12} or 5% Dang Gui injection. Each point is injected 0.5 ml.

(3) **Pricking Method**: There are three points above Changqiang (GV 1) for selection. They are located 0.5 cun, 1 cun, one and half cun above Changqiang (GV 1) successively. Prick the subcutaneous muscular fibre, once a week, three treatments are taken as one course.

27. Dizziness

The mild case can be relieved by closing one's eyes, while the serious case has an illusion of bodily movement with rotatory sensation like in a sailing boat, and even accompanied by nausea, vomiting, sweating, and falling down.

The symptom is mostly seen in hypertension, arteriosclerosis, neurosis, and otogenic dizziness.

Etiology and Pathogenesis

There are three causes of dizziness. They are hyperactivity of the liver-Yang, deficiency of Qi and blood, interior retention of phlegm dampness.

The liver is analogized as wind and wood, the liver is characterized by movement of ascending, worry, anxiety, or anger can consume the liver Yin, resulting in hyperactivity of liver-Yang, which may disturb the clear mind and cause dizziness. Kidney is the congenital foundation, and it stores essence and manufactures marrow. Deficiency of congenital foundation, deficiency of kidney essence, over sexual intercourse, old age, or chronic diseases with damaged kidney may lead to deficiency of kidney essence, so that the kidney can not produce the marrow. Since brain is taken as the sea of marrow, the deficiency of marrow may result in dizziness.

The heart and spleen are damaged by mental stress in case of a weak constitution after a disease. The damaged spleen fails to produce Qi and blood, leading to deficiency. In case the brain is poorly nourished by Qi and blood, dizziness occurs.

In a fat person with generally abundant phlegm dampness, irregular food intake and overwork damage the spleen, impairing its function in transportation and transformation and leading to production of dampness and phlegm. The stagnant phlegm and Qi may impede the ascending of clear Yang and descending of the turbid Yin, and thus dizziness occurs.

Differentiation
(1) Hyperactivity of the Liver-Yang
Main Manifestations: Dizziness aggravated by anger or excitement, flushed face, red eyes, bitter taste in mouth, tinnitus, dreamy sleep, red tongue proper with yellow coating, string-taut, rapid pulse.

Treatment
Principle: The points of Liver Meridian, Gallbladder Meridian, Kidney Meridian are selected as the main points to nourish Yin and pacify liver-Yang. Reinforcing and reducing manipulations are applied with either one first according to the condition of the dizziness.

Prescription: Fengchi (GB 20), Xingjian (LR 2), Taichong (LR 3), Taixi (KI 3), Sanyinjiao (SP 6).

Explanation: Fengchi (GB 20) is to pacify the liver Yang and to eliminate wind so as to clear the mind and the vision. Xingjian (LR 2) is the Ying-(Spring) point and is used to reduce the liver-fire, to remove the bitter taste in the mouth. Taichong (LR 3) is used to pacify liver. Taixi (KI 3) is used to nourish the kidney. Sanyinjiao (SP 6) is used to nourish the liver and kidney, the common function of three points is to pacify liver-Yang and nourish Yin.

(2) **Deficiency of Qi and Blood**

Main Manifestations: Dizziness accompanied by weakness, pallor, pale lips, palpitation, insomnia, tongue proper is pale, pulse is thready and weak, loss of consciousness happens in severe cases.

Treatment

Principle: The points of Governor Vessel, Conception Vessel, Spleen and Stomach Meridians are selected as the main points with reinforcing in combination with moxibustion to replenish Qi and blood.

Prescription: Baihui (GV 20), Guanyuan (CV 4), Zusanli (ST 36), Fenglong (ST 40), Sanyinjiao (SP 6).

Explanation: Baihui (GV 20) is located at the vertex. Moxibustion is used to Baihui (GV 20) can make Qi and blood ascend to the head to nourish the brain and check dizziness. Moxibustion to Guanyuan (CV 4) is used to strengthen the primary-Qi. Sanyinjiao (SP 6), Zusanli (ST 36) and Fenglong (ST 40) are for invigorating the spleen and stomach to produce Qi and blood.

(3) **Interior Retention of Phlegm Dampness**

Main Manifestations: Dizziness with heaviness of the head and suffocating sensation in the chest, nausea, profuse sputum, heavy feeling of body somnolence, tongue coating is white and sticky, pulse is soft, rolling.

Treatment

Principle: The points of Conception Vessel, Stomach and Bladder Meridians are selected as the main points with even manipulation to eliminate dampness, and resolve phlegm.

Prescription: Zhongwan (CV 12), Quchi (LI 11), Fenglong (ST 40), Sanyinjiao (SP 6).

Additional Points

Neiguan (PC 6) for chest congestion and nausea.

Explanation: Spleen is a source of phlegm manufacturd, Zhongwan (CV 12) is the Front-(Mu) point of Stomach Meridian, it can be used to strengthen the spleen and stomach to resolve phlegm and stop dizziness. Quchi (LI 11), Hegu (LI 4) are used to descend the upward perversion of damp phlegm so as to clear the mind and the vision. Fenglong (ST 40) is the Luo-(Connection) point of Stomach Meridian, it can nourish the spleen and stomach, and is the main point for resolving the phlegm, combining with Sanyinjiao (SP 6), it can strengthen the spleen and stomach, so as to resolve the phlegm. Neiguan (PC 6) is the Luo-(Connecting) point of the Pericardium Meridian with the function of relaxing the chest, regulating Qi and harmonizing the stomach to stop vomiting.

Alternative Treatment
(1) **Scalp Acupuncture**
Vertigo and hearing area. Insert No. 30, 1.5 cun needle to the periosteum, fast swirl for two minutes stop for five minutes rest, later rotate needle for another two minutes, again such manipulation is done for thirty minutes totally once a day, ten treatments make one course.

(2) **Ear Acupuncture**
Pt. Infratragic Apex, Pt. End of inferior Antihelix Crus, Pt. Herat, Pt. Shenmen, needling once a day, ten treatments are taken as one course. One week break before the next course.

(3) **Cutenous Needling**
Baihui (GV 20), Taiyang (EX-HN 5), Yintang (EX-HN 3) Jiaji (EX-B2) points. One or two treatments per day with mild stimulation, five to ten treatments are taken as one course.

28. Melancholia

Melancholia is a general term for disorder resulting from emotional depression and stagnation of Qi. The main symptoms are mental disorders like laughing without reasons, crying, singing, sighing or dematia, silence, sudden aphasia, blindness, stuffiness in the chest, hiccup, difficulty in swallowing, even sudden loss of consciousness, numbness and pain in the limbs, paralysis, and trembling. Most of the patients are young women. The disease is similar to hysteria and meno-pause syndrome in modern medicine.

Etiology and Pathogenesis
Generally speaking, melancholia is caused by emotional injuries resulting in disharmony of the activity of Zang-organs. As said in Chapter 28 of *Miraculous Pivot*: "Grief, sorrow, worry and anxiety disturb the mind, and the disturbance of the mind will affect all the five Zang and six Fu organs."

Differentiation

(1) Depression of the Qi in the Liver

Main Manifestations: Mental depression, distending pain in the chest and hypochondriac regions, epigastric distension, belching, abdominal distension, poor appetite, abnormal bowel movement, irregular menstruation. thin and sticky tongue coating, string-taut pulse.

(2) Transformation of Depressed Qi into Fire

Main Manifestations: Irritability, hot temper, headache, red eyes, tinnitus, constipation, red tongue with yellow coating, string-taut and rapid pulse.

(3) Stagnation of Phlegm Qi (also known as globus hystericus).

Main Manifestations: Feeling of a lump choking in the throat, hard to expectorate it out or swallow it, stuffiness in the chest, thin, sticky tongue coating, string-taut, rolling pulse.

(4) Insufficiency of Blood (also known as hysteria)

Main Manifestations: Grief without reasons, capricious joy or anger, suspicions, liability to get frightened, palpitation, irritability, insomnia, or sudden distress of chest, hiccup, sudden aphonia, convulsion or loss of consciousness in severe cases, thin white coating, string-taut, thready pulse.

Treatment

Principle: The main points are selected form Pericardium Meridian, Liver Meridian and Spleen Meridians, even movement or reinforcing with moxibustion method is applicable.

Prescription: Taichong (LR 3), Neiguan (PC 6), Sanyinjiao (SP 6).

Additional Points:

Depression of liver Qi: Tanzhong (CV 17), Zhongwan (CV 12).

Transmission of depressed Qi into fire: Xingjian (LR 2), Zhigou (TE 6), Xiaxi (GB 43). Stagnation of phlegm and Qi: Tiantu (CV 22), Tanzhong (CV 17), Fenglong (ST 40), Insufficiency of blood: Shenmen (HT 7), Zusanli (ST 36)

Explanation: Heart, liver and spleen are involved in melancholia. Taichong (LR 3) is the Yuan-(Primary) point of the Liver Meridian to smooth liver-Qi and remove depression, it refers to earth in five elements, therefore, the point is also good for tonifying spleen and stomach and resolving phlegm. Neiguan (PC 6) is the Luo-(Connection) point of the Pericardium Meridian to connect with

Triple Energizer Meridian, it is good for relaxing the chest and regulating Qi; Sanyinjinao (SP 6) is for tonifying spleen and stomach, regulating liver and benefiting kidney. All the points used together are to smooth liver, remove depression, tonify spleen, resolve phlegm and calm down the mind. Tanzhong (CV 17) is the converging point of Qi to regulate Qi and relax chest; Zhongwan (CV 12), Zusanli (ST 36) are good for harmonizing stomach and reducing the perversion of Qi. Three points used together are for strengthening the function of smoothing liver and regulating Qi. Xingjiao (LR 2) is for reducing liver-fire, Xiaxi (GB 43) is for reducing liver-fire. Zhigou (TE 6) is for reducing Triple Enrgizer fire. Three points used together are for reducing liver-fire. Zhigou (TE 6) is for reducing Triple Energizer fire. Three points used together are for reducing fire so as to strengthen the function of smoothing liver-Qi and eliminate depression. Tiantu (CV 22) is for reducing Qi and resolving phlegm. Fenglong (ST 40) is for tonifying spleen and stomach so as to resolve phlegm; Tanzhong (CV 17) is for regulating Qi, relaxing chest. Three points used together are for strengthening the function of resolving phlegm and eliminating masses. Shenmen (HT 7) is good for calming down the mind, Zusanli (ST 36) is for tonifying Qi and blood, two points used together are to strengthen the function of calming down the mind and tonifying blood.

Alternative Treatment
(1) Ear Acupuncture
Selection of Points: Pt. Heart. Pt. Brain. Pt. Subcortes.
Method: Mild stimulation is applied, retain needles for 20 minutes.
(2) Electric Acupuncture
Selection of Points: During the attack: Shuigou (GV 26), Hegu (LI 4), Neiguan (PC 6), Shenmen (HT 7), Zusanli (ST 36), Taichong (LR 3)

Non-attacking period: Neiguan (PC 6), Shenmen (HT 7), Zusanli (ST 36), Sanyinjiao (SP 6).

Hysterical paralysis: Add Quchi (LI 11) and Yanglingquan (GB 34).

Method: To select sparse-dense wave or continuous wave, to give strong stimulation during the attack for 5—10 minutes for each treatment; to apply mild or moderate stimulation in non-attacking period depending on patients intolerance, 10—20 minutes for each treatment, to give treatment once a day or every other day. Ten times make a course.

(3) **Cutaneous Needle**

Selection of Points: Governor Vessel and Bladder Meridian on the nape and back.

Method: Tap mildly till skin turns light red, once a day or every other day, 10 times make a course.

(4) **Point Injection**

Selection of Points: Xinshu (BL 15), Ganshu (BL 18), Pishu (BL 20), Jianshi (PC 5), Zusanli (ST 36)

Method: Inject mixed Vitamin B1 and Vitamin B12 injection, 0.1 — 0.5 ml for each point, once every other day.

29. Obesity

The standard body weight (kg) = body height(cm) — 100. Obesity refers to excessive adipose tissues. The diagnosis of obesity may be made by the body weight which exceeds the standard body weight by 10 — 20%. The fat on the neck, low abdomen and buttocks is obviously excessive. Obesity is manifested by disorder of metabolism like fatigue, lassitude, hidrosis and various neurosis, headache, palpitation, and abdominal distention. The modern medicine holds that obesity is closely related to cerebrovascular diseases, cardiovascular diseases, hypertension, arteriosclerosis and diabetes. Obesity may speed aging and cause various diseases. The disease includes simple and secondary obesity.

Etiology and Pathogenesis

(1) **Overtaking Greasy Food**: Accumulation of fat will affect the transportation and transformation of spleen to cause retention of phlegm damp in the interior which results in obesity.

(2) **Dysfunction of Lung in Descending**: Failure of warming function of kidney, retention of damp heat in the interior result in obesity.

Differentiation

(1) **Dysfunction of Spleen in Transportation and Transformation**

Main Manifestations: Poor appetite, weak constitution, loosen stools, flaccid muscles, fat body, flabby tongue, weak, soft and moderate pulse.

(2) **Retention of Damp Heat in the Interior**

Main Manifestations: Large amount of eating, constipation, thirst, foul breath, tense muscles, fat body, red tongue with sticky coating, rolling, rapid pulse.

(3) Derangement of Thoroughfare and Conception Vessels

Main Manifestations: Fat neck and buttocks, lumbar pain, weakness of legs, irregular menstruation with less amount of menstrual flow, pale, flabby tongue, deep, thready pulse.

Treatment

Principle: The points are mainly selected from Stomach and Spleen Meridians to tonify stomach and spleen and resolve phlegm-damp and promote bowel movement by even needling.

Prescription: Quchi (LI 11), Zusanli (ST 36), Sanyinjiao (SP 6), Tianshu (ST 25), Liangqiu (ST 34) and Gongsun (SP 4)

Explanation: Obesity results from retention of phlegm-damp in the interior including spleen, stomach and large intestine. Gonsun (SP 4) and Sanyinjiao (SP 6) are good for tonifying spleen and stomach so as to promote transportation and transformation and eliminate phlegm-damp; Zusanli (ST 36) and Liangqiu (ST 34) are to promote digestion, Quchi (LI 11) and Tianshu (ST 25) are to promote bowel movement so as to eliminate damp-phlegm from large intestine. All the points used together aim at body weight reduction.

Alternative Treatment

Ear Acupuncture

① **Selection of Points**: Pt. Endocrine, Pt. Ovary, Pt. Brain point, Pt. Hungry point, Pt. Ear-Shenmen, Pt. Spleen, Pt. Stomach and Pt. Sympthatic N.

Method: Reducing manipulation with strong stimulation is applied without retaining needles or with retaining for about 20 minutes. Six points are selected in each treatment. Two ears are used alternatively or at same time, once a day, ten treatments make a course.

② **Selection of Points**: Pt. Stomach, Pt. Lung, Pt. Hungry Point

Method: Embedding method is applied on one point. Press the point before feeling hungry or during meal.

③ **Selection of Points**: Disorder of Endocrine: Pt. Endocrine, Pt. Thalamus, Pt. Ovary, Pt. Brain point.

Hypeorexia: Pt. Hungry point, Pt. Thirsty point, Pt. Spleen, Pt. Stomach.

Somnolence: Pt. Thalamus, Pt. Ear-Shenmen

Method: Select 4—6 points in each treatment, five treatments for a course, one week break between two courses.

30. Headache

Headache is a subjective symptom. It can occur in various acute and chronic diseases. This section only deals in detail with headache as the predominant symptom.

Headache frequently happens in hypertension, intracranial tumor, neuro-headache, migraine, disorders of five sensory organs and infectious febrile diseases.

Etiology and Pathogenesis

The head is the highest place of the body where Qi and blood of Zang-Fu organs and Yang meridians of foot and hand gather as well as Governor Vessel which dominates all the Yang of the body flow up. That's why the head is regarded as the converging place of all the Yang.

(1) Invasion of various pathogens and endogenic diseases may directly or indirectly cause derangement of Qi and blood, obstruction of meridians and collaterals on the head, leading to headache. Six exogenous pathogens can attack the vertex and inhibit the flowing of lucid Yang.

(2) Dysfunction of liver in maintaining the free flow of Qi and prolonged depression will turn into heat which may go up and disturb the head; Yin deficiency of liver and kidney may lead to hyperactivity of liver-Yang.

(3) Constitutional weakness, deficiency of Qi and blood as well as malnutrition of brain may result in headache.

Differentiation

(1) Invasion of Pathogenic Wind into Meridians and Collaterals

Main Manifestations: Headache occurs on exposure to wind. The pain may extend to the nape and back. It is a violent, boring and fixed pain, string-taut pulse, white, thin tongue coating. The type is also called "head wind".

(2) Hyperactivity of Liver-Yang

Main Manifestations: Headache, vertigo, severe pain on bilateral sides of the head, irritability, hot temper, insomnia, red face, bitter taste in the mouth, string-taut pulse, red tongue with yellow coating.

(3) Insufficiency of Qi and Blood

Main Manifestations: Lingering headache, dizziness, vertigo, lassitude, lustreless face, pain relieved by warmth and aggravated by cold, overstrain or mental stress, weak, thready pulse, thin, white tongue coating.

Treatment
Principle: Headache can be caused by invasion of pathogenic wind in meridians, hyperactivity of liver-Yang and insufficiency of Qi and blood. The points are selected in the local area or based on the distributions of the meridians involved.

Prescription: Baihui (GV 20), Fengchi (GB 20), Taiyang (EX-HN 5).

Additional Points
Frontal Headache (Yangming Headache): Yangbai (GB 14), Yintang (EX-HN 3), Cuanzhu (BL 2), Hegu (LI 4) and Neiting (ST 44).

Temporal Headache (Shaoyang headache): Penetrating needle from Touwei (ST 8) to Shuaigu (GB 8), Waiguan (TE 5) and Zulinqi (GB 41).

Occipital Headache (Taiyang headache): Tianzhu (BL 10), Dazhui (GV 14), Houxi (SI 3) and Jinmen (BL 63).

Parietal Headache (Jueyin headache): Sishencong (EX-HN 1), Taichong (LR 3), Neiguan (PC 6) and Yongquan (KI 1).

Invasion of pathogens: Add Hegu (LI 4), Lieque (LU 7).

Hyperactivity of liver-Yang: Add Taichong (LR 3), Sanyinjiao (SP 6).

Deficiency of Qi and blood: Add Qihai (CV 6), Zusanli (ST 36) and Pishu (BL 20).

Explanation
The prescription is made by the local points and distal points on the affected meridians to promote the Qi circulation in the meridians so as to stop pain. The Liver Meridian goes to the vertex, The Gallbladder Meridian distributes on the bilateral sides of the headache. Fengchi (GB 20), Shugu (BL 65) and Touwei (ST 8) together with the distal points e.g. Taichong (LR 3) and Zulinqi (GB 41) are selected to pacify the liver-Yang; Pishu (BL 20), Zusanli (ST 36), Hegu (LI 4) and Sanyinjiao (SP 6) are good for promoting digestion so as to produce enough blood which may nourish the marrow. As a result, the sea of marrow is fully filled and pain is relieved.

Alternative Treatment

(1) **Cutaneous Needle**

Tap the region from Taiyang (EX-HN 5) to Yintang (EX-HN 3) and pain area to cause bleeding, then use cupping. The way is good for headache due to invasion of pathogenic wind and hyperactivity of liver-Yang.

(2) **Ear Acupuncture**

Selection of Points: Pt. Occiput, Pt. Forehead, Pt. Brain, Pt. Ear-shenmen.

Method: Select 2—3 points, retain needles for 20—30 minutes, to stimulate needles once every five minutes or to embed needles for 3—7 days. Bleeding is given for the obstinated headache on the vein on the back of the ear.

Remarks

Acupuncture can receive very good result for headache. But the causative factors of headache are various. If there is no effect, pain becomes worse gradually, the further check up should be given to prevent from incorrect diagnosis.

31. Facial Pain

Facial pain is a kind of severe pain occurring in transient paroxysms in a certain facial region It mostly occurs in one side of the forehead, maxillary region or mandibular region. The onset is abrupt like an electric shock, and the pain in cutting, burning and intolerable, Frequent recurrence denotes a chronic disease. In most cases, it starts after middle age in women.

Facial pain refers to trigeminal neuralgia in modern medicine.

Etiology and Pathogenesis

(1) **Invasion of Pathogenic Wind and Cold**

Pathogenic wind and cold attack the meridians on the face to cause contracture of them and obstruct the circulation of Qi and blood. As a result, pain occurs abruptly.

(2) **Stagnation of Fire of the Liver and Stomach**

The fire transformed from stagnated liver-Qi and the heat resulting from improper food intake and accumulation of food lead to the fire of liver and stomach flaring to the face. Finally, the facial pain results.

(3) **Excessive Fire due to Yin Deficiency**

Constitutional Yin deficiency and over sex consuming essence may cause excessive fire due to Yin deficiency. As a result, the facial pain occurs.

Besides, the facial pain can be induced by disorders of teeth, mouth, ear, nose and mental disorders.

Differentiation
(1) Invasion of Pathogenic Wind and Cold

Main Manifestations: Abrupt onset of pain occurs like an electric shock. The pain is cutting, burning and intolerable, but transient and paroxysmal. Each attack lasts a few seconds or one to two minutes. It may occur several times a day. A trigger point can be found on the face. The disease is accompanied by the local spasm, lacrimation, nasal discharge and salivation as well as the exterior symptoms and string-taut, tense pulse.

(2) Stagnation of Fire of the Liver and Stomach

Main Manifestations: Besides the characters of pain in last type, it combines with irritability, hot temper, thirst, constipation, yellow, dry coating and string-taut, rapid pulse.

(3) Excessive Fire due to Yin Deficiency

Main Manifestations: Insidious pain, emaciation, malar flush, soreness in the lumbar region, lassitude, pain aggravated by fatigue, thready, rapid pulse, red tongue with little coating.

Treatment
Principle: The points are selected from the local area and the distal along the course of the affected meridians, and punctured by reducing manipulation with filiform needles combining with continuous rotation.

Prescription: Pain at supraorbital region: Yangbai (GB 14), Yuyao (EX-HN 4), Cuanzhu (BL 2), Taiyang (EX—HN 5), Hegu (LI 4).

Pain at maxillary region: Sibai (ST 2), Quanliao (ST 18), Yingxiang (LI 20), Hegu (LI 4).

Pain at mandibular region: Xiaguan (ST 7), Jiache (ST 6), Daying (ST 5), Jiachengjiang (EX), Hegu (LI 4).

Additional Points
Invasion of Pathogenic Wind and Cold: Fengchi (GB 20), Stagnation of fire in the liver and stomach: Taichong (LR 3), Neiting (ST 44).

Excessive Fire due to Yin Deficiency: Zhaohai (KI 6), Sanyinjiao (SP 6).

Explanation: The local points can promote the circulation of Qi in the meridians on the face and reduce excess so as to stop pain. Hegu (LI 4) and Neiting (ST 44) can reduce stomach heat, Waiguan (TE 5) and Taichong (LR 3) can reduce heat from liver and gallbladder, Fengchi (GB 20) can eliminate wind so as to stop pain, while Zhaohai (KI 6) and Sanyinjiao (SP 6) can nourish Yin so as to reduce fire.

Alternative Treatment
(1) Ear Acupuncture

Selection of Points: Pt. Cheek, Pt. Maxillary, Pt. Mandibullar, Pt. Ear—Shenmen

Method: Select 2—3 points in each treatment, retain the needles for 20—30 minutes, rotate needles once every five minutes, or embed needle.

(2) Points Injection

Method: Inject Vitamin B_{12} or B_2, 1‰ procaine on the tender points, 0.5—1ml for each point, to inject once every two to three days.

Remarks
Acupuncture is effective to trigeminal neuralgia. The causative factors of secondary trigeminal neuralgia and trigeminal neural paralysis should be searched so as to give proper treatments.

32. Pain in Hypochondriac Region

Hypochondriac pain is a subjective symptom on the unilateral or bilateral sides of the body. The liver is located below the ribs, gallbladder attaches to the liver, besides, both Liver and Gallbladder Meridians supply the hypochondriac regions. Therefore, the occurrence of hypochondriac pain is closely concerned with disorders of liver and gallbladder.

The disease is commonly seen in acute or chronic disorders of liver, gallbladder and pleurae, sternocostal injury and intercostal neuralgia.

Etiology and Pathogenesis
(1) Stagnation of Liver-Qi

The liver is located in the hypochondriac region, its meridian distributes on the bilateral sides of the hypochondriac regions. The emotional depression will lead to dysfunction of liver in maintaining free flow of Qi, and obstruction of the meridian. The hindered circulation of Qi in the meridian results in hypochondriac pain.

(2) Deficiency of Essence and Blood

Deficiency of blood fails to nourish Liver Meridian.

(3) Traumatic Injury

Sprain and contusion may cause blood stasis in the meridians, resulting in hypochondriac pain.

Differentiation

(1) Stagnation of Liver-Qi

Main Manifestations: Distending pain in one side or bilateral hypochondriac regions, which is related to the emotional changes without fixed place sturriness in the chest, sighing, poor appetite, bitter taste in the mouth, thin and white coating, string-taut pulse.

(2) Stagnation of Qi and Blood

Main Manifestations: Stabbing pain in the hypochondriac regions with fixed place, pain aggravated by pressure and being severe at night, dark and purplish tongue, deep and hesitant pulse.

(3) Insufficiency of Liver-Yin

Main Manifestations: Dull and lingering pain in the hypochondriac regions, dizziness, vertigo, dry mouth, irritability, red tongue with little coating, weak or thready and rapid pulse.

Treatment

Principle: The main points are selected from Liver and Shaoyin Meridians combining with local and Back-(Shu) points. Reducing method is applied for excess syndrome, reinforcing or even manipulation is for deficiency syndrome.

Prescription: Zhigou (TE 6), Yanglingquan (GB 34), Qimen (LR 14), Taichong (LR 3).

Additional Points

Stagnation of Qi and Blood: Geshu (BL 17), Sanyinjiao (SP 6)

Insufficiency of liver-Yin: Ganshu (BL 18), Shenshu (BL 23), Zusanli (ST 36), Sanyinjiao (SP 6).

Explanation: Qimen (LR 14) which is the Front-(Mu) point of liver, Taichong (LR 3) which is Yuan-(Source) point and Zhigou (TE 6) and Yanglingquan

(GB 34) can promote the circulation of Qi in the Liver and Gallbladder Meridians so as to stop pain. The converging point of blood, Geshu(BL 17) combining with Sanyinjiao (SP 6) can activate the circulation of blood and eliminate stagnation. Ganshu(BL 18) Shenshu(BL 23) combining with Taichong (LR 3) can nourish essence and blood, regulate liver function so as to stop pain, Zusanli(ST 36) and Sanyinjiao (SP 6) can strengthen the function of spleen and stomach in manufacturing Qi and blood.

Alternative Treatment
(1) Cutaneous Needling

Tap the affected area and then apply cupping. The method is suitable for hypochondriac pain due to overstrain and traumatic injury with effects of stopping, pain and eliminating stagnation.

(2) Ear Acupuncture

Pt. Chest, Pt. Ear-Shenmen, Pt. Liver.

Method: Select 2—3 points on the affected side, puncture them during the attack of pain and retain the needles for 20—30 minutes.

Remarks
(1) During the acupuncture treatment of hypochondriac pain, the related examinations should be processed. It is necessary to treat the causative factors.

(2) Application of Huatuojiaji points of the corresponding segments gives gratifying effect to relieve pain in the treatment of intercostal neuralgia.

33. Lumbago

Lumbago, also called "pain in the lumbar and spinal regions." The pain can be located on the spine or one side or both sides of the spine. It is one of the main common symptoms in the clinic. Lumbago is closely associated with disorders of kidney for the lumbus is considered as the palace of the kidney.

The disease is commonly seen in soft tissues injury of lumbar region, muscular rheumatism and disorders of spinal column and internal organs.

This section only deals with lumbago due to cold and damp, sprain and kidney deficiency.

Etiology and Pathogenesis
(1) Lumbago due to Cold and Damp

It results from invasion of wind and cold, or sitting or lying on the damp place of being caught by rain and walking in the river or exposing to wind after sweating. As a result, the Qi circulation in the meridians is blocked due to pathogenic wind, cold and damp, then leading to pain.

(2) **Lumbar Strain**

Overstress on the lumbar region or traumatic injury due to sprain and contusion may injure the circulations of Qi and blood in the meridians, which leads to stagnation of Qi and blood, then lumbago results.

(3) **Lumbago due to Kidney Deficiency**

Oversex and consumption of essential Qi may lead to lumbago due to kidney deficiency.

Differentiation

(1) **Lumbago due to Cold and Damp**

Main Manifestations: Lumbago occurring after exposure to cold and damp, cold pain and heavy sensation in the dorsolumbar region, limitation of rotation, extension and flexion of the back, pain radiating downward to the buttocks and low limbs, the symptoms aggravated in the rainy days. The pain can not be relieved by lying position, white and sticky tongue coating, deep, weak or deep, slow pulse.

(2) **Lumbago due to Strain**

Main Manifestations: History of lumbar sprain, stiffness and pain in the lumbar region with fixed place, limited extension and flexion of the lumbar region in the mild case, limited rotation of the back in the severe cases, pain aggravated by pressure, light red or purplish, dark tongue, string-taut or hesitant pulse.

(3) **Lumbago due to Kidney Deficiency**

Main Manifestations: Dull pain and weakness in the lumbar region, lassitude, repeated attack, pain aggravated by strain and alleviated by rest in bed. In case of kidney-Yang deficiency, cold hands and feet, cramp in the lower abdomen, feeling cold in the lumbar region; in case of Yin deficiency, feverish in the chest, palms and soles, irritability, insomnia, dry mouth and throat, pale tongue, deep and slow pulse or red tongue, thready and rapid pulse.

Treatment

Principle: Points are mainly selected from Bladder Meridian and Governor Vessel. Needling and moxibustion are applied based on excess or deficiency.

Prescription: Shenshu (BL 23), Yaoyangguan (GV 3), Jiaji (EX-B 2), Weizhong (BL 40)

Additional Points
Cold and damp: Dachangshu (BL 25), Guanyuanshu (BL 26)
Kidney Yang deficiency: Mingmen (GV 4), Yaoyan (EX-B 7)
Kidney Yin deficiency: Zhishi (BL 52), Taixi (KI 3)
Overstrain: Shugou (GV 26), Yaotondian (EX-UE 7), Ashi Point.

Explanation: Since lumbus is the seat of the kidney, Shenshu (BL 23) is selected to tonify kidney-Qi, with moxibustion to eliminate cold and damp; Yaoyangguan (GV 3) is the local point, Weizhong (BL 40) is one of the four general points, which is the distal point for pain in the lumbar region and back; Dachangshu (BL 25) and Guanyuanshu (BL 26) are selected to eliminate wind and cold, promote the circulation in the meridian so as to stop pain, Mingmen (GV 4) and Yaoyan (EX-B 7) are punctured together with moxibustion to tonify kidney-Yang and essence; Zhishi (BL 52) and Taixi (KI 3) are for nourishing kidney-Yin, Governor Vessel goes in the spine, Shuigou (GV 26) is the distal point on the affected meridian for stiffness and pain in the spine; Yaotong (EX) is the effective extral point for lumbago due to sprain.

Alternative Treatment
(1) Pricking and Cupping

Tap the pain area and Weizhong (BL 40) by cutaneous needle to cause bleeding, then apply cupping. The method is applicable for lumbago due to cold and damp and chronic lumbar strain.

(2) Points Injection

Inject the cutaneous layer of the pain points by 5—10ml 10% glucose injection mixed with 100 mg Vitamin B 1 or compound Danggui (Radix Angelicae Sinensis) injection. Injection is applied once every other day, ten treatments for a course.

Remarks

Remarkable effect can be achieved by acupuncture for various lumbago. But in case of lumbago due to spinal tuberculosis of tumor, it is not suitable to puncture the focus, the treatment should aim at etiology.

34. Blockage Syndromes (Bi Syndromes)

Blockage syndromes are the syndromes characterized by obstruction of Qi and blood in meridians due to invasion of external pathogens and manifested by pain, swelling, heaviness and numbness of the limbs, and limitation of movement.

Blockage syndromes may include rheumatic fever, rheumatic arthritis, rheumatoid arthritis, fibrositis, neuralgia and gout.

Etiology and Pathogenesis

Blockage syndromes are caused by weakness of defensive Qi, dysfunction of the pores, when one is wet with perspiration and exposed to the wind, wading in water or dwelling in damp places for a long time. So the meridians and collaterals are obstructed by wind, cold and damp pathogens. The results are blockages syndromes. *Plain Question Bi Chapter* said "When wind, cold and dampness together invade to the body, the result is blockage syndromes."

There are different types of Bi syndromes, such as wandering Bi (in which wind predominates), painful Bi (in which cold predominates), fixed Bi (in which dampness predominates) and wind damp heat Bi (in which wind, cold and dampness turn into heat).

Differentiation

(1) Wandering Bi

Main Manifestations: Wandering pain in the joints, especially the wrists, elbows, knees and ankles, limitation of movement, chills and fever, thin and sticky tongue coating, superficial and tight or superficial and slow pulse.

(2) Painful Bi

Main Manifestations: Severe pain in all of the body or in the joints, alleviated by warmth and aggravated by cold, with fixed localization, but no local redness and hotness, thin and white tongue coating, string-taut and tense pulse.

(3) Fixed Bi

Main Manifestations: Numbness and heavy sensation of the limbs, soreness and fixed pain of the joints, aggravated on cloudy and rainy days, white and sticky tongue coating and soft pulse.

(4) Heat Bi

Main Manifestations: Arthragra involving one or several joints, local redness, swelling and excruciating pain with limitation of movement, accompanied by fever and thirst, yellow tongue coating, rolling and rapid pulse.

Treatment

Principle: The selection of the local points along the meridians is applied and points according to the syndrome are mainly selected. Ashi points are used together. Filiform needles are used for wandering Bi and heat Bi syndromes, reducing manipulation with shallow method. Subcutaneous needles may also be applied. For painful Bi; it needs prolonged retaining of the needles. It is better to use moxibustion of warm needles. Fixed Bi may also be treated by combined acupuncture and moxibustion, or together with cupping.

Prescription: Pain in the scapula: Jianyu(LI 15), Jianliao (TE 14), Naoshu (SI 10).

Pain in the elbow: Quchi (LI 11), Hegu (L 14), Tianzong(SI 11), Chize(LU 5), Waiguan(TE 5).

Pain in the wrist: Yangchi(TE 4), Waiguan (TE 5), Yangxi(LI 5), Wangu (GB 12).

Pain in the lumbar region: Renzhong (GV 26), Shenzhu(GV 12), Yaoyangguan (GV 3)

Pain in the hip joint: Huantiao (GB 30), Juliao (GB 29), Xuanzhong (GB 39). Pain in the thigh region: Zhibain (BL 54), Chengfu (BL 36), Yanglingquan (GB 34).

Pain in the knee joint: Dubi(ST 35), Liangqiu (ST 34), Yanglingquan (GB 34), Xiyangguan(GB 33).

Pain in the ankle: Shenmai(BL 62), Zhaohai (K 16), Kunlun (BL 60), Qiuxu (GB 40).

Wandering Bi: Geshu (BL 17), Xuehai (SP 10), Sanyinjiao (SP 6).

Painful Bi: Shenshu (BL 23), Guanyuan (CV 4)

Fixed Bi: Zusanli(ST 36), Shangqiu(SP 5), Yanglingquan(GB 34)

Heat Bi: Dazhui (GV 14), Quchi(LI 11)

Explanation: The above prescriptions are formulated on the basis of the different types of Bi syndromes. Wandering Bi is due to exogenous wind, Geshu (BL 17), Xuehai (SP 10), Sanyinjiao (SP 6), have the function of activating and nourishing the blood. The selection is based on the principle: "Wind will be naturally eliminated if blood circulates smoothly." Fixed Bi can select Zusanli (ST 36), Yinlingquan (SP 9), Shangqiu (SP 5), because damp water is obstructed. It is the basic principle to eliminate dampness. To select this point is in order to strengthen the function of spleen and stomach. Guanyuan (CV 4), Shenshu (BL 23), strengthen the kidney-fire and to relieve the cold, Dazhui (GV 14), Quchi (LI 11) are used to relieve the heat and release the exterior. The above prescriptions are formulated by the selection of the local and distal points on the meridians supplying the diseased areas. The principle of the treatment is to remove obstruction from the meridians and collaterals and to regulate Ying (nutrient Qi) and Wei (defensive Qi) for elimination of wind, cold and dampness. Shallow or deep insertion should be used and depend on the location and depth of diseases, depend on symptoms and signs to use the different manipulation and therapies.

Alternative Treatments
(1) Cupping
Heavily tapping to induce slight bleeding along the two sides of the spine or the local area of the affected joint plus cupping is often used for treatment of pain of the joints.

(2) Point Injection
Danggui, Fangfeng, Weiling are used to inject to shoulder, wrist, hip joint, knee points 0.5—1ml can be injected. Pay attention, don't inject the joint cavity, once injection every one to three days. Ten treatments are taken as one course. Don't use too many points for each treatment.

Remarks
(1) Acupuncture is effective in treatment: For rheumatoid arthritis, the pain is insidious, so long term treatment is needed.
(2) Bisyndromes have to be distinguished with bone tuberculosis and bone tumor in order to avoid incorrect treatment.

35. Wry Face
Wry face showed by deviation of eye and mouth means facial paralysis. It

mostly occurs in winter and autumn. It can occur in patients of any ages, but mostly at the age of twenty to forty, and more frequently in males.

Deviation of eye and mouth is divided into peripheral facial paralysis and central facial paralysis. The causative factor and clinical manifestations are quite different. The first type is caused by facial neuritis, the second type is caused by cerebrovascular disease or the tumour of brain. Here we only discuss peripheral facial paralysis.

Etiology and Pathogenesis

Deviation of the eye and the mouth is due to paralysis of the facial muscles caused by the attack of pathogenic wind and cold on Yangming and Shaoyang Meridians, which leads to malnutrition of the muscle and the meridians.

Differentiation

Sudden onset, one side of face numbness even the muscles paralysis, inability to frown, the eye can not be closed, salivation, shallow of mouth groove, deviate of the angle of the mouth, inability to swallow, in the affected side, inability to frown, raise the eyebrow, show the teeth or blow out the cheek, and in some cases, pain in the mastoid region or headache, poor sense of taste, sensitive hearing. Chronic case may have contracture of the atrophied muscles, mouth can be pulled to the affected side. It is named paradoxical wrying of face.

Treatment

Principle: The points both of Large Intestine and Stomach Meridians are mainly selected, and also the points of Triple Energizer and Gallbladder Meridians. The penetrating method can be used for the points on the face.

Prescription: Yangbai(GB 14), Sibai(ST 2), Cuanzhu(BL 2), Xiaguan (ST 7), Quanliao (SI 18), Juliao (ST 3), Dicang(ST 4), to Jiache (ST 6), Hegu (LI 4), Zusanli(ST 36).

Additional Points

Level of groove of nose: Yingxiang(LI 20)

Level of the philtrum: Renzhong (GV 26), deviation of the groove of the lip Chengjiang(CV 24)

Pain of the mastoid region: Fengchi(GB 20), Yifeng (TE 17), Waiguan (TE

5)

Explanation: Hegu(LI 4), Zusanli(ST 36) are used to promote the circulation of Qi of Large Intestine and Stomach Meridians, and they can eliminate pathogenic wind from the head and facial region. Yifeng(TE 17), Fengchi(GB 20), Waiguan(TE 5) can eliminate pathogenic wind from Triple Energizer and Gallbladder Meridians and to stop pain. Yangbai (GB 14), Sibai(ST 2), Cuanzhu (BL 2), Xiaguan(ST 7), Quanliao (SI 18), Juliao(ST 3), Dicang(ST 4), Jiache (ST 6) are the local points, they can promote the Qi of affected side.

Alternative Treatment
(1) The Cutaneous or Tapping Needing

Yangbai(GB 14), Taibai(SP 3), Sibai(ST 2), Qianzheng(EX) can be punctured by cutaneous or tapping needle, use the small cup for cupping in five-ten minutes, once every other day. This method is used for the new case, or numbness, feeling of facial paralysis.

(2) Point Injection

Selection of Points Yifeng(TE 17), Qianzheng(EX) are injected by Vitamin B_1 one hundred milligram or B_{12} one hundred. Each point is injected 0.5ml, once every day or every other day. Above these points can be changed each other.

(3) Paste Herbs on Points

Points Xiaguan is pasted with Ma Qianzi powder about one to two minutes, every two to three days. Change new paste. General speaking, four to five treatments are needed.

Remarks

(1) There are peripheral facial paralysis and central facial paralysis. Differentiation is necessary for these two types.

(2) For new cases, stimulation can't be too strong.

(3) During the treatment, avoid wind cold to affect the face. Massage and warming application are helpful.

(4) To prevent infection of the eye, the patient can use eyeshade and eye drop two to three times a day.

36. Atrophy-Syndromes (Wei Syndromes)

The Wei syndrome is characterized by flaccidity or atrophy of the limbs with motor impairment. It is also called "flaccid lame", the leg is usually involved.

The Wei syndrome is seen in polyneuritis, sequelae of poliomyelitis, early acute myelitis, myasthenia gravis, hysterical paralysis, and peripheral paralysis.

Etiology and Pathogenesis

(1) Burning Heat from the Lung

The muscular flaccidity or atrophy of the limb results from malnourishment of the tendons due to exhaustion of body fluid. This condition may be caused by exogenous pathogenic heat, attacking the lung.

(2) Damp-Heat

Exogenous pathogenic damp invades Yangming Meridian, the muscles and tendons become flaccid. So bones and joints can not move.

(3) Deficiency of Yin in Liver and Kidney

Deficiency of Yin in liver and kidney is caused by chronic illness, oversex, resulting in deficiency of Yin in liver and kidney.

(4) Trauma

The muscles and tendons are poorly nourished, and become flaccid.

Differentiation

(1) Heat in the Lung

Main Manifestations: Muscular flaccidity of the lower limbs with motor impairment, accompanied by fever, cough, irritability, thirst, scanty and brownish urine, reddened tongue with yellow coating, thready and rapid or rolling pulse.

(2) Damp-Heat

Main Manifestations: Flaccid or slightly swollen legs, a little hot feeling and fullness in the chest and epigastric region, painful urination, hot and brownish urine, yellow, sticky tongue coating, soft and rapid pulse.

(3) Deficiency of Yin of the Liver and Kidney

Main Manifestations: Muscular flaccidity of the lower limbs with motor impairment, combined with soreness and weakness of the lumbar region, spermatorrhea, prospermia, leukorrhoea, dizziness, blurred vision, reddened tongue, thready and rapid pulse.

(4) Trauma

Main Manifestations: History of trauma, flaccid paralytic limbs may be accompanied with incontinence of urine and feces, relaxed or hesitant pulse, pink or dark purplish tongue with thin white coating.

Treatment

Principle: Main points are selected from the Large Intestine and Stomach Meridians. The Large Intestine Meridian is mostly selected for upper extremity. The points of Stomach Meridian are mostly selected for lower extremity. For heat in the lung and damp heat, only punctured with reducing manipulation in combination with cutaneous or tapping needling by pricking. Reinforcing manipulation is used for deficiency of Yin of liver and kidney.

Prescription: Upper extremity: Jianyu(LI 15), Quchi(LI 11), Hegu(LI 4), Waiguan(TE 5)

Lower extremity: Biguan (ST 31), Huantiao (GB 30), Xuehai (SP 10), Liangqiu (ST 34), Zusanli (ST 36), Yanglingquan (GB 34), Jiexi (ST 41), Xuanzhong (GB 39)

Additional Points

Heat in the lung: Chize(LU 5), Feishu(BL 13).

Damp-heat: Pishu(BL 20), Yinlingquan(SP 9).

Deficiency of Yin in the liver and kidney: Ganshu(BL 18), Shenshu(BL 23).

Trauma: Huatuojiaji points can be used for affected area,

Incontinence of urine: Zhongji(CV 3), Sanyinjiao(SP 6),

Incontinence of feces: Dachangshu(BL 25), Ciliao(BL 32).

Explanation: Main points are selected from Yangming Meridians, according to *Plain Question* one chapter of Wei said "To treat Wei syndrome, only select the points from Yangming Meridians. Yanglingquan (GB 34) and Xuanzhong (GB 39), the converging points of tendon and marrow respectively are added to enhance the effect of nourishing the tendons and bones. Feishu(BL 13) and Chize (LU 5) are used to dissipate heat from the lung. Pishu(BL 20) and Yinlingquan (SP 9) eliminate damp heat. Ganshu(BL 18) and Shenshu (BL 23) are chosen to tonify the Yin in the liver and kidney. Huatuojiaji (points are selected to regulate Qi in the Governor vessel. Zhongji(CV 3), and Sanyinjiao (SP 6) are taken to adjust the Qi in the kidney and bladder. Dachangshu (BL 25), and Ciliao (BL 32), improve the function of the large intestine.

Alternative Treatment

(1) **Cutaneous or Tapping Needling**

Pricking method by cutaneous or tapping needling on above Yangming points. Jiaji points (three—five) vertebrae on upper limb. Jiaji points (thirteen—twenty one) vertebrae on lower limb. On the affected side do pricking method more and again.

(2) **Point Injection**

Selection of Points: Jianyu (LI 15), Quchi (LI 11), Shousanli (LI 10), Waiguan (TE 5), Biguan (ST 31), Zusanli (ST 36), Yanglingquan (GB 34), Juegu (GB 39), Vitamin B1 100 milligram, B6 50 milligram, B12 100 are given and inject on above-mentioned points, 2—4 points each time. 0.5—1ml injection on each point each time, once every other day, ten treatments are taken as one course.

Remarks

(1) Since the Wei syndrome needs a long period of treatment, the patients should cooperate with the doctor during the treatment. The results are individual.

(2) It is necessary to check up to make clear location and causative factors.

(3) During the period of treatment, medicine, massage and physical therapy can be used together to get better result.

4. With the help of doctor, the patient needs more functional exercise. It is very important.

Section 2 Gynecological and Pediatric Diseases

1. Irregular Menstruation

Irregular menstruation refers to the abnormal changes of menstrual cycle, quantity and color of bleeding accompanied by other symptoms. The common conditions are predated and postdated menstruation and irregular menstrual cycle. It is often found in menstrual disorders due to hypophyseal or ovarian dysfunctions.

Etiology and Pathogenesis

(1) **Predated Menstruation**

It is mainly caused by fire transformed from long-standing Qi stagnation due to mental depression or worrying, or by the accumulation of heat in uterus so covery of menses and easing of pain. Ciliao(BL 32) is an empirical point for dysmenorrhea.

(2) Deficient Syndrome

Principle: Points of Conception Vessel and the Back-(Shu) Points of spleen and kidney are mainly prescribed. Reinforcing technique with filiform needles is applied and moxibustion likewise.

Prescription: Guanyuan(CV 4), Pishu (BL 20), Shenshu (BL 23), Zusanli (ST 36) and Sanyinjiao (SP 6).

Explanation: Guanyuan(CV 4), the crossing point of Conception Vessel with three Foot-Yin Meridians in combination with Shenshu(BL 23) can be performed with moxibustion to warm the Lower-Energizer and to regenerate essence and blood so that Thoroughfare Vessel and Conception Vessel are warmed and furnished. Pishu(BL 20), Zusanli (ST 36) and Sanyinjiao(SP 6) in all are beneficial to reinforce spleen and stomach so as to replenish Qi and blood. When Qi and blood are sufficient, uterus and collaterals can be nourished and the flow is smooth in Thoroughfare Vessel and Conception Vessel, so the dysmenorrhea is eased.

Alternative Treatment

(1) Point Injection

Method: 1 millilitre of 1% procaine injection is injected subcutaneously into Shangliao (BL 31) and Ciliao (BL 32) once daily.

(2) Ear Acupuncture

Selection of Points: Pt. Uterus, Pt. Ovary, Pt Intertragus, and Pt. Kidney.

Method: 2 to 4 points are selected in each session. Needles are rotated to give moderate or intense stimulation and retained for 15 to 20 minutes. Embedding of needles in the points is also applicable.

Remarks

(1) Good personal hygiene: during the period, emotional stress is avoided. Exposure to cold and excessive intake of cold or raw food are prevented.

(2) Since there are various causative factors for dysmenorrhea, gynaecological examination is necessary in order to ensure the diagnosis.

3. Amenorrhea

Amenorrhea occurs around the age of 14 in healthy females. If the menarche does not occur over the age of 18, or the regular menstrual cycle has been established, but the menstruation has been suppressed over the period of 3 months excluding pregnancy and lactation, the conditions are known as amenorrhea which is often caused by neurological or psychiatric factors and ovarian or endocrine dysfunctions.

Etiology and Pathogenesis

The disease is classified into two types, deficiency and excess.

(1) Exhaustion of Blood

Generating function of spleen and stomach is lessened due to multiparity, over anxiety, constitutional debility, and physical weakness caused by chronic illness. so Yin and blood are consumed, leading to the exhaustion in the source of blood, thus amenorrhea results.

(2) Stagnation of Blood

Pathogenic cold guesting in the womb due to the invasion of cold and excessive cold diet, or disturbance of the Qi circulation because of the mental depression may give rise to blood stagnation in meridians, so the stagnation brings about amenorrhea.

Differentiation

On the basis of etiology, symptoms and pulse, amenorrhea is classified into exhaustion of blood and stagnation of blood.

(1) Exhaustion of Blood

Main Manifestations: Postdated menstrual period with the decrease and eventually the suppression of bleeding. Chronic case may be accompanied by sallow complexion, lassitude, dizziness, blurred vision, anorexia, loose stool, dry skin, pale tongue with white coating and slowish weak pulse which signify the deficiency of Qi and blood. Secondly, the condition can be also associated with dizziness and tinnitus. soreness and weakness of lower back and knees, dryness in mouth and throat, feverish feeling of palms and soles, tidal fever, night sweating, pale tongue with scanty coating and wiry, thready pulse which indicates the insufficiency of essence and blood.

(2) Stagnation of Blood

Main Manifestations: Suppression of menses for months, distending pain in lower abdomen intolerable with pressure, masses or lumps found in the lower abdomen, distention and fullness in the chest and costal region, dark-purplish sides of tongue or purple spots visible on the tongue, and deep, tense pulse.

Treatment

(1) Exhaustion of Blood

Principle: Points of Conception Vessel and Back-(Shu)points are prescribed as principal points which are manipulated with reinforcing technique in combination with moxibustion.

Prescription: Guanyuan (CV 4), Ganshu (BL 18), Pishu (BL 20), Shenshu (BL 23), Zusanli (ST 36) and Sanyinjiao (SP 6).

Explanation: Seeing that spleen is the acquired foundation and responsible for food digestion and the transformation of refined nutrients into Qi and blood which efficiently maintain the sufficiency of blood source and the subsequent normal flow of menses. Pishu (BL 20), Zusanli (ST 36) and Sanyinjiao (SP 6) are recommended to tonify spleen and stomach. Kidney is the congenital foundation and vigorous kidney-Qi may sustain the essence and blood, so Shenshu (BL 23) and Guanyuan (CV 4) are devoted to the reinforcement of Kidney-Qi. Ganshu (BL 18) serves to replenish liver-blood, as liver stores blood. At length, spleen, liver and kidney are efficacious to fulfill their respective functions of controlling blood, storing blood and storing essence, and Thoroughfare Vessel and Conception Vessel are abundantly nourished, so menstruation recovers.

(2) Stagnation of Blood

Principle: Points of Conception Vessel, Spleen and Liver Meridians are mostly prescribed. Reducing technique is employed.

Prescription: Zhongji (CV 3), Guilai (ST 29), Xuehai (SP 10), Taichong (LR 3), Hegu (LI 4) and Sanyinjiao (SP 6).

Explanation: Zhongji (CV 3), the crossing point of Conception Vessel with three Foot Yin Meridians, serves to regulate Thoroughfare and Conception Vessels and to smooth the flow in Lower-Energizer. Guilai (ST 29), selected as a local point, is employed to disperse the blood stagnation in the uterus. Xuehai (SP 10) from spleen and Taichong (LR 3) belonging to Liver Meridians play the role of freeing the flow of liver-Qi to dissolve the stagnation. Hegu (LI 4) and Sanyinjiao (SP 6) regulate Qi and blood and enable them to descend so as to reopen the menstruation.

Alternative Treatment

(1) Ear Acupuncture

Selection of Points: Pt. Uterus, Pt Endocrine, Pt. Liver, Pt. Spleen, Pt, Kidney, Pt. Ear-Shenmen, Pt. Subcortex and Pt. Ovary.

Method: 2 or 3 points in each session. Apply moderate stimulation. One session for every second day. One course consists of ten sessions. Embedding of needles in the points is also applicable.

(2) Cutaneous Needling

The cutaneous needle is used to tap gently or moderately the course of Governor Vessel and Bladder Meridian on the lumbosacral region, once daily. One treating course is composed of ten sessions.

Remarks

(1) Amenorrhea must be differentiated from early gestation.

(2) At the same time of acupuncture therapy, relevant examinations are essential to determine the etiology and to provide corresponding measures.

4. Uterine Bleeding

Nonperiodic uterine bleeding is called "Beng" and "Lou". A sudden and drastic onset that will be massive amount of bleeding is known as Beng while a slow onset with slight but persistent dripping of blood is named as Lou. Beng and Lou are intertransmutable as the emergent haemostatic, treatment may sometimes change the heavy running to the dripping of blood and the long-standing dripping may also develop to the bursting of excessive bleeding. This disease occurs mostly in the pubescent and menopausal females.

Etiology and Pathogenesis

The occurrence of the disease is principally caused by the harm of Thoroughfare and Conception Vessels and dysfunctions of the liver and spleen.

(1) Unfirmness due to Kidney Deficiency

Kidney functions in storation. Indulgent sexual intercourse undermines the kidney, and subsequently deplenishes Thoroughfare and Conception Vessels. Then blood and vessels become metablized and blood discharges from uterus beyond the menstruation.

(2) Transformation of Fire from Liver Stagnation

Mental depression makes the liver-Qi unable to flourish leading to the stagnation of Qi and blood which is transformed into fire. Liver fails in the function of storing blood. The pathogenic heat extravagates the blood.

(3) Spleen-Qi Deficiency

Spleen is weakened by irregular intake of diet and over anxiety. Then spleen fails in restraining blood, resulting in continuous dripping of blood as a mild case or bursting out of excessive bleeding as the severe condition.

Uterine bleeding is classified into excessive and deficient syndromes.

Differentiation
(1) Excessive Heat Syndrome

Main Manifestations: Sudden excessive vaginal bleeding or persistent dripping of blood, deep red in color, associated with irritability, insomnia, dizziness, red tongue with yellow coating and rapid pulse.

(2) Qi Deficiency Syndrome

Main Manifestations: Sudden bursting of blood in massive quantity, or continuous slight bleeding which are light red, thin, lassitude, sluggish limbs, shortness of breath, reluctance to speak, anorexia, pale tongue and thready weak pulse.

Treatment

Principle: Points of Conception Vessel and Spleen Meridian are prescribed as primary points. Reducing technique is used for excessive heat syndrome and moxibustion is inapplicable. Reinforcing technique and heavy dosage of moxibustion are applied to the deficient cold syndrome.

Prescription: Guanyuan(CV 4), Sanyinjiao (SP 6) and Yinbai(SP 1).

Additional Points

Excessive heat: Xuehai(SP 10) and Shuiquan(KI 5).
Yin deficiency: Neiguan(PC 6) and Taixi(KI 3)
Qi deficiency: Pishu (BL 20) and Zusanli(ST 36)
Collapse: Baihui(GV 20) and Qihai (CV 6) with moxibustion.

Explanation: The prescription acts chiefly to regulate and reinforce the flow of Qi in Thoroughfare and Conception Vessels and subsidiarily to clear heat and disperse the stagnation. Guanyuan (CV 4), the convergent point of Conception

Vessel with Thoroughfare Vessel and three Foot-Yin Meridians, serves to reinforce Qi in Thoroughfare and Conception Vessels so as to enhance the ability to stabilize and restrain the overflow of uterine blood. Sanyinjiao(SP 6), the crossing point of three Foot-Yin Meridians, is a major point for gynaecological disorders because of the action of building up spleen and strengthening its blood-restraining function. Yinbai(SP 1), the Jing-(Well)point of Spleen Meridian is used frequently in the the treatment of uterine bleeding. For a heat syndrome, Xuehai (SP 10)and Shuiquan (KI 5)are employed to reduce heat from blood on the purpose of arresting the overflowing blood. Zusanli(ST 36)and Pishu(BL 20)beneficial to replenishing Qi in Middle-Energizer, are supplemented to the syndrome of Qi deficiency, in the view that vigorous Qi is capable of restraining blood. Neiguan (PC 6)and Taixi(KI 3)are combined to nourish the heart and kidney aiming at the elimination of deficient heat. Moxibustion on Baihui(GV 20)and Qihai (CV 6)invigorates primary Qi to prevent Yang from collapse.

Alternative Treatment
(1)Ear Acupuncture

Selection of Points: Pt. Uterus, Pt. Subcortex, Pt. Endocrine, Pt. Ovary and Pt. Aadrenal Gland.

Method: Tender spots are punctured. Needles are retained for one or two hours. Needles are manipulated during the retention.

(2)Scalp Acupuncture

Bilateral Reproduction Zone is punctured with needle-rotating method for 3 to 5 minutes. The rotation is repeated for 2 more times with 5 minutes interval.

Remarks

(1)Menopausal females who undergo persistent uterine bleeding must be examined by gynaecologists to rule out tumours.

(2) When collapse occurs after heavy loss of blood, emergency measures must be given promptly.

5. Morbid Leukorrhea

Morbid leukorrhea is characteristic of constantly increased vaginal discharge and is seen in various diseases e. g. vaginitis, cervicitis, pelvic inflammation, and cervical carcinoma.

Etiology and Pathogenesis

Morbid leukorrhea is chiefly caused by the instability of Conception Vessel and the incapability of restraining of Belt Vessel. The consequence is the downward running or dampness and turbid fluid.

(1) Spleen Deficiency

Irregular food intake and over fatigue impair spleen and stomach which fail in the function of transportation and transformation, causing down flow of the accumulated dampness, hence leukorrhea results. The yellowish leukorrhea is ascribed to the damp-heat in spleen while the whitish is related to deficiency and cold.

(2) Yang Deficiency of the Spleen and Kidney

Weakness of kidney-Yang brings about the coexistent Yang deficiency in kidney and spleen, so water and dampness can not be transformed but run downward, thus leukorrhea occurs.

Differentiation

(1) Spleen Deficiency

Main Manifestations: Excessive white or yellowish leukorrhea which is sticky, odourless and persistent, sallow complexion or pallor, lassitude, anorexia, loose stools, edema of lower limbs, pale tongue with white sticky coating, and slowish, weak pulse.

(2) Damp-Heat

Main Manifestations: Profuse yellow leukorrhea which is sticky and malodorous, itching of vulva, constipation, dark and short urination, yellow and sticky tongue coating, and soft rapid pulse, or yellow and sanguineous leukorrhea, bitter taste, dryness in throat, irritability and feverishness, palpitation, insomnia, hot temper, yellow tongue coating, and wiry, rapid pulse.

(3) Kidney Deficiency

Main Manifestations: Large quantity of leukorrhea which is clear, thin and persistent, pain of lower back so severe as being broken, coldness in lower abdomen, frequent clear and profuse urination, loose stools, pale tongue with thin and white coating and deep pulse.

Treatment

Principle: Points of Conception Vessel, Spleen and Kidney Meridians are mainly selected. Reducing technique is used for damp heat and moxibustion is contraindicated. Deficiency of spleen and kidney is treated with even technique in combination with large dosage of moxibustion.

Prescription: Daimai(GB 26), Zhongji (CV 3), Ciliao (BL 32), Qihai (CV 6), Sanyinjiao (SP 6) and Taichong (LR 3).

Additional Points

Damp-heat: Xingjian (LR 2), and Yinlingquan(SP 9).

Spleen deficiency: Guanyuan(CV 4) and Zusanli (ST 36).

Kidney deficiency: Shenshu(BL 23), Guanyuan (CV 4), Fuliu (KI 7), and Dahe(KI 12).

Itching of vulva: Ligou (LR 5).

Sanguineous leukorrhea: Xuehai(SP 10).

Severe heat: Quchi (LI 11).

Explanation: Reducing manipulation on Zhongji (CV 3), the Front-(Mu) point of Bladder, can clear the damp-heat from Lower-Energizer. Daimai (GB 26), a crossing point of Gallbladder Meridian with Belt Vessel can consolidate the firmness of Belt Vessel and is a major point for leukorrhea. Ciliao (BL 32) selected as a local point is for suppressing leukorrhea and eliminating the damp-heat Sanyinjiao(SP 6) and Taichong (LR 3) are cooperated to reinforce the spleen so as to remove dampness and to reduce the fire from the liver. The combination is to reinforce the spleen so as to remove dampness and to reduce the fire from the liver. The combination of Yinlingquan(SP 9) and Zusanli (ST 36) can reinforce spleen to drain the dampness. Shenshu(BL 23), Guanyuan(CV 4), Dahe(KI 12) and Fuliu(KI 7), the combination between the adjacent and distant points can invigorate kidney-Yang to restore storing and sealing function of kidney, so Conception Vessel is firm and Belt Vessel is able to restrain hence the suppression of leukorrhea. Ligou(LR 5) clears damp-heat from Liver Meridian. Xuehai (SP 10) eliminates heat from blood. Quchi(LI 11) is supplemented to reduce heat when the heat is severe. They may assist each other to elevate the therapeutic effect.

Alternative Treatment

(1) **Ear Acupuncture**

Selection of Points: Pt. Uterus, Pt. Ovary, Pt. Endocrine, Pt. Urinary Bladder, and Pt. Kidney.

Method: 3 to 5 points are selected each time. The needles are retained for 15 to 20 minutes.

(2) Moxibustion with Moxa Stick

Selection of Points: Mingmen (GV 4), Shenque (CV 8), Zhongji (CV 3), Yinbai (SP 1), and Sanyinjiao (SP 6).

Method: Fumigating the points with moxa sticks for 5 minutes for each, once every second day, and one treating course consists of ten to fifteen sessions. The method is applicable to the deficiency and cold syndrome.

Remarks

(1) Acupuncture has certain effect in treating leukorrhea. In case of yellow and sanguineous leukorrhea, gynaecological examination must be given.

(2) Personal hygiene is important and the vulva has to be kept clean.

6. Prolapse of Uterus

Normally, the uterus is situated in the midpelvis and is anteverted and anteflexed. The fundus of uterus is at the level of the symphasis pubis and the uterine cervix is at the level with ischial spine. Whenever the uterus moves longitudinally downward along the vagina, and is lower than the level of ischial spine or even worse, protruding from the vaginal orifice, the condition is known as prolapse of uterus.

Etiology and Pathogenesis

The disorder is due to the constitutional debility, over exertion after delivery when Qi and blood do not get recovered, and multiparity which undermines Qi, so the deficient Qi sinks, and the uterine collaterals are flaccid and unable to restrain the uterus.

Differentiation

(1) Qi Deficiency

Main Manifestations: An object sinking in vagina, or moving down to the vaginal orifice, or protruding from the orifice as much as several inches, light red and goose-egg-like; subjective feeling of dragging down in the lower abdomen, lassitude, fatigue, palpitation, shortness of breath, frequent urination, profuse leukorrhea, pale tongue with thin coating and weak pulse.

(2) Kidney Deficiency

Main Manifestations: An object protruding from the vaginal orifice, soreness and weakness in lumbar region and legs, feeling dragging-down in the lower abdomen, dryness in vagina, frequent urination, dizziness, tinnitus, light red tongue and deep, weak pulse.

Treatment

Principle: Points of Conception and Governor Vessel are mainly prescribed. Reinforcing technique is applied. Moxibustion is used jointly.

Prescription: Baihui(GV 20), Guanyuan(CV 4), Qihai(CV 6), Zigong(EX-CA 1), and Zhongwan(CV 12).

Additional Points

Qi deficiency: Zusanli (ST 36) and Sanyinjiao (SP 6).

Kidney deficiency: Dahe (KI 12) and Zhaohai (KI 6)

Explanation: The prescription aims at elevating Yang-Qi and consolidating the fixing of the uterus. Baihui(GV 20), situated at the vertex is selected in view of that "A lower disease is treated with the selection of upper points" and "sinking conditions are elevated". Qihai (CV 6) and Guanyuan(CV 4) are used to replenish Qi so as to strengthen the stability. Zigong (EX-CA 1) is an efficacious extra point for this disease. Zhongwan(CV 12) is beneficial to Qi in the Middle-Energizer. Qi deficiency is supplemented with Zusanli(ST 36) and Sanyinjiao (SP 6) which act to build up the spleen and to replenish Qi in the Middle-Energizer. Dahe(KI 12) and Zhaohai (KI 6) are combined for kidney deficiency, to they are capable of tonifying kidney-Qi to enhance the stability of uterus.

Alternative Treatment

(1) Point Injection

Selection of Points: Pishu (BL 20), Ganshu (BL 18), Tituoxue (EX), and Weibao(EX).

Method: Each point is injected with 0.5 to 1 ml of 5% angelica injection, once for every second day on both sides alternatively. Only when the needle is thrusted 0.8 to 1 cm deep, the medicine is injected. One course consists of ten sessions.

(2) Electric Acupuncture

Selection of Points: Zigong(EX-CA 1) and Zusanli(ST 36)

Method: Zusanli(ST 36) is punctured with reinforcing manipulation. Zigong (EX-CA 1) is inserted with a 2-cun filiform needle obliquely toward the uterus until the patient feels upward drawing of the uterus associated with the soreness and distention in the lumbar region and the vulva. The electric apparatus is connected with the needles for 15 to 20 minutes.

(3) Scalp Acupuncture

Bilateral Reproduction Zone and Foot-Motor-Sensory Zone are selected. Needle-rotating technique is performed. Retention of needle ranges from 15 to 20 minutes.

Remarks

(1) Acupuncture has certain effect in treating prolapse of uterus in various degrees.

(2) Medication can be combined to those with constitutional fragility or secondary infection.

(3) Heavy physical exertion should be avoided. The patient is required to exercise the levatory ani muscle.

7. Morning Sickness

Morning sickness refers to the symptom-complex of nausea, vomiting dizziness, anorexia, or immediate vomitus on the intake of food, occurring in the first few months of pregnancy. It is the most common disorder in early pregnancy, severe vomiting may bring about emaciation, or other complications to the gravida.

Morning sickness is chiefly caused by the original weakness of stomach-Qi and the fetal Qi invasion to the stomach. Stomach-Qi, therefore, is unable to descend, but perversively ascend.

Etiology and Pathogenesis

(1) Weakness of the Spleen and Stomach

Stomach-Qi is primarily deficient. When the conception starts, menstruation is suppressed so the sea of blood does not discharge. Qi in Thoroughfare Vessel becomes vigorous and rushes upward to attack stomach. Stomach-Qi fails to descend and rises together with the Qi of Thoroughfare Vessel, thus the sickness takes place.

(2) Disharmony between the Liver and Stomach

After the conception, Yin and blood concentrate on nourishing the fetus. Liver blood is decreased and consequently Liver-Yang becomes predominant to over-act on the stomach. Stomach-Qi can not descend but adversely ascend, hence the disease occurs.

Differentiation
(1) Weakness of the Spleen and Stomach
Main Manifestations: In the first few months of gestation, nausea, vomiting of clear liquid or undigested food immediately after food intake, distention and fullness in the epigastrium, lassitude, sleepiness, pale tongue with white coating, and rolling forceless pulse.

(2) Disharmony between the Liver and Stomach
Main Manifestations: In the early gestation, vomiting of bitter or sour liquid, stuffiness in epigastrium, pain in costal region, belching, sighing, mental depression, dizziness, distention of eyes, yellowish tongue coating, and wiry rolling pulse.

Treatment
Principle: The points of Stomach Meridian, Conception Vessel, and Pericardium Meridian are selected as primary points. Even technique is applied to tonify the spleen, pacify the stomach, smooth the liver and disperse the stagnation so as to bring down the perversion of ascending Qi and to stop vomiting.
Prescription: Zhongwan (CV 12), Neiguan (PC 6), and Zusanli (ST 36).

Additional Points
Weakness of spleen and stomach: Gongsun (SP 4).

Disharmony between liver and stomach: Tanzhong (CV 17), and Taichong (LR 3).

Explanation: Zhongwan (CV 12) pacifies stomach to bring down the perversion of Qi and regulates the flow of Qi in Triple Energizer, as it is the converging point of Fu-organs, the Front (Mu) Point of stomach from which all the Fu-organs receives Qi and the convergent points of Conception Vessel, Small Intestine, Triple Energizer and Stomach Meridians. Zusanli (ST 36), the He-(Sea) point of Stomach Meridian is to restore the descending of Qi and is also a major systemic tonic point and the sovereign point for insufficiency of Qi and blood. Zusanli (ST 36) is combined with Zhongwan (CV 12) to reinforce the spleen, pacify the stomach, replenish Qi and blood and lower the perversion of Qi to cease vomiting. Neiguan (PC 6), the Luo-(Connecting) point of Pericardium Meridian, acts to regulate Qi, remove the stuffiness of chest, pacify the stomach and bring down the perversion so as to stop vomiting. In combination with Zhongwan (CV 12), it enhances the regulation of Qi flow in Triple Energizer. Gongsun (SP 4) is used to tonify the spleen and harmonize the stomach when there is weakness of spleen and stomach, for it is the Lou-(Connecting) point of Spleen Meridian. As one of the Eight Confluent Points connecting Thoroughfare Vessel, Gongsun (SP 4) replenishes Qi and makes the perversive Qi down in Thoroughfare Vessel known as "the sea of blood" and "the sea of Twelve Meridians", originated in the uterus. Disharmony between liver and stomach is supplemented with Tanzhong (CV 17) for which is the Front-(Mu) Point of Pericardium Meridian and the converging point of Qi, no doubt beneficial to regulating Qi and activating blood and invigorating the flow of Qi in Triple-Energizer to relieve the symptoms of distending pain in hypochondrium, belching, sighing, and mental depression, Taichong (LR 3), the Yuan-(Primary) Point of Liver Meridian, works to soothe liver, disperse liver-Qi stagnation, harmonize stomach and decline the perversion of Qi.

Remarks

(1) In early pregnancy, the fetus is not yet stabilized, so less points are prescribed. The needling should be gentle so as not to disturb the fetal Qi.

(2) The patient is kept quiet and rest in bed, cold, raw and greasy foot is prohibited. Frequent small-meals are beneficial to stomach-Qi.

8. Malposition of Fetus

Malposition of fetus refers to the abnormal position of fetus in uterus after 30 weeks of gestation which occurs mainly in multipara or gravidas with lax wall of abdomen. The gravida has no subjective symptoms, only can the obstetric examination ensure the diagnosis. The commonly-seen conditions include breech and transverse presentations.

Etiology and Pathogenesis

Uterine collaterals are linked with kidney. Constitutional kidney deficiency and the undermining of kidney by oversex or multiparity may give rise to the insufficiency of essence and blood. Furthermore, after conception, essence and blood are fully engaged in supporting the fetus and unable to sustain the uterus through the uterine collatesals, so the fetus is not maintained in normal position.

Differentiation
Usually the gravida complains of no subjective symptoms and obstetric examination is needed to make the diagnosis.

Treatment
Prescription: Zhiyin(BL 67) on both sides.

Performance: In the treatment, the patient unties the belt, sits in an armchair or lies supine on a bed. Moxibustion is given with mox stick on the points, 15 to 20 minutes each side, once or even twice daily until the malposition is corrected. According to number of reports, the success rate is over 80%. The effect is better in multipara than in primipara. The optimal success time is seven months of gestation. It is fairly unsatisfactory over eight months of pregnancy, needling is applied by some physicians but moxibustion is more employed.

Remarks
Malposition of fetus can be caused by various factors, so careful examination is necessary. If it is due to contracted pelvis, or uterine deformity, other relevant treating measures should be considered.

9. Protracted Labour
After the onset of pariturition, if the whole birth process exceeds 24 hours, it is known as protracted labor, was called "difficult labor" or "difficulty of labor" in ancient times.

Etiology and Pathogenesis
It is mainly due to the nervousness of primigravidas, or premature delivery which brings on early rupture of membranes and heavy loss of blood, or uterine inertia resulting from physical weakness with insufficiency of Qi and blood.

Differentiation
(1) **Deficiency of Qi and Blood**
Main Manifestations: Dull labor pain in the lower abdomen, forceless drag-

ging down and bulging sensation, large amount of light red heamorrhage, arrested labor process, pallor, lassitude, palpitation, shortness of breath, pale tongue, and weak pulse.

(2)Stagnation of Qi and Blood
Main Manifestations: Severe pain in the abdomen extending to the lower back, slight amount of dark red heamorrhage, retarded labor process, dark-purplish complexion, mental depression, distention and fullness in the epigastrium and chest, nausea, vomiting, dark red tongue and deep, forceful pulse.

Treatment
Principle: The points of Spleen and Large Intestine Meridians are prescribed as primary points.

Reinforcing technique is employed to the deficiency and reducing technique for the excess.

Prescription: Hegu(LI 4), Sanyinjiao(SP 6), Zhiyin(BL 67) and Duyin (EX-LE 11).

Additional Points
Deficiency of Qi and blood: Zusanli(ST 36) and Fuliu(KI 7)
Stagnation of Qi and blood: Taichong(LR 3) and Jianjing(GB 21).

Explanation: Hegu (LI 4), the Yuan-(Primary) point of Large Intestine Meridian accelerates and regulates the flow of Qi and activates the blood circulation to remove the stagnation. Sanyinjiao (SP 6), the crossing point of Three Foot-Yin Meridians, animates Qi circulation to eliminate stasis, and replenishes Qi and blood. Zhiyin(BL 67), the Jing-(Well) point of Bladder Meridian, and Duyin (EX-LE 11) are combined to enhance the oxytocic efficacy. Deficiency of Qi and blood is supplemented with Zusanli(ST 36) which builds up spleen and stomach to generate Qi and blood, and with Fuliu (KI 7) which reinforces kidney to strengthen the uterine contraction. Taichong (LR 3) and Jianjing (GB 21) are devoted to the stagnation of Qi and blood, for the formers can accelerate the flow of Qi to promote the circulation of blood, and the latter can regulate Qi and help parturition.

Alternative Treatment
Ear Acupuncture

Selection of Points: Pt. Uterus, Pt. Subcortex, Pt. Endocine, Pt, Kidney and Pt. Bladder.

Method: The points are needled with moderate stimulation. The needles are rotated in every 5 minutes.

Remarks

Acupuncture possesses oxytocic effect in treating protracted labour due to uterine inertia. The conditions caused by uterine deformity and contracted pelvis should be treated with other methods.

10. Insufficient Lactation (Appendix: Delactation)

Lactation starts in the gravida 2 or 3 days after the delivery. If there is insufficient lactation or even total absence of lactation, it is known as hypogalactia, or galactischia.

Etiology and Pathogenesis

(1) **Deficiency of Qi and Blood**

Milk is transformed from Qi and blood, but the transformation may fail because of Qi and blood deficiency which results from physical fragility of the gravida with dysfunction of transportation and transformation in spleen and stomach, and from the heavy loss of blood in the labor.

(2) **Liver-Qi Stagnation**

Emotional disturbance such as worry, anxiety and stress may impede the flow of Qi, so the circulation in the meridians is stagnated, hence the lack of lactation takes place.

Differentiation

(1) **Deficiency of Qi and Blood**

Main Manifestations: Insufficiency of lactation, even complete absence of milk after delivery, or decrease of lactation during the breast feeding period, no distending pain present in breasts, pallor, dry skin, palpitation, lassitude, poor appetite, loose stools, pale tongue with scanty coating and thready, weak pulse.

(2) **Liver-Qi Stagnation**

Main Manifestations: Suppression of lactation, distention and pain in breasts, mental depression, stuffiness in chest, pain in the costal region, distention and fullness in the epigastrium, decrease of appetite, light red tongue and wiry pulse.

Treatment
Principle: The points of Stomach Meridian are selected as principal points. Reinforcing technique and moxibustion are employed to the deficiency of Qi and blood and reducing or even technique is applied to liver-Qi stagnation.

Prescription: Rugen(ST 18), Tanzhong(CV 17), and Shaoze(SI 1).

Additional Points
Qi and blood deficiency: Pishu(BL 20), Zusanli(ST 36) and Sanyinjiao (SP 6).

Liver-Qi stagnation: Qimen (LR 14), Neiguan (PC 6) and Taichong(LR 3).

Explanation: The Stomach Meridian runs through the breast. Rugen (ST 18), a point of the meridian and situated at the breast, is recommended to regulate the flow of Qi to promote the lactation. Tanzhong (CV 17), the converging point of Qi, can regulate Qi and enhance lactation. Shaoze(SI 1) is the sovereign point for lactation deficiency. Pishu(BL 20), Zusanli(ST 36) and Sanyinjiao(SP 6) can tonify spleen and stomach so as to generate blood for the transformation of milk. Qimen (LR 14) and Taichong (LR 3) serve to regulate the flow of liver-Qi and disperse the stagnation. Neiguan (PC 6) is used together to regulate Qi and remove the stuffiness from the chest for the recovery of lactation.

Alternative Treatment
Ear Acupuncture
Selection of Points: Pt. Mammary Gland, Pt. Endocrine, Pt. Chest and Pt. Adrenal Gland.

Method: Find the tender spots. Rotate needles for several minutes. or embed needles from one day to one week.

Remarks
To treat insufficient lactation, good nutrition and adequate fluid intake are also necessary.

Appendix Delectation
Acupuncture is also applicable to delectation if breast feeding will not be

given after delivery.

Selection of Points: Zulinqi(GB 41)and Guangming (GB 37)

The points are punctured in combination with subsequent moxibustion for 10 minutes, once a day, continuously for three to five sessions.

11. Acute Infantile Convulsion

Acute infantile convulsion is one of the acute paediatric diseases with manifestations of coma, convulsion of limbs, lockjaw, and opisthotonus. It occurs mainly in those under 3 years, and is named as acute convulsion because of the sudden onset and the drastic symptoms.

This illness is often seen in disorders such as infantile hyperpyrexia, meningitis, encephalitis, hypocalcemia, atelencephaeia and epilepsy.

Etiology and Pathogenesis
(1) Invasion of Exogenous Seasonal Pathogens

Infants are fragile physically and of Qi and the constitution is of pure Yang character. When the exogenous seasonal pathogens invades the body, Yang-Qi fails in dispersion, but accumulates as internal heat which stirs up liver wind.

(2) Accumulation of Phlegm-Fire

The spleen and stomach are impaired by irregular intake or milk or food. Distribution of fluid is disturbed. Water in the body is stagnated and condensed as phlegm which accumulates and turns into heat, bringing on wind.

(3) Drastic Fright

Drastic fright may also give rise to sudden onset of convulsion.

Differentiation

Main Manifestations: In the beginning, there are high fever, flushed face, invotunlary motion of head, tongue and teeth, disturbed sleep, cry and fear on the waking, irritability, restlessness of limbs. When aggravated, there appear unconsciousness, gazing of eyes, lockjaw, persistent or intermittent contraction and tremor of limbs, gasping for breath, constipation, dark urine, superficial, rapid or wiry, rolling pulse, and blue-purplish finger crease.

Treatment

Principle: Points of Governor Vessel and Large Intestine Meridians are primarily selected and these from Liver Meridian are prescribed as secondary points. Superficial puncture is applied without retention of needles. Reducing technique of bleeding with three-edged needle is used.

Prescription: Shuigou (GV 26), Yintang (EX-HN 3), Shixuan (EX-UE 11), Hegu (LI 4) and Taichong (LR 3).

Additional Points
High fever: Dazhui (GV 14) and Quchi (LI 11).
Copious sputum: Lieque (LU 7) and Fenglong (ST 40).
Lockjaw: Jiache (ST 6) and Hegu (LI 4)

Explanation: The prescription aims at easing the convulsion by means of subduing wind, Shuigou (GV 20) and Yintang (EX-HN 3), situated in Governor Vessel, play the role of resuscitation and easing convulsion. Bleeding applied at Shixuan (EX-UE 11) serves to reduce pathogenic heat from various meridians. The combination of Hegu (LI 4) and Taichong (LR 3) is known as 4-gate points which are effectual to treat infantile convulsion, Dazhui (GV 14) and Quchi (LI 11) are supplemented to reduce the excessiveness of Yang heat for the condition of high fever. Liegue (LU 7), the Lou-(Connecting) point of Lung Meridian, and Fenglong (ST 40), that of Stomach Meridian, possess the efficacy of regaining the dispersion of Lung-Qi to remove the sputum. For lockjaw, Hegu (LI 4) and Jiache (ST 6) act to relax the mouth and cheek.

Alternative Treatment
Ear Acupuncture
Selection of Points: Pt. Sympathetic Nerve, Pt. Ear-Shenmen, Pt. Subcortex, Pt. Brain Point, and Pt. Heart.

Method: Strong stimulation is applied. Needles are retained for one hour.

Remarks
Acupuncture has a fair effect in relieving the convulsion, however the causes must be determined and relevant etiotropic therapies should be administered.

12. Chronic Infantile Convulsion

Chronic infantile convulsion is also known as "chronic spleen wind" with manifestations of convulsion, emaciation, diarrhea, etc. It is a serious condition and usually occurs in children under 3 years old after severe illness or with deficiency in Middle-Energizer due to chronic diseases.

Etiology and Pathogenesis

Chronic infantile convulsion mainly occurs after severe vomiting and diarrhea or is caused by weakness of spleen and stomach leading to insufficient source of transformation, over-administration of medicines with drastic cold or purgative property which over-act on spleen and stomach and deplete Yang in Middle-Energizer, febrile diseases which consume Yin with consequent insufficiency of kidney-Yin and liver blood, hence the stirring-up of internal wind, and acute convulsion protracted by improper treatment.

Differentiation

Main Manifestations: Sallow complexion, emaciation, lassitude, tiredness, sluggish or cold limbs, feeble breath, depressed fentanel, opening of eyes and intermittent contraction of limbs with lethargy. Greenish loose stools. tarsal and facial edema, deep slow and forceless pulse and pale tongue are due to spleen Yang deficiency. Lassitude, irritability, flushed face, completely or partially uncoated tongue, and deep, thready and rapid pulse are due to Yin deficiency of liver and kidney.

Treatment

Principle: The points of Conception Vessel and Stomach Meridian and Back-(Shu)Points are primarily selected. Reinforcing technique and moxibustion are applied.

Prescription: Zhongwan(CV 12), Zhangmen(LR 13), Qihai(CV 6), Tianshu(ST 25), Zusanli(ST 36), Taichong (LR 3), Pishu(BL 20), Weishu(BL 21), Ganshu(BL 18)and Shenshu(BL 23).

Explanation: Zhongwan (CV 12), the converging point of Fu-organs, and Zusanli(ST 36), the He-(Sea)Point of Stomach Meridian are selected to build up the spleen and stomach so as to support the acquired foundation. Zhangmen(LR 13), the Front-(Mu)Point of spleen is to tonify spleen Yang. Qihai(CV 6) serves to enhance the Primary Qi for strengthening the transportation and transformation function. Tianshu(ST 25), the Front-(Mu)Point of Large Intestine Meridian, is performed with moxibustion to warm the cold and reinforce the deficiency of spleen and stomach and to assist the transportation and transformation to cure loose stools. Taichong (LR 3), the Yuan-(Primary) Point of Liver Meridian, nourish liver blood to subside the wind. Pishu (BL 20), Weishu (BL 21), Ganshu (BL 18) and Shenshu (BL 23) are devoted to invigorating the spleen and kidney and soothing liver for the subsidence of wind. In brief, the prescription is of efficacy to warm and tonify spleen and stomach and to consolidate the genuine source so as to calm down the wind.

Alternative Treatment
Cutaneous needling
Primary points: Dazhui (GV 14), Shenzhu (GV 12), Qihai (CV 6), Zusanli (ST 36), Weishu (BL 21), Pishu (BL 20), and Jiaji (EX-B 2) from T5 to L2.

Secondary points: Guanyuan (CV 4), Baihui (GV 20), Zhangmen (LR 13), and Tianshu (ST 25).

Remarks
Chronic infantile convulsion seems comparable to chronic cerebrospinal meningitis. Acupuncture can only relieve the symptoms of the disease. Western and traditional Chinese medicines should be used together at the same time.

13. Infantile Diarrhea
Infantile diarrhea is characterized by the increase in frequency of defecation with loose or watery stools, and is a common pediatric disease occurring all year around, especially in summer and autumn.

Etiology and Pathogenesis
Infants have frail spleen and stomach which can be easily impaired by the improper nursing and irregular or unclean diet. The function of transportation and transformation is impaired, giving rise to the failure of digesting food and drink which therefore are not separated but discharged all through the large intestine, thus diarrhea results. The endogenous damage from improper diet is one of the principal causes for infantile diarrhea. In addition, due to the fragility of Zang-Fu organs in infants, the occasional invasion of exogenous pathogens may also directly disturb spleen and stomach and bring on dysfunction in transportation and transformation, consequently the disease occurs.

Differentiation
Main Manifestations: Abdominal distention, borborygmus, and persistent

abdominal pain followed by the instant desire to empty the bowel and being alleviated after the diarrhea, several times of defecation a day with sour and putrid feces, or with undigested food, frequence of belching, anorexia, sticky tongue coating, and rolling, forceful pulse. All the symptoms indicate the syndrome of overfeeding. Yellow odorous loose stools, abdominal pain, fever, thirst, burning sensation at the anus, dark and short urination, yellowish sticky tongue coating and rolling rapid pulse signify the syndrome of damp heat.

Treatment

Principle: Points are mainly selected from Stomach Meridian. Needles are not retained.

Prescription: Tianshu(ST 25), Shangjuxu(ST 37) and Sifeng(EX-UE 10).

Additional Points

Diarrhea due to overfeeding: Jianli(CV 11) and Qihai(CV 6)

Damp-heat diarrhea: Quchi(LI 11), Hegu(LI 4) and Yinlingquan(SP 9).

Explanation: Tianshu(ST 25), serving as the Front-(Mu)Point of Large Intestine Meridian, and Shangjuxu(ST 37), the lower He-(Sea)Point of Large Intestine Meridian are used in combination to regulate the intestines and relieve diarrhea. Sifeng(EX-UE 10) is to promote the digestion, and invigorate the transportation so as to relieve the retention of food and diarrhea. Jianli(CV 11) and Qihai(CV 6) are used to build up spleen and stomach, to relieve food retention, and distention. Quchi(LI 11) and Hegu(LI 4) serve to clear heat. Yinlingquan(SP 9) is used in combination to dispel dampness and relieve diarrhea.

Remarks

(1) Be aware that severe diarrhea is apt to develop into the critical condition with depletion of Yin and Yang, and further the collapse of Qi and exhaustion of Yin.

(2) During the treatment, food should be restricted. Only small amount of light diet is given.

14. Children's Malnutrition

Children's malnutrition is a pediatric disease characterized by emaciation, sparse hair, distention of belly, protruding blue veins, parorexia, and lassitude.

It may occur in the conditions of underfeeding and inadequate diet, and in the disease e.g. chronic diarrhea, intestinal parasitosis, and tuberculosis.

Etiology and Pathogenesis

The factors of irregular food intake, early cessation of nursing, improper feeding, inadequated care after illness, medication, and parasitosis may impair the functions of spleen and stomach and consume body fluid, resulting in the failure of digesting. Long-standing stagnation of undigested food will turn into heat and bring about malnutrition.

Differentiation

Main Manifestations: Progressing onset, and at the beginning, there are slight fever, or afternoon tidal fever, dry mouth, abdominal distention, diarrhea with foul and putrid feces, rice-water-like urine, irritable crying, and anorexia. Later, there appear internal stagnation with distending belly, protruding navel, sallow complexion, emaciation, dry and scaly skin, sparse hair, sticky and dirty tongue coating or absence of coating and weak pulse all of which are ascribed to the deficiency of spleen and stomach. The abnormal appetite with irregularity of hunger and satiety and the parorexia are due to the parasitosis.

Treatment

Principle: The points of Spleen and Stomach Meridians are principally selected. Superficial puncture is performed without retention of needles.

Prescription: Xiawan(CV 10), Zusanli(ST 36), Taibai(SP 3) and Sifeng(EX-UE 10).

Additional Points

Parasitosis: Baichongwo (EX-LE 3).

Tidal fever: Dazhui(GV 14).

Bloodletting is applicable at Pishu (BL 20), Weishu (BL 21) and Ganshu (BL 18).

Explanation: The etiological cause for this disease is the dysfunction of transportation and transformation in spleen and stomach which form the acquired foundation. Xiawan(CV 10), situated at the lower outlet of the stomach, is used to remove the retention and stagnation. Zusanli (ST 36), the Lower He-(Sea) Point of Stomach Meridian, serves to build up the earth for replenishing Qi in

Middle-Energizer. Taibai(SP 3), the Yuan-(Primary)Point of Spleen Meridian, is to reinforce spleen and to remove the stagnation. Sifeng(EX-UE 10)is an efficacious extra point for the malnutrition. Baichongwo(EX) is the sovereign point for parasitosis. Bleeding at Pishu(BL 20), Weishu (BL 21)and Ganshu (BL 18) is beneficial to invigorate Qi of spleen and stomach to recover the transportation and transformation.

Remarks

(1)Children with malnutrition must take diet regularly. Excessive intake of rich food and the variability between overfeeding and underfeeding are avoided.

(2)During the weaning, the weaning must be provided with adequate nourishment.

(3)If the malnutrition results from parasitosis or tuberculosis, the primary diseases should be treated.

15. Infantile Paralysis

Infantile paralysis is categorized to "Wei-Syndrome" in traditional Chinese medicine. The disease stated here is the sequela of poliomyelitis.

Etiology and Pathogenesis

This disease is caused mainly by the invasion of pathogenic wind, dampness and heat. The epidemic pathogens attack spleen and stomach through nose and mouth and accumulate to turn into heat which wander in the meridians and stagnate their flow. Consequently, the circulation of Qi and blood gets inactive and is unable to nourish the tendons, vessels and muscles, thus the paralysis of limbs occurs. The illness in a long run will give rise to the deficiency of Qi and blood and undermine liver and kidney. Tendons and muscles wither. Therefore, in the later stage, the disease is manifested by flaccid tendons, atrophic muscles and deformed bones.

Differentiation

Main Manifestations: The chief complaint of the disease is paralysis which is manifested with paralytic and flaccid limbs, mainly lower limbs of one side, or with hemiplegia, paralysis may also occur in other muscles e. g. intercostal muscles and diaphragm, and the condition is severe. In a chronic case, muscles in the affected part get atrophic with deformity of trunk, so the paralysis is refractory.

Treatment

Principle: Points of Yangming Meridians are principally selected and local points from the affected regions are supplemented. Either reducing or reinforcing technique is applied according to the character of the disease.

Prescription: Upper limb paralysis: Jianyu(LI 15), Quchi(LI 11), Waiguan (TE 5), Hegu(LI 4), Dazhui(GV 14) and Tianzhu(BL 10).

Lower limb paralysis: Huantiao(GB 30), Biguan(ST 31), Zusanli(ST 36), Yanglingquan(GB 34), Xuanzhong(GB 39), Kunlun(BL 60), Sanyinjiao(SP 6), Jiexi (ST 41)and Jiaji(EX-B2) from L1 to L5.

Abdominal muscle paralysis: Liangmen(ST 21), Tianshu(ST 25), Daimai (GB 26)and Guanyuan(CV 4).

Additional Points

Back knee: Chengfu(BL 36), Weizhong(BL 40) and Chengshan(BL 57).
Inversion of foot: Fengshi(GB 31) and Shenmai(BL 62).
Exversion of foot: Taixi(KI 3) and Zhaohai(KI 6).
Drop of wrist: Yangchi(TE 4) and Zhongquan(EX-UE 3).

Explanation: In the prescription, points of Yangming Meridians are mostly selected on the basis of forty-fourth chapter of *Plain Question* that Yangming meridians are mainly recommended to treat Wei-syndrome "Yanglingquan(GB 34), the converging point of tendons and Xuanzhong(GB 39), the converging point of marrow can enhance the nourishment of tendons and bones. Other component points are local or adjacent ones and used to regulate the flow of Qi in meridians by removing the obstruction and stagnation. Jiaji(EX-B2), the extra points serving to regulate the Zang-Fu organs and clear meridians, are also used as local points.

Alternative Treatment
(1)**Cutaneous Needling**

The points can follow the above-mentioned points. The treatment is given once daily or every second day. One course consists of ten to fifteen sessions.

(2)**Embedding of Thread(Catgut) in Acupoints**

The above-mentioned points are referred.

Remarks
Since the oral live pollomyelitis vaccine is employed for the prevention of the disease in the recent years, the incidence is markedly reduced. The sequela of the disease must be treated as early as possible and functional exercises can be combined. Plastic surgery is considered to these with serious deformity of joints.

16. Mumps

Mumps is an acute communicable disease characterized by abrupt onset and painful swelling in the parotid region. The modern medical term is known as epidemic parotitis.

The disease is mainly caused by epidemic wind and heat. The pathogens enter the body via mouth and nose and stay in Shaoyang collaterals, inactivating the circulation of Qi and blood, and bringing on stagnation in the parotid region.

Differentiation
Main Manifestations: In a mild case, there is pain in the parotid region followed by swelling which will gradually disappear in several days if no other complications occur. In a severe case, chills and fever, headache, and vomiting can be present at the onset, Subsequently there appear heat, redness and swelling in the parotid region unilaterally or bilaterally which cause difficulty in chewing. When the disease is aggravated, high fever, irritability, thirst, swelling of testis, yellow and sticky tongue coating, and superficial, rapid or rolling pulse can be seen.

Treatment
Principle: Points of Triple Energizer and Large Intestine Meridians are mainly selected. Superficial needling with reducing technique is performed.

Prescription: Yifeng(TE 17), Jiache(ST 6), Waiguan(TE 5), Quchi(LI 11) and Hegu(LI 4).

Additional Points
Chills and fever: Lieque(LU 7)
High fever: Dazhui(GV 14) and Twelve Jing-(Well) points.
Painful swelling of testis: Taichong(LR 3) and Ququan(LR 8)

Explanation: The focus of disease involves the Shaoyang Meridians. Yifeng (TE 17) is the convergent point of Hand and Foot Shaoyang Meridians and is able to split the local stagnation of Qi and blood. Yangming Meridians run up to the face, so Jiache (ST 6), Quchi (LI 11) and Hegu (LI 4) are used to reduce pathogenic heat for antitoxidity. Waiguan (ST 5), is a distant point beneficial to the flow of Qi in Shaoyang Meridians to attain the efficacy of clearing heat and resolving swelling. Lieque (LU 7) serves to disperse wind and expel pathogenes. Dazhui (GV 14) and Twelve Jing-(Well) Points are employed to eliminate heat. Taichong (LR 3) and Ququan (LR 8) work to restore the flow of Qi in the Jueyin Meridians.

Alternative Treatment
Rush-Pith Fire Moxibustion
Method: The hair at Jiaosun (TE 20) on the affected side is cut. The rush pith soaked with sesame oil is ignited to burn the point swiftly. The fire is removed as soon as the sound of burning skin is heard. The moxibustion is given once or twice. If the swelling is not yet resolved, the treatment is repeated the next day.

Remarks

(1) Acupuncture has satisfactory effect in treating mumps. When there appear severe complications, adequate therapeutic measures should be combined.

(2) Since the onset, the patient should be isolated until the swelling has completely gone.

(3) In the epidemic season, Jiache (ST 6) and Hegu (LI 4) can be punctured twice daily for prophylaxis of the disease.

Section 3 External Diseases

1. Urticaria

Urticaria, known in traditional Chinese medicine as "wind wheal" or "hidden rash", is a common skin disease characterized by the eruption of bright red or pale wheals with itching and in most cases is evanescent in the short time after the acute onset.

Etiology and Pathogenesis
(1) Invasion of pathogenic wind: The loose pores are invaded by pathogenic wind which accumulates in the skin and muscles, hence the disease occurs.

(2) Accumulation of heat in stomach and intestines can neither be discharged nor be dissipated, but stagnated in skin and muscles.

(3) Parasitosis in intestines: The disease develops due to the constitution, overintake of sea food, or the parasites in intestines.

Differentiation
Main Manifestations: The disease may occur in any part of the body but mostly in the medial aspect of arms and thighs. There is an abrupt onset with the eruption of wheals in various sizes and shapes, but mainly in close aggregation. The eruption can be popular, evanescent in one place and rising in another, associated with intense itching, and aggravated or alleviated by the change of weather. Both the appearance and disappearance of the eruption are swift and no marks are left after the vanishing. When it occurs in the throat, there may appear dyspnea nausea, vomiting, abdominal pain and diarrhea are present when stomach and intestines are involved.

Treatment
Principle: Points of Large Intestine and Spleen Meridians are mainly prescribed. Reducing technique is applied.
Prescription: Quchi(LI 11), Hegu(LI 4), Xuehai(SP 10), Geshu(BL 17), Weizhong(BL 40) and Tianjing(TE 10).

Additional Points
Dyspnea: Tiantu(CV 22).
Nausea and vomiting: Neiguan(PC 6).
Abdominal pain and diarrhea: Tianshu(ST 25)

Explanation: The disease is due to the stagnation of pathogenic wind in the exterior, so Quchi(LI 11) and Hegu(LI 4) are selected to clear the Yangming and to remove the stagnation from the exterior. Xuehai(SP 10), efficacious to disorders of blood, serves in combination with Quchi(LI 11) and Hegu (LI 4) to dissipate the pathogenic wind, and to eliminate the heat from blood with reducing technique. Weizhong (BL 40), known as "cleft point of blood", and Geshu (BL 17), the converging point of blood are beneficial to the hidden rashes resulting from the insidious heat in blood. Tianjing (TE 10), the He-(Sea) Point of Triple Energizer Meridian, is employed to regulate the flow in Triple-Energizer so as to eliminate the stagnated heat.

Alternative Treatment
Ear Acupuncture
Selection of Points: Pt. Ear-Shenmen, Pt. Lung, Pt. Occipitus, Pt. Endocrine and Pt. Adrenal Gland.

Method: Needles are rotated and retained for 15 to 30 minutes. Or scratching puncture, or intravenous bleeding at the retroauricular veins is given at the back auricle, once daily.

Remarks
Acupuncture has satisfactory effect in the treatment of urticaria. To chronic cases, the etiology must be confirmed and relevant treatment is given. The above-mentioned therapy can be taken as reference in the treatment of cutaneous pruritus.

2. Acne

It is a facial skin disease characterized by pellet-like pustules, from which the white-oily powder-like substance can be squeezed out. The disease is also known in Traditional Chinese Medicine as "alcohol horn" or "acne of lung wind", and is apt to occur on the face and in few cases on the chest and back in both male and female youth. It is considered that the occurrence is mainly due to the heat in blood.

Etiology and Pathogenesis
(1) Overintake of greasy food leads to the stagnation of damp heat in spleen and stomach, which steams the face, causing acne.

(2) Lung Meridian is accumulated with heat and is invaded by pathogenic wind. The wind and heat steam the face, hence the disease results.

(3) The hot body is suddenly exposed to cold or soaked in cold water, so the blood and heat are coagulated on the head and face, bringing on the disease.

Differentiation

Main Manifestations: At the onset, there is a comedo as big as the pintip, or the millet, from which linear cream can be squeezed out. Subsequently, a pustule develops on the top of the comedo and is hardened, slightly painful and scarring.

Treatment

Principle: Points from Pericardium and Bladder Meridians are primarily selected. Reducing technique is employed to eliminate the excessiveness of heat and the toxicity.

Prescription: Yuji(LU 10), Zhongfu(LU 1), Feishu(BL 13) and Hegu (LI 4).

Explanation: Lung dominates skin and hair. Yuji(LU 10), the Ying-(Spring) point of Lung Meridian, and Zhongfu (LU 1), the Front-(Mu) Point of Lung Meridian are used together to reduce the heat from lung. Feishu (BL 13) serves to restore the dispersion of lung-Qi so as to remove the stagnation from skin and hair. Hegu(LI 4) regulates the flow of Qi to clear the heat and to soothe the exterior. Four points used together attain the effect of clearing lung, reducing heat and eliminating toxin.

Alternative Treatment

(1) Electric Acupuncture

Selection of Points: Quchi(LI 11), Hegu(LI 4), Dazhui(GV 14), Feishu(BL 13), Zusanli(ST 36) and Sanyinjiao (SP 6).

Method: After the arrival of Qi, the needles in 2 or 3 points are connected with electric apparatus for 20 minutes, once daily. One course consists of twenty sessions.

(2) Ear Acupuncture

Selection of Points: Pt. Lung, Pt. Ear-Shenmen, Pt. Sympathetic Nerve, Pt. Endocrine, and Pt. Subcortex.

Performance: Points are given routine sterile procedure, and then stuck with Semen Vaccariae and fixed with plaster. The patient is required to press the points 5 times a day, 3 minutes each time as hard as the feeling of slight pain. Two ears are alternated, five sessions form a course.

(3) Red-Hot Needling

Selection of Points: Geshu(BL 17), Feishu(BL 13) and Dazhui(GV 14).

Performance: The needle is burnt red, and thrusted into the points swiftly as deep as 0.2 to 0.3 cun. Once for every second day. One course is composed of ten sessions.

(4) Autohemo Injection

Selection of Points: Zusanli(ST 36), one side or both sides.

Performance: The amount of 4 ml of blood is abstracted from the patient and immediately injected into the point 2 millilitres each side, once weekly. One course consists of five sessions.

3. Erysipelas

Erysipelas is an acute contagious skin disease which is characterized by the onset of sudden reddening of skin. It may occur in any part of the body, therefore is named with various terms in Traditional Chinese Medicine, e.g. "erysipelas of head fire", "red immigrant erysipelas" and "shank erysipelas."

Etiology and Pathogenesis

The disease is due to the accumulation of damp heat in spleen and stomach, invasion of exogenous wind heat giving birth to heat in blood which stagnates in skin and muscles, and the entering of toxic matters via lesions of skin. The occurrence on face and head is mostly caused by wind heat while that on the lower limbs is mostly related to damp heat.

Differentiation

Main Manifestations: There is a rapid onset with red hot and painful lesion of the skin which is cloud-like and circumscribed, but soon spreads to all around. The color in the middle of the lesion gets healed with desquamation in several days. If chills, fever, headache, red tongue with thin and yellowish coating and superficial and rapid pulse are present, it is a syndrome of wind heat. If there are fever, irritability, thirst, stuffiness in chest, poor appetite, constipation, dark urine, sticky and yellow tongue coating, and soft rapid pulse, it is a syndrome of damp heat. High fever, vomiting, unconsciousness, delirium, and occasional convulsion of limbs symbolize the syndrome of internal transmission of toxicity.

Treatment

Principle: Points of Large Intestine and Spleen Meridians are mainly prescribed. Reducing technique or bloodletting in the local region is applied.

Prescription: Quchi(LI 11), Hegu(LI 4), Quze(PC 3), Weizhong(BL 40), Xuehai(SP 10) and Ashi points.

Additional Points

Wind heat: Fengchi(GB 20)

Damp-heat: Zusanli(ST 36) and Yinlingquan(SP 9).

Fever: Dazhui (GV 14).

Internal transmission of toxin: Twelve Jing-(Well) points, and Laogong(PC 8).

Constipation: Zhigou (TE 6).

Explanation: Quchi(LI 11) and Hegu(LI 4) serve to disperse the wind heat from Yangming. Reducing Xuehai(SP 10) and Weizhong(BL 40) and bleeding applied at Quze(PC 3) and Ashi points aim at clearing heat from blood. Zusanli (ST 36) and Yinlingquan(SP 9) eliminate damp-heat. Bloodletting at the Twelve Jing-(Well) points and reducing Laogon(PC 8) are efficacious to reduce heat and clear heart for resuscitation. Reducing Dazhui(GV 14) and Fengchi(GB 20) is able to eliminate heat and relieve the exterior. Zhigou(TE 6) can clear heat and move the bowels.

Alternative Treatment
Bleedletting plus Cupping

Method: The focus of redness and swelling is punctured with a three-edged needle in a leopard-spot way, or is tapped with a cutaneous needle for bloodletting. Cupping is given after the needling, once or twice a day.

Remarks

Disinfection should be stressed in acupuncture for erysipelas in order to prevent infection. If there appear ulceration, septicemia and pyemia due to spreading of infection, integrated treatment with both Traditional Chinese Medicine and western medicine must be given.

4. Herpes Zoster

This is a skin disease characterized by the eruption of vesicles running together like a string of beads associated with excruciating pain. It often occurs around the waist or on the chest and face mostly in spring and autumn.

Etiology and Pathogenesis
The disease is caused by the stagnated fire in Liver Meridian and the accumulated damp heat in spleen and stomach. The invasion of exogenous pathogenic heat stirs up the liver fire and enables the damp heat to steam and infiltrate the skin and the collaterals, bringing on the herpes.

Differentiation
Main Manifestations: At the onset, there are sharp pain and flushing of skin girdle-like in the local region associated with slight fever, fatigue and anorexia. Then there appear patches of vesicles in the size of mung bean or soybean which are sanguineous or pustular and lined bandlike. The eruption occurs in most cases, unilaterally in the costal region and sometimes on the face and head. In 2 to 3 weeks, the vesicles will dry up and form crusts and after the decrustation, the vesicles are healed almost, always without scarring. In few cases, the residual pain will extend for period of time.

Treatment
Principle: Points are mainly prescribed from the affected meridians. Local points are combined, reducing technique is applied.

Prescription: Quchi(LI 11), Hegu(LI 4), Xuehai(SP 10), Weizhong(BL 40), Yinlingquan(SP 9) and Taichong(LR 3).

Manipulation: The head and the tail of the eruption are distinguished. A three-edged needle is employed to thrust 4 or 5 times 0.5 cun away from both ends and several times more on both sides of the eruption according to its extent, slight bleeding is given. Then the above-mentioned points are punctured. Needles are retained for 20 minutes. The treatment is given once daily.

Explanation: Bleeding with three-edged needle around the focus serves to clear pathogenic toxins. Quchi(LI 11) and Hegu(LI 4) are used to disperse wind heat. Xuehai(SP 10) and Weizhong(BL 40) clear heat from blood. Yinlingquan(SP 9) and Taichong(LR 3) can eliminate damp heat from liver and gallbladder.

Alternative Treatment

Ear Acupuncture

Selection of Points: Corresponding tender points, Pt. Lung, Pt. Liver, Pt. Intertragus, and Pt. Infratrgic Apex.

Method: 2 to 3 points are punctured with intense stimulation by rotation of needles. Retain the needles for 20 to 30 minutes.

Remarks

Acupuncture has marked analgesic effect in the treatment of herpas zoster. Surgical measures must be taken to few cases with complicate purulent infection.

5. Boils

Boil is a common acute surgical disease occurring often on the face and the tip or fingers. At the onset, it is small-sized and deeply-seated with the root as hard as a nail. According to its location and the form, it has different names e. g. "philtrum boil" when located at the median groove of the upper lip "snake—head boil" when situated at the finger tip, and "red-thread boil" if a red line extends proximately from the boil.

Etiology and Pathogenesis

The disease is usually due to over-intake of spicy and greasy food which gives birth to the accumulation of heat in Zang-Fu organs and generation of endogenous toxin, or contamination of skin which results in the invasion of exogenous toxin inactivating the circulation of Qi and blood and remaining in interstitial tissue. It would be critical if the toxin is so vigorous as to run through the meridians to attack the internal organs.

Differentiation

Main Manifestations: At the onset, it appears like a yellowish or purplish grain of millet, or is a blister or pustule with a hard base, associated with numbness, itching and mild pain. Then there are redness, swelling, burning sensation and intense pain usually accompanied by chills and fever. Then the presence of high fever. irritability, dizziness, vomiting, unconsciousness, red tongue with yellow coating and rapid pulse signifies the toxicity of the boil, intoxicating the interior and it is known as "septic boil".

Treatment

Principle: Points of Governor Vessel and Large Intestine Meridians are mainly prescribed. Reducing technique or bleeding with three-edged needle is applied.

Prescription: Shenzhu (GV 12), Lingtai (GV 10), Hegu (LI 4) and Weizhong (BL 40).

Additional Points

Some points are supplemented in accordance with the meridians involved by the focus of the boil, e. g. boil on the face: Shangyang (LI 1) and Quchi (LI 11); on the tip of index finger: Quchi (LI 11) and Yingxiang (LI 20), on temporal region: Yanglingquan (GB 34) and Zuquaoyin (GB 44), on the fourth or fifth toe: Yanglingquan (GB 34) and Tinghui (GB 2); and the red-thread boil is punctured by pricking the red line from the proximal end to the focus on the purpose to eliminate the toxic blood.

Explanation: The Governor Vessel governs all the Yang meridians, so Shenzhu (GV 12) and Lingtai (GV 10), the empirical points for boils are reduced to disperse and discharge the excessive toxic fire from the Yang meridians. Yangming Meridians are abundant in Qi and blood, Hegu (LI 4), the Yuan-(Primary) point of Large Intestine Meridian is reduced to eliminate the toxic fire from Yangming and especially recommendable to the boils on face and lips. Weizhong (BL 40), the He-(Sea) Point of Bladder Meridian is bled to clear heat from blood. Supplementary points are selected for the treatment in light of the principle that "the illness is treated where the meridian is opened up."

Alternative Treatment

Pricking MethodMethod: Papular nodules are found on both sides of the spine and pricked with a thick needle, once daily.

Remarks

(1) At the early stage, the boil is prohibited from squeezing and pricking. Acupuncture and cupping are neither appropriate to the focus. Surgical incision is contraindicated to the red hardened swelling for the avoidance of spreading infection.

(2) The critical condition of septic boil must be administered with instant e-

mergency measures. The suppuration of boil should be treated by surgeons.

(3) Eruptive food like fishes, shrimps, crabs is prohibited.

6. Breast Abscess

Breast abscess is an illness in traditional Chinese medicine referring to the acute purulent disease of breast which occurs mainly in breast feeding women, but seldom in gravidas.

The term is equivalent to acute mastitis in modern medicine.

Etiology and Pathogenesis
(1) Liver-Qi Stagnation

Depression, anxiety, and anger may lead to liver Qi stagnation.

(2) Accumulation of Heat in Stomach Meridian

Overfeeding of rich food results in the accumulation of heat in Stomach Meridian.

(3) Lesion of the Nipple

The breaking of skin in the nipple is susceptible to the invasion of exogenous toxic fire into the breast which blocks the collaterals and inactivates the lactation. The toxic fire is mixed with the stagnated milk, forming the swelling and abscess.

Differentiation

Main Manifestations: Red painful swelling of breast develops after delivery. At the beginning, there are a lump in the breast, swelling, distending pain, difficult ejaculation of milk, chills and fever, headache, nausea, and irritable thirst, but purulency has not been formed yet. If the lump is enlarged, associated with bright redness, and throbbing pain, the suppuration develops.

Treatment

Principle: The points of Liver, Gallbladder and Stomach Meridians are mainly selected. Reducing technique is applied.

Prescription: Jianjing (GB 21), Tanzhong (CV 17), Rugen (ST 18), Shaoze (SI 1), Zusanli (ST 36) and Taichong (LR 3)

Additional Points

Chills and fever: Hegu(LI 4) and Waiguan(TE 5).

Distending pain of the breast: Zulinqi(GB 41)

Explanation: Since the breast abscess is caused by stomach fire and liver stagnation, Taichong(LR 3) is selected to soothe liver and disperse the stagnation and Zusanli(ST 36) and Rugen(ST 18) serve to reduce the stomach fire and remove the accumulation from Yangming. Tanzhong(CV 17) is used to regulate the flow of Qi and resolve the stagnation for the renewal of lactation. Jianjing (GB 21), is able to regulate Qi in chest and costal region, is a sovereign point for breast abscess. Shaoze(SI 1) is an empirical point for the disease. Hegu(LI 4) clears heat from Yangming. Waiguan(TE 5), connecting with Yang Link Vessel, is indicated to chills and fever. Zulinqi(GB 41) is capable of activating the distribution of Qi and blood, is used to open up the stagnation of milk so as to ease the distending pain of the breast.

Alternative Treatment

(1) Moxibustion

Before the suppuration, the focus is stuck with smashed garlic and white scallion stalk over which moxibustion is given with moxa stick for 10 to 20 minutes, once or twice daily.

(2) Cupping

After the suppuration, cupping with glass jars in proper size is performed on the eroded wound to suck out the pus.

7. Intestinal Abscess

Intestinal abscess is an acute abdominal disease with abscess occurring in the intestines. In ancient literatures, it is classified into large-intestinal abscess and small-intestinal abscess according to the location of pain. If the pain is around Tianshu(ST 25), it is called "Large-intestinal abscess" while the pain around Guanyuan(CV 4) is known as "small-intestinal abscess". Since the disease is symptomized by the limitation of right leg extension, it is also named "leg-contraction intestinal abscess."

This disease is equivalent to the acute appendicitis in modern medicine.

Etiology and Pathogenesis

The disease is mainly caused by irregular food intake, food retention, profuse cold and raw diet, disturbance by cold and dampness, running after big meal. These factors bring on the dysfunction of transportation in the intestines with accumulation of damp heat which stagnates the flow of Qi and blood. The stagnation is integrated with heat giving birth to the erosion of blood and tissues, thus the suppuration occurs.

Differentiation
Main Manifestations: Firstly, there is epigastric or periumbilical pain which soon moves down to the right lower quadrant. The pain is localized, intensified by pressure and accompanied by limited extention of right leg, chills and fever, nausea, vomiting, constipation, dark urine, thin, yellowish sticky tongue coating, and rapid forceful pulse. The presence of excruciating pain intolerable with pressure, tenseness of belly, palpable lump found in the local region of abdomen, high fever, spontaneous sweating, and surging and rapid pulse indicates a severe condition.

Treatment
Principle: Points from Large Intestine Meridian and Stomach Meridians are chiefly prescribed. Reducing technique is applied with needles retained for 20 to 40 minutes. The treatment is given usually once or twice a day, but once every four hours for the severe cases.

Prescription: Tianshu (ST 25), Lanwei (EX-LE 7), Quchi (LI 11) and Shangjuxu (ST 37).

Additional Points
Fever: Dazhui (GV 14) and Hegu (LI 4)
Vomiting: Neiguan (PC 6) and Zhongwan (CV 12)

Explanation: Lanwei (EX-LE 7) is a sovereign point for the treatment of intestinal abscess. Shangjuxu (ST 37), the lower He-(Sea) Point of Large Intestine and Tianshu (ST 25), the Front-(Mu) Point of Large Intestine Meridian are used together to eliminate the accumulation of damp-heat from the intestines, invigorate the flow of Qi and relieve pain. Quchi (LI 11), the He-(Sea) Point of Large Intestine Meridian, serves to clear the intestines and reduce the accumulated heat. Dazhui(GV 14) and Hegu(LI 4) are combined to enhance the antipyretic action and Zhongwan(CV 12)and Neiguan (PC 6) are supplemented to pacify the stomach for arresting the nausea.

Alternative Treatment
(1)**Point Injection**
Selection of Points: Lanwei(EX-LE 17) and tender spot in the lumbar region.
Method: 5 ml of 10% glucose injection are injected into the points as deep as 0.5 to 0.8 cun, once daily.

(2)**Ear Acupuncture**
Selection of Points: Pt. Appendix, Pt. Inferior Antihelix Curs, Pt. Large Intestine, and Pt. Ear-Shenmen.
Method: Intermittent rotation of the needles is applied, and continue the needle retention for 2 or 3 hours.

Remarks
(1)Acupuncture has good effect in treating simple appendicitis. When the symptoms are severe with the tendency towards perforation or necrosis of the appendix, surgical measures must be given instantly.
(2)The above-mentioned points can be also used to treat chronic appendicitis, once daily or every second day. Moxibustion with moxa stick or indirect moxibustion with ginger slice can be applied in the local region.

8. Goiter

Goiter is an illness symptomized by the enlargement or marked bulkiness of the neck and is popularly called "big neck" disease. It is characterized by diffuse swelling or lump in the neck, absence of skin discoloration, pain and ulceration, and difficulty of resolution.

The disease corresponds to simple goiter and hyperthyroidism.

Etiology and Pathogenesis
The disease is mainly due to anger, anxiety, sorrow, or mental depression. The emotional reaction gives rise to the stagnation of Qi. The long-standing stagnation will aggregate the fluid into phlegm and bring on blood stasis. So the stag-

nated Qi, phlegm and stasis are mixed together in the neck, thus the goiter occurs. Besides, inadaptability to the environment of location may be also a causative factor.

Differentiation
Main Manifestations: Growth of the diffuse swelling in the neck is painless, not circumscribed, and no skin discoloration. In some cases, it is big and drooping and usually changed with emotions. If the swelling is severe, there may appear dyspnea and hoarse voice. There can be also stuffiness in chest, palpitation, shortness of breath, tremor of fingers, irritability, hot temper, perspiration, exophthalmos, and wiry, rolling, rapid pulse.

Treatment
Principle: Points of Triple Energizer and Large Intestine Meridians are mostly prescribed. Reducing technique is applied with filiform needles.
Prescription: Naohui(TE 13), Tianding(LI 17), Tintu(CV 22), Tianrong(SI 17), Hegu(LI 4) and Zusanli(ST 36).

Additional Points
Liver Qi stagnation: Tanzhong(CV 17) and Taichong(LR 3)
Palpitation: Neiguan(PC 6) and Shenmen(HT 7)
Exophthalmos: Sizhukong(TE 23), Cuanzhu(BL 2), Jingming(BL 1) and Fengchi(GB 20).
Irritability, hot temper and sweating: Fuliu(KI 7) and Sanyinjiao(SP 6).

Explanation: Naohui(TE 13), the crossing point of Triple Energizer and Yang Link Vessel is punctured to open the Qi in Triple Energizer Meridian so as to clear the accumulation in the meridian. Since Yangming Meridians run through the neck. Hegu(LI 4) and Zusanli(ST 36) can regulate the flow in the meridian to disperse the aggregation of Qi, blood and turbid phlegm. Tiantu(CV 22), Tianrong(SI 17) and Tianding(LI 17), all situated at the neck are local points, being employed to activate the circulation of Qi and blood to resolve the stasis and phlegm. Tanzhong(CV 17), the converging point of Qi and Taichong (LR 3), the Yuan-(Source) point of Liver Meridian are used to soothe liver and to regulate its Qi. Neiguan(PC 6) can nourish the heart, calm down the mind and ease the palpitation. Sizhukong(TE 23), Cuanzhu(BL 2), and Jingming(BL 1), the local points of eyes, and Fengchi(GB 20) communicating with eyes, are used together to regulate Qi and blood in the orbital region on the purpose of relieving the bulging eyes. Fuliu(KI 7) and Sanyinjiao(SP 6) serve to replenish Yin and to suppress Yang aiming at the treatment of irritability, hot temper and profuse sweating.

Alternative Treatment
Ear Acupuncture
Selection of Points: Pt. Ear-Shenmen, Pt. Subcortex, Pt. Endocrine, and the corresponding points to the affected area.

Method: 2 to 3 points are selected each time, one session daily. These points are applicable to the simple goiter. Heart, Spleen, Brain points are supplemented to hyperthyroidism.

Remarks
(1) It is fairly effective to resolve the lump by means of surrounding needling around the goiter in combination with a perpendicular thrust in the centre of the goiter.

(2) When acupuncture is used to treat simple goiter, iodine can be orally taken to enhance the therapeutic effect. Surgical operation can be taken into consideration in case of prominent enlargement of the thyroid resulting in pressure symptoms. In the condition of hyperthyroidism, the presence of hyperpyrexia, vomiting, delirium, and thready, rapid pulse reveals the thyroid crisis, emergency measures must be given promptly.

9. Sprain and Contusion(Appendix: Torticollis)

Sprain and contusion refer to the injuries of soft tissues such as skin muscles, tendons and ligaments, at limbs, joints and body trunk without fracture, dislocation and skin wound. The folk name is "injury of tendons."

Clinical manifestations include swelling and pain in the injured area.

Etiology and Pathogenesis
Due to ill posture of carrying heavy things, improper movement, falling, bruising, traction and over-twisting, tendons, and joints are injured, the circulation of Qi and blood is stagnated in the local region and meridians and collaterals

are obstructed.

Differentiation
Main Manifestations: Swelling and pain with redness or ecchymosis in the injured area because of the obstruction. A new injury with slight swelling and tenderness indicates a mild condition while remarkable swelling and redness with motor impairment of joints signifies a serious case. An old injury has not marked swelling but has the repeated recurrence in case of the invasion by exogenous pathogenic wind, cold and dampness. The injury occurs mainly in the shoulder, elbow, wrist, back hip, knee and ankle.

Treatment
Principle: Points are mainly selected from the injured area. Reducing technique is applied. Moxibustion or warming-needling method is recommendable to the old injury.

Prescription: Shoulder: Jianyu(LI 15), Jianliao(TE 14)and Jianzhen(SI 9) Elbow: Quchi(LI 11), Xiaohai(SI 8), Tianjing(TE 10)Wrist: Yangchi(TE 4), Yangxi(LI 5)and Yanggu(SI 5)Back: Shenshu(BL 23), Yaoyangguan(GV 3)and Weizhong(BL 40)Hip: Huantiao(GB 30), Zhibian(BL 54)and Chengfu(BL 36) Knee: Xiyan(EX—LE 5), Liangqiu(ST 34)and Xiyangguan(GB 33)Ankle: Jiexi (ST 41), Kunlun(BL 60)and Qiuxu(GB 40)Neck: Tianzhu(BL 10), Fengchi(GB 20), Dazhu(BL 11)and Houxi(SI 3)

Explanation: Local and adjacent points are usually prescribed for sprain and contusion to activate Qi and blood and open up meridians so as to restore the function of the injured tissues. Local and distant points of the involved meridians can be used together for severe cases.

Alternative Treatment
(1)**Bleeding plus Cupping**
Method: Forceful tapping with a cutaneous needle is performed on the tender area until the extravagation of blood occurs, and then cupping is given. The method is applicable to a new injury with remarkable swelling, an old injury with long-standing blood stasis, and invasion of collaterals by pathogenic cold.
(2)**Point Injection**

Method: 10 ml of 10% glucose of mixed with 100 mg Vitamin B_1 injection is injected into the tender muscle bundle and it is required that the needling sensation should be propagated to the same orientation as the pain radiates. The injection is once daily or for every second day and is appropriate to the acute lumbar sprain.

(3) **Ear Acupuncture**

Selection of Points: Tender spots corresponding to the injured part. Subcortex, Ear-Shenmen, and Adrenal Gland.

Method: Moderate or intense stimulation. Needles are retained for 10 to 30 minutes, once a day or every second day. Applicable to acute sprain anywhere with noticeable analgesic effect.

Remarks

(1) Acupuncture has an definite effect in treating sprain. Fracture, dislocation and breaking of ligaments must be ruled out.

(2) Massage and medication can be used together when necessary.

Appendix: Torticollis

Torticollis, also known as "tendon injury of neck", here or refers to what is caused by bad position of sleep, or by the invasion of exogenous wind cold to the neck and back, which gives rise to the obstruction of Qi and blood in the local meridians.

Main Manifestations: Getting up in the morning, referred pain occurs on one side of the nape and upper back, even radiating to the homolateral shoulder and upper arm, and associated with motor impairment of the neck.

Treatment

Principle: Points of Governor Vessel and Taiyang Meridians are mainly prescribed. Reducing technique is applied. Moxibustion is also applicable after acupuncture.

Prescription: Dazhui(GV 14), Tianzhu(BL 10), Jianwaishu(SI 14), Juegu (GB 39), and Houxi(SI 3).

Additional Points

Limitation of flexion and extension: Kunlun(BL 60) and Lieque(LU 7)

Difficult rotation of neck: Zhizheng(SI 7)

Cupping can be given on the affected area. In addition, Laozhen(EX) can be applied alone.

Remarks

(1) Acupuncture has a fair effect for torticollis. Massage and hot pad can be applied after acupuncture.

(2) The height of pillow should be properly adjusted and exposure to cold should be avoided to prevent the recurrence.

Section 4   Diseases and Syndromes of the Eye, Ear, Nose, Throat and Mouth.

1. Tinnitus and Deafness

Both tinnitus and deafness are auditory disturbances, which can be caused by various diseases. Tinnitus is characterized by ringing sound in the ears felt by the patient and deafness is loss of hearing. Because of the similarities between these two conditions in etiology and treatment, they are discussed together.

Etiology and Pathogenesis

(1) Excess of Liver and Gallbladder

Excess of liver and gallbladder fire is caused by fury and fright with upward rush of fire of the liver and gallbladder that obstructs the Qi circulation in Shaoyang Meridians.

(2) Invasion by Exogenous Pathogenic Wind

Deafness and tinnitus are caused by exogenous pathogenic wind blocking the orifice.

(3) Deficiency of Kidney-Essence

Deficiency of the kidney Qi and failure of essential Qi to ascend to the ear. Deafness and tinnitus can be divided into two types.

Differentiation

(1) Excess Type

Main Manifestations: Sudden deafness, distention sensation and constant ringing in the ear that can not be relieved by obstruction of the meatus. In the case of upward perversion of pathogenic wind fire of the liver and gallbladder, there are distention in heat, flushed face, dry throat, irritability and hot temper, wiry pulse in the case of invasion by exogenous pathogenic wind, there are headache, aversion to cold, fever, superficial and rapid pulse.

(2) Deficiency Type

Main Manifestations: Hard hearing after chronic disease, intermittent tinnitus like singing of the cicada, aggravated by strain and alleviated by pressing to close the meatus, dizziness, soreness and aching of the lower back, and knees, spermatorrhea, excessive leukorrhea, thready pulse of deficiency type.

Treatment

Principle: The points of Triple Energizer and Gallbladder Meridians are used as main points, which are punctured by filiform needles with reducing manipulation for the excess and reinforcing manipulation for the deficiency. Moxa can be used on the local acupoints with small size cones.

Prescription: Yifeng(TE 17), Tinghui(GB 2), Xiaxi(GB 43), Zhongzhu(TE 3).

Additional Points

For fire preponderance in the liver and gallbladder, Taichong(LR 3), Zulinqi(GB 41) are added, for invasion of exogenous pathogenic wind, Waiguan(TE 5), Hegu(LI 4), for deficiency of kidney Shenshu(BL 23), Mingmen(GV 4), Guanyuan(CV 4), Taixi(KI 3).

Explanation: The Triple Energizer and Gallbladder Meridians travel to the anterior and posterior of the ear region, so points of these meridians are used, e.g. Zhongzhu(TE 3), Yifeng(TE 17) from Triple Energizer Meridian, Tinghui(GB 2) and Xiaxi(GB 43) from Gallbladder Meridian. Those are used together to regulate the Qi circulation in meridians, and serve as the main prescription for deafness and tinnitus, for excessive fire of liver and gallbladder to select Taichong(LR 3) of Liver Meridian, Zulinqi(GB 41) of Gallbladder Meridian to eliminate the fire of liver and gallbladder, according to the theory of the points which are located in upper part of body, using to treat the problem in the lower part of the body, and reducing manipulation used for the excess. Waiguan(TE 5), Hegu(LI 4) expel pathogenic wind. Shenshu(BL 23), Mingmen(GV 4), Guanyuan(CV 4) reinforce the primary Qi of kidney so as to conduct the essential Qi to the ear.

Alternative Treatment

(1) **Points Injection**

Selection of Points: Tinggong(SI 19), Yifeng(TE 17), Shenshu(BL 23), Wangu(GB 12).

Method: Select scopolamine injection and either of the bilateral point, 5 ml for each point. In case of 100μ Vitamin B_{12} each point 0.2—0.5ml is injected. Depth of needle insertion is 0.5—1cm.

(2) **Scalp Acupuncture**

To select vertigo and hearing areas on both sides, to manipulate needles intermittently, to retain needles for twenty minutes. To apply the treatment once every other day. This method is used for neural deafness and tinnitus and declining of hearing.

Deafness and tinnitus may be present in various diseases. Acupuncture has a good effect for neural deafness and tinnitus.

2. Congestion, Swelling and Pain of the Eye

Congestion, swelling and pain of the eye is an acute condition in various external eye disorders. The main symptoms are redness of the eye, swelling of the eyelids and pain of the eye.

Popular terms are "hong yan" and "huo yan". In the classic literature of Traditional Chinese Medicine. It is named as "feng re yan", "bao feng ke re", "tian xing chi yan", etc. According to the causes, acute or severe symptoms and epidemicity, this condition is involved in acute conjunctivitis, pseudomenbranous conjunctivitis, epidemic kerato-conjunctivitis.

Etiology and Pathogenesis

(1) **Exogenous Pathogenic Wind Heat**

This condition is mostly due to exogenous pathogenic wind heat causing obstruction of Qi circulation in the meridians.

(2) **Preponderancing of Fire in the Liver and Gallbladder**

This condition is due to preponderance of fire in liver and gallbladder which flares up along the related meridians, causing Qi stagnation and blood stasis in the meridians.

Differentiation

Main Manifestations: Congestion, swelling and pain of the eye, photophobia, lacrimation and sticky discharge. In the case of wind heat, there occur headache, fever, superficial and rapid pulse. In the case of preponderance of fire in the liver and gallbladder, there are bitter taste in the mouth, irritability with feverish feeling, constipation and string-taut pulse.

Treatment
Principle: The points of Large Intestine, Liver Meridians are used as main points, to disperse wind heat with filiform needles by reducing manipulation.
Prescription: Jingming (BL 1), Fengchi (GB 20), Taiyang (EX-HZ 5), Hegu (LI 4), Xingjian (LR 2).

Additional Points
Wind heat: Waiguan (TE 5)
Fire preponderance in the liver: Taichong (LR 3)
Explanation: The liver has its opening in the eyes, Shaoyang, Yangming and Taiyand Meridians all run up to the eye region. Therefore, Fengchi (GB 20), and Hegu (LI 4) are used to regulate the Qi circulation of the Yangming and Shaoyang Meridians in order to dispel wind and heat, Jingming (BL 1) is where the Taiyang and Yangming Meridians meet, and is used to disperse the local accumulated heat. Xingjian (LR 2), the Ying-(Spring) Point of the Liver Meridian can conduct the Qi of the Jueyin Meridian downward so as to remove the heat from the liver. Taiyang, the adjacent point to the eye region is pricked to bleed to reduce heat and relieve swelling. In case of wind heat, Waiguan (TE 5) is used to clear away the heat from eyes and head, the Yuan-(Primary) Point of the Liver Meridian, is selected to clear the fire from the liver and gallbladder.

Alternative Treatment
(1) **Ear Acupuncture**
Selection of Points: Pt. Eye, Pt. Eye No. 1, Pt. Eye No. 2, Pt. Liver.
Method: Retain needles for twenty minutes, rotate the needles intermint-tently, pricking method can be used on the veins on the ear apex or on the posterior of the ear.
(2) **Pricking Method**
This method can be used on the tender point between two scapulars or on the points with 0.5 cun lateral to Dazhui (GV 14). This method is used for acute conjunctivitis.

Remarks

In case of puncturing the point which is located inside of the eye orbit, the strict sterilization of the needles, slow insertion, gentlen rotation and no lifting and thrusting needle are required to prevent from infection or bleeding.

3. Rhinorrhea with Turbid Discharge

Rhinorrheat with turbid discharge is accompanied by nasal obstruction and loss of smelling. Other names are "Brain Ooze", "Brain Leaks." It is mostly seen in chronic rhinitis and chronic nasosinusitis.

Etiology and Pathogenesis

This disease is caused by the exogenous wind cold attacking the lung. The exogenous wind cold may transform into heat and disturb the nose, or the lung is directly attacked by wind heat, leading to dysfunction of the lung in dispersing, then the pathogenic Qi goes upward to block the nose. The third condition is that the pathogenic factors have been eliminated, but the rest of heat is still disturbing the nose.

Differentiation

Main Manifestations: Yellow fetid nasal discharge, nasal obstruction, loss of smelling, accompanied by dizziness, distention in forehead, poor memory, red tongue with yellow sticky coating, rapid pulse.

Treatment

Principle: The points of the Lung Meridian and Large Intestine Meridian are selected as the main points punctured by filiform needles with reducing manipulation to clear heat and to smooth the flow of the lung Qi, and to expel pathogenic wind heat to stop the nasal discharge.

Prescription: Chize(LU 5), Lieque(LU 7), Hegu(LI 4), Yingxiang(LI 20), Fengchi(GB 20), Zusanli(ST 36).

Explanation: Chize(LU 5), the water point of Lung Meridian, has function to reduce the heat from lung. Lieque (LU 7), is the Luo-(Connecting) point of Lung Meridian, and it is exteriorly-interiorly corresponding to the Large Intestine Meridian, and Large Intestine Meridian goes upward to the nose, when Lieque(LU 7), combines with Yingxiang (LI 20). Both of them can be used to promote the nose, reduce heat and stop discharge. Hegu(LI 4), Fengchi(GB 20) are used to smooth the flow of the lung-Qi and to release the exterior. Zusanli

(ST 36), is the He-(Sea) point of Stomach Meridian, the Stomach Meridian starts from nose, Zusanli(ST 36)can be used to nourish spleen and stomach, and also can tonify Qi and blood, to resolve the turbid phlegm, to reduce the dysfunction of Qi. It is an effective point for the chronic nasal disorders.

Alternative Acupuncture
Ear Acupuncture
Selection of Points: Pt. Internal Nose, Pt. Infratragic Apex, Pt. Lung, Pt. Forehead.
Method: Slight stimulation is applied, retain the needles for twenty minutes.

4. Epistaxis

Epistaxis means the bleeding in nose. The blood doesn't circulate in the normal way. As a result, the blood comes out from the nose. It can be caused by trauma, nasal disorders, acute febrile diseases, hypertension, liver cirrhosis, blood disorders and retrograde menstruation.

Etiology and Pathogenesis
Epistaxis is caused by the blood heat that damages the Luo Vessels. The lung-Qi flows up to the nose. The Stomach Meridian starts on the nose, and Large Intestine Meridian stops on the nose. If wind heat is accumulated in the lung or pathogenic fire in Yangming, they would rush upward to the nose. If there is Yin deficiency leading to upflaring of the asthenic fire, then the fire will be obstructed in lung. All of these cause heat to rush out of vessels, resulting in epistaxis.

Differentiation
(1)**Extreme Heat in the Lung and Stomach**
Main Manifestations: Epistaxis accompanied by fever, cough, red tongue, superficial and rapid pulse, or dryness, thirst with preference for cold drink, constipation, foul breath, red tongue with yellow coating, forceful and rapid pulse.
(2)**Deficiency of Yin with Preponderance of Fire**
Main Manifestations: Epistaxis accompanied by flush cheek, dryness of the mouth, feverish of the palms and soles, night sweating, afternoon fever, red tongue proper, thready and rapid pulse.

Treatment

Principle: The points of Large Intestine Meridian and Governor Vessel are selected as the main points. The reducing manipulation is applied to clear off the heat and stop bleeding for extreme heat in the lung and stomach. The even manipulation is used to nourish Yin and descend the fire for deficiency of Yin with preponderance of fire.

Prescription: Yingxiang (LI 20), Hegu (LI 4), Shangxing (GV 23).

Additional Points

Heat in the lung: Shaoshang (LU 11), heat in the stomach: Neiting (ST 44), deficiency of Yin with preponderance of fire: Zhaohai (KI 6).

Explanation: Yingxiang (LI 20) can help the nose and also it is the Vessel Point of Large Intestine Meridian. Hegu (LI 4) is used to clear off heat and stop bleeding. Shangxing (GV 23) is a point of Governor Vessel, and Governor Vessel controls all the Yang meridians. To reduce Shangxing (GV 23), is in order to reduce the heat from Yang. Kongzui (LU 6), the Xi-(Cleft) point of the Lung Meridian, the function of this point is to stop the blood. Neiting (ST 44), is a Ying-(Spring) point and water point of the Stomach Meridian. It is good for eliminating the stomach fire, Zhaohai (KI 6), has the function of nourishing Yin and reducing fire. All of these points have the common function to eliminate heat and stop nose bleeding.

5. Toothache

Toothache is a common ailment. It may occur due to wind fire, stomach fire, deficiency fire and dental caries. It is commonly seen in acute and chronic pulpitis, dental caries, peridental abscess and pericoronitis.

Etiology and Pathogenesis

Toothache is mainly caused by the tooth damaged by fire heat. The Large Intestine and Stomach Meridians go into the upper and lower gums, toothache may be due to flaring up along the meridian of the pathogenic heat in Yangming Meridian or from exogenous pathogenic wind heat that attacks and accumulates in Yangming Meridian. The stomach fire flaring up along the meridian, or deficiency of the kidney-Yin with flaring up of the asthenic fire may also give rise to toothache. Sometimes toothache is due to dental caries caused by overintake of sour, sweet food, and dirty accumulation on the teeth.

Differentiation
(1) Toothache due to Stomach-Fire
Main Manifestations: Severe toothache accompanied by foul breath, thirst, constipation, yellow tongue coating, forceful and rapid pulse.
(2) Toothache Caused by Wind Fire
Main Manifestations: Acute toothache with gingival swelling accompanied by chills and fever, superficial and rapid pulse.
(3) Toothache due to Deficiency of Kidney
Main manifestations: Dull pain comes and goes, loose teeth, absence of foul breath, red tongue, thin tongue body, thready and rapid pulse.

Treatment
Principle: The points of Large Intestine and Stomach Meridians are selected. Reducing manipulation is applied to eliminate heat and stop pain. For toothache due to wind fire, points of Triple Energizer meridian are added. The reducing manipulation is applied to dispel wind and clear off heat, for toothache caused by deficiency of Kidney, the points of Kidney Meridian are added. The even manipulation is applied to nourish Yin and lower the fire.

Prescription: Hegu(LI 4), Neiting(ST 44), Xiaguan(ST 7).

Additional Points

For toothache caused by wind fire: Yifeng(TE 17), Yemen(TE 2), for toothache due to deficiency: Taixi(KI 3).

Explanation: The Large Intestine Meridian goes into the lower teeth, the Stomach Meridian goes into upper teeth, so Hegu(LI 4), Jiache(ST 6), two points are selected, the combination of both of these two points is used to clear fire from Yangming Meridians for both upper and lower toothache, Neiting(ST 44) is the Ying-(Spring) Point and water point can clear stomach fire, it is combined with the local point Jiache(ST 6) to treat the lower toothache.

Yemen(TE 2) is the Ying-(Spring) point of Triple Energizer Meridian. It is combined with Yifeng(TE 17), the distal and local points can clear wind and fire, to stop toothache caused by wind fire. Taixi(KI 3), is the Yuan-(Source) point of Kidney Meridian. It is used to nourish Yin of kidney and lower the asthenic fire. It is used to stop toothache.

Alternative Treatment

Ear Acupuncture

Selection of Points: Pt. Shenmen, Pt. Subcortex, Pt. Toothache Point.

Method: Strong stimulation, retain the needles for 20 to 30 minutes.

6. Sore Throat with Swelling

Sore throat with swelling is a disease which is redness in throat. In TCM theory, "Hou Bi", "Ru E", "Hou Tong", all belong to sore throat. Wind heat, phlegm fire and Yin deficiency are the three causative factors. It is divided into deficiency and excess types.

It is mostly seen in acute tonsilitis, acute pharyngitis, simple laryngitis and peritonsillar abscess.

Etiology and Pathogenesis

(1) Sore throat caused by exogenous pathogenic wind heat that scorches the lung system and then is obstructed in the throat.

(2) Sore throat caused by over pungent food intake leads to stomach fire flarring upward, and fluid consumed, so the phlegm fire is obstructed in throat.

(3) Sore throat of deficiency of kidney-Yin that fails to flow upward and moisten the throat.

(1) **Sore Threat of Excess of Heat**

Differentiation

Main Manifestations: Abrupt onset with swelling pain in the throat, chills, fever, headache, thirst, constipation, tongue is red, tongue coating is thin and yellow, superficial and rapid pulse.

Treatment

Principle: The points of Lung Meridian, Stomach Meridian are selected as the main points, reducing manipulation is used to disperse wind and heat.

Prescription: Shaoshang(LU 11), Hegu(LI 4), Neiting(ST 44), Tianrong(SI 17).

Explanation: Pricking Shaoshang(LU 11) to let a few drops of blood out is used to clear off the heat from the lung and stop pain. Hegu(LI 4), disperses exterior pathogens from the Lung Meridian and the accumulated heat from Yangming Meridians, Neiting(ST 44), the Ying-(Spring) Point of the Stomach Meridian reduces heat in the stomach. Tianrong(SI 17) is a local point used to ease sore throat.

(2) Sore Throat of Deficiency of Yin

Main Manifestations: Gradual onset of dry throat, slightly congested throat with intermittent pain or pain during swallowing after too much speaking, the pain in the throat onset, hot sensation in the palms and soles, dryness of throat more marked at night, red and furless tongue, thready and rapid pulse.

Treatment

Principle: The points of Kidney Meridian and Lung Meridian are selected as main points to nourish Yin and descend fire to stop pain with reinforcing manipulation.

Prescriptions: Zhaohai (KI 6), Lieque (LU 7), Lianquan (CV 23), Futu (ST 32).

Explanation: Zhaohai (KI 6), Lieque (LU 7), a pair of the eight confluent points, relieve sore throat by leading the asthenic fire downward. Lieque (LU 7), eliminates the fire from the lung. Zhaobai (KI 6) nourishes kidney-Yin. Combination of the two points reduces fire and nourishes the fluid. They are the main points for sore throat. Lianquan (CV 23), is the local point near to throat, the function of Lianquan (CV 23), is to moisten the throat fluid. Futu (ST 32) relieves sore throat and pain.

Alternative Treatment
Ear Acupuncture
Selection of Points: Pt. Throat, Pt. Tonsil, Pt. Helix 1—6
Method: Moderate or strong stimulation is applied, retains needles in one hour. The treatment is given once a day.

7. Blindness with Insidious Onset

Blindness with insidious onset is a chronic eye disorder marked by gradual declination of vision. At the early stage, there is only blurring of vision, it is called "Shi Zhan Hun Miao" in Chinese, but in the later stage, the eyesight may be totally lost. It is mostly due to deficiency of the kidney and liver-Yin, deficiency of Qi and blood and stagnation of liver-Qi. It is mostly seen in optic atrophy.

Etiology and Pathogenesis

(1) Deficiency of the liver and kidney-Yin leads to consumption of the essence and blood that nourish the eyes.

(2) Dysfunction in transportation and transformation of the spleen due to irregular diet and overstrain results in inadequate supply of the essential nutrition for the eyes.

(3) Dysfunction of liver with stagnation of Qi and blood in emotional troubles causes failure of the essential Qi to flow upwards to nourish the eyes.

Differentiation
(1) Deficiency of the Liver and Kidney
Main Manifestations: Blurred vision, tinnitus, nocturnal spermatorrhea aching of the lower back, thready and weak pulse, red tongue, scanty coating.

(2) Deficiency of Qi and Blood
Main Manifestations: Blurred vision, weakness of breath, disinclination to talk, lassitude, poor appetite, loose stools, thready and weak pulse, pale tongue with thin, white coating.

(3) Stagnation of the Liver-Qi
Main Manifestations: Blurred vision, distention in both hypochondriac regions, dizziness, vertigo, bitter taste in the mouth, dry throat, string-taut pulse.

Treatment
Principle: The points of Kidney Meridian and Spleen Meridian are selected as the main points. To reinforce the liver and kidney and nourish Qi and blood by reinforcing manipulation for deficiency of the liver and kidney-Yin and deficiency of Qi and blood. The even manipulation is applied to the same points to remove the stagnation of the liver-Qi.

Prescriptions: Fengchi (GB 20), Jingming (BL 1), Qiuhou (EX-HN 7), Guangming (GB 37).

Additional Points
Deficiency of liver and kidney: Taichong (LR 3), Taixi (KI 3), Ganshu (BL 18), Shenshu (BL 23).

Deficiency of Qi and Blood: Zusanli (ST 36), Sanyinjiao (SP 6).

Stagnation of liver-Qi: Qimen (LR 14), Taichong (LR 13), Neiguan (PC 6).

Explanation: The Gallbladder Meridian and Bladder Meridian connect with eye region. So Fengchi (GB 20), Guangming (GB 37), Jingming (BL 1) are selected to regulate the Qi circulation in the meridians and to improve the eyesight. Qiuhou (EX-HN 7) is an extra point, effective for eye diseases. Ganshu (BL 18),

Shenshu(BL 23), Taixi(KI 3), Taichong(LR 3) are used to reinforce the Yin of the liver and kidney, Zusanli(ST 36), Sanyinjiao(SP 6) reinforce Qi and blood, Qimen(LR 14), Taichong(LR 3), Neiguan(PC 6) remove stagnation of liver-Qi.

Alternative Treatment
Ear Acupuncture
Selection of Points: Pt. Eye, Pt. Liver, Pt. Kidney, Pt. Spleen, Pt. Heart, Pt. Eye No 1, Pt. Eye No 2.

Method: Three to four points are punctured in each treatment. Moderate stimulation is used, retain needles for 20 to 30 minutes. Ten treatments are taken as one course.

8. Myopia

Myopia refers to normal vision for near sights while blurred vision for far sights. In ancient times, it is called "the syndrome of ability for near sights while aversion to far sights." The main causative factors are congenital deficiency, deficiency of liver and kidney and bad habits of vision. The disease is commonly seen in myopia, amblyopia and astigmatism.

Etiology and Pathogenesis
(1) Strain of Eyes

The liver stores blood, opens into the eyes, the vision results from the nourishment of eyes by the blood. Prolonged watching TV, reading in the dim or extreme bright light or lying in the bed or on bus, and prolonged reading will injure the blood.

The failure of the liver blood flowing up to nourish the eyes, thus, results in myopia.

(2) Insufficiency of Liver and Kidney

It can be caused by various reasons. Insufficiency of Yin essence leads to that kidney essence that fails to infuse the eyes.

(3) Improper Food Intake

Indulgence of certain food injures the spleen and stomach. Qi and blood can not be produced abundantly. Failure of the nourishment of the eyes leads to myopia.

Differentiation

(1) Injury of Blood Due to Over-Reading

Main Manifestations: Vision is gradually declining, soreness and distention of the eyes which is relieved by rest. The tongue and pulse are normal.

(2) Insufficiency of Liver and Kidney

Main Manifestations: Vision is declining gradually, dryness of eyes, dizziness, insomnia, poor memory, soreness and weakness of the lumbar region, red tongue and thready pulse.

(3) Deficiency of Spleen and Stomach

Main Manifestations: Myopia, indulgence of certain food, preference to cold food, sallow complexion or with insect spots, lassitude, poor memory, pale tongue, weak pulse indicating insufficiency of Qi and blood.

Treatment

Principle: The points are mainly selected from Bladder Meridian and Gallbladder Meridian to tonify the liver and kidney, benefit Qi and brighten the eyes by reinforcing manipulation.

Prescription: Fengchi (GB 20), Guangming (GB 37), Jingming (BL 1), Chengqi (ST 1) to the inner canthus, Ganshu (BL 18), Shenshu (BL 23), and Hegu (LI 4).

Explanation: The liver stores blood which nourish the eyes for the vision, the liver and gallbladder are corresponded externally and internally. There are Fengchi (GB 20), Guangming (GB 37), and Ganshu (BL 18) are selected. Shenshu (BL 23) is for tonifying liver and kidney so as to make the liver blood and kidney essence go up to nourish the eyes. Jingming (BL 2) is the crossing point of Bladder, Stomach, Small Intestine Meridians, Yin Heel and Yang Heel Vessels; Hegu (LI 4), the Yuan-(Primary) point of Large Intestine Meridian which has profused Qi and blood. The above-mentioned three points are used together to benefit Qi and blood so as to brighten the eyes.

Alternative Treatment

(1) Ear Acupuncture:

Selection of Points: Pt. Liver, Pt. Kidney, Pt. Urinary Bladder, Pt. Spleen, Pt. Heart, Pt. Eye, Pt. Eye No. 1 and Pt. Eye No 2.

Method: 3—4 points are selected with moderate stimulation. The needles are retained for 30 minutes. The treatment is given once every other day. Ten treatments make a course. Embed seed, press the points 3—4 times per day, change the points every five days.

(2)Plum-Blossom Needle

Tapping is applied around the eyes and Fengchi(GB 20),and Dazhui(GV 14), once a day, ten treatments make a course. Tapping with electricity can also be applied.

针 灸 学

付 炎 学

绪　言

　　针灸学是以中医理论为指导，运用针刺和艾灸防治疾病的一门临床学科。它是祖国医学的重要组成部分，其内容包括经络、腧穴、针灸方法及临床治疗四个部分。

　　针灸具有适应症广、疗效明显、操作方便、经济安全等优点，数千年来深受广大劳动人民的欢迎，对中华民族的繁衍昌盛作出了巨大的贡献。

　　针灸学是我国历代劳动人民及医学家在长期与疾病作斗争中创造和发展起来的。远在文字创造前针灸即已萌芽，当时的古人生活于洪荒大地，与鸷鸟猛兽相搏食，不能无病，一旦患病，往往会本能地用手或石片抚摩、捶击体表某一部位，有时竟使疾病获得缓解，经过长期的经验积累，逐步形成砭石治病的方法。1963年，内蒙古自治区多伦旗头道洼在新石器时代遗址出土了一根磨制的石针，据鉴定，认为是针法的原始工具砭石，因此，砭石的起源，可远溯到距今一万年至四千年前的新石器时代。

　　随着冶金术的发明，针具也得到不断的改进，由古代的石针、骨针、竹针而改变为铜针、铁针、金针、银针等金属制针，代替砭石之法，直到现在改进为不锈钢针。1978年，在内蒙古自治区达拉特旗树林召公社的出土文物中首次发现一根"青铜针"。1968年在河北满城发掘的西汉刘胜墓，内有金制、银制医针九根。制作颇为精细，证明了金属制针的不断进步。

　　灸法的产生是在火的发现与使用以后，人们发现身体某一部位的病痛受到火的烘烤而感到舒适或缓解，通过长期的实践，从各种树枝施灸发展到艾灸，形成了灸法。《素问·异法方宜论》说："藏寒生满病，其治宜灸焫。"即指此言，随着后世医学的进步发展为多种多样的灸法。

　　由于针灸用具材料的逐步改革，提高了针灸治疗效果，有力地促进了针灸学术的发展。

　　针灸学术的发展经历了一个漫长的过程。1973年湖南长沙市马王堆三号汉墓出土的医学帛书中，有两种古代经脉的著作，即"足臂十一脉灸经"、"阴阳十一脉灸经"。其中叙述了十一脉的循行分布、病候表现及灸法治疗。经初步考证，其著作年代早于《黄帝内经》，经络学说的早期面貌于此可见一斑。

　　至《黄帝内经》对经络、腧穴、针灸方法以及适应症、禁忌症等，都作了比较详细的论述，其中尤以《灵枢》所载针灸理论更为丰富而有系统，故《灵枢》又称"针经"。可见当时针灸学已经比较成熟，为后世针灸学术的发展奠定了理论基础。

　　现存最早的针灸专著除《灵枢》外首推晋代皇甫谧的《针灸甲乙经》，作者参考《内经》、《明堂孔穴针灸治要》(已佚)，论述了脏腑经络学说；依照头、面、胸、腹、背等部位记述腧穴，在《内经》的基础上发展和确定了349个腧穴的位置、主治及操作，介绍了针灸手法、宜忌和常见病的治疗，这是继《内经》之后针灸学的又一次总结，在针灸发展史上起了承前启后的作用。东晋葛洪著《肘后备急方》所录针灸医方109条，其中99条是灸方，引起了人们对灸法的重视，使灸法与针法一样得到了发展。唐代孙思邈在《千金方》中说明了"阿是穴"的取法和应用，并绘制了"明堂三人图"，分别把人体正面、背面及侧面的十二经脉、奇经八脉用不同的颜色绘出，尤其值得推崇的是提出灸法预防疾病的方法,为预防医学作出了贡献。

此后唐王焘在其所著的《外台秘要》中,全面介绍了灸法,为推广灸法起到了积极作用。隋唐设"太医署"来掌管医学教育,针灸成为其中一个专门学科,内设针博士、针助教、针师等从事教学工作,足见当时对针灸的重视。北宋王惟一编撰了《铜人腧穴针灸图经》,叙述了经络、腧穴等内容,并考证了354个腧穴,全书曾刻在石碑上,竖于汴京(今河南开封),供针灸学习者拓印和阅读。次年,还设计铸造了两座铜人,是我国最早的针灸模型,对辨认经穴与教学起了很大作用。元代滑伯仁认为任督二脉虽属奇经,但有专穴,宜与十二经并论,总结为十四经,著《十四经发挥》,系统阐述了经络的循行路线和有关腧穴,对后人研究腧穴很有裨益。明代是针灸发展昌盛的朝代,杨继洲以家传《卫生针灸玄机秘要》为基础,汇集了历代针灸著作,并结合实践经验撰写了《针灸大成》,内容丰富,是继《内经》、《甲乙经》之后对针灸学的又一次总结,直到今天它仍是学习针灸的主要参考著作。当时还有陈会的《神应经》,徐凤的《针灸大全》,高武的《针灸聚英》,汪机的《针灸问对》,李时珍的《奇经八脉考》等,蔚为大观,诸家各有所长,形成不同流派,相互争鸣,促进了针灸的发展。到了清代虽然也有吴谦等编著的《医宗金鉴·刺灸心法》及廖润鸿的《针灸集成》等书问世,但很少新义,至清代末叶,针灸走向衰落。于1822年竟以"针刺火灸,究非奉君所宜"的荒谬理论,下令停止太医院使用针灸,废止针灸科,一般"儒医"也注重汤药而轻针灸,鸦片战争失败以后,帝国主义入侵,在各地设立教会医院和医学院校,排斥攻击中国医药学,使中医事业包括针灸学更趋衰落。

新中国成立以后,由于党的中医政策的实施,祖国医学获得了新生,带来了针灸事业的复兴与繁荣。全国各地先后成立了中医学院,中医院,设置了针灸专业和专科,并建立了专门研究机构,使针灸在教学、医疗科研等方面都获得了巨大的成就。

三十多年来编撰出版了大量针灸著作。全国高等医药院校使用了统一的针灸教材,开展了对《内经》、《难经》、《甲乙经》、《针灸大成》的校释工作,在全国各报刊发表的针灸论文资料不下万篇。为学习针灸创造了良好的条件,大大丰富了针灸医学的内容。

针灸的临床工作有较大的进展,治疗病种不断扩大。临床实践证明,针灸对内、外、妇、儿等科300多种病症的治疗有不同程度的效果,对其中100种左右的病症有较好或很好的疗效。针灸治疗心脑血管疾病、胆道结石,细菌性痢疾等,不仅用科学的方法肯定了疗效,而且用现代生理学、生化学、微生物学、免疫学等阐明其作用机理,积累了大量的资料。六十年代以来,我国医学界采用针刺麻醉,成功地进行了多种外科手术,为麻醉方法增加了新的内容,引起了世界各国学者的普遍重视,推动了针灸医学的发展。

近年通过多学科的大协作,深入研究针灸治病原理,证明针灸对机体各系统功能有调整作用,能增强机体的抗病能力。针灸镇痛原理的研究已深入到神经细胞、电生理学和神经递质如脑腓肽等分子生化学水平。

经络的研究经过大量普查,不仅肯定了循经感传的客观存在,而且从循经感传现象出现的规律、客观指标及测定方法等方面进行了研究,为经络实质的探讨提供了重要的线索。同时,不少地区还开展了对针刺手法的研究工作,并取得了初步的成绩。

几千年来,针灸医学不仅对我国人民的保健事业起过重大的作用,而且很早就流传到国外,对其他一些国家的医疗保健事业也作出了一定的贡献。约在公元六世纪,针灸医学传入朝鲜,并以《针灸甲乙经》等书为教材。公元562年,我国吴人知聪携带《明堂图》、《针灸甲乙经》到日本。公元701年,日本在医学教育中开始设置针灸科,至今还开办针灸大专学校,深受日本人士的欢迎。公元十七世纪末叶,针灸又传到欧洲。有些国家除设有针灸专科外,还成立了研究针灸医学的专门机构,并多次召开国际针灸学术会议。我国一些省市设立了国际针灸培训基地,为世界各国培训了大批针灸医生。目前,全世界已有一百多个国家正在使用和研究针灸。我国独特的针灸医学已成为世界医学的重要组成部分,并将产生积极的广泛的影响。

继承和发扬祖国医学遗产,除运用中医理论广泛开展教学、医疗、科研等工作外,应用现代科学研究经络的实质与针灸治病的原理,是有志于研究祖国医学者的重要任务。只要我们努力运用辩证唯物主义观点,勇于实践,针灸医学必然会取得更丰硕的成果,为人类的保健事业作出更大的贡献。

上篇 经络腧穴

第一章 经络总论

经络是经脉和络脉的总称,是人体联络、运输和传导的体系。经,有路径的含义,经脉贯通上下,沟通内外,是经络系统中的主干;络,有网络的含义,络脉是经脉别出的分支,较经脉细小,纵横交错,遍布全身。《灵枢·脉度》说:"经脉为里,支而横者为络,络之别者为孙。"

经络内属于脏腑,外络于肢节,沟通于脏腑与体表之间,将人体脏腑组织器官联系成为一个有机的整体;并借以行气血,营阴阳,使人体各部的功能活动得以保持协调和相对的平衡。针灸临床治疗时的辨证归经,循经取穴,针刺补泻等,无不以经络理论为依据。《灵枢·经别》说:"夫十二经脉者,人之所以生,病之所以成,人之所以治,病之所以起,学之所始,工之所止也。"说明经络对生理、病理、诊断、治疗等方面的重要意义。

经络学说是研究人体经络系统的循行分布、生理功能、病理变化及其与脏腑相互关系的一种理论,多少年来一直指导着中医各科的诊断与治疗,其与针灸学科关系尤为密切。

第一节 经络学说的形成

经络学说是我国劳动人民通过长期的医疗实践,不断观察总结而逐步形成的。根据文献分析,其形成途径如下:①"针感"等传导的观察:针刺时产生酸、麻、重、胀等感应,这种感应常沿着一定路线向远部传导;②腧穴疗效的总结:主治范围相似的腧穴往往有规律地排列在一条路线上;③体表病理现象的推理:某一脏器发生病变,在体表相应部位可有压痛、结节、皮疹、色泽改变等现象,也是发现经络系统的途径之一;④解剖,生理知识的启发:古代医家通过解剖,在一定程度上认识了内脏的位置、形态及某些生理功能,观察到人体分布着很多管状和条索状结构,并与四肢联系,观察到某些脉管内血液流动的现象。

以上几点表明,发现经络的途径是多方面的,各种认识互相补充,相互佐证,相互启发从而使人们对经络认识逐步完善,从现存文献来看,经络学说在二千多年前已基本形成。

第二节 经络系统的组成

经络系统是由经脉和络脉组成的。其中经脉包括十二经脉和奇经八脉,以及附属于十二经脉的十二经别、十二经筋、十二皮部。络脉有十五络脉、浮络、孙络等。其基本内容列表如下:

表1-1 经络系统表

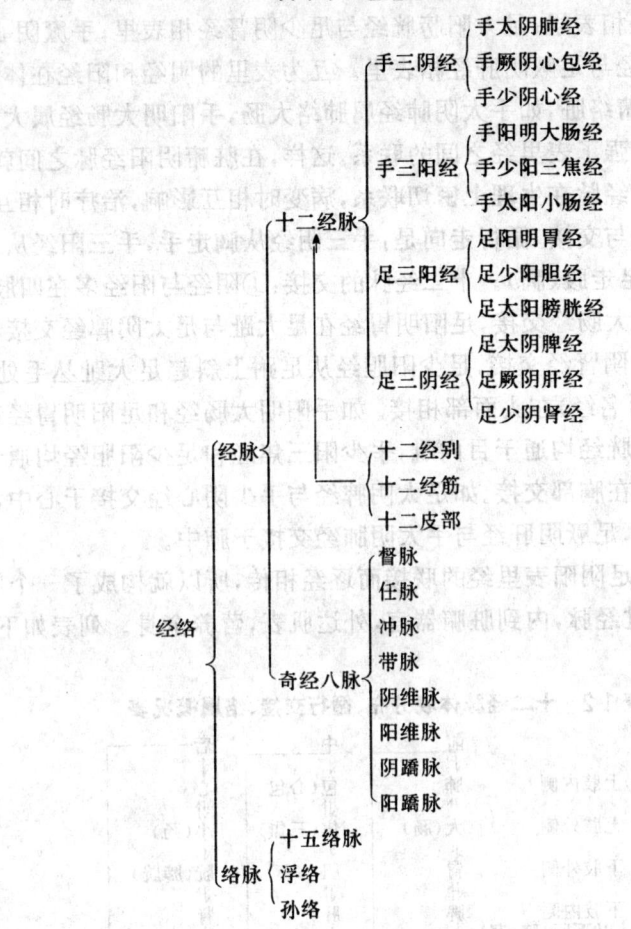

```
                          ┌ 手太阴肺经
              ┌ 手三阴经 ┤ 手厥阴心包经
              │          └ 手少阴心经
              │          ┌ 手阳明大肠经
              │ 手三阳经 ┤ 手少阳三焦经
     ┌ 十二经脉┤          └ 手太阳小肠经
     │        │          ┌ 足阳明胃经
     │        │ 足三阳经 ┤ 足少阳胆经
     │        │          └ 足太阳膀胱经
     │        │          ┌ 足太阴脾经
     │        └ 足三阴经 ┤ 足厥阴肝经
     │                   └ 足少阴肾经
经脉 ┤ 十二经别
     │ 十二经筋
     │ 十二皮部
     │          ┌ 督脉
     │          │ 任脉
     │          │ 冲脉
经络┤          │ 带脉
     └ 奇经八脉┤ 阴维脉
                │ 阳维脉
                │ 阴跷脉
                └ 阳跷脉
            ┌ 十五络脉
     络脉  ┤ 浮络
            └ 孙络
```

1. 十二经脉

十二经脉即手三阴经(肺、心包、心)、手三阳经(大肠、三焦、小肠)、足三阳经(胃、胆、膀胱)、足三阴经(脾、肝、肾)的总称。它们是经络系统的主体,故又称为"正经"。

十二经脉的名称是根据脏腑、手足、阴阳而定的。它们分别隶属于十二脏腑,各经都用其所属脏腑的名称,结合循行于手、足、内、外、前、中、后的不同部位,根据阴阳学说而给予不同名称,如将其中隶属于六腑,循行于四肢的外侧的经脉称为阳经。将其中隶属于五脏,循行于四肢内侧的经脉称为阴经,并根据阴阳衍化的道理分为三阴、三阳,这样就出现了手太阴肺经,手阳明大肠经等十二经脉名称。

十二经脉在体表的分布规律:它们左右对称地分布于头面、躯干和四肢,纵贯全身。六条阴经分布于四肢的内侧和胸腹,其中上肢的内侧是手三阴经,下肢的内侧是足三阴经;六条阳经分布于四肢外侧和头面,躯干,其中上肢的外侧是手三阳经,下肢的外侧是足三阳经。手足三阳经在四肢的排列是阳明在前,少阳在中,太阳在后。手三阴经在上肢的排列是太阴在前,厥阴在中,少阴在后。足三阴经在小腿下部及足背,其排列是厥阴在前,太阴在中,少阴在后,至内踝上八寸处足厥阴与足太阴交叉,而成为太阴在前、厥阴在中,少阴在后。

十二经脉的表里络属关系:十二经脉,内属于脏腑,脏与腑有表里相合的关系,阴经与阳经有表里络属关系。即手太阴肺经与手阳明大肠经相表里；足阳明胃经与足太阴脾经相表里；手少阴心经与手太阳小肠经相表里；足太阳膀胱经与足少阴肾经相表里；手厥阴心包经与手少阳三焦经相表里；足少阳胆经与足厥阴肝经相表里。互为表里的阴经和阳经在体内有属络关系，即阴经属脏络腑，阳经属腑络脏，如手太阴肺经属肺络大肠，手阳明大肠经属大肠络肺等等；在四肢又通过络脉的衔接加强了表里经之间的联系。这样，在脏腑阴阳经脉之间就形成了六组表里络属关系。互为表里的经脉在生理上密切联系，病变时相互影响，治疗时相互为用。

十二经脉的循行走向与交接。循行走向是：手三阴经从胸走手，手三阳经从手走头，足三阳经从头走足，足三阴经从足走腹（胸）。十二经脉的交接：①阴经与阳经多在四肢部衔接。如手太阴肺经在食指与手阳明大肠经交接，足阳明胃经在足大趾与足太阴脾经交接，足太阳膀胱经从足小趾斜趋足心与足少阴肾经交接，足少阳胆经从足跗上斜趋足大趾丛毛处与足厥阴肝经交接。②阳经与阳经（指同名经）在头面部相接。如手阳明大肠经和足阳明胃经都通过于鼻旁，手太阳小肠经与足太阳膀胱经均通于目内眦，手少阳三焦经和足少阳胆经均通于目外眦。③阴经与阴经（即手足三阴经）在胸部交接。如足太阴脾经与手少阴心经交接于心中，足少阴肾经与手厥阴心包经交接于胸中，足厥阴肝经与手太阴肺经交接于肺中。

由于十二经脉通过手足阴阳表里经的联接而逐经相传，所以就构成了一个周而复始，如环无端的传注体系，气血通过经脉，内到脏腑器官，外达肌表，营养全身。列表如下：

表1-2 十二经脉体表分布、循行交接、络属概况表

	前	中	后
上肢内侧	肺	包（心包）	心
上肢外侧	大（肠）	焦（三焦）	小（肠）
下肢外侧	胃	胆	胱（膀胱）
下肢内侧（八寸以下肝、脾、肾）	脾	肝	肾

2. 奇经八脉

奇经八脉是督脉、任脉、冲脉、带脉、阴维脉、阳维脉、阴跷脉、阳跷脉的总称，它们与十二正经不同，既不直属脏腑，又无表里配合关系，"别道奇行"，故称"奇经"。

八脉中的督、任、冲脉皆起于胞中，同出会阴，称为"一源三岐"，其中督脉行于腰背正中，上至头面；任脉行于胸腹正中，上抵颏部；冲脉与足少阴肾经相并上行，环绕口唇，带脉起于胁下，环行腰间一周。阴维脉起于小腿内侧，沿腿股内侧上行，至咽喉与任脉会合。阳维脉起于足跗外侧，沿腿膝外侧上行，至项后与督脉会合。阴跷脉起于足跟内侧，随足少阴等经上行，至目内眦与阳跷脉会合。阳跷脉起于足跟外侧，伴足太阳等经上行。至目内眦与阴跷脉会合，沿足太阳经上额，于项后会合足少阳经。

奇经八脉交错地循行分布于十二经之间，其作用主要体现于两个方面。其一，沟通了十二经脉之间的联系。奇经八脉将部位相近，功能相仿的经脉联系起来，达到统摄有关经脉气血、协调阴阳的作用。督脉与六阳脉有联系，称为"阳脉之海"。具有调节全身阳经经气的作用；任脉与六阴经有联系，称为"阴脉之海。"具有调节全身诸阴经经气的作用；冲脉与任、督脉，足阳明，足少阴等经有联系，故有"十二经之海"、"血海"之称，具有涵蓄十二经气血的作用；带脉约束联系了纵行躯干部的诸条足经;阴阳维脉联系阴经与阳经,分别主管一身之表里;阴阳蹻脉主持阳动阴静,共司下肢运动与寤寐。其二,奇经八脉对十二经气血有蓄积和渗灌的调节作用。当十二经脉及脏腑气血旺盛时,奇经八脉能加以蓄积,当人体功能活动需要时,奇经八脉又能渗灌供应。

冲、带、蹻、维六脉腧穴,都寄附于十二经与任、督脉之中,惟任、督二脉各有其所属腧穴,故与十二经相提并论,合称为"十四经"。十四经具有一定的循行路线,病候及所属腧穴,是经络系统的主要部分,在临床上是针灸治疗及药物归经的基础。十四经分布如图1-1。

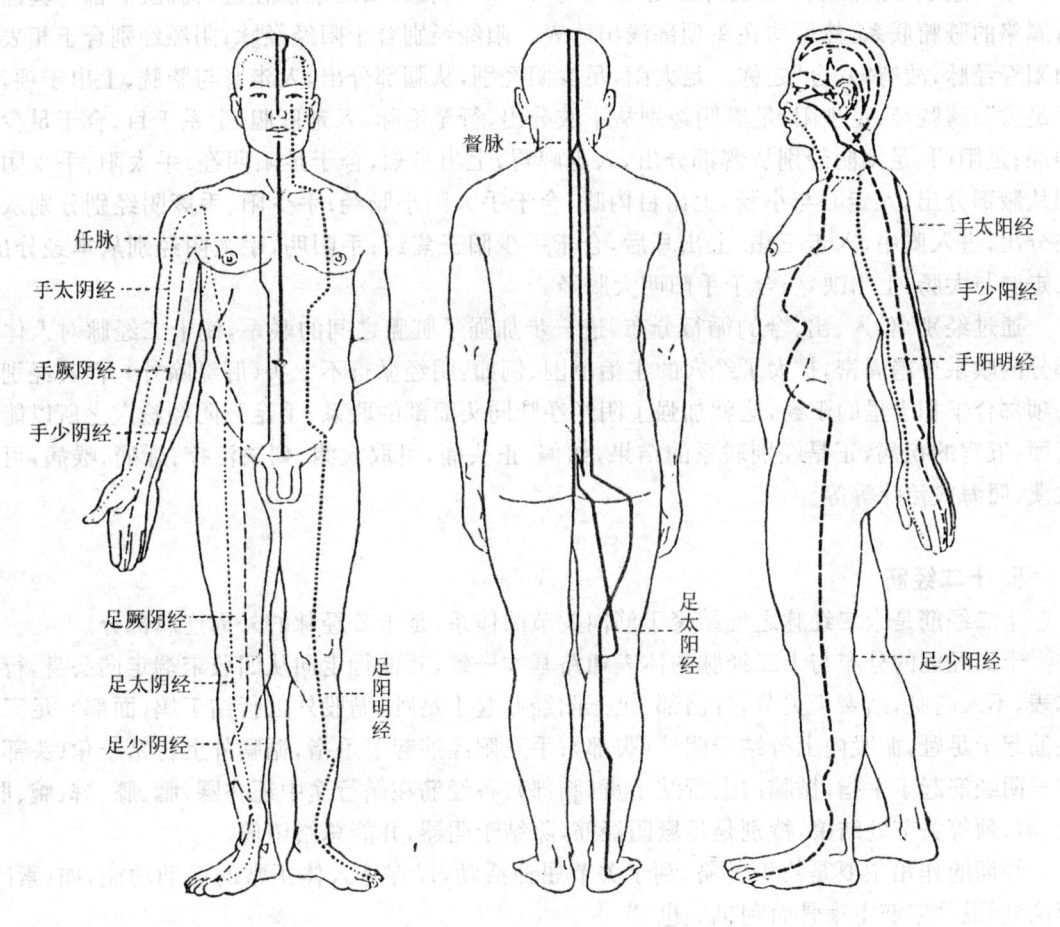

图1-1 十四经循行分布示意图

图例 ——手足太阳、少阴经 ---手足少阳、厥阴经 ……手足阳明、太阴经

3. 十五络脉

十二经脉和任、督二脉各自别出一络,加上脾之大络,共计十五条,称为"十五络",分别以十五络所发出的腧穴命名。

十二经的络脉都由肘膝关节以下的本经分出,走向其相表里的脉;任脉的络脉从鸠尾分出,散布于腹部;督脉别络从长强分出,散布于头部,左右别走足太阳经;脾之大络从大包分出,散布于胸胁。全身络脉中,十五络较大,络脉中浮行于浅表部位的称为"浮络"。络脉中最细小的分支称为"孙络",遍布全身,难以计数。

十二经的络脉加强了阴阳表里经之间的联系;任脉别络沟通了腹部经气;督脉别络沟通了背部经气;脾之大络沟通了侧胸部经气。孙络细小密布,其作用主要是输布气血以濡养全身组织。

4. 十二经别

十二经别是十二正经离、入、出、合的别行部分,是正经别行深入体腔的支脉。

十二经别多从四肢肘膝上下的正经离别,再深入胸腹。阳经经别在进入胸腹后都与其经脉所属络的脏腑联系,然后均在头项部浅出体表。阳经经别合于阳经经脉;阴经经别合于相表里的阳经经脉,故有"六合"之称。足太阳,足少阴经别,从腘部分出,入走肾与膀胱,上出于项,合于足太阳膀胱经;足少阳,足厥阴经别从下肢分出,行至毛际,入走肝胆,上系于目,合于足少阳胆经;足阳明、足太阴经别从髀部分出,入走脾胃,上出鼻頞,合于足阳明经;手太阳、手少阴经别从腋部分出,入走心与小肠,上出目内眦,合于手太阳小肠经;手少阳、手厥阴经别分别从本经分出,进入胸中,入走三焦,上出耳后,合于手少阳三焦经;手阳明,手太阴经别从本经分出,入走肺与大肠,上出缺盆,合于手阳明大肠经。

通过经别离、入、出、合的循行分布,进一步加强了脏腑之间的联系,使十二经脉对人体各部分的联系更趋周密,扩大了经穴的主治范围。例如:阴经循行不上头(肝经除外),但其经别在头项部合于相表里的阳经,这就加强了阴经经脉同头面部的联系,手足三阴经腧穴之所以能治头面、五官的疾病,正是经别联系的结果,如偏、正头痛,可取太渊、列缺治疗;牙痛,喉病,可取太溪、照海穴治疗等等。

5. 十二经筋

十二经筋是十二经脉之气结聚于筋肉关节的体系,是十二经脉的外周连属部分。

十二经筋的分布与十二经脉的体表通路基本一致,其循行走向从四肢末端走向头身,行于体表,不入内脏,结聚于关节,骨骼部。足三阳经筋起于足趾,循股外上行结于鸠(面部);足三阴经筋起于足趾,循股内上行结于阴器(腹部);手三阳经筋起于手指,循臑外上行结于角(头部);手三阴经筋起于手指,循臑内上行结于贲(胸部)。各经筋在循行途中还在踝、腘、膝、髀、腕、肘、腋、肩、颈等关节处结聚,特别是足厥阴经筋,除结于阴器,并能总络诸筋。

经筋的作用主要是约束骨骼,利于关节屈伸活动,以保持人体正常的运动功能,如《素问、痿论》所说:"宗筋主束骨而利机关也。"

6. 十二皮部

十二皮部是十二经脉功能活动反映于体表的部位,也是络脉之气散布之所在。《素问·皮部论》说:"凡十二经络脉者,皮之部也。"

十二皮部的分布区域,是以十二经脉在体表的分布范围为依据的,《素问·皮部论》指出:"欲知皮部,以经脉为纪者,诸经皆然。"

由于十二皮部居于人体最外层,所以是机体的卫外屏障。

上述十二经脉,奇经八脉、十二经别、十二经筋和十二皮部等共同组成经络系统,成为不可分割的整体。

第三节　经络的根结、标本与气街、四海

经络学说除了前面介绍的内容外,还有根结、标本与气街、四海等理论。它是从另一个角度来说明经络与人体各部的联系。

《灵枢·根结》指出,足六经的"根"在四肢末端的井穴,"结"在头、胸、腹的一定部位。(见表1-3)窦汉卿《标幽赋》则进一步指出十二经脉的"四根"、"三结",即十二经脉以四肢为"根",以"头、胸、腹三部为"结"。

《灵枢·卫气》论述了十二经的标与本,大体上"本"在四肢,"标"在头面躯干,其范围较"根""结"为广。(见表1-4)

表1-3　足六经根结表

经脉	根	结
太阳	至阴	睛明
阳明	厉兑	头维
少阳	足窍阴	听宫
太阴	隐白	中脘
少阴	涌泉	廉泉
厥阴	大敦	玉堂、膻中

表1-4　十二经标本部位表

经脉		本部	标部
足三阳	太阳	足跟至跟以上五寸中一段	眼
	少阳	足窍阴	耳前
	阳明	厉兑	颈、颊、顽颡部
足三阴	少阴	交信	背俞与舌下两脉
	厥阴	足背	背俞
	太阴	内踝至踝上四寸一段	背俞与舌本
手三阳	太阳	腕背	眼之上一寸
	少阳	中渚	耳后、耳上角至目外眦
	阳明	肘部	鼻旁
手三阴	太阴	寸口部	腋内动脉
	少阴	锐骨之端	背俞
	厥阴	掌后两筋之间二寸中	腋下三寸

十二经的"根"与"本","结"与"标"位置相近或相同,它们的意义也相似,根者,本者,部位在下,皆经气始生始发之地,为经气之所出;结者,标者,部位在上,皆为经气归结之所。

标本根结的理论补充说明了经气的流注运行情况。《灵枢·经脉》、《灵枢·逆顺肥瘦》、《灵枢·营气》等篇所论述的十二经脉逐经循环传注的体系,使气血周流不息,营养全身;而标本根结理论不仅说明了人体四肢与头身的密切联系,而且更强调四肢为经气的根与本。在临床上,针刺这些部位的腧穴,易于激发经气、调节脏腑经络的功能,所以,四肢肘、膝关节以下的腧穴主治病症的范围较远较广,不仅能治局部病,而且能治远离腧穴部位的脏腑、头面,五官病等。

气街是指经气聚集通行的共同道路。《灵枢·卫气》说："胸气有街,腹气有街,头气有街,胫气有街。"

气街部位多为"结"与"标"的部位,基于这一理论,分布于头身的腧穴可以治疗局部和内脏疾患,部分腧穴又可治疗四肢病症。

《灵枢·海论》提出人有四海:脑为髓海,膻中为气海,胃为水谷之海,冲脉为十二经之海,又称血海。

四海的部位与气街类似,髓海位于头部;气海位于胸部;水谷之海位于上腹部;血海位于下腹部。各部相互联系,主持全身气血津液。

脑部髓海,为神气的本源,脏腑经络功能活动的主宰;胸部为气海,宗气所聚之处,推动肺的呼吸和心血的运行;胃为水谷之海,是营气、卫气的化源;冲脉起于胞宫,胞宫为血室,与月经关系密切,故为血海。《难经》载"脐下,肾间动气者",为十二经之根本,是为原气,通过三焦布于五脏六腑,是人体生命活动的原动力。宗气、卫气、营气、原气共同构成人体的真气(正气),真气行于经络者称为经气或脉气。因此,四海的理论进一步明确了经气的组成和来源。

第四节　经络的生理功能及经络学说在临床上的应用

1. 经络的生理功能

经络具有联系作用:人之五脏六腑、四肢百骸、五官九窍、皮肉筋骨等组织器官,虽各有不同的生理功能,但又共同进行着有机的整体活动,使机体的内、外、上下保持着协调统一,构成一个有机的整体。这种联系和有机配合主要是经络系统的联系作用完成的。《灵枢·海论》说:"夫十二经脉者,内属于腑脏,外络于肢节。"

经络具有营养作用:《灵枢·本藏》说:"经脉者,所以行血气而营阴阳,濡筋骨,利关节者也。"指出经络具有运行气血、调节阴阳、和濡养全身的作用。人体的各个脏腑组织器官均需要气血的温养濡润,才能发挥其正常作用。气血是人体生命活动的物质基础,必须依赖经络的传注,才能输布周身。

经络具有固卫作用:由于经络能"行血气而营阴阳"。营气运行于脉中,卫气运行于脉外,使营卫之气密布于周身,加强了机体的防御能力,起到了抗御外邪,保卫机体的作用。《灵枢·本藏》说:"卫气和则分肉解利,皮肤调柔,腠理致密矣。"

2. 经络学说在临床上的应用

经络用于诊断:经络所通,异常可现。由于每条经脉都有一定的循行路线和联系一定的脏腑组织器官,因此,临床上可根据疾病的症状,结合经络循行的部位和所联系的脏腑,作为辨证归经的依据。例如头痛一证,痛在前额,多与阳明有关,痛在两侧,多与少阳有关,痛在颈项,多与太阳有关,痛在巅顶,多与厥阴有关。此外,在经脉循行路线上出现的异常,如过敏,压痛,结节、条索等,也是诊断疾病的依据。如阑尾炎患者,可在胃经的上巨虚穴出现过敏,压痛,胆囊炎患者,可在胆经的阳陵泉穴附近出现压痛等。临床上常采用循经按压,电测等方法进行诊断。

经络用于治疗:经络所过,主治可及。针灸治病,主要是通过针刺或艾灸腧穴以疏通气血调节脏腑的的功能,针灸选穴,应根据"经脉所过,主治可及"的原则,循经选穴,即某一经或某脏腑有病时,选病经的穴位进行治疗。如《四总穴歌》:"肚腹三里留,腰背委中求,头项寻列缺,面口合谷收"就是循经取穴的例子。

此外,依据皮部与经络脏腑的密切联系,临床上还采用梅花针叩刺皮肤;皮内埋针;刺络放血等方法治疗脏腑经络病证。

第五节 十二经脉的循行与病候

1. 手太阴肺经

《灵枢·经脉》:肺手太阴之脉,起于中焦,下络大肠,还循胃口,上膈属肺,从肺系横出腋下,下循臑内,行少阴心主之前,下肘中,循臂内上骨下廉,入寸口,上鱼,循鱼际,出大指之端;其支者,从腕后,直出次指内廉,出其端(图1-2)。

是动则病,肺胀满,膨膨而喘咳,缺盆中痛,甚则交两手而瞀,此为臂厥;是主肺所生病者,咳,上气喘喝,烦心胸满,臑臂内前廉痛厥,掌中热。气盛有余则肩背痛,风寒汗出中风,小便数而欠;气虚则肩背痛,寒,少气不足以息,溺色变。

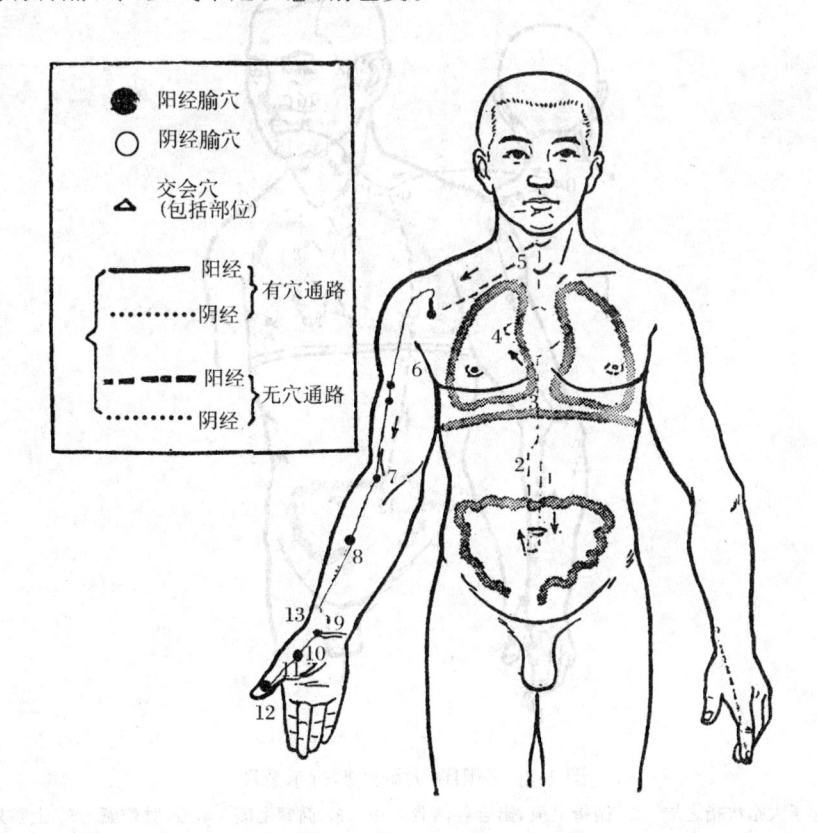

图1-2 手太阴肺经循行示意图
1. 起于中焦,下络大肠　2. 还循胃口　3. 上膈　4. 属肺　5. 从肺系横出腋下　6. 下循臑内,行少阴、心主之前　7. 下肘中　8. 循臂内上骨下廉　9. 入寸口　10. 上鱼　11. 循鱼际　12. 出大指之端　13. 其支者,从腕后直出次指内廉,出其端
图例　——本经有穴通络　……本经无穴通路　○本经腧穴　●常用腧穴△他经腧穴

2. 手阳明大肠经

《灵枢·经脉》：大肠手阳明之脉，起于大指次指之端，循指上廉，出合谷两骨之间，上入两筋之中，循臂上廉，入肘外廉，上臑外前廉，上肩，出髃骨之前廉，上出于柱骨之会上，下入缺盆，络肺，下膈属大肠。

其支者，从缺盆上颈，贯颊，入下齿中，还出挟口，交人中，左之右，右之左，上挟鼻孔（图1-3）。

是动则病，齿痛，颈肿，是主津液所生病者，目黄，口干，鼽衄，喉痹，肩前臑痛，大指次指痛不用。气有余则当脉所过者热肿；虚，则寒栗不复。

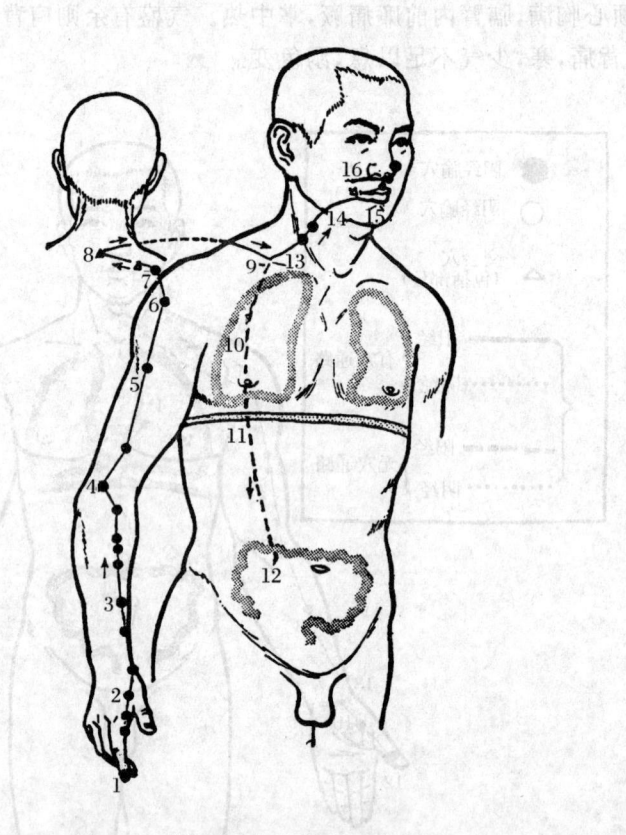

图1-3 手阳明大肠经循行示意图

1. 起于大指次指之端 2. 循指上廉，出合谷两骨之中 3. 循臂上廉 4. 入肘外廉 5. 上臑外前廉 6. 上肩 7. 出髃骨之前廉 8. 上出于柱骨之会上 9. 下入缺盆 10. 络肺 11. 下膈 12. 属大肠 13. 其支者，从缺盆上颈 14. 贯颊 15. 入下齿中 16. 还出挟口，交人中，左之右，右之左，上挟鼻孔

3. 足阳明胃经

胃足阳明之脉,起于鼻,交頞中,旁纳太阳之脉,下循鼻外,入上齿中,还出挟口,环唇,下交承浆,却循颐后下廉,出大迎,循颊车、上耳前,过客主人前,循发际,至额颅。

其支者,从大迎前,下人迎,循喉咙,入缺盆,下膈,属胃,络脾。

其直者,从缺盆下乳内廉,下挟脐,入气街中。

其支者,起于胃口,下循腹里,下至气街中而合。以下髀关,抵伏兔,下膝髌中,下循胫外廉,下足跗,入中指内间。

其支者,下膝三寸而别,下入中指外间。

其支者,别跗上,入大指间,出其端。(图1-4)

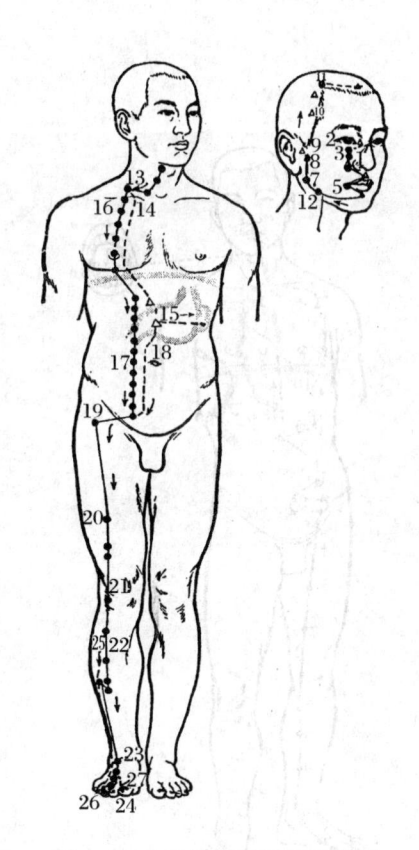

图1-4 足阳明胃经循行示意图

1. 起于鼻,交頞中 2. 旁纳太阳之脉 3. 下循鼻外 4. 入上齿中 5. 还出挟口环唇 6. 下交承浆 7. 却循颐后下廉出大迎 8. 循颊车 9. 下耳前,过客主人 10. 循发际 11. 至额颅 12. 其支者,从大迎前,下入迎,循喉咙 13. 入缺盆 14. 下膈 15. 属胃络脾 16. 其直者,从缺盆下乳内廉 17. 下挟脐,入气街中 18. 其支者,起于胃口,下循腹里,下至气街中而合 19. 以下髀关 20. 抵伏兔 21. 下膝膑中 22. 下循胫外廉 23. 下足跗 24. 入中指(按:指应作趾,以下足经均同)内间(按应作次指处间) 25. 其支者,下廉三寸而别 26. 下入中指外间 27. 其支者,别跗上,入大指间,出其端是动则病,洒洒振寒,善呻数欠颜黑,病至则恶人与火,闻木声则惕然而惊,心欲动,独闭户塞牖而处;甚则欲上高而歌,弃衣而走;贲响腹胀,是为骭厥。

是主血所生病者,狂,疟,温淫、汗出、鼽衄、口㖞、唇胗、颈肿、喉痹、大腹水肿、膝髌肿痛,循膺、乳、气街、股、伏兔、骭外廉、足跗上皆痛,中指不用。

气盛,则身以前皆热,其有余于胃,则消谷善饥,溺色黄;气不足则身以前皆寒栗;胃中寒则胀满。

4. 足太阴脾经

《灵枢·经脉》脾足太阴之脉,起于大指之端,循指内侧白肉际,过核骨后,上内踝前廉,上踹内,循胫骨后,交出厥阴之前,上膝股内前廉,入腹属脾络胃,上膈、挟咽,连舌本,散舌下。

其支者,复从胃,别上膈、注心中。(图1-5)

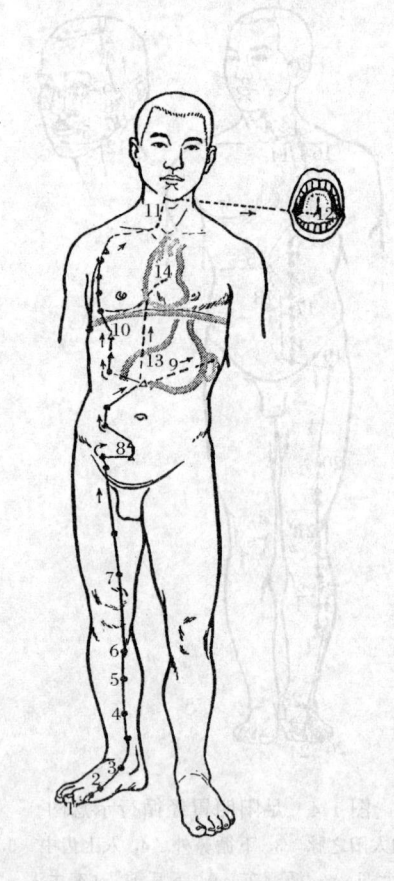

图 1-5 足太阴脾经循行示意图

1. 起于大指之端,循指内侧白肉际 2. 过核骨后 3. 上内踝前廉 4. 上踹内 5. 循胫骨后 6. 交出厥阴之前 7. 上膝股内前廉 8、9. 入腹属脾络胃 10. 上膈 11. 挟咽 12. 连舌本散舌下 13. 其支者,复人胃别上膈 14. 注心中是动则病:舌本强,食则呕,胃脘痛,腹胀善噫,得后与气则快然如衰,身体皆重。

是主脾所生病者,舌本痛,体不能动摇,食不下,烦心,心下急痛,溏、瘕、泄、水闭,黄疸,不能卧,强立股膝内肿厥,足大指不用。

5. 手少阴心经

《灵枢·经脉》心手少阴之脉,起于心中,出属心系,下膈,络小肠。

其支者,从心系,上挟咽,系目系。

其直者,复从心系却上肺,下出腋下,下循臑内后廉,行太阴心主之后,下肘内,循臂内后廉,抵掌后锐骨之端,入掌内后廉,循小指之内出其端。(图1-6)

是动则病,嗌干,心痛,渴而欲饮,是为臂厥。

是主心所生病者,目黄,胁痛,臑臂内后廉痛厥,掌中热痛。

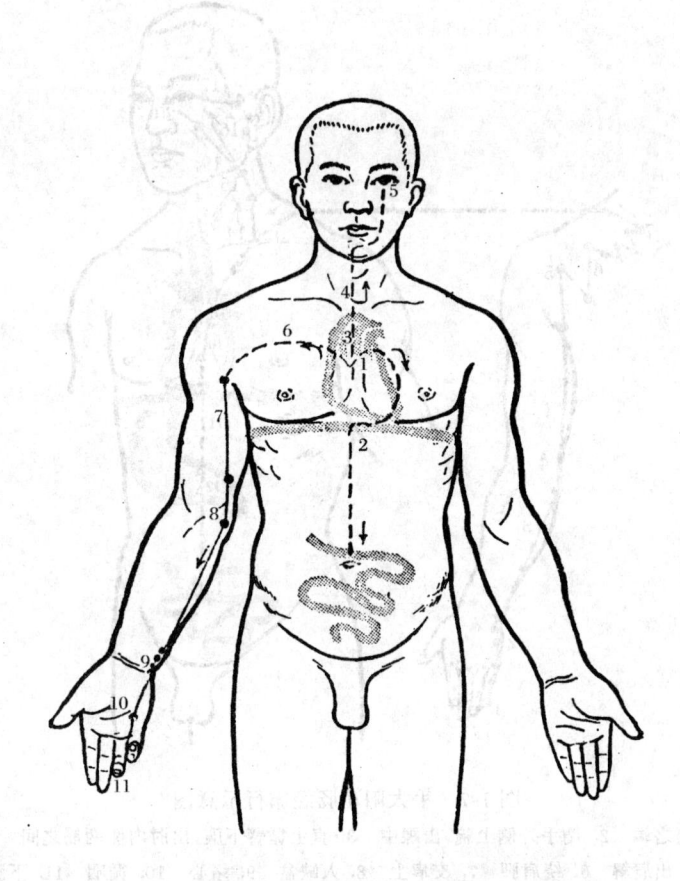

图1-6 手少阴心经循行示意图

1. 起于心中 2. 下膈,络小肠 3. 其支者,从心系 4. 上挟咽 5. 系目系 6. 其支者,复从心系却上肺,下出腋下 7. 下循臑内后廉,行太阴、心主之后 8. 下肘内,循臂内,循臂内后廉 9. 抵掌后锐骨之端 10. 入掌内后廉 11. 循小指之内,出其端

6. 手太阳小肠经

《灵枢·经脉》小肠手太阳之脉,起于小指之端,循手外侧上腕,出踝中,直上循臂骨下廉,出肘内侧两筋之间,上循臑外后廉,出肩解,绕肩胛,交肩上,入缺盆,络心,循咽下膈抵胃属小肠。

其支者,从缺盆,循颈上颊,至目锐眦,却入耳中。

其支者,别颊,上䪼,抵鼻,至目内眦,(斜络于颧)。(图1-7)是动则病,嗌痛,颔肿不可以顾,肩似拔、臑似折。

是主液所生病者,耳聋、目黄,颊肿、颈、颔、肩、臑肘、臂外后廉痛。

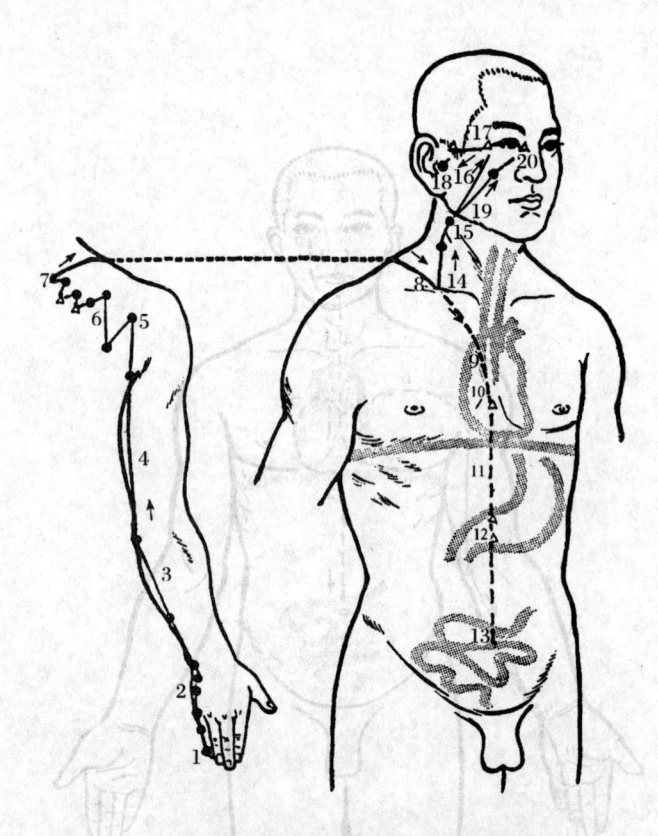

图1-7 手太阳小肠经循行示意图

1. 起于小指之端 2. 循手外侧上腕,出踝中 3. 直上循臂下廉,出肘内侧两筋之间 4. 上循臑外后廉 5. 出肩解 6. 绕肩胛 7. 交肩上 8. 入缺盆 9. 络心 10. 循咽 11. 下膈 12. 抵胃 13. 属小肠 14. 其支者,从缺盆 15. 循颈 16. 上颊 17. 至目锐眦 18. 却入耳中 19. 其支者,别颊上䪼,抵鼻 20. 至目内眦,斜络于颧

7. 足太阳膀胱经

《灵枢·经脉》膀胱足太阳之脉,起于目内眦,上额,交巅。

其支者,从巅至耳上角。

其直者,从巅入络脑,还出别下项,循肩髆内,挟脊抵腰中,入循膂,络肾属膀胱。

其支者,以腰中,下挟脊,贯臀,入腘中。

其支者,从髆内左右别下贯胛,挟脊内,过髀枢,循髀外后廉下合腘中,以下贯腨内,出外踝之后,循京骨,至小指外侧。图(1-8)

是动则病,冲头痛,目似脱,项如拔,脊痛,腰似折、髀不可以曲,腘如结,踹如裂,是为踝厥。

是主筋所生病者,痔,疟,狂,癫疾,头囟项痛,目黄,泪出,鼽衄,项,背,腰,尻,腘,踹,脚,皆痛,小指不用。

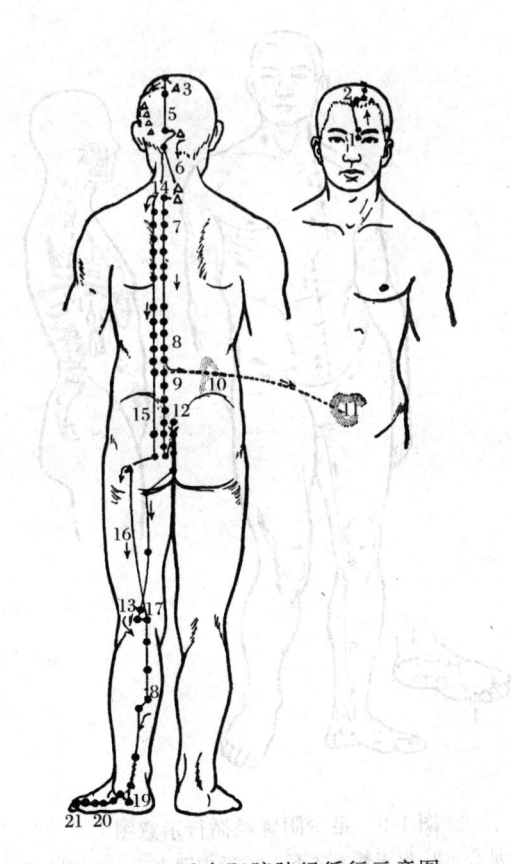

图 1-8 足太阳膀胱经循行示意图

1. 起于目内眦 2. 上额 3. 交巅 4. 其支者,从巅至耳上角 5. 其直者,从巅入络脑 6. 还出别下项 7. 循肩髆内,挟脊 8. 抵腰中 9. 入循膂 11. 属膀胱 12. 其支者,从腰中下挟脊贯臀 13. 入腘中 14. 其支者,从髆内左右,别下贯胛,挟脊内 15. 过髀内 19. 出外踝之后 20. 循京骨 21. 至小指外侧

8. 足少阴肾经

《灵枢·经脉》肾足少阴之脉,起于小指之下,邪走足心,出于然谷之下,循内踝之后,别入跟中,以上踹内,出腘内廉,上股内后廉,贯脊属肾络膀胱。

其直者,从肾,上贯肝,膈,入肺中,循喉咙,挟舌本。

其支者,以肺出,络心,注胸中。(图1-9)

是动则病,饥不欲食,面如漆柴,咳唾则有血,喝喝而喘,坐而欲起,目䀮䀮如无所见,心如悬若饥状,气不足则善恐,心惕惕如人将捕之,是为骨厥。

是主肾所生病者,口热,舌干、咽肿,上气,嗌干及痛,烦心,心痛,黄疸,肠澼,脊,股内后廉痛,痿,厥,嗜卧,足下热而痛。

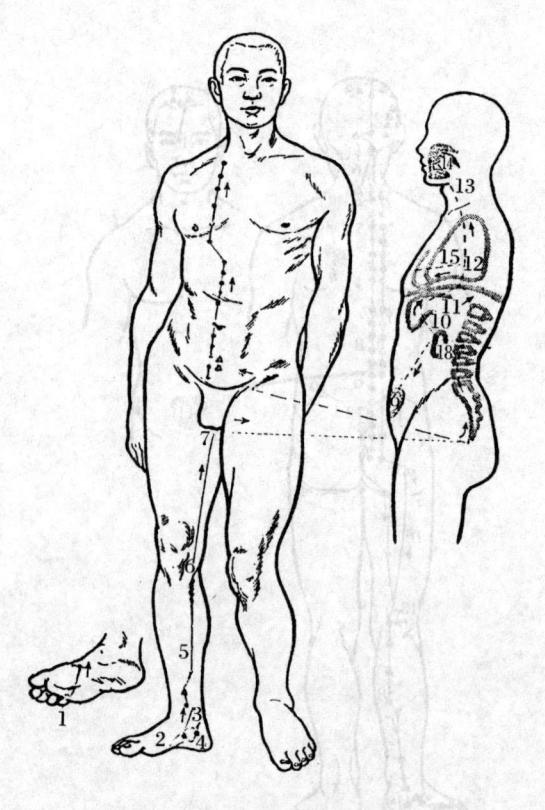

图1-9 足少阴肾经循行示意图

1. 起于小指之下,邪走足心 2. 出于然谷之下 3. 循内踝之后 4. 别入跟中 5. 以上踹(按:踹应作腨) 6. 出腘内廉 7. 上股内后廉 8. 贯脊属肾 9. 络膀胱 10. 其直者,上肾 11. 上贯肝膈 12. 入肺中 13. 循喉咙 14. 挟舌本 15. 其支者,从肺出络心,注胸中

9. 手厥阴心包经

《灵枢·经脉》心主手厥阴心包络之脉，起于胸中，出属心包络，下膈，历络三焦。

其支者，循胸出胁，下腋三寸，上抵腋下，循臑内，行太阴少阴之间，入肘中，下臂，行两筋之间，入掌中，循中指，出其端。

其支者，别掌中，循小指次指出其端。（图1-10）

是动则病，手心热，臂、肘挛急，腋肿，甚则胸胁支满，心中憺憺大动，面赤，目黄，喜笑不休。

是主脉所生病者，烦心，心痛，掌中热。

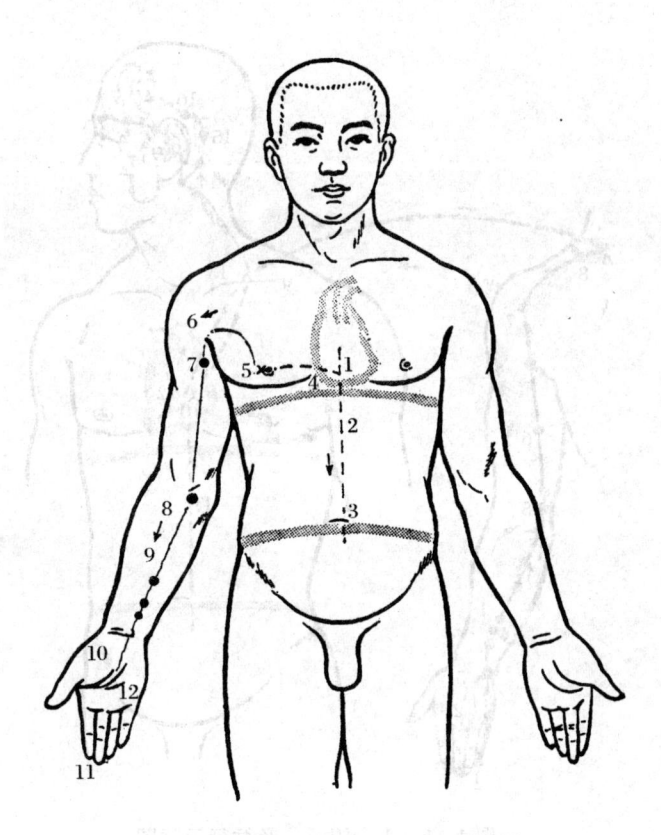

图1-10 手厥阴心包经循行示意图

1. 起于胸中，出属心包络 2. 下膈 3. 历络三焦 4. 其支者，循胸 5. 出胁，下腋三寸 6. 下抵下腋下 7. 循臑内，行太阴少阴之间 8. 入肘中 9. 下臂，行两筋之间 10. 入掌中 11. 循中指，出其端 12. 其支者，别掌中，循小指次指，出其端

10. 手少阳三焦经

《灵枢·经脉》三焦手少阳之脉，起于小指次指之端，上出两指之间，循手表腕，出臂外两骨之间，上贯肘，循臑外上肩，而交出足少阳之后，入缺盆，布膻中，散络心包，下膈，循属三焦。

其支者，从膻中，上出缺盆，上项，系耳后，直上出耳上角，以屈下颊至𩒱。

其支者，从耳后，入耳中，出走耳前，过客主人前，交颊，至目锐眦。（图1-11）

是动则病，耳聋，浑浑淳淳，嗌肿，喉痹。

是主气所生病者，汗出，目锐眦痛，颊肿，耳后，肩，臑，肘，臂外皆病，小指次指不用。

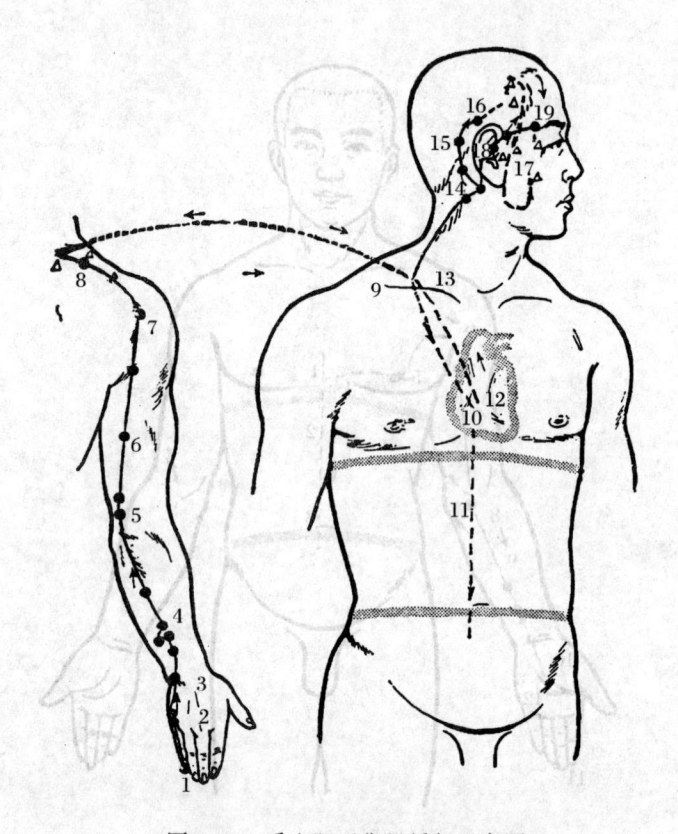

图1-11 手少阳三焦经循行示意图

1. 起于小指次指之端 2. 上出两指之间 3. 循手表腕 4. 出臂外两骨之间 5. 上贯肘 6. 循臑外 7. 上肩 8. 而交出足少阳之后 9. 入缺盆 10. 布膻中，散络心包 11. 下膈，循属三焦 12. 其支者促膻中 13. 上出缺盆 14. 上项 15. 系耳后直上 16. 出耳上角 17. 以屈上颊至𩒱 18. 其支者，从耳后入耳中，出走耳前，过这各主人前，交颊 19. 至目锐眦

11. 足少阳胆经

《灵枢、经脉》胆，足少阳之脉，起于目锐眦，上抵头角，下耳后，循颈，行手少阳之前，至肩上，却交出手少阳之后，入缺盆。

其支者，从耳后，入耳中，出走耳前，至目锐眦后。

其支者，别锐眦，下大迎，合于手少阳，抵于䪼，下加颊车，下颈，合缺盆，以下胸中，贯膈，络肝，属胆，循胁里，出气街，绕毛际，横入髀厌中。

其直者，从缺盆下腋，循胸过季胁，下合髀厌中，以下循髀阳，出膝外廉，下外辅骨之前，直下抵绝骨之端，下出外踝之前，循足跗上，入小指次指之间。

其支者，别跗上，入大指之间，循大指岐骨内，出其端，还贯爪甲，出三毛。（图1-12）

是动则病，口苦，善太息，心胁病，不能转侧，甚则面微有尘，体无膏泽，足外反热，是为阳厥。

是主骨所生病者，头痛，颔痛，目锐眦痛，缺盆中肿痛，腋下肿，马刀侠瘿，汗出振寒，疟，胸胁、肋、髀、膝外至胫、绝骨、外踝前，及诸节皆痛，小指次指不用。

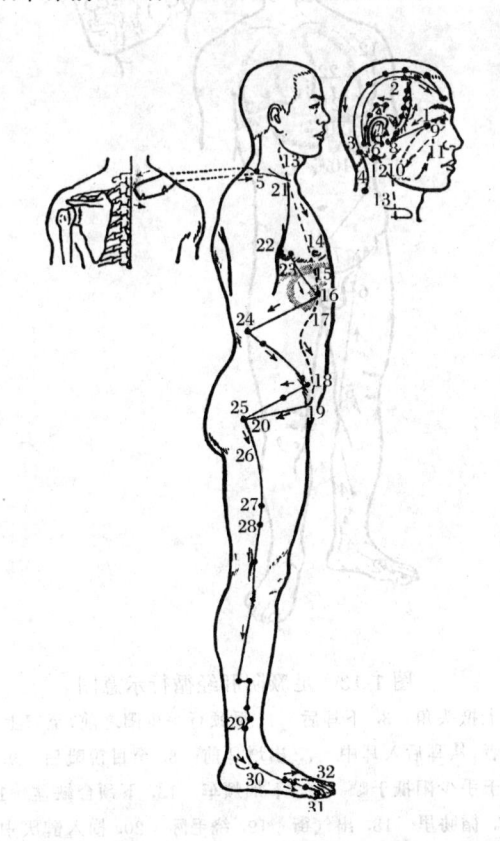

图1-12 足少阳胆经循行示意图

1.起于大指丛毛之际 2.上循足跗上廉 3.去内踝一寸 4.上踝八寸，交出太阴之后 5.上腘内廉 6.循股阴 7.入毛中 8.过阴器 9.抵小腹 10.挟胃属肝络胆 11.上贯膈 12.布胁肋 13.循喉咙之后 14.上入颃颡 15.连目系 16.上出额 17.与督脉会于巅 18.其支者，从目系，下颊里 19.环唇内 20.其支者，复人肝 21.别贯膈 22.上注肺

12. 足厥阴肝经

《灵枢·经脉》肝,足厥阴之脉,起于大指丛毛之际,上循足跗上廉,去内踝一寸,上踝八寸,交出太阴之后,上腘内廉,循股阴,入毛中,过阴器,抵小腹,挟胃属肝络胆,上贯膈,布胁肋,循喉咙之后,上入颃颡,连目系,上出额,与督脉会于巅。

其支者,从目系,下颊里,环唇内。

其支者,复从肝,别贯膈,上注肺。(图1-13)

是动则病,腰痛不可以俛仰,丈夫㿉疝,妇人少腹肿,甚则嗌干,面尘脱色。

是主肝所生病者,胸满,呕逆,飧泄,狐疝,遗溺,闭癃。

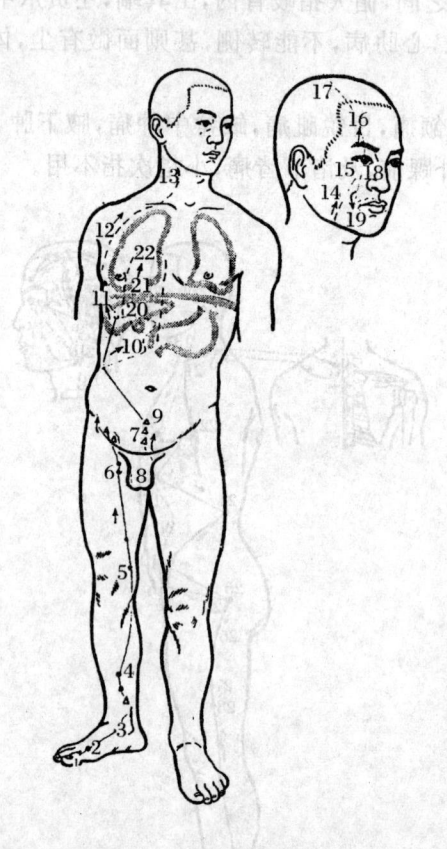

图1-13 足厥阴肝经循行示意图

1. 起于目锐眦 2. 上抵头角 3. 下耳后 4. 循颈行手少阳之前,至肩上却交出手少阳之后 5. 入缺盆 6. 其支者,从耳后入耳中 7. 出走耳前 8. 至目锐眦后 9. 其支者,别目锐眦 10. 下大迎 11. 合于手少阳抵于䪼 12. 下加颊车 13. 下颈合缺盆 14. 以胸中贯膈 15. 络肝 16. 属胆 17. 循胁里 18. 出气街 19. 绕毛际 20. 横入髀厌中 21. 其直者,从缺盆 22. 下腋 23. 循胸 24. 过季胁 25. 下合髀厌中 26. 以下循髀阳 27. 出膝外廉 28. 下外辅骨之前 29. 直下抵绝骨之端 30. 下出外踝之前循跗上 31. 入小指次指之间 32. 其支者,别跗上,入大指之间,循大指岐骨内出其端还贯爪甲,出三毛

第六节 奇经八脉的循行、病候及交会腧穴

1. 督脉

循行：①起于小腹内，下出于会阴部，②向后行于脊柱的内部，③上达项后风府，进入脑内，④上行巅顶，⑤沿前额下行至鼻柱。（图1-14）

主要病候：脊柱强痛，角弓反张等症。

交会腧穴：长强、陶道、大椎、哑门、风府、脑户、百会、水沟、神庭。

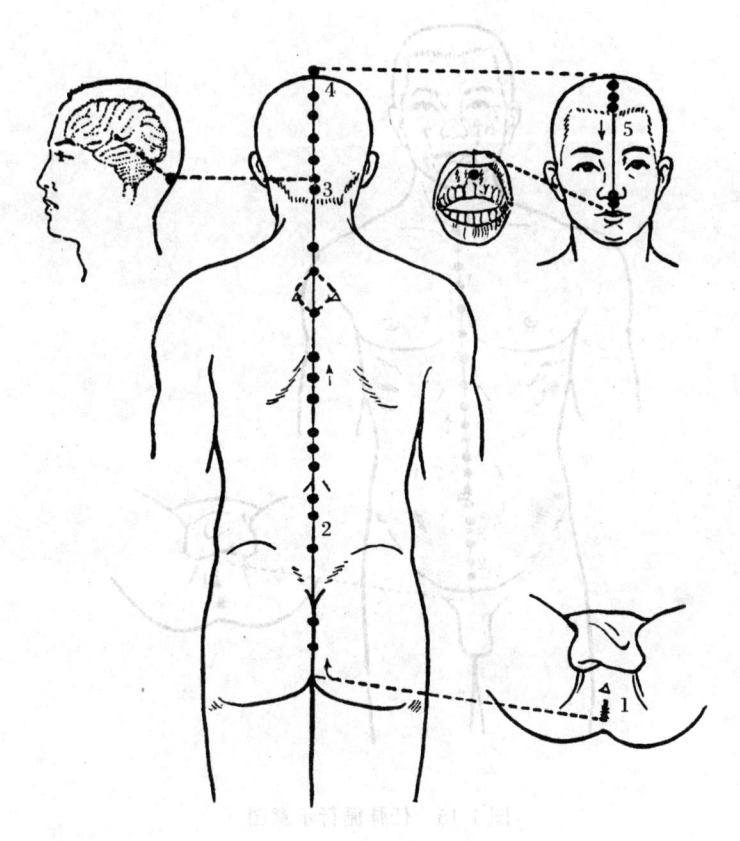

图1-14 督脉循行示意图
1. 起于下极之输 2. 并于脊里 3. 上至风府，入脑 4. 上巅 5. 循额，至鼻柱

2. 任脉

循行：①起于小腹内，下出会阴部，②向上行于阴毛部，③沿着腹内，向上经过关元等穴，④到达咽喉部，⑤再上行环绕口唇，⑥经过面部，⑦进入目眶下（承泣穴属足阳明胃经）（图 1-15）

主要病候：疝气，带下，腹中结块等证。

交会腧穴：会阴、曲骨、中极、关元、阴交、下脘、中脘、上脘、天突、廉泉、承浆。

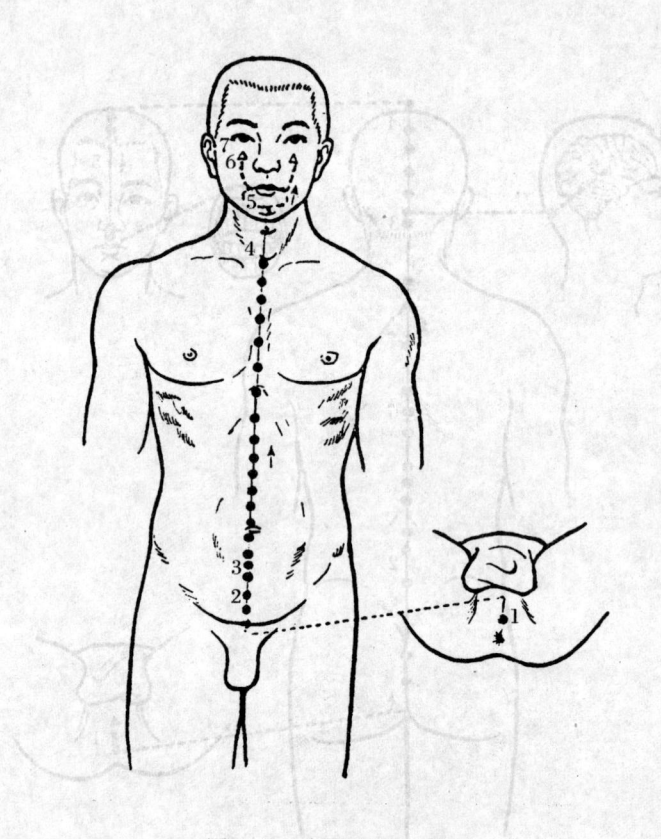

图 1-15 任脉循行示意图
1. 起于中极之下 2. 以上毛部 3. 循腹里，上关元 4. 至咽喉 5. 上颐 6. 循面 7. 入圆

3. 冲脉

循行：①起于小腹内，下出于会阴部，②向上行于脊柱内，③其外行者经气冲与足少阴经交会，沿着腹部两侧，④上达咽喉，⑤环绕口唇。（图1-16）

主要病候：腹部气逆而拘急。

交会腧穴：会阴，阴交；气冲；横骨，大赫，气穴，四满、中注，肓俞，商曲、石关、阴都、通谷、幽门。

4. 带脉

循行：①起于季胁部的下面，斜向下行到带脉、五枢，维道穴，②横行绕身一周。（图1-17）

主要病候：腹满，腰部觉冷如坐水中。

交会腧穴：带脉、五枢、维道。

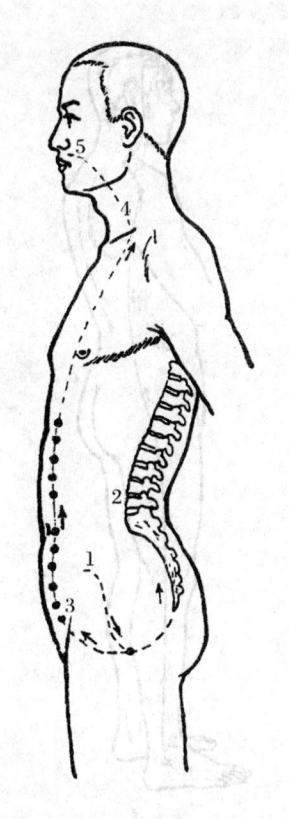

图1-16 冲脉循行示意图 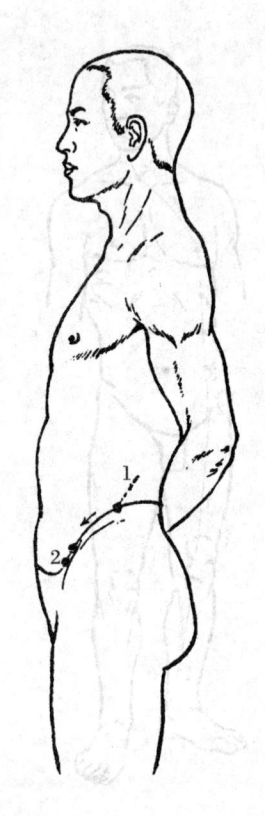　　　　图1-17 冲脉循行示意图

5. 阴维脉

循行：①起于小腿内侧，②沿大腿内侧上行到腹部，③与足太阴经相合，④过胸部，⑤与任脉会于颈部。（图1-18）

主要病候：心痛，忧郁。

交会腧穴：筑宾；府舍、大横、腹哀；期门；天突、廉泉。

6. 阳维脉

循行：①起于足跟外侧，②向上经过外踝，③沿足少阳经上行髋关节部，④经胁肋后侧，⑤从腋后上肩，⑥至前额，⑦再到项后，合于督脉。（图1-19）

主要病候：恶寒发热，腰疼。

交会腧穴：金门；阳交；臑俞；天髎；肩井；头维；本神、阳白、头临泣、目窗、正营、承灵、脑空、风池；风府、哑门。

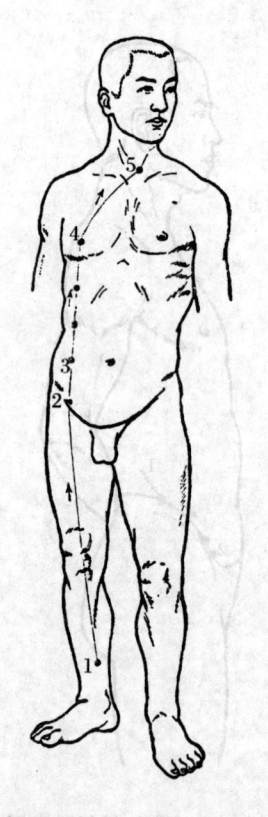

图1-18 阴维脉循行示意图　　　　图1-19 阳维脉循行示意图

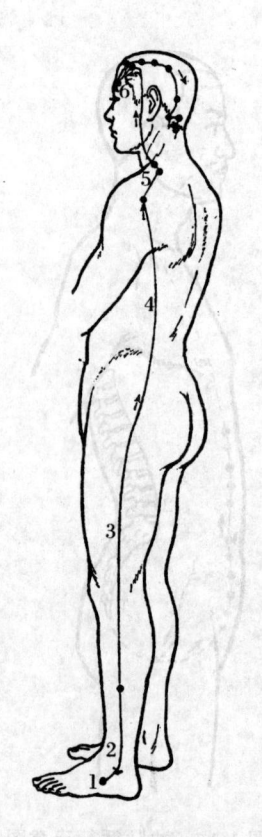

7. 阴跷脉

循行：①起于足舟骨的后方②上行内踝的上面，③直上沿大腿内侧，④经过阴部，⑤向上沿胸部内侧，⑥进入锁骨上窝，⑦上经人迎的前面，⑧过颧部，⑨到目内眦，与足太阳经和阳跷脉相会合。（图1-20）

主要病候：多眠、癃闭，足内翻等证。

交会腧穴：照海、交信；睛明。

8. 阳跷脉

循行：①起于足跟外侧，②经外踝上行腓骨后缘，沿股部外侧和胁后上肩，过颈部上挟口角，进入目内眦，与阴跷脉会合，再沿足太阳经上额，③与足少阳经合于风池。（图1-21）

主要病候：目痛从内眦始，不眠，足外翻等证。

交会腧穴：申脉、仆参、跗阳；居髎；臑俞、肩髃、巨骨；天髎；地仓、巨髎、承泣；睛明；风池。

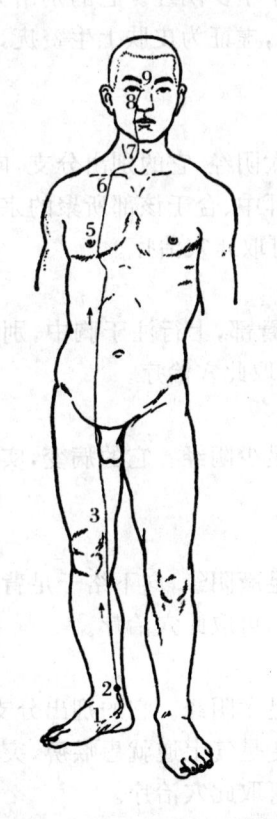

图1-20 阴跷脉循行示意图 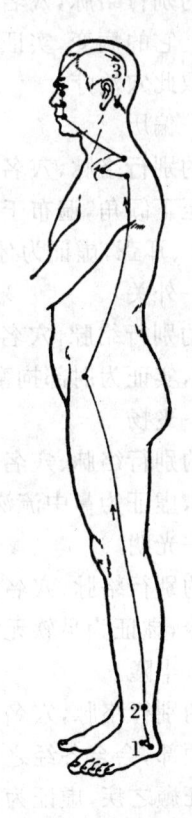　　　图1-21 阳跷脉循行示意图

第七节　十五络脉的穴名、循行、病候及治疗

手太阴络—列缺

手太阴经的别行络脉,穴名列缺,起于腕后桡侧的筋骨缝中,与手太阴本经并行,直入手掌中,散布于大鱼际部。它的病变:实证:手腕锐骨和掌中发热;虚证:呵欠频作,小便失禁或频数。治疗:列缺。穴在腕后一寸半处,别行于手阳明经。

手少阴络—通里

手少阴经的别行络脉,穴名通里,距腕一寸,别而上行,沿着手少阴本经入于心中,系于舌根,会属于目系。它的病变,实证:为胸中支满阻隔,虚证为不能言语,可取通里治疗,通里别行于手太阳经。

手厥阴络—内关

手厥阴经的别行络脉,穴名内关,在距腕二寸的两筋间,别行手少阳经。它沿着手厥阴本经上系于心包,连络于心系,它的病变,实证为心痛,虚证为头项强,可取此穴治疗。

手太阳络—支正

手太阳经的别行络脉,穴名支正,在腕上五寸,向内注于手少阴经。它的别出分支,上行肘部,络于肩髃穴。它的病变,实证为骨节弛缓,肘部不能活动,虚证为皮肤上生赘疣,小的象手指上的痂疥。可取此穴治疗。

手阳明络—偏历

手阳明经的别行络脉,穴名偏历,距腕三寸,别行于手太阴经。它的别出分支,向上沿臂部,经肩髃穴上行至下颌角,遍布于齿中,再别出分支,上行入耳中、合于该部所聚的宗脉。它的病变,实证为龋齿、耳聋,虚证为牙齿寒冷酸楚、内闭阻隔。可取此穴治疗。

手少阳络—外关

手少阳经的别行络脉,穴名外关,距腕二寸,向外绕行臂部,上行注于胸中,别行合于手厥阴经,它的病变,实证为肘部拘挛,虚证为肘部弛缓不收,可取此穴治疗。

足太阳络—飞扬

足太阳经的别行络脉、穴名飞扬,距外踝七寸,别行于足少阴经。它的病变,实证为鼻塞流涕,头背部疼痛,虚证为鼻中流涕出血,可取此穴治疗。

足少阳络—光明

足少阳经的别行络脉、穴名光明,距外踝五寸,别行于足厥阴经,向下络于足背。它的病变,实证为足胫厥冷,虚证为足软无力不能行走,坐而不能起立,可取此穴治疗。

足阳明络—丰隆

足阳明经的别行络脉,穴名丰隆,距外踝八寸,别行于足太阴经。它的别出分支,沿胫骨外缘上行络于头项部,会合各经之气,向下络于咽喉。它的病变是气上逆就患喉痹,突然失音不能言语。实证为狂癫之疾,虚证为足缓不收,胫部肌肉萎缩,可取此穴治疗。

足太阴络—公孙

足太阴经的别行络脉,穴名公孙,在足大趾本节后一寸,别行于足阳明经。它的别出分支,入腹络于肠胃,其气上逆则为霍乱。实证为肠中剧痛,虚证为鼓胀之疾,可取此穴治疗。

足少阴络—大钟

足少阴经的别行络脉、穴名大钟,在内踝后面,绕过足跟而别行于足太阳经。它的别出分支,与足少阴本经并行向上而至于心包下,向外贯穿腰脊。它的病变,气上逆则为烦闷,实证为小便不利,虚证为腰痛。可取此穴治疗。

足厥阴络—蠡沟

足厥阴经的别行络脉,穴名蠡沟,距内踝五寸,别行于足少阳经。它的别出分支,经过胫部上至睾丸,终结于阴茎。它的病变,气上逆就睾丸肿大,突患疝气。实证为阴茎挺长,虚证为阴部暴痒,可取此穴治疗。

任脉络—尾翳

任脉的别行络脉,穴名尾翳(即鸠尾穴),在剑突下面,散布于腹中。它的病变,实证为腹部皮肤疼病,虚证为腹部皮肤瘙痒,可取此穴治疗。

督脉络—长强

督脉的别行络脉,穴名长强,依着脊骨上行项部,散布于头上,再向下到两肩胛之间分左右别行于足太阳经,入而贯穿于脊骨中。它的病变,实证为脊柱强直而难于俯仰,虚证为头重难支而从身体的高处摇摆不定,此皆挟脊之脉有病,可取此穴治疗。

脾之大络—大包

脾的大络,穴名大包,在渊腋穴下3寸,散布于胸胁部。它的病变,实证为全身皆痛,虚证为周身骨节松弛无力。此一络脉象网罗样绕络周身,如现血瘀,可取此穴治疗。

第二章　腧穴总论

第一节　腧穴的基本概念

　　腧穴,是人体脏腑经络之气输注于体表的部位,这些部位不是孤立于体表的点,而是与内部的脏腑器官相通,外部多当筋肉或骨骼之间的凹陷处,因其功能上内外互相输通,位置上又以孔隙为主,所以称为"腧穴"。腧,又写作"俞"、"输"。含有转输的意义;穴,具有孔隙的意义。腧穴即指针灸施术的部位,包括十四经穴、经外奇穴和阿是穴,历代针灸文献上所说的"气穴"、"气府"、"节"、"会"、"骨空"、"脉气所发"、"砭灸处"、"穴位"、"穴道"等,都是腧穴的别称。

第二节　腧穴的发展与分类

　　腧穴的发展:腧穴是我国古代人民在长期的抗病活动中陆续发现和逐步积累起来的。它的发展经过了以痛为腧、定位命名和分类归经等阶段。初期的针灸治病,没有确定的腧穴,只是在病痛的局部进行针灸,这就叫"以痛为腧"。随着医疗经验的积累,肯定了一些腧穴的疗效和位置,才加以定位和命名,以便推广应用,这是腧穴的定位和命名阶段。后来针灸继续发展,应用腧穴增多,治疗范围扩大,于是,人们把某些治疗作用相类似、感传路线比较一致的腧穴加以归纳,这就进入了分类归经阶段。现在所介绍的经穴,就属于这一类腧穴。

　　腧穴的分类:腧穴可分为经穴、经外奇穴和阿是穴三类。凡是属于十四经上的腧穴都叫经穴,它们是腧穴的主要部分,共 361 个穴名;在原有十四经腧穴以外的,但对某些疾病有一定疗效的穴则叫经外奇穴;此外,临床上有根据压痛点定穴,又不属于原有的经穴和经外奇穴的,则称阿是穴、天应穴、不定穴等,这类腧穴既无名称,又无固定位置,而是以压痛点或病痛在体表的反应点作为针灸的部位。阿是穴多位于病变附近,也可在病变较远的部位。

第三节　腧穴的命名

　　腧穴的名称,不仅有其医学意义,也是我国古代灿烂文化的一部分,《千金翼方》指出:"凡诸孔穴,名不徒设,皆有深意。"了解腧穴命名的意义,有助于熟悉腧穴的部位及主治作用。依据所在部位的有:腕旁的腕骨、乳下的乳根、脊间的脊中等。依据治疗作用的有:治目疾的睛明、光明;治水肿的水分、水道;治脏腑疾患的肺俞、心俞、肝俞等。结合中医学理论的有:上肢外侧的阳溪、阳池、阳谷;上肢内侧的阴郄;肺俞、心俞之旁的魄户、神堂;三阴交、百会;气海、血海等穴。利用天体地貌的有:承山、大陵、商丘、水沟;上星、日月、太乙等。参照动植物名称的有:膝下的犊鼻、胸腹部的鸠尾、眉端的攒竹等。借助建筑物名称的有:神阙、印堂、志室、库房等。

第四节 腧穴的作用

诊断作用：人体有病时就会在腧穴上有所反应而做为针灸临床诊断的依据。如胃肠疾患的人常在足三里、地机等穴出现过敏压痛，有时并可在五至八胸椎附近触到软性异物；患有肺脏疾患的人，常在肺俞、中府等穴有压痛、过敏及皮下结节。因此，临床上常用指压背俞穴、募穴、郄穴、原穴的方法，察其腧穴的压痛、过敏、肿胀、硬结、凉、热，以及局部肌肉的隆起，凹陷坚实虚软程度，皮肤的色泽、瘀点、丘疹、脱屑等来协助诊断。

近来，在利用腧穴协助诊断方面又有新的发展，如耳廓中耳穴的测定，对原穴用导电量的测定，对十二井穴用知热感度的测定等等。通过仪器对这些腧穴的测定，可以在一定程度上反应经络、脏腑、组织器官的病变，为协助诊断增添了新的内容。

治疗作用：

①近治作用　这是一切腧穴主治作用所具有的共同特点。这些腧穴均能治疗该穴所在部位及邻近组织、器官的病症。如眼区的睛明、承泣、四白、瞳子髎，均能治疗眼病；耳区的听宫、听会、耳门、翳风诸穴，皆能治疗耳病；胃部的中脘、建里、梁门诸穴，皆能治疗胃病等。

②远治作用　这是十四经腧穴主治作用的基本规律。在十四经腧穴中，尤其是十二经脉在四肢肘、膝关节以下的腧穴，则不仅能治疗局部病症，而且还可以治疗本经循行所及的远隔部位的脏腑、组织、器官的病症，有的甚至具有影响全身的作用。例如：合谷穴不仅能治疗手腕部病症，而且还能治疗颈部和头面部病症，同时，还能治疗外感病的发热；足三里穴不仅能治疗下肢病症，而且对调整整个消化系统的功能，甚至对人体防卫、免疫反应方面都具有很大的作用。

③特殊作用　临床实践证明，针刺某些腧穴，对机体的不同状态可起双向的良性调整作用。例如：泄泻时，针刺天枢能止泻；便秘时，针刺天枢又能通便。此外，腧穴的治疗作用还具有相对的特异性，如大椎退热，至阴矫正胎位等，均是其特殊的治疗作用。

第五节 特定穴的概念和分类

特定穴是指若干类具有特殊治疗作用的经穴。由于它们的主治功能不同，因此各有特定的名称和含义。共有十类。

1. 五输穴

五输穴即十二经脉分布在肘、膝关节以下的井、荥、输、经、合穴，简称"五输"，其分布次序是根据标本根结的理论，从四肢末端向肘膝方向排列的。古代医家把经气在经脉中运行的情况，比作自然界的水流，以说明经气的出入和经过部位的深浅及其不同作用。如经气所出，象水的源头，称为"井"；经气所溜，象刚出的泉水微流，称为"荥"；经气所注，象水流由浅入深，称为"输"；经气所行，象水在通畅的河中流过，称为"经"；最后经气充盛，由此深入，进而汇合于脏腑，恰象百川汇合入海，称为"合"。

《难经·六十八难》："井主心下满，荥主身热，输主体重节痛，经主喘咳寒热，合主逆气而泄。"概括了五输穴的主治范围。十二经各有一个井穴，因多位于赤白肉际处，故井穴具有交通阴阳气血的作用，多用于急救，有开窍醒神，消炎镇痛之效；各经荥穴均可退热；输穴多用于止痛,兼治身体沉重由水湿所致者;经穴主治外感病,咳嗽,哮喘;合穴治六腑病,如呕吐、泄泻、头晕、头胀,可将上逆之气向下引。

井穴还用于诊断:井穴是各经的"根"穴,日本针灸家用燃着的线香熏烤井穴,分析井穴对热的敏感程度,以确定各经的虚实,此法叫知热感度测定法。

古人根据脏腑的不同作用,把其分属五行,即肝、胆属木,心、小肠属火,脾、胃属土,肺、大肠属金,肾、膀胱属水。又将五腧穴也分属五行。《难经·六十四难》指出:"阴井木,阳井金,阴荥火,阳荥水,阴输土,阳输木,阴经金,阳经水,阴合水,阳合土。"据此,又根据五行的相生规律及疾病的不同表现,制定出"虚则补其母,实则泻其子"的治疗方法,即补母泻子法。具体应用又有本经补母泻子法,子午流注纳子法和异经补母泻子法。(表2-5、表2-6)

表2-5 六阴经五输穴五行配属表

六阴经	井(木)	荥(火)	输(土)	经(金)	合(水)
肺(金)	少商	鱼际	太渊	经渠	尺泽
肾(水)	涌泉	然谷	太溪	复溜	阴谷
肝(木)	大敦	行间	太冲	中封	曲泉
心(火)	少冲	少府	神门	灵道	少海
脾(土)	隐白	大都	太白	商丘	阴陵泉
心包(相火)	中冲	劳宫	大陵	间使	曲泽

表2-6 六阳经五输穴五行配属表

六阳经	井(金)	荥(水)	输(木)	经(火)	合(土)
大肠(金)	商阳	二间	三间	阳溪	曲池
膀胱(水)	至阴	通谷	束骨	昆仑	委中
胆(木)	足窍阴	侠溪	足临泣	阳辅	阳陵泉
小肠(火)	少泽	前谷	后溪	阳谷	小海
胃(土)	厉兑	内庭	陷谷	解溪	足三里
三焦(相火)	关冲	液门	中渚	支沟	天井

2. 原穴、络穴

"原"即本源,原气之意。原穴是脏腑原气经过和留止的部位。十二经脉在四肢各有一个原穴,又名"十二原"。在六阳经,原穴单独存在,排列在输穴之后,六阴经则以输为原。"络"即联络之意,络脉从经脉分出的部位各有一个腧穴叫络穴。络穴具有联络表里两经的作用。十二经的络穴皆位于四肢肘膝关节以下,加之任脉络穴鸠尾位于腹,督脉络穴长强位于尾骶部,脾之大络大包穴位于胸胁,共十五穴,故称为"十五络穴"。

2.1. 原穴

一、用于诊断:《灵枢·九针十二原》:"五脏有疾也,应出十二原,十二原各有所出,明知其源,睹其应,而知五脏之害矣。"目前,应用经络测定仪,测量各经原穴的导电情况,分析各经的虚实,以协助诊断脏腑疾病。其读数与井穴知热感度的读数相反,数字大表示脏腑实证。

二、用于治疗:《灵枢·九针十二原》:"五脏有疾也,当取之十二原"。原穴可调整脏腑经络的功能,既可补虚,又可泻实,原穴对脏腑疾病有很好的疗效,可单用,亦可与相表里的络穴配用,叫原络配穴法。因此法是以病经的原穴为主,表里经的络穴为客,所以又叫主客原络配穴。

2.2. 络穴

一、用于诊断:《灵枢·经脉》:"凡此十五络者,实则必见,虚则必下,视之不见,求之上下,人经不同,络脉异所别也。"当经脉有病时,有时会在络穴所在的络脉上出现酸痛、麻木、硬结及颜色改变,可帮助诊断疾病。

二、用于治疗:一是络穴主治络脉病,如手少阴经别络,实则胸中支满,虚则不能言语,可取通里穴治疗。(详见络脉病候)。二是一络通二经,即络穴不仅治本经病,也能治其相表里经的病症,如手太阴络穴列缺,即能治肺经之咳嗽、气喘,又可治大肠经的牙痛、头项强痛等症。三是络穴治疗慢性病,特别是脏腑的慢性疾病,古人有"初病在经,久病在络"之说,即指久病不愈时,其病理产物气血痰湿等常由经入络,故凡一切内伤疾病或脏腑久病均可取络穴治疗。对于络脉之实证,用浅刺放血的方法治疗。(表 2-7)

表 2-7 原络穴表

经脉	肺	大肠	胃	脾	心	小肠	膀胱	肾	心包	三焦	胆	肝	任	督	脾大络
原穴	太渊	合谷	冲阳	太白	神门	腕骨	京骨	太溪	大陵	阳池	丘墟	太冲			
络穴	列缺	偏历	丰隆	公孙	通里	支正	飞扬	大钟	内关	外关	光明	蠡沟	鸠尾	长强	大包

3. 背俞穴、募穴

背俞穴是脏腑之气输注于背腰部的腧穴;募穴是脏腑之气汇聚于胸腹部的腧穴。它们均分布于躯干部,与脏腑有密切关系。

3.1. 背俞穴

一、用于诊断:《灵枢·背俞》:"则欲得而验之,按其处,应在中而痛解,乃其俞也。"《难经·六十七难》:"阴病行阳,俞在阳。"指出五脏有病常在背俞穴上出现反应,按压背俞穴可以协助诊断。

二、用于治疗:治五脏病。《素问·长刺节论》:"迫脏刺背,背俞也。"是说背俞穴对于五脏病针刺具有直接作用。《素问·阴阳应象大论》:"阴病治阳"也说明五脏有病可以取相应的背俞穴进行治疗。背俞穴不但可治与脏腑有关的疾病,还可治疗与本脏腑有关的五官九窍、皮肉筋骨病。如肝俞既能治肝病,又治目疾(肝开窍于目)、筋脉挛急(肝主筋,肝藏血);肾俞治肾病,又可治与肾有关的耳聋耳鸣(肾开窍于耳,肾和则耳能闻五音)、阳痿(肾藏精、主生殖)及骨髓病(肾主骨生髓)。背俞穴可单用,亦可配募穴,叫俞募配穴法。

3.2. 募穴

一、用于诊断：《难经·六十七难》"阳病行阴,故令募在阴"指出六腑有病（阳病）常在胸腹部的募穴上出现异常,指压募穴,可协助诊断,亦可与背俞穴互参诊病,即所谓"审募而察俞,察俞而诊募"。

二、用于治疗：募穴可治本脏腑病及阳经经络病症,《素问·阴阳应象大论》"阳病治阴"即指六腑病及阳经经络病可取募穴治疗。如胃脘痛取中脘；腹痛、腹泻取天枢；膀胱经之坐骨神经痛取中极等。（表2-8）

2-8 脏腑俞募穴表

脏腑	背俞穴	募穴
肺	肺俞	中府
大肠	大肠俞	天枢
胃	胃俞	中脘
脾	脾俞	章门
心	心俞	巨阙
小肠	小肠俞	关元
膀胱	膀胱俞	中极
肾	肾俞	京门
心包	厥阴俞	膻中
三焦	三焦俞	石门
胆	胆俞	日月
肝	肝俞	期门

4. 八会穴

"会"即聚会之意,八会穴即脏、腑、气、血、筋、脉、骨、髓的精气聚会的八个腧穴,故称八会穴,分布于躯干部和四肢部。

用于治疗：八会穴与其所属的八种脏器组织的生理功能有密切关系,各治疗与八者相关的疾病,尤其是八者的慢性虚弱性疾病。如脏会章门主治五脏疾患,尤以肝脾多用；腑会中脘主治六腑病,尤以胃及大肠效优；筋会阳陵泉主治筋病、半身不遂、肩臂疼痛、拘挛瘫痪、痿痹多用；髓会悬钟主治下肢瘫痪、痿软无力、贫血、疼痛等；骨会大杼主治骨病,以周身骨节疼痛,尤其是颈肩背及四肢骨痛效佳；血会膈俞主治血病,吐血、衄血、咳血、便血、痔血、尿血、崩漏、贫血以及外伤出血、瘀血等；气会膻中主治气机不利的各种疾患,如胸闷、气短、噎膈、哮喘、郁证、呕逆嗳气等；脉会太渊主治脉管病,如脉管炎、无脉症、动脉硬化等。

5. 郄穴

"郄"有空隙之意,郄穴是各经经气深集的部位。十二经脉、阴蹻、阳蹻、阴维、阳维脉各有一个郄穴,共十六个郄穴。多分布于四肢肘、膝关节以下。（表2-9）

表 2-9　十六郄穴表

阴经	郄穴	阳经	郄穴
手太阴肺经	孔最	手阳明大肠经	温溜
手厥阴心包经	郄门	手少阳三焦经	会宗
手少阴心经	阴郄	手太阳小肠经	养老
足太阴脾经	地机	足阳明胃经	梁丘
足厥阴肝经	中都	足少阳胆经	外丘
足少阴肾经	水泉	足太阳膀胱经	金门
阴维脉	筑宾	阳维脉	阳交
阴蹻脉	交信	阳蹻脉	跗阳

一、诊断：脏腑有病可按压郄穴，以协助诊断。

二、治疗：因郄穴为气血深藏之处，一般情况下，邪不可干，如果郄穴出现异常，说明病邪已深，表现必然急、重，故郄穴可用于本经循行和所属脏腑的急症、痛症、炎症以及久治不愈的疾病。阴经郄穴有止血作用，如孔最止咯血。中都止崩漏、阴郄止吐血衄血等。阳经郄穴偏于止痛，如急性腰痛取养老，急性胃脘痛取梁丘等。郄穴可以单用，亦可与会穴合用，叫郄会取穴法，如梁丘配中脘治急性胃病；孔最配膻中治气逆吐血等。

6. 下合穴

下合穴是指手足三阳六腑之气下合于足三阳经的六个腧穴，故称下合穴。主要分布于下肢膝关节附近。

下合穴是治疗六腑病的重要穴位，《灵枢·邪气脏腑病形》曰："合治内府。"如足三里治胃脘痛；下巨虚治泄泻；上巨虚治肠痈；阳陵泉治蛔厥；委阳、委中治三焦气化失常引起的癃闭、遗尿等。

7. 八脉交会穴、交会穴

八脉交会穴是指奇经八脉与十二经脉之气相交会的八个腧穴，故称"八脉交会穴"。它们分布于腕踝关节上下。（表 2-10）

表 2-10　八脉交会穴

经属	八穴	通八脉	会合部位
足太阴 手厥阴	公孙 内关	冲脉 阴维	胃、心、胸
手少阳 足少阳	外关 足临泣	阳维 带脉	目外眦、颊、颈、耳后、肩
手太阳 足太阳	后溪 申脉	督脉 阳蹻	目内眦、项、耳、肩胛
手太阴 足少阴	列缺 照海	任脉 阴蹻	胸、肺、膈、喉咙

交会穴是指两经以上的经脉相交会合处的腧穴,多分布于躯干部。

八脉交会穴应用很广,李梴在《医学入门》中说:"八法者,奇经八穴为要,乃十二经之大会也,周身三百六十穴,统于手足六十六穴,六十六穴又统于八穴。"由于奇经与正经的经气以此八穴相通,所以此八穴既能治奇经病,又能治正经病,如公孙通冲脉,因公孙为脾经穴,故公孙既能治脾经病,又能治冲脉病;内关通阴维脉,又为手厥阴心包经穴,故内关既可治心包经病,又可治阴维为病。余穴类推。八脉交会穴临床上常采用上下相应配穴法,且针时常交叉针穴。公孙、内关治胃心胸疾病及疟疾;后溪、申脉治内眼角、耳、项、肩胛部及恶寒发热症;外关、足临泣、治外眼角、耳、颊、肩及寒热往来病症;列缺、照海治咽喉、胸膈、肺及阴虚内热等病症。

全身交会穴很多,交会穴不但治本经病,还能治所交会经脉的病症。如中极、关元是任脉穴位,又与足三阴经交会,因此,这二穴既可治任脉病,又可治足三阴经疾病;大椎是督脉经穴,又与手足三阳经交会,因此,它既可治督脉病,又治诸阳经引起的全身性疾病;三阴交是脾经穴,又与肝、肾二经交会,因此,三阴交既可治脾经病,又治肝肾经疾病。

各经主要交会穴:

一、肺经:

中府:手、足太阴之会

二、大肠经:

肩髃:手阳明、阳蹻之会

迎香:手、足阳明之会

三、胃经:

承泣:足阳明、阳蹻、任脉之会

地仓:阳蹻、手足阳明之会

下关:足少阳、阳明之会

头维:足少阳、阳明、阳维之会

四、脾经:

三阴交:足太阴、少阴、厥阴之会

大横:足太阴、阴维之会

腹哀:足太阴、阴维之会

五、小肠经

颧髎:手太阳、少阳之会

听宫:手足少阳、手太阳之会

六、膀胱经

睛明:手足太阳、阴阳蹻、足阳明之会

大杼:手、足太阳之会

风门:督脉、足太阳之会

七、肾经

大赫、气穴、四满、中注、肓俞、商曲、石关、阴都、腹通谷、幽门:足少阴、冲脉之会。

八、心包经

天池:手厥阴、足少阳之会

九、三焦经

翳风：手、足少阳之会
角孙：手、足少阳、手阳明之会

十、胆经

瞳子髎：手太阳、手足少阳之会
阳白：足少阳、阳维之会
头临泣：足太阳、少阳、阳维之会
风池：足少阳、阳维之会
肩井：手足少阳、阳维之会
日月：足太阴、少阳之会
带脉：足少阳、带脉之会
环跳：足少阳、太阳之会

十一、肝经

章门：足厥阴、少阳之会
期门：足厥阴、太阴、阴维之会

十二、任脉

承浆：足阳明、任脉之会
廉泉：阴维、任脉之会
天突：阴维、任脉之会
上脘：任脉、足阳明、手太阳之会
中脘：手太阳、少阳、足阳明、任脉之会
下脘：足太阴、任脉之会
阴交：任脉、冲脉之会
关元：足三阴、任脉之会
中极：足三阴、任脉之会
会阴：任、督、冲三脉之会

十三：督脉

神庭：督脉、足太阳、阳明之会
水沟：督脉、手足阳明之会
百会：督脉、足太阳之会
脑户：督脉、足太阳之会
风府：督脉、阳维之会
哑门：督脉、阳维之会
大椎：督脉、手足三阳之会☆
陶道：督脉、足太阳之会

☆出《铜人》。《甲乙》无"手、足"二字

第六节 腧穴的定位方法

腧穴的定位方法有三种。

①体表标志法 可分为固定标志和活动标志两种:固定标志是指各部由骨节和肌肉所形成的突起或凹陷、五官轮廓、发际、指(趾)甲、乳头、脐窝等。例如:于腓骨小头前下方定阳陵泉;三角肌止点部定臂臑;眉头定攒竹;两眉之中间定印堂;两乳头之中间定膻中等;活动标志是指各部的关节、肌肉、肌腱、皮肤随着活动而出现的空隙、凹陷、皱纹等。例如:听宫在耳屏与下颌关节之间,微张口呈凹陷处;曲池在屈肘时,肘横纹外侧端凹陷处。

②骨度折量法:此法是以体表骨节为标志,将全身不同的部位规定成一定的长度或宽度,再等分折量的定位方法,因此法是等分折量,因此不论是男、女、老、幼、高、矮、胖、瘦都很适用。常用的骨度分寸列表如下:(表2-11)(图2-22)

表2-11 "骨度"折量寸表

部位	起止点	折量寸	度量表	说明
头面部	前发际正中→后发际正中	12	直寸	用于确定头部经穴的纵向距离
	眉间(印堂)→前发际正中	3	直寸	用于确定前后发际不明时及头部经穴的纵向距离
	第七颈椎棘突下(大椎)→后发际正中	3	直寸	
	眉间(印堂)→后发际正中→第七颈椎棘突下(大椎)	18	直寸	
	额角(头维)之间	9	横寸	用于确定头前部经穴的横向距离
	两乳突之间	9	横寸	用于确定头后部经穴的横向距离
胸腹胁部	胸骨上窝→胸剑联合中点	9	直寸	用于确定胸部任脉穴的纵向距离
	胸剑联合中点→脐中	8	直寸	用于确定上腹部经穴的纵向距离
	脐中→耻骨联合上缘	5	直寸	用于确定下腹部经穴的纵向距离
	两乳头之间	8	横寸	用于确定胸腹部经穴的横向距离
	腋窝顶点→第11肋游离端	12	直寸	用于确定胁肋部经穴的纵向距离
背腰部	肩胛骨内缘→后正中线	3	横寸	用于确定背腰部经穴的横向距离
	肩峰外缘→后正中线	8	横寸	用于确定肩背部经穴的横向距离
上肢部	腋前后纹头→肘横纹(平肘尖)	9	直寸	用于确定上臂部经穴的纵向距离
	肘横纹(平肘尖)→腕掌(背)侧横纹	12	直寸	用于确定前臂部经穴的纵向距离
下肢部	耻骨联合上缘→股骨内上髁上缘	18	直寸	用于确定下肢内侧足三阴经穴的纵向距离
	胫骨内侧髁下方→内踝尖	13	直寸	
	股骨大转子→腘横纹	19	直寸	用于确定下肢外、后侧足三阳经经穴的纵向距离(臀沟→腘横纹相当14寸)
	腘横纹→外踝尖	16	直寸	用于确定下肢外、后侧足三阳经穴的纵向距离

③指寸定位法:这是指利用患者本人手指的宽度以量取腧穴的方法。

拇指同身寸:以患者拇指的指间关节的宽度作为一寸。(图2-23)

中指同身寸:以患者的中指中节桡侧两端纹头之间的距离作为一寸。

横指同身寸(一夫法):患者手四指并拢,以中指中节横纹为准,其四指的宽度作为三寸。

在具体取穴时,医生应当在骨度折量定位法的基础上,参照被取穴对象自身的手指进行比量,并结合一些简便的活动标志,以确定经穴的标准部位。

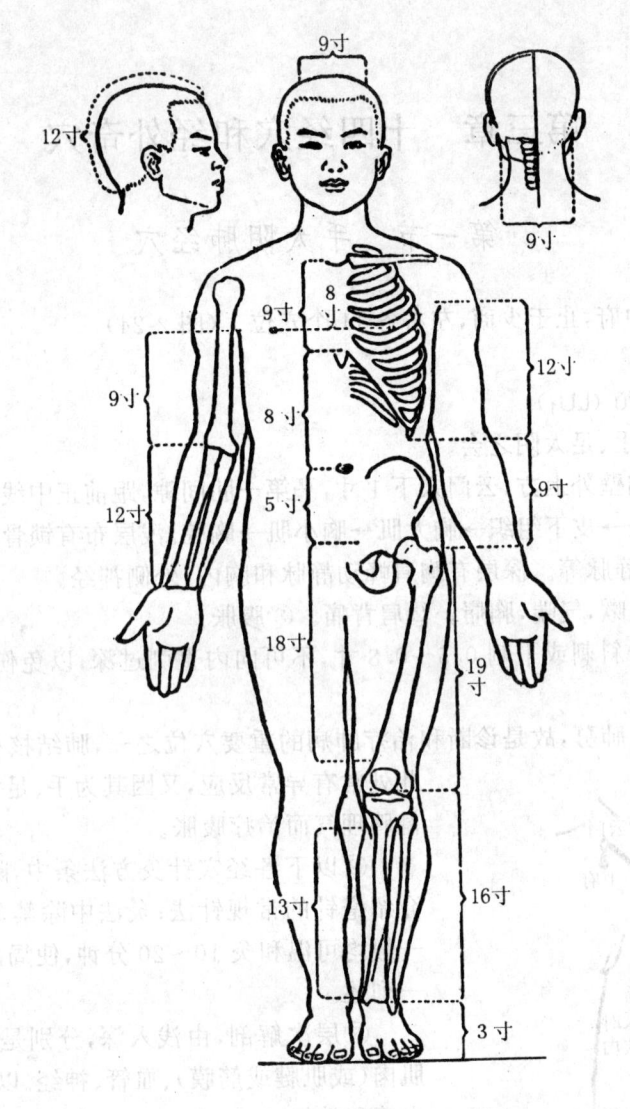

图 2-22　常用骨度分寸示意图

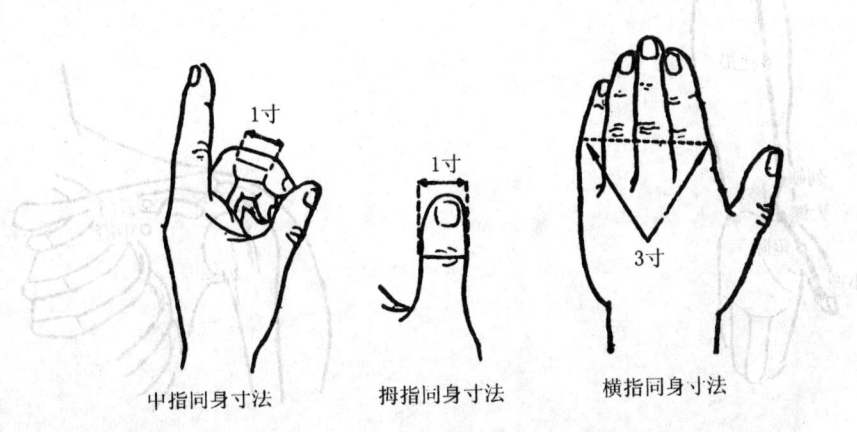

中指同身寸法　　拇指同身寸法　　横指同身寸法

图 2-23　拇指同身寸法

第三章 十四经穴和经外奇穴

第一节 手太阴肺经穴

本经经穴起于中府，止于少商，左右各11个穴位。（图2-24）

1. 中府 Zhōng fǔ （LU₁）

【类别】肺募穴，手、足太阴之会。

【体表定位】在胸壁外上方，云门穴下1寸，平第一肋间隙，距前正中线6寸。（图2-25）

【层次解剖】皮肤→皮下组织→胸大肌→胸小肌→胸腔。浅层布有锁骨上中间神经、第一肋间神经外侧皮支、头静脉等。深层有胸肩峰动静脉和胸内、外侧神经。

【主治病证】①咳嗽，气喘，胸痛。②肩背痛。③腹胀。

【针灸方法】向外斜刺或平刺0.5～0.8寸，不可向内直刺过深，以免伤及肺脏，造成气胸；温和灸10～20分钟。

【附注】①本穴是肺募，故是诊断和治疗肺病的重要穴位之一，肺结核和支气管哮喘病人，此处常有异常反应，又因其为手、足太阴之会穴，故又能健脾理气而治疗腹胀。

②以下各经穴针灸方法条中，除禁针穴外，一般仅介绍毫针的常规针法；灸法中除禁灸穴及特殊灸法外，一般均可温和灸10～20分钟，使局部皮肤发红，不再一一列述。

③层次解剖，由浅入深，分别是皮肤→皮下组织→肌肉（或肌腱或筋膜）、血管、神经。以下各穴只写穴下的血管和神经。

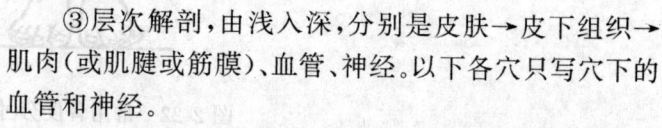

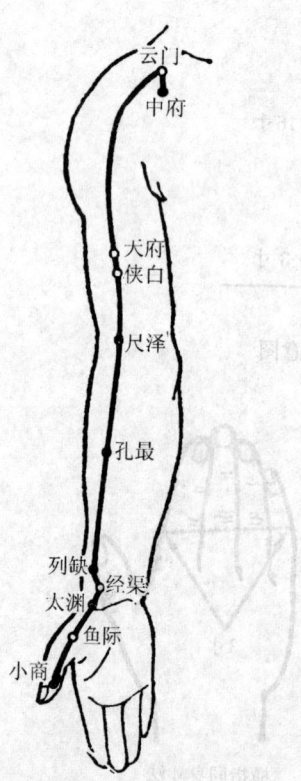

图2-24 肺经经穴总图

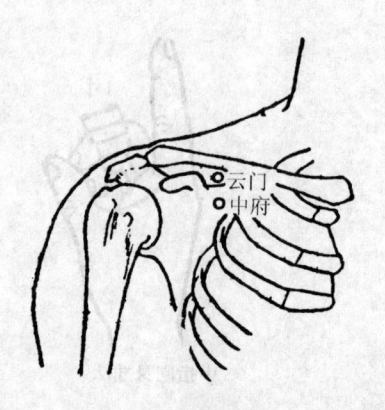

图2-25

2. 云门 Yún mén (LU₂)

【体表定位】在胸壁的外上方,肩胛骨喙突上方,锁骨下窝凹陷处,距前正中线6寸。(图2-25)

【层次解剖】深层有腋动脉及臂丛神经的外侧支。

【主治病证】①咳嗽,气喘。②胸痛,肩背痛。

【针灸方法】向外斜刺0.5~0.8寸,不可向内侧深刺,以免伤及肺脏。

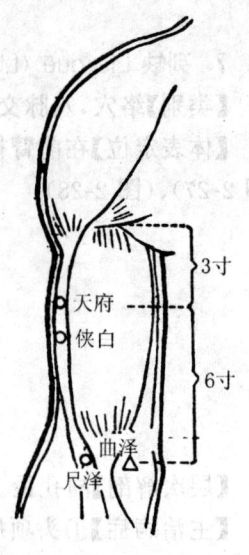

3. 天府 Tiān fǔ (LU₃)

【体表定位】在上臂内侧面,肱二头肌桡侧缘,腋前纹头下3寸处。(图2-26)

【层次解剖】有头静脉及肱动、静脉肌支。分布着臂外侧皮神经。

【主治病症】①鼻衄。②咳嗽,气喘。③肩及上肢内侧疼痛。

【针灸方法】直刺0.5~1寸。

4. 侠白 Xiá bái (LU₄)

【体表定位】在上臂内侧面,肱二头肌桡侧缘,腋前纹头下4寸。(图2-26)

【层次解剖】血管、神经分布同天府穴。

【主治病症】①咳嗽,气喘,烦满。②干呕。③上臂内侧痛。

【针灸方法】直刺0.5~1寸。

5. 尺泽 Chǐ zé (LU₅)

【类别】合穴。

【体表定位】在肘横纹中,肱二头肌腱桡侧凹陷处。(图2-26)

【层次解剖】有头静脉及桡神经。

【主治病症】①咳嗽,气喘,咳血,潮热,胸部胀满。②咽喉肿痛。③急性腹痛吐泻。④小儿惊风。⑤肘臂挛急。

【针刺方法】①直刺0.8~1.2寸。②治急性腹痛吐泻时在穴位的头静脉上放血。

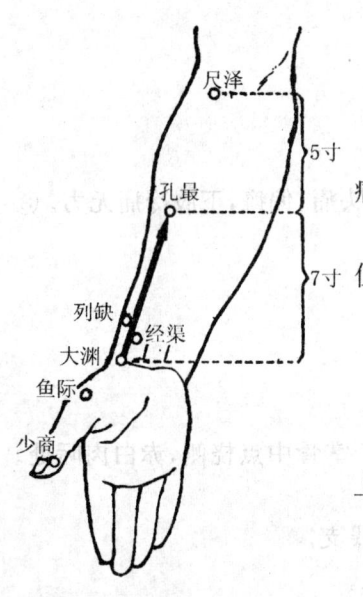

6. 孔最 Kǒng zuì (LU₆)

【类别】郄穴。

【体表定位】在前臂掌面桡侧,当尺泽与太渊连线上,腕横纹上7寸。(图2-27)

【层次解剖】有头静脉、桡动脉及桡神经浅支。

【主治病症】①急性咳血,痔疮出血,鼻衄,咳嗽气喘。②咽喉肿痛。③热病无汗。④前臂疼痛。

【针灸方法】直刺0.5~1寸。

7. 列缺 Liè quē (LU₇)

【类别】络穴，八脉交会穴通任脉。

【体表定位】在前臂桡侧缘，桡骨茎突上方，腕横纹上1.5寸，当肱桡肌与拇长展肌腱之间。（图2-27）、（图2-28）

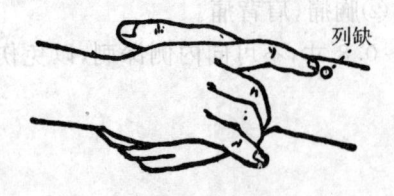

图 2-28

【层次解剖】同孔最。

【主治病症】①头项病：外感所致的偏正头痛，项强，口眼歪斜，牙痛，咽喉肿痛，咳嗽气喘。②泌尿生殖系统疾病：阴茎痛，尿血，遗精。③腹胀。④拇食指无力。

【针灸方法】向上斜刺0.3~0.5寸。

8. 经渠 Jīng qú (LU₈)

【类别】经穴。

【体表定位】在前臂掌面桡侧，桡骨茎突与桡动脉之间凹陷处，腕横纹上1寸。（图2-27）

【层次解剖】同孔最。

【主治病症】①咳嗽，气喘，胸痛，咽喉肿痛。②手腕痛。

【针灸方法】避开桡动脉，直刺0.3~0.5寸。《甲乙经》：不可灸。

9. 太渊 Tài yuān (LU₉)

【类别】原穴，输穴，八会穴（脉会）。

【体表定位】在腕掌侧横纹桡侧，桡动脉搏动处。（图2-27）

【层次解剖】有桡动脉及桡神经浅支。

【主治病症】①咳嗽痰多，气喘乏力。②血管性疾病：无脉症，头痛，偏瘫，下肢冷痛无力。③手腕痛。④呃逆。

【针灸方法】避开动脉直刺0.3~0.5寸。

10. 鱼际 Yú jì (LU₁₀)

【类别】荥穴。

【体表定位】在拇指本节（第一掌指关节）后凹陷处，约当第一掌骨中点桡侧，赤白肉际处。（图2-27）

【层次解剖】有拇指静脉回流支及正中神经掌皮支和桡神经浅支。

【主治病症】①哮喘。②咽喉肿痛，发热，失音。③咳嗽，咳血。

【针灸方法】向掌心方向刺0.5~0.8寸。

11. 少商 Shào shāng(LU₁₁)

【类别】井穴。

【体表定位】在手拇指桡侧,距指甲角0.1寸(指寸)。(图2-27)

【层次解剖】有动、静脉网,桡神经和正中神经形成的末梢神经网。

【主治病症】①咽喉肿痛,咳嗽,鼻衄。②发热。③昏迷,癫狂。④指端麻木。

【针灸方法】向上斜刺0.1寸,或点刺出血。

第二节 手阳明大肠经穴

本经经穴起于商阳,止于迎香,左右各20穴。(图2-29)

1. 商阳 Shāng yáng (LI₁)

【类别】井穴。

【体表定位】在食指末节桡侧,距指甲角0.1寸(指寸)。(图2-30)

【层次解剖】同少商。

【主治病症】①咽喉肿痛,牙痛。②热病昏迷。③食指端麻木。④耳聋。

【针灸方法】浅刺0.1寸,或点刺出血。

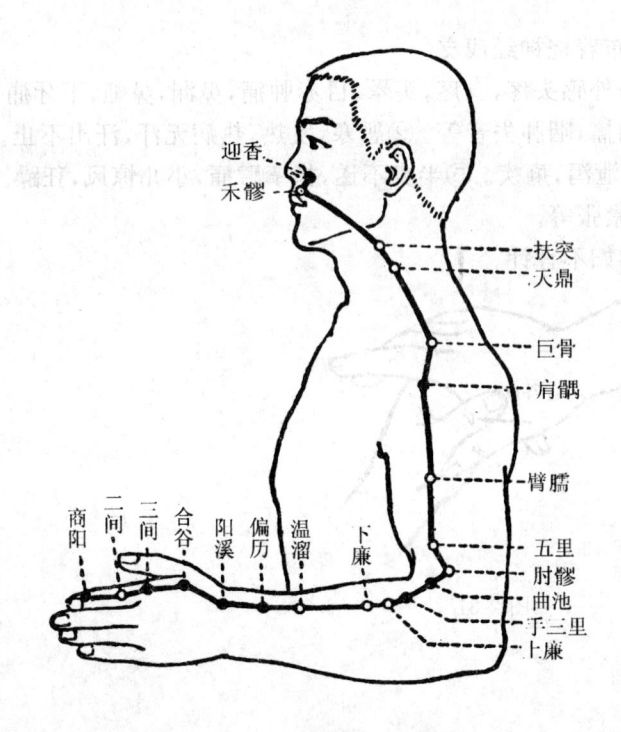

图2-29 大肠经经穴总图

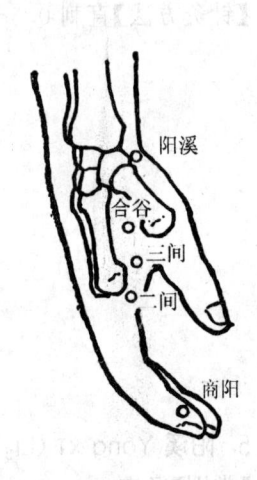

图2-30

2. 二间 Èr jiān (LI₂)

【类别】荥穴。

【体表定位】微握拳,在手食指本节(第二掌指关节)前,桡侧凹陷处。(图2-30)

【层次解剖】有指背及指掌侧动、静脉。分布有桡神经及正中神经的分支。

【主治病症】①牙病,咽喉肿痛。②目赤痛,食指关节肿痛。

【针灸方法】直刺0.2～0.3寸。

3. 三间 Sān jiān (LI₃)

【类别】输穴。

【体表定位】微握拳,在手食指本节(第二掌指关节)后,桡侧凹陷处。(图2-30)

【层次解剖】同二间。

【主治病症】①目痛,齿痛,咽喉肿痛。②身热,手背及手指红肿疼痛。

【针灸方法】直刺0.5～0.8寸。

4. 合谷 Hé gǔ (LI₄) 别名虎口

【类别】原穴。

【体表定位】在手背,第一、二掌骨间,当第二掌骨桡侧的中点处。(图2-30)

简便取法:以一手的拇指指间关节横纹,放在另一手拇、食指之间的指蹼缘上,当拇指尖下是穴。(图2-31)

【层次解剖】有手背静脉网。分布着桡神经浅支。

【主治病症】①头面一切疾患。如外感头疼,身疼,头晕,目赤肿痛,鼻渊,鼻衄,下牙痛,牙关紧闭,耳聋,痄腮,面肿,面瘫,面肌抽搐,咽肿失音等。②恶寒,发热,热病无汗,汗出不止。③痛经,经闭,滞产。④胃痛,腹痛,便秘,泄泻,痢疾。⑤半身不遂,指挛臂痛,小儿惊风,狂躁。⑥疔疮,瘾疹,疥疮。⑦各种疼痛及精神紧张等。

【针灸方法】直刺0.5～1寸。孕妇不宜针。

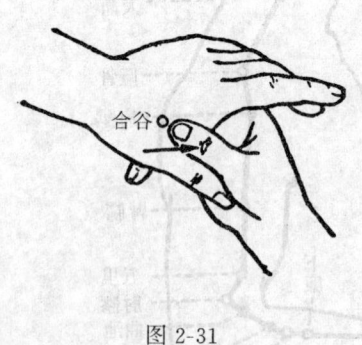

图2-31

5. 阳溪 Yáng xī (LI₅)

【类别】经穴。

【体表定位】在腕背横纹桡侧,手拇指向上翘起时,当拇短伸肌腱与拇长伸肌腱之间的凹陷

中。(图 2-30)
【层次解剖】有头静脉、桡动脉、桡神经浅支。
【主治病症】①前头痛,目赤肿痛,牙痛。②手腕无力。
【针灸方法】直刺 0.5～0.8 寸。

6. 偏历 Piān lì (LI$_6$)
【类别】络穴。
【体表定位】屈肘,在前臂背面桡侧,当阳溪与曲池连线上,腕横纹上 3 寸。(图 2-32)
【层次解剖】有头静脉及桡神经浅支。
【主治病症】①龋齿,耳聋,面瘫。②水肿,手背酸痛。
【针灸方法】直刺或斜刺 0.5～0.8 寸。

7. 温溜 Wēn liú (LI$_7$)
【类别】郄穴。
【体表定位】屈肘,在前臂背面桡侧,当阳溪与曲池连线上,腕横纹上 5 寸。(图 2-32)
【层次解剖】有桡动脉支,头静脉,前臂背侧皮神经。
【主治病症】①急性腹痛,肠鸣,肩背酸痛。②面瘫,面肿。
【针灸方法】直刺 0.5～1 寸。

8. 下廉 Xià lián (LI$_8$)
【体表定位】屈肘,在前臂背面桡侧,当阳溪与曲池的连线上,肘横纹下 4 寸。(图 2-32)
【层次解剖】同温溜。
【主治病症】①腹胀,腹痛。②肘臂痛。
【针灸方法】直刺 0.5～1 寸。

9. 上廉 Shàng lián (LI$_9$)
【体表定位】屈肘,在前臂背面桡侧,当阳溪与曲池的连线上,肘横纹下 3 寸。(图 2-32)
【层次解剖】同温溜。
【主治病症】①半身不遂,肩臂酸痛,手臂麻木。②腹痛,肠鸣。
【针灸方法】直刺 0.5～1 寸。

10. 手三里 Shǒu sān lǐ (LI$_{10}$)
【体表定位】屈肘在前臂背面桡侧,当阳溪与曲池的连线上,肘横纹下 2 寸。(图 2-32)
【层次解剖】有桡返动脉的分支及桡神经深支。
【主治病症】①腹痛,腹泻。②上肢不遂。③止痛,弹拨此穴可消除针刺不当引起的酸胀感。
【针灸方法】直刺 0.8～1.2 寸。

11. 曲池 Qū chí (LI$_{11}$)
【类别】合穴。

【体表定位】在肘横纹外侧端,屈肘,当尺泽与肱骨外上髁连线中点。(图2-32)
【层次解剖】有桡返动脉分支,前臂背侧皮神经,深层为桡神经。
【主治病症】①一切热病,发烧,咽痛,疟疾。②半身不遂,肩痛不举,膝关节肿痛。③头痛,头晕,目赤肿痛,视物不清,牙痛。④月经不调,风疹,湿疹,荨麻疹,丹毒。⑤腹痛吐泻。⑥癫狂。⑦瘰疬。
【针灸方法】直刺1.0～1.5寸。治瘰疬针尖平刺上透臂臑穴。

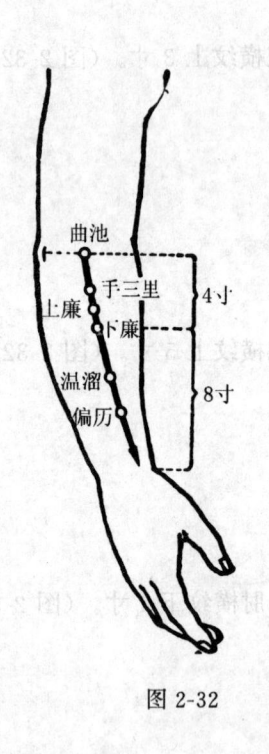

图2-32

图2-33

12. 肘髎 Zhǒu liáo (LI₁₂)

【体表定位】在臂外侧,屈肘,曲池上方1寸,当肱骨边缘处。(图2-33)
【层次解剖】有桡侧副动脉及前臂背侧皮神经,内侧深层为桡神经。
【主治病症】肘臂部酸痛,麻木,挛急。
【针灸方法】直刺0.5～1.0寸。

13. 手五里 Shǒu wǔ lǐ (LI₁₃)

【体表定位】在臂外侧,当曲池与肩髃连线上,曲池上3寸处。(图2-33)
【层次解剖】同肘髎。
【主治病症】①肘臂挛痛。②瘰疬。
【针灸方法】避开动脉,直刺0.5～1.0寸。

14. 臂臑 Bì nào (LI₁₄)

【体表定位】在臂外侧,三角肌止点处,当曲池与肩髃的连线上,曲池上7寸。(图2-33)

【层次解剖】深层有肱深动脉,分布着臂背侧皮神经,深层有桡神经。
【主治病症】①目疾:畏光,焦灼感,重感,红肿疼痛,视力减弱,辨色模糊等。②瘰疬,肩臂痛。
【针灸方法】直刺或向上斜刺0.8～1.5寸。

15. 肩髃 Jiān yú (LI₁₅)
【类别】手阳明与阳蹻脉交会穴。
【体表定位】在肩部三角肌上,臂外展或向前平伸时,当肩峰前下方凹陷处。(图2-33 2-34)
【层次解剖】有旋肱后动脉及锁骨上神经。
【主治病症】①上肢不遂,肩痛不举。②瘰疬,风疹。
【针灸方法】直刺或向下斜刺0.8～1.5寸。

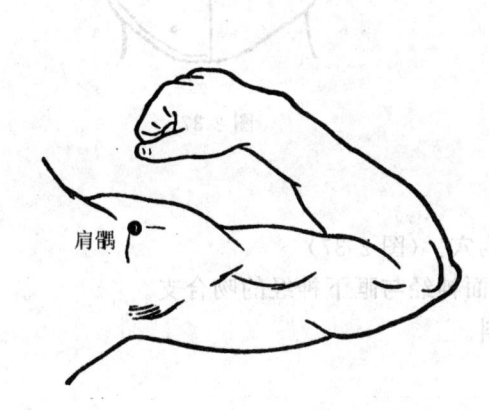

图 2-34 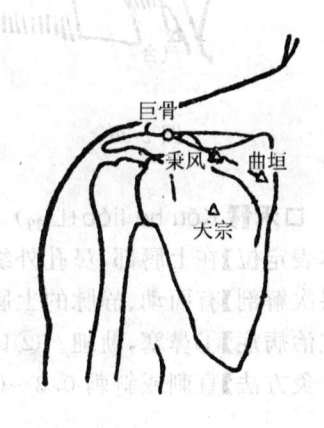   图 2-35

16. 巨骨 Jù gǔ (LI₁₆)
【类别】手阳明与阳蹻脉交会穴。
【体表定位】在肩上部,当锁骨肩峰端与肩胛冈之间凹陷处。(图2-35)
【层次解剖】深层有肩胛上动、静脉及锁骨上神经后支。
【主治病症】肩背疼痛,上肢抬举不利。
【针灸方法】直刺或微斜向外下方刺,进针0.5～1.0寸。

17. 天鼎 Tiān dǐng (LI₁₇)
【体表定位】在颈外侧部,胸锁乳突肌后缘,当喉结旁,扶突与缺盆连线中点。(图2-36)
【层次解剖】有颈外浅静脉,深层为膈神经。
【主治病症】①暴喑。②咽喉肿痛,瘰疬,瘿气。
【针灸方法】直刺0.5～0.8寸。

18. 扶突 Fú tū (LI₁₈)
【体表定位】在颈外侧部,结喉旁,当胸锁乳突肌的胸骨头与锁骨头之间。(图2-36)

【层次解剖】深层内侧有颈升动脉及膈神经、舌下神经。
【主治病症】①呃逆。②上肢不遂,肩痛不举。③咽喉肿痛,瘰疬,瘿气。
【针灸方法】直刺0.5~0.8寸。

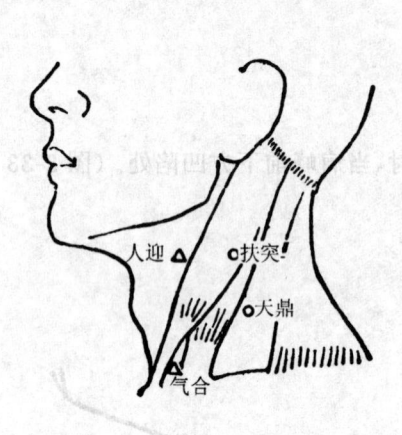

图 2-36

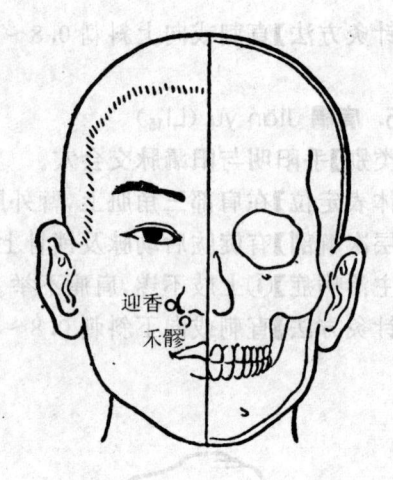

图 2-37

19. 口禾髎 Kǒu hé liáo（LI₁₉）

【体表定位】在上唇部,鼻孔外缘直下,平水沟穴。（图 2-37）
【层次解剖】有面动、静脉的上唇支。分布着面神经与眶下神经的吻合支。
【主治病症】①鼻塞,鼽衄。②口噤,口眼歪斜。
【针灸方法】直刺或斜刺0.3~0.5寸。

20. 迎香 Yíng xiāng（LI₂₀）

【类别】手、足阳明交会穴。
【体表定位】在鼻翼外缘中点旁,当鼻唇沟中。（图 2-37）
【层次解剖】同口禾髎。
【主治病症】①鼻塞,鼽衄。②口㖞,面痒。③胆道蛔虫症。
【针灸方法】斜刺或平刺0.3~0.5寸。不宜灸。

第三节 足阳明胃经

本经经穴起于承泣,止于厉兑,左右各四十五穴。（图 2-38）

1. 承泣 Chéng qì（ST₁）

【类别】足阳明、阳蹻、任脉交会穴。
【体表定位】在面部、鼻孔直下当眼球与眶下缘之间。（图 2-39）
【层次解剖】有眶下动、静脉的分支及眼动、静脉的分支,分布着眶下神经分支、动眼神经下支及面神经肌支。
【主治病症】①目赤肿痛,流泪,夜盲。②眼睑瞤动,口眼㖞斜。

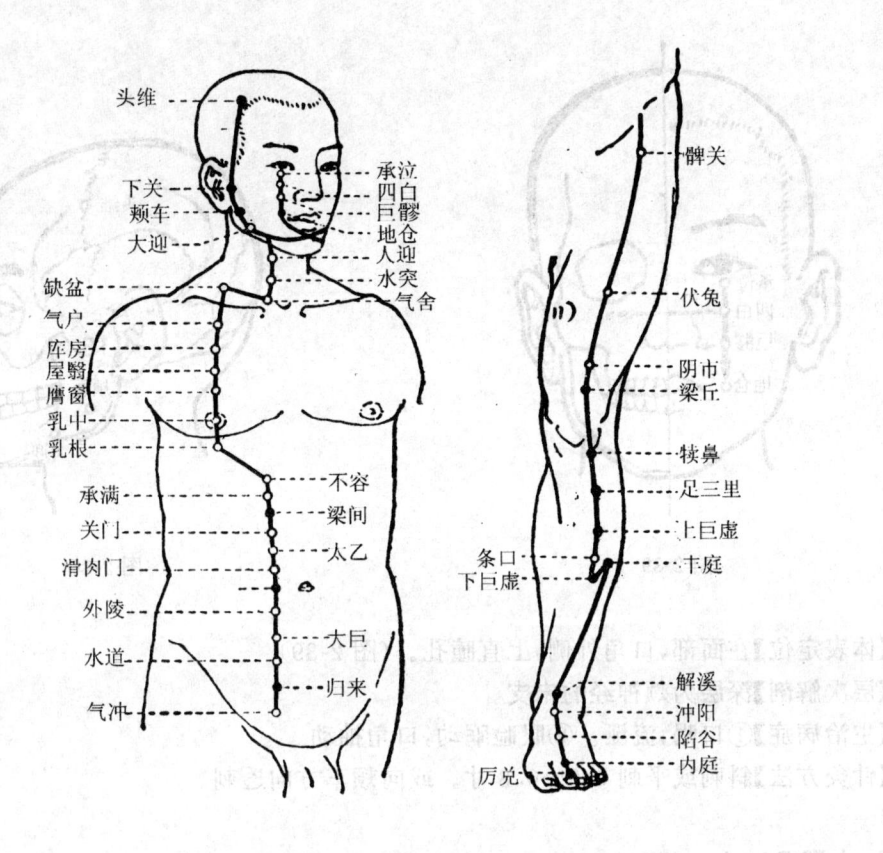

图 2-38 胃经经穴总图

【针灸方法】以左手拇指向上轻推眼球,紧靠眶缘缓慢直刺0.5～1.5寸,不宜提插,以防刺破血管引起血肿。禁灸。

2. 四白 Sì bái (ST₂)

【体表定位】在面部,瞳孔直下,当眶下孔凹隐处。(图2-39)

【层次解剖】同承泣穴。

【主治病症】①近视,目翳,目赤痒痛。②眼睑瞤动,口眼㖞斜。③面痛。

【针灸方法】治近视向内眼角平刺或直刺2～3分,一般不灸。

3. 巨髎 Jù liáo (ST₃)

【类别】足阳明、阳蹻之会。

【体表定位】在面部,瞳孔直下,平鼻翼下缘处,当鼻唇沟外侧。(图2-39)

【层次解剖】同承泣。

【主治病症】①口眼㖞斜,眼睑瞤动。②鼻衄,牙痛,唇颊肿。

【针灸方法】斜刺或平刺0.3～0.5寸。

4. 地仓 Dì cāng (ST₄)

【类别】手、足阳明、阳蹻之会。

图 2-39　　　　　　　　　图 2-40

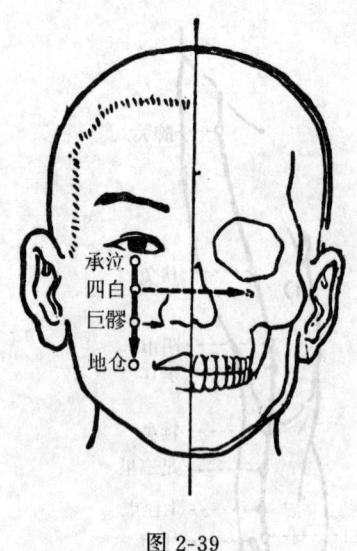

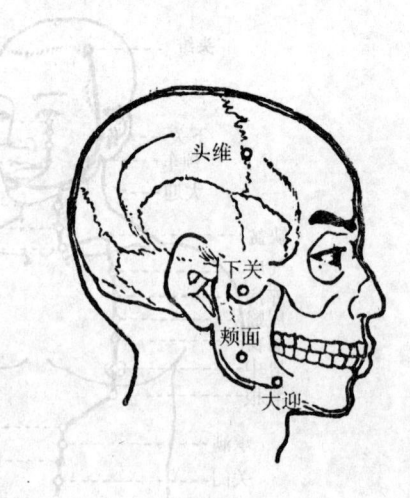

【体表定位】在面部,口角外侧,上直瞳孔。(图 2-39)
【层次解剖】深层为颊神经的末支。
【主治病症】①口㖞,流涎。②眼睑瞤动,口角抽动。
【针灸方法】斜刺或平刺 0.5～0.8 寸。或向颊车方向透刺。

5. **大迎** Dà yíng (ST$_5$)

【体表定位】在下颌角前方,咬肌附着部的前缘,面动脉博动处。(图 2-40)
【层次解剖】前方有面动、静脉。分布着面神经和颊神经。
【主治病症】①颊肿,牙痛。②口㖞,口噤。
【针灸方法】避开动脉,斜刺或平刺 0.3～0.5 寸。

6. **颊车** Jiá chē (ST$_6$)

【体表定位】在面颊部,下颌角前上方约一横指(中指),当咀嚼时咬肌隆起,按之凹陷处。(图 2-40)
【层次解剖】有咬肌动脉。耳大神经、面神经及咬肌神经。
【主治病症】①颊肿,口㖞。②下牙痛,牙关紧急,张口困难。
【针灸方法】直刺 0.3～0.5 寸,平刺 0.5～1 寸,或向地仓透刺。

7. **下关** Xià guān (ST$_7$)

【类别】足阳明、少阳之会。
【体表定位】在面部耳前方,当颧弓与下颌切迹所形成的凹陷中。(图 2-40)
【层次解剖】有面横动、静脉,最深层有颌动、静脉。布有面神经颧支及耳颞神经分支。
【主治病症】①耳聋,耳鸣。②牙痛,鼻塞。③口眼㖞斜,张口困难,面痛。
【针灸方法】直刺 0.5～1 寸。

8. 头维 Tóu wéi (ST$_8$)

【类别】足阳明足少阳、阳维之会。

【体表定位】在头侧部,当额角发际上0.5寸,头正中线旁4.5寸。(图2-40)

【层次解剖】有颞浅动、静脉的额支。分布着耳颞神经之分支及面神经颞支。

【主治病症】①头痛,头晕目眩。②眼痛,迎风流泪,视物不明,眼睑瞤动。

【针灸方法】平刺0.5~1寸。《甲乙》:禁不可灸。

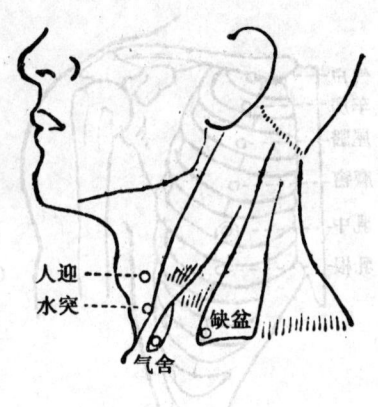

图2-41

9. 人迎 Rén yíng (ST$_9$)

【类别】足阳明、少阳之会。

【体表定位】在颈部,结喉旁,当胸锁乳突肌的前缘,颈动脉搏动处。(图2-41)

【层次解剖】当颈内、外动脉的分支处。深层为颈动脉球及交感神经干。

【主治病症】①咽喉肿痛,瘰疬,瘿气。②哮喘,咳血。③高血压,中风偏瘫。④膝关节疼痛。

【针灸方法】避开颈总动脉,直刺0.3~0.8寸。《甲乙》:禁不可灸。《素注》:刺过深杀人。

10. 水突 shuǐ tū (ST$_{10}$)

【体表定位】在颈部,胸锁乳突肌的前缘,当人迎与气舍连线的中点。(图2-41)

【层次解剖】有颈总动脉及交感干。

【主治病症】①咽喉肿痛。②咳嗽气喘。

【针灸方法】直刺0.3~0.8寸。

11. 气舍 Qì shè (ST$_{11}$)

【体表定位】在颈部,当锁骨内端的上缘,胸锁乳突肌的胸骨头与锁骨头之间。(图2-41)

【层次解剖】深部为颈总动脉。分布着锁上神经前支。

【主治病症】①胸满咳喘,呼吸困难。②瘿瘤,瘰疬,颈项强痛。

【针灸方法】直刺0.3~0.5寸。本经气舍至乳根诸穴,深部有大动脉及肺、肝等重要脏器,不可深刺。

12. 缺盆 Quē pén (ST$_{12}$)

【体表定位】在锁骨上窝中央,距前正中线4寸。(图2-41)

【层次解剖】上方有颈横动脉,深层有臂丛神经。

【主治病症】①咳嗽,气喘,咽喉肿痛。②缺盆中痛,瘰疬。

【针灸方法】直刺或斜刺0.3~0.5寸。《图翼》:孕妇禁针。

13. 气户 Qì hù (ST$_{13}$)

【体表定位】在胸部,当锁骨中点下缘,距前正中线4寸。(图2-42)

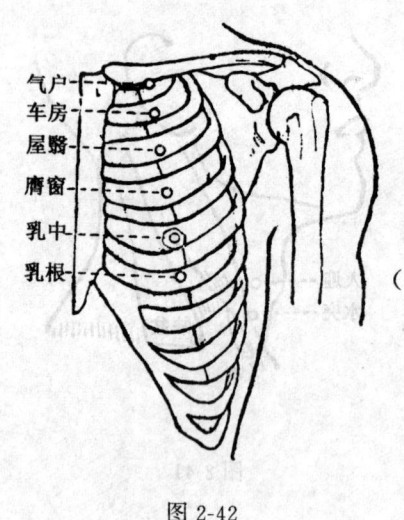

【层次解剖】有胸肩峰动、静脉分支,分布着胸前神经分支。
【主治病症】①咳喘。②胸痛胀满。
【针灸方法】斜刺或平刺 0.5～0.8 寸。

14. 库房 Kù fáng (ST₁₄)
【体表定位】在胸部,当第一肋间隙,距前正中线 4 寸。(图 2-42)
【层次解剖】同气户穴。
【主治病症】①咳喘。②胸胁胀痛。
【针灸方法】斜刺或平刺 0.5～0.8 寸。

15. 屋翳 Wū yì (ST₁₅)
【体表定位】在胸部,当第二肋间隙,距前正中线 4 寸。

图 2-42

(图 2-42)
【层次解剖】同气户穴。
【主治病症】①咳喘。②胸胁胀痛,乳痈。
【针灸方法】斜刺或平刺 0.5～0.8 寸。

16. 膺窗 Yīng chuāng (ST₁₆)
【体表定位】在胸部,当第三肋间隙,距前正中线 4 寸。(图 2-42)
【层次解剖】有胸外侧动、静脉。分布有胸前神经分支。
【主治病症】①咳喘。②胸胁胀痛,乳痈。
【针灸方法】斜刺或平刺 0.5～0.8 寸。

17. 乳中 Rǔ zhōng (ST₁₇)
【体表定位】在胸部,当第四肋间隙,距前正中线 4 寸,乳头中央。(图 2-42)
【层次解剖】第四肋间神经前皮支及外侧皮支。
【附注】本穴不针不灸,只作胸腹部腧穴的定位标志。

18. 乳根 Rǔ gēn (ST₁₈)
【体表定位】在胸部,乳头直下,乳房根部,第五肋间隙,距前正中线 4 寸。(图 2-42)
【层次解剖】有肋间动、静脉分支及第五肋间神经分支。
【主治病症】①乳痈,乳汁少。②胸痛,咳喘。
【针灸方法】斜刺或平刺 0.5～0.8 寸。

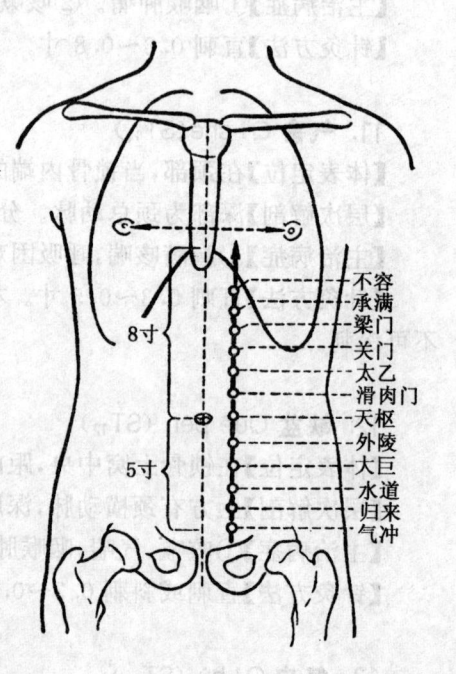

图 2-43

19. 不容 Bù róng (ST₁₉)
【体表定位】在上腹部,脐中上6寸,距前正中线2寸。(图2-43)
【层次解剖】有第七肋间动、静脉分支,分布有第七肋间神经分支。
【主治病症】①胃痛,呕吐。②食欲不振,腹胀。
【针灸方法】直刺0.5~0.8寸。

20. 承满 Chéng mǎn (ST₂₀)
【体表定位】在上腹部,脐中上5寸,距前正中线2寸。(图2-43)
【层次解剖】同不容穴。
【主治病症】胃痛,呕吐,食欲不振,腹胀。
【针灸方法】直刺0.5~0.8寸。

21. 梁门 Liáng mén (ST₂₁)
【体表定位】在上腹部,脐中上4寸,距前正中线2寸。(图2-43)
【层次解剖】有第八肋间动、静脉分支及第八肋间神经分支。
【主治病症】胃痛,呕吐,食欲不振,腹胀,泄泻。
【针灸方法】直刺0.8~1.2寸。

22. 关门 Guān mén (ST₂₂)
【体表定位】在上腹部,脐中上3寸,距前正中线2寸。(图2-43)
【层次解剖】同梁门穴。
【主治病症】①腹胀,腹痛,肠鸣泄泻。②水肿。
【针灸方法】直刺0.8~1.2寸。

23. 太乙 Tài yǐ (ST₂₃)
【体表定位】在上腹部,脐中上2寸,距前正中线2寸。(图2-43)
【层次解剖】有第八、九肋间动、静脉分支及第八、九肋间神经分支。
【主治病症】①癫狂。②心烦。③吐舌。
【针灸方法】直刺0.8~1.2寸。

24. 滑肉门 Huá ròu mén (ST₂₄)
【体表定位】在上腹部,脐中上1寸,距前正中线2寸。(图2-43)
【层次解剖】有第九肋间动、静脉分支及第九肋间神经分支。
【主治病症】①癫狂,呕逆。②吐舌,舌强。
【针灸方法】直刺0.8~1.2寸。

25. 天枢 Tiān shū (ST₂₅)
【类别】大肠募穴。

【体表定位】在腹中部,距脐中旁2寸。(图2-43)
【层次解剖】有第十肋间动、静脉分支及第十肋间神经分支。
【主治病症】①腹胀肠鸣,绕脐痛,便秘,泄泻,痢疾。②月经不调,癥瘕,痛经,闭经。
【针灸方法】直刺1~1.5寸。《千金方》:孕妇不可灸。

26. 外陵 Wài líng (ST26)
【体表定位】在下腹部,脐中下1寸,距前正中线2寸。(图2-43)
【层次解剖】同天枢穴。
【主治病症】腹痛,疝气,痛经。
【针灸方法】直刺1~1.5寸。

27. 大巨 Dà jù (ST27)
【体表定位】在下腹部,脐中下2寸,距前正中线2寸。(图2-43)
【层次解剖】有第十一肋间动、静脉分支及第十一肋间神经。
【主治病症】①小腹胀痛,小便不利。②疝气。③遗精,早泄。
【针灸方法】直刺1~1.5寸。

28. 水道 Shuǐ dào (ST28)
【体表定位】在下腹部,脐中下3寸,距前正中线2寸。(图2-43)
【层次解剖】有肋下动、静脉分支及第十一肋间神经分布。
【主治病症】①小腹胀满,小便不利。②痛经,不孕,疝气。③便秘。
【针灸方法】直刺1~1.5寸。

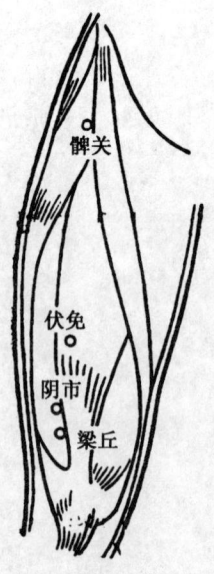

29. 归来 Guī Lái (ST29)
【体表定位】在下腹部,脐中下4寸,距前正中线2寸。(图2-43)
【层次解剖】布有髂腹下神经。
【主治病症】①阴挺,月经不调,闭经,白带。②疝气,腹痛。
【针灸方法】直刺1~1.5寸。

30. 气冲 Qì chōng (ST30)
【体表定位】在腹股沟稍上方,脐中下5寸,距前正中线2寸。(图2-43)
【层次解剖】有腹壁浅动、静脉分支及髂腹股沟神经。
【主治病症】①疝气。②月经不调,不孕。③阳痿,阴肿。
【针灸方法】直刺0.5~1寸。

31. 髀关 Bì guān (ST31)
【体表定位】在大腿前面,髂前上棘与髌底外侧端的连线上,屈股时,平会阴,居缝匠肌外侧凹陷处。(图2-44)
【层次解剖】深层有旋股外侧动、静脉分支,股外侧皮神经。

图2-44

【主治病症】①下肢痿痹，中风偏瘫。②腰膝冷痛。
【针灸方法】直刺1～2寸。

32. 伏兔 Fú tù (ST$_{32}$)
【体表定位】在大腿前面，髂前上棘与髌底外侧端的连线上，髌底上6寸。（图2-44）
【层次解剖】有股外侧皮神经分布。
【主治病症】下肢不遂，腰膝冷痛。
【针灸方法】直刺1～2寸。

33. 阴市 Yīn shì (ST$_{33}$)
【体表定位】在大腿前面，髂前上棘与髌底外侧端的连线上，髌底上3寸。（图2-44）
【层次解剖】有股外侧皮神经分布。
【主治病症】①腿膝冷痛，屈伸不利。②疝气，腹胀，腹痛。
【针灸方法】直刺1～1.5寸。

34. 梁丘 Liáng qiū (ST$_{34}$)
【类别】郄穴。
【体表定位】屈膝，在大腿前面，髂前上棘与髌底外侧端的连线上，髌底上2寸。（图2-44）
【层次解剖】同阴市穴。
【主治病症】①急性胃痛，乳痈。②膝关节肿痛，下肢不遂。
【针灸方法】直刺0.5～1寸。

35. 犊鼻 Dú bí (ST$_{35}$)
【体表定位】屈膝，在膝部，髌骨与髌韧带外侧凹陷中。（图2-45）
【层次解剖】有膝关节动、静脉网及腓总神经关节支。
【主治病症】膝关节肿痛，屈伸不利。
【针灸方法】向后内斜刺0.5～1寸。

36. 足三里 Zú sān lǐ (ST$_{36}$)
【类别】合穴，本穴有强壮作用，为保健要穴。
【体表定位】在小腿前外侧，当犊鼻下3寸，距胫骨前缘一横指（中指）。（图2-45）
【层次解剖】有胫前动、静脉，分布着腓肠外侧皮神经及隐神经的分支，深层为腓深神经。
【主治病症】①胃痛，呕吐，噎膈，腹胀，肠鸣，泄泻，消化不良，痢疾，便秘，腹痛，乳痈。②虚劳羸瘦，心悸气短，纳差乏力，头晕失眠。③咳嗽气喘。④膝关节疼痛，中风偏瘫，脚气水肿。⑤癫狂。
【针灸方法】直刺1～2寸。

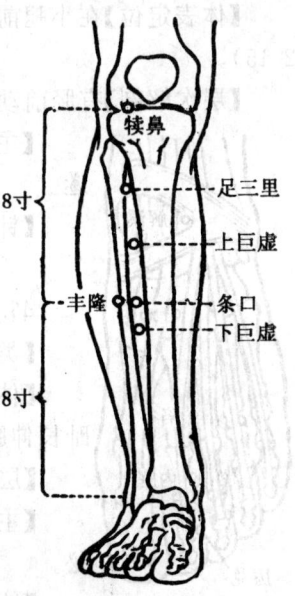

图2-45

37. 上巨虚 Shàng jù xū (ST₃₇)

【类别】大肠下合穴。

【体表定位】在小腿前外侧,当犊鼻下6寸,距胫骨前缘一横指(中指)。(图2-45)

【层次解剖】同足三里。

【主治病症】①肠痈,腹痛,肠鸣,便秘,泄泻。②下肢痿痹,脚气。

【针灸方法】直刺1~1.5寸。

38. 条口 Tiáo kǒu (ST₃₈)

【体表定位】在小腿前外侧,当犊鼻下8寸,距胫骨前缘一横指(中指)。(图2-45)

【层次解剖】同足三里。

【主治病症】①肩周冷痛,抬举困难。②下肢痿痹,跗肿,转筋。

【针灸方法】直刺1~1.5寸。

39. 下巨虚 Xià jù xū (ST₃₉)

【类别】小肠下合穴。

【体表定位】在小腿前外侧,当犊鼻下9寸,距胫骨前缘一横指(中指)。(图2-45)

【层次解剖】有胫前动、静脉。分布着腓浅神经分支及腓深神经。

【主治病症】①小腹痛,腰脊痛引睾丸。②泄泻,痢疾。③下肢痿痹。

【针灸方法】直刺1~1.5寸。

40. 丰隆 Fēng lóng (ST₄₀)

【类别】络穴。

【体表定位】在小腿前外侧,当外踝尖上8寸,条口外,距胫骨粗隆前缘二横指(中指)。(图2-45)。

【层次解剖】有胫前动、静脉分支。分布着腓浅神经。

【主治病症】①咳嗽,痰多,哮喘。②癫狂,癫痫。③头痛,眩晕。④下肢不遂。

【针灸方法】直刺1~1.5寸。

41. 解溪 Jiě xī (ST₄₁)

【类别】经穴。

【体表定位】在足背与小腿交界处的横纹中央凹陷中,当拇长伸肌腱与趾长伸肌腱之间。(图2-46)

【层次解剖】有胫前动、静脉。分布着腓浅神经及腓深神经。

【主治病症】①踝关节疼痛,下肢痿痹。②头痛,眩晕,癫狂。③腹胀,便秘。

【针灸方法】直刺0.5~1寸。

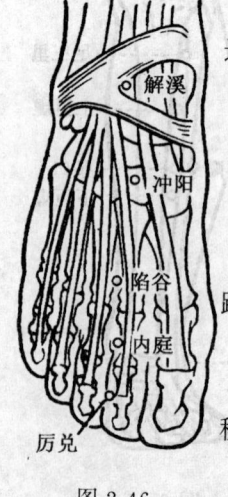

图2-46

42. 冲阳 Chōng yáng (ST₄₂)
【类别】原穴。
【体表定位】在足背最高处,当拇长伸肌腱与趾长伸肌腱之间,足背动脉搏动处。(图 2-46)
【层次解剖】有足背动、静脉,深层为腓深神经。
【主治病症】①胃疼,腹胀。②足背肿痛。③面肿牙痛,口眼㖞斜。
【针灸方法】直刺 0.2～0.5 寸。

43. 陷谷 Xiàn gǔ (ST₄₃)
【类别】输穴。
【体表定位】在足背,当第二、三跖骨结合部前方凹陷处。(图 2-46)
【层次解剖】有足背静脉网及足背内侧皮神经。
【主治病症】①上眼肌无力,睁眼困难。②面浮身肿,足背肿痛。
【针灸方法】直刺或斜刺 0.5～1 寸。

44. 内庭 Nèi tíng (ST₄₄)
【类别】荥穴。
【体表定位】在足背,当二、三趾间,趾蹼缘后方赤白肉际处。(图 2-46)
【层次解剖】同陷谷穴。
【主治病症】①上牙痛,咽喉肿痛,口㖞,鼻衄。②腹胀,便秘,胃痛。③足背肿痛。
【针灸方法】直刺或斜刺 0.5～0.8 寸。

45 厉兑 Lì duì (ST₄₅)
【类别】井穴。
【体表定位】在足第二趾末节外侧,距趾甲角 0.1 寸(指寸)。(图 2-46)
【层次解剖】有趾背动、静脉形成的动、静脉网。分布着腓浅神经的趾背神经。
【主治病症】①面肿,牙痛,鼻衄,咽痛。②梦魇,癫狂。
【针灸方法】浅刺 0.1 寸。

第四节　足太阴脾经穴

本经经穴起于隐白,止于大包,左右各 21 穴。(图 2-47)

1. 隐白 Yǐn bái (SP₁)
【类别】井穴。
【体表定位】在足大趾末节内侧,距趾甲角 0.1 寸(指寸)。(图 2-48)
【层次解剖】有趾背动脉及腓浅神经的细小分支。
【主治病症】①月经过多,崩漏,便血,尿血。②腹胀。③癫狂,梦魇,惊风。
【针灸方法】浅刺 0.1 寸。

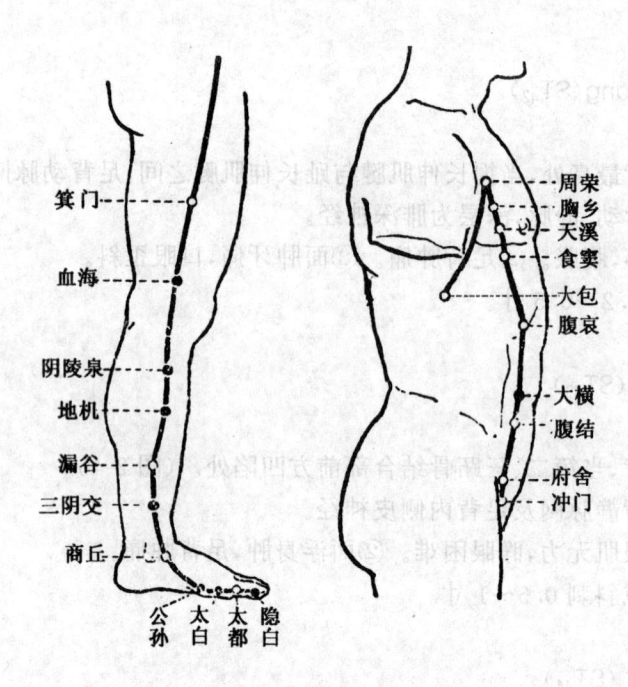

图 2-47 脾经经穴总图

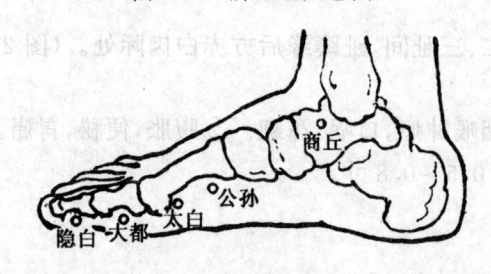

图 2-48

2. 大都 Dà dū (SP$_2$)

【类别】荥穴。

【体表定位】在足内侧,当足大趾本节(第一跖趾关节)前下方赤白肉际凹陷处。(图 2-48)

【层次解剖】有足底内侧动静脉的分支,及趾底固有神经。

【主治病症】①胃痛,便秘。②热病无汗。

【针灸方法】直刺 0.3～0.5 寸。

3. 太白 Tài bái (SP$_3$)

【类别】输穴,原穴。

【体表定位】在足内侧缘,当足大趾本节(第一跖趾关节)后下方赤白肉际凹陷处。(图 2-48)

【层次解剖】有足底内侧动脉的分支,及隐神经分支。

【主治病症】①胃病,腹胀,腹痛,泄泻,痢疾。②肢倦,身重。③心痛。

【针灸方法】直刺 0.5～0.8 寸。

4. 公孙 Gōng Sūn（SP₄）

【类别】络穴,八脉交会穴通冲脉。

【体表定位】在足内侧缘,当第一跖骨基底部的前下方。(图2-48)

【层次解剖】有跗内侧动脉及隐神经分支。

【主治病症】①急性胃脘痛,胃脘堵闷,不思饮食,绕脐腹痛,泄泻,便血。②心痛,胸闷,胁胀。③月经不调,胎衣不下,产后血晕。

【针灸方法】直刺0.6~1.2寸。

5. 商丘 Shāng qiū（SP₅）

【类别】经穴。

【体表定位】在足内踝前下方凹陷中,当舟骨结节与内踝尖连线的中点处。(图2-48)

【层次解剖】有跗内动脉及小腿内侧皮神经。

【主治病症】①足踝疼痛。②痔疾。③腹胀,泄泻,便秘。

【针灸方法】直刺0.5~0.8寸。

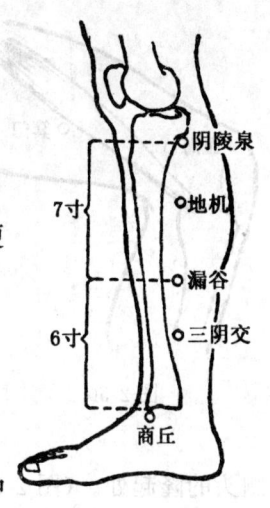

图2-49

6. 三阴交 Sān yīn jiāo（SP₆）

【类别】足太阴、少阴、厥阴经交会穴

【体表定位】在小腿内侧,当足内踝尖上3寸,胫骨内侧缘后方。(图2-49)

【层次解剖】有大隐静脉及隐神经,深层后方有胫神经。

【主治病症】①月经不调,痛经,崩漏,赤白带下,经闭,癥瘕,阴挺,难产,产后血晕,恶露不尽,久不成孕,梦遗,遗精,阳痿,早泄,阴茎痛,疝气,睾丸缩腹。②遗尿,尿闭,水肿,小便不利。③脾胃虚弱,肠鸣,腹胀,泄泻,足痿,脚气,肌肉疼痛。④皮肤病,湿疹,荨麻疹。⑤失眠,头痛头晕,两胁下痛等。

【针灸方法】直刺1~1.5寸,孕妇禁针。

7. 漏谷 Lòu gǔ（SP₇）

【体表定位】在小腿内侧,当内踝尖与阴陵泉的连线上,距内踝尖6寸。

【层次解剖】同三阴交穴。

【主治病症】①肠鸣腹胀。②下肢痿痹。

【针灸方法】直刺1~1.5寸。

8. 地机 Dì jī（SP₈）

【类别】郄穴。

【体表定位】在小腿内侧,当内踝尖与阴陵泉的连线上,阴陵泉下3寸。(图2-49)

【层次解剖】深层有胫后动、静脉。神经分布同三阴交。

【主治病症】①腹痛,泄泻。②小便不利,水肿。③月经不调,痛经,遗精,阳痿,腰痛。

【针灸方法】直刺1~2寸。

517

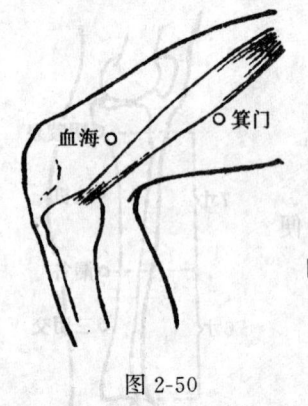

9. 阴陵泉 Yīn líng quán（SP₉）

【类别】合穴。

【体表定位】在小腿内侧,当胫骨内侧后下方凹陷处。(图2-49)

【层次解剖】深层有胫后动、静脉及胫神经。

【主治病症】①小便不利或失禁,水肿。②腹胀,泄泻,黄疸。③膝内侧疼痛。④阴茎痛,痛经,妇人阴痛等。

【针灸方法】直刺1～2寸。

图2-50

10. 血海 Xuè hǎi（SP₁₀）

【体表定位】屈膝,在大腿内侧,髌底内侧端上2寸,当股四头肌内侧头的隆起处。(图2-50)

【层次解剖】有股动、静脉肌支及股前皮神经。

【主治病症】①月经不调,崩漏,经闭。②瘾疹,湿疹,丹毒。

【针灸方法】直刺1～1.5寸。

11. 箕门 Jī mén（SP₁₁）

【体表定位】在大腿内侧,当血海与冲门连线上,血海上6寸。(图2-50)

【层次解剖】有大隐静脉,深部有隐神经。

【主治病症】①腹股沟肿痛。②小便不利,遗尿。

【针灸方法】避开动脉,直刺0.5～1寸。

12. 冲门 Chōng mén（SP₁₂）

【类别】足太阴、厥阴经交会穴。

【体表定位】在腹股沟外侧,距耻骨联合上缘中点3.5寸,当髂外动脉的外侧。(图2-51)

【层次解剖】内侧为股动脉。当股神经经过处。

【主治病症】①疝气,腹痛。②崩漏,带下。

【针灸方法】避开动脉,直刺0.5～1寸。

13. 府舍 Fǔ shè（SP₁₃）

【类别】足太阴、厥阴、阴维脉交会穴。

【体表定位】在下腹部,当脐下4寸,冲门上方0.7寸,距前正中线4寸。(图2-51)

【层次解剖】分布着髂腹股沟神经。

【主治病症】疝气,腹痛。

【针灸方法】直刺1～1.5寸。

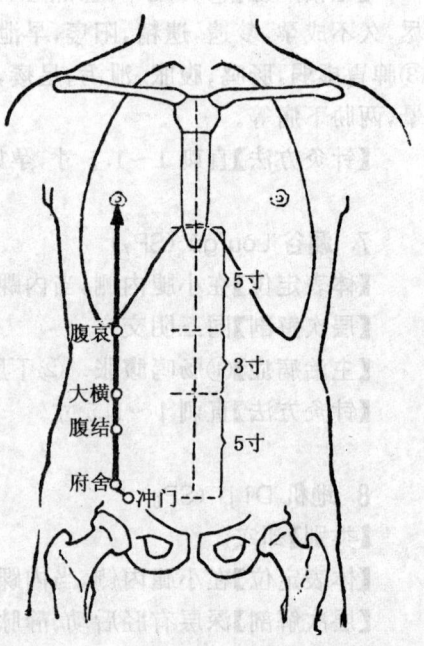

图2-51

14. 腹结 Fǔ jié (SP₁₄)

【体表定位】在下腹部,大横下 1.3 寸,距前正中线 4 寸。(图 2-51)

【层次解剖】有第十一肋间动、静脉及第十一肋间神经。

【主治病症】①绕脐腹痛,腹胀,泄泻,便秘。②疝气。

【针灸方法】直刺 1～2 寸。

15. 大横 Dà héng (SP₁₅)

【类别】足太阳、阴维脉交会穴。

【体表定位】在腹中部,距脐中 4 寸。(图 2-51)

【层次解剖】有第十肋间动、静脉及第十肋间神经。

【主治病症】泄泻,便秘,腹痛。

【针灸方法】直刺 1～2 寸。

16. 腹哀 Fù āi (SP₁₆)

【类别】足太阴、阴维脉交会穴。

【体表定位】在上腹部,当脐中上 3 寸,距前正中线 4 寸。(图 2-51)

【层次解剖】有第八肋间动、静脉及第八肋间神经。

【主治病症】腹痛,肠鸣,消化不良。

【针灸方法】直刺 1～1.5 寸。

17. 食窦 Shí dòu (SP₁₇)

【体表定位】在胸外侧部,当第五肋间隙,距前正中线 6 寸。(图 2-52)

【层次解剖】有胸腹壁静脉分布着第五肋间神经外侧皮支。

【主治病症】①胸胁胀痛,翻胃,食入即吐。②腹胀水肿,黄疸。③老人大便不禁。

【针灸方法】斜刺或向外平刺 0.5～0.8 寸。本经食窦至大包诸穴,深部为肺脏,不可深刺。

18. 天溪 Tiān xī (SP₁₈)

【体表定位】在胸外侧部,当第四肋间隙,距前正中线 6 寸。(图 2-52)

【层次解剖】有第四肋间动、静脉,及第四肋间神经外侧皮支。

【主治病症】①胸胁疼痛,咳嗽。②乳痈,乳汁少。

【针灸方法】斜刺或向外平刺 0.5～0.8 寸。

19. 胸乡 Xiōng xiāng (SP₁₉)

【体表定位】在胸外侧部,当第三肋间隙,距前正中线 6 寸。

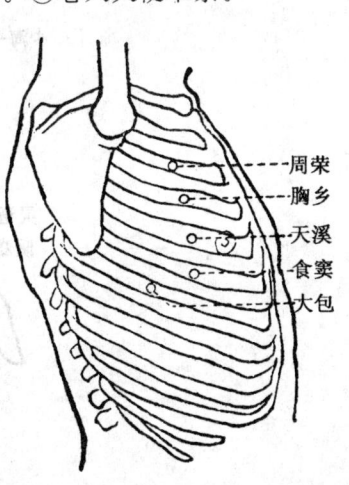

图 2-52

(图 2-52)

【层次解剖】有第三肋间动、静脉及第三肋间神经外侧皮支。
【主治病症】胸胁胀痛。
【针灸方法】斜刺或向外平刺 0.5～0.8 寸。

20. 周荣 Zhōu róng（SP$_{20}$）

【体表定位】在胸外侧部,当第二肋间隙,距前正中线 6 寸。(图 2-52)
【层次解剖】有第二肋间动、静脉及第二肋间神经外侧皮支。
【主治病症】咳嗽,胸胁胀满。
【针灸方法】斜刺或向外平刺 0.5～0.8 寸。

21. 大包 Dà bāo（SP$_{21}$）

【类别】脾之大络。
【体表定位】在侧胸部,腋中线上,当第六肋间隙处。(图 2-52)
【层次解剖】有第七肋间动、静脉及第七肋间神经。
【主治病症】①全身疼痛,四肢无力。②气喘,胸胁痛。
【针灸方法】斜刺或向后平刺 0.5～0.8 寸。

第五节　手少阴心经穴

本经经穴起于极泉,止于少冲,左右各 9 穴(图 2-53)

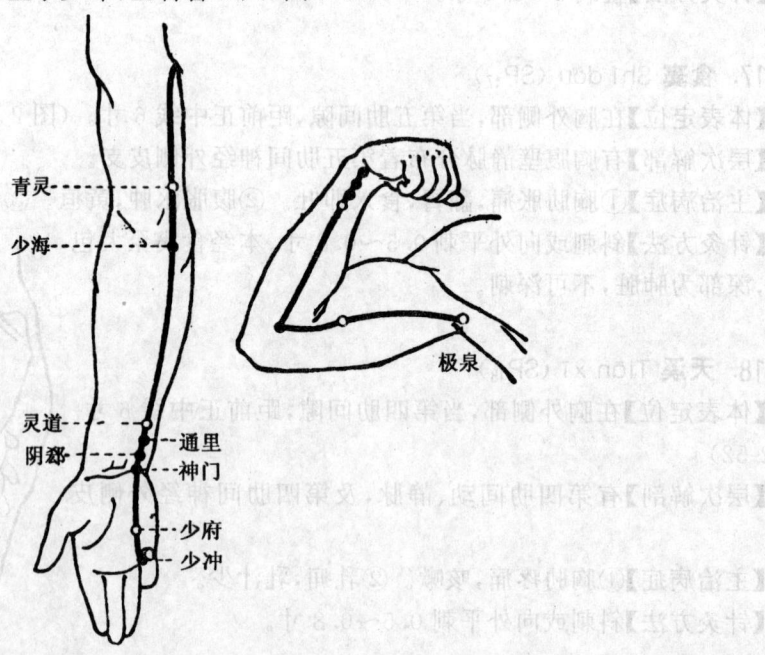

图 2-53

1. 极泉 Jí quán (HT₁)

【体表定位】在腋窝顶点,腋动脉搏动处。(图 2-53)

【层次解剖】外侧为腋动脉,穴下为尺神经、正中神经。

【主治病症】①胸闷气短,心痛心悸,悲愁不乐。②中风偏瘫,肩臂疼痛,胸胁胀痛。

【针灸方法】避开腋动脉,直刺或斜刺 0.3～0.5 寸。

2. 青灵 Qīng líng (HT₂)

【体表定位】在臂内侧,当极泉与少海的连线上,肘横纹上 3 寸,肱二头肌的内侧沟中。(图 2-54)

【层次解剖】有贵要静脉及尺神经。

【主治病症】心痛,胁痛,肩臂痛。

【针灸方法】直刺 0.5～1 寸。

图 2-54

3. 少海 Shào hǎi (HT₃)

【类别】合穴。

【体表定位】屈肘,在肘横纹内侧端与肱骨内上髁连线中点处。(图 2-54)

【层次解剖】有贵要静脉及前臂内侧皮神经。

【主治病症】①心痛,肘臂挛痛,麻木,手颤。②瘰疬,腋胁痛。

【针灸方法】直刺 0.5～1 寸。

4. 灵道 Líng dào (HT₄)

【类别】经穴。

【体表定位】在前臂掌侧,当尺侧腕屈肌腱的桡侧缘,腕横纹上 1.5 寸(图 2-55)

【层次解剖】有尺动脉及臂内侧皮神经。

【主治病症】心痛,暴喑。

【针灸方法】直刺 0.3～0.5 寸。

5. 通里 Tōng lǐ (HT₅)

【类别】络穴。

【体表定位】在前臂掌侧,当尺侧腕屈肌腱的桡侧缘,腕横纹上 1 寸。(图 2-55)

【层次解剖】同灵道穴。

【主治病症】①暴喑,舌强不语,腕臂痛。②心悸,怔忡。

【针灸方法】直刺 0.3～0.5 寸。

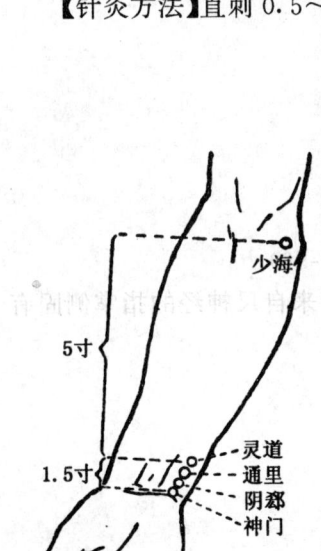

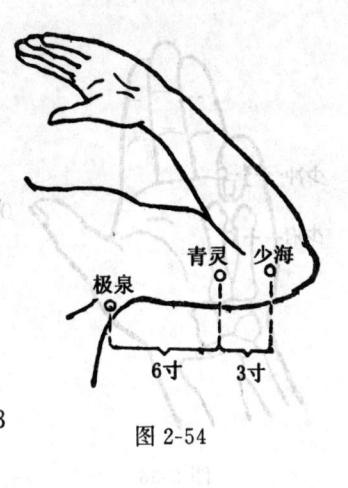

图 2-55

6. 阴郄 Yīn xì (HT₆)
【类别】郄穴。
【体表定位】在前臂掌侧,当尺侧腕屈肌腱的桡侧缘,腕横纹上0.5寸。(图2-55)
【层次解剖】同灵道。
【主治病症】①心痛,惊悸。②骨蒸盗汗。③吐血,衄血,暴喑。
【针灸方法】直刺0.3~0.5寸。

7. 神门 Shén mén (HT₇)
【类别】输穴,原穴。
【体表定位】在腕部,腕掌横纹尺侧端,尺侧腕屈肌腱的桡侧凹陷处。(图2-55)
【层次解剖】同灵道穴。
【主治病症】①失眠健忘。②心痛,惊悸,心烦,胸痛。③癫狂痫证,呆痴。
【针灸方法】直刺0.3~0.5寸。

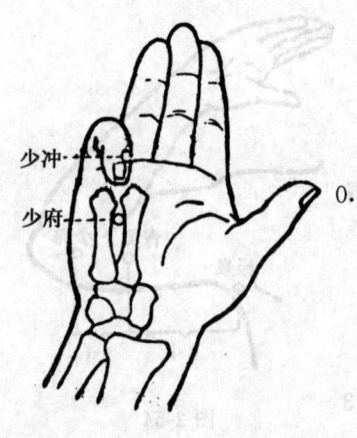

图2-56

8. 少府 Shào fǔ (HT₈)
【类别】荥穴。
【体表定位】在手掌面,第四、五掌骨之间,握拳时,当小指尖处。(图2-56)
【层次解剖】有指掌侧总动、静脉,及指掌侧总神经。
【主治病症】①阴痒痛。②小指挛痛。③心悸,胸痛。
【针灸方法】直刺0.3~0.5寸。

9. 少冲 Shào chōng (HT₉)
【类别】井穴。
【体表定位】在手小指末节桡侧,距指甲角0.1寸(指寸)。(图2-56)
【层次解剖】有指掌侧固有动、静脉所形成的动、静脉网,分布着来自尺神经的指掌侧固有神经。
【主治病症】①心悸,心痛,胸胁痛。②癫狂,热病,昏迷。
【针灸方法】浅刺0.1寸或点刺出血。

第六节 手太阳小肠经穴

本经经穴起于少泽,止于听宫,左右各19穴。(图2-57)

1. 少泽 Shào zé (SI₁)
【类别】井穴。
【体表定位】在手小指末节尺侧,距指甲角0.1寸(指寸)。(图2-58)

【层次解剖】有动、静脉网及尺神经分支。

【主治病症】①热病，中风，昏迷。②乳汁少，乳痛。③咽喉肿痛，目翳头痛。

【针灸方法】浅刺 0.1 寸或点刺出血。

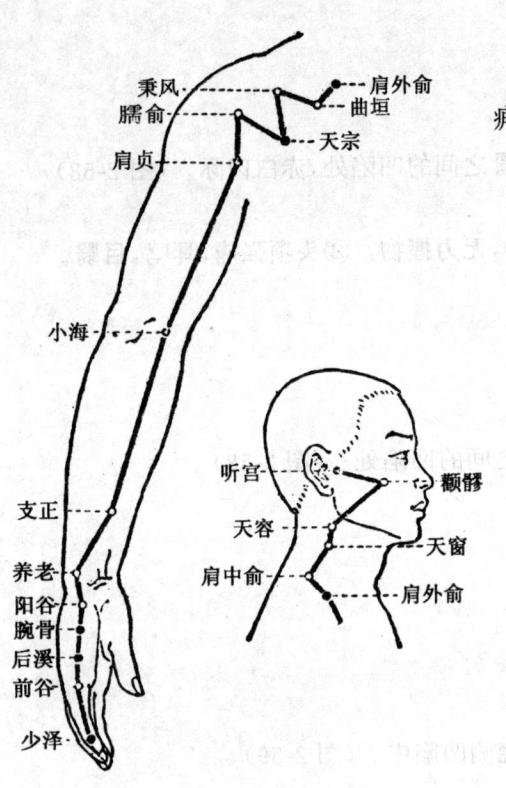

图 2-57 小肠经经穴总图

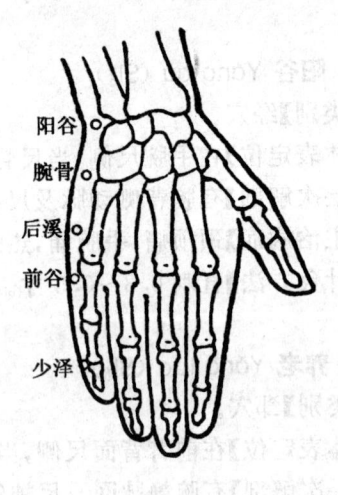

图 2-58

2. **前谷** Qián gǔ (SI$_2$)

【类别】荥穴。

【体表定位】在手尺侧，微握拳，当小指本节（第五掌指关节）前的掌指横纹头赤白肉际。（图 2-58）

【层次解剖】有指背动、静脉及指背神经分支。

【主治病症】①手指麻木。②发热，头痛，耳鸣。③小便短赤。

【针灸方法】直刺 0.3～0.5 寸。

3. **后溪** Hòu xī (SI$_3$)

【类别】输穴，八脉交会穴通督脉。

【体表定位】在手掌尺侧，微握拳，当小指本节（第五掌指关节）后的远侧掌横纹头赤白肉际。（图 2-58）

【层次解剖】有指背侧动、静脉及尺神经手背支。

【主治病症】①头项强痛，疟疾，腰骶痛，手指及肘臂挛急。②癫狂，痫证。③耳聋，目赤。④盗汗。

【针灸方法】直刺 0.5～1 寸。

4. 腕骨 Wàn gǔ (SI₄)

【类别】原穴。

【体表定位】在手掌尺侧,当第五掌骨基底与钩骨之间的凹陷处,赤白肉际。(图 2-58)

【层次解剖】有手背静脉网及尺神经手背支。

【主治病症】①黄疸,消渴。②腰腿痛,指挛腕痛,无力握物。③头项强痛,耳鸣,目翳。

【针灸方法】直刺 0.3～0.5 寸。

5. 阳谷 Yáng gǔ (SI₅)

【类别】经穴。

【体表定位】在手腕尺侧,当尺骨茎突与三角骨之间的凹陷处。(图 2-58)

【层次解剖】有腕背侧动脉及尺神经手背支。

【主治病症】颈项痛,手腕痛,热病。

【针灸方法】直刺 0.3～0.5 寸。

6. 养老 Yǎng lǎo (SI₆)

【类别】郄穴。

【体表定位】在前臂背面尺侧,当尺骨小头近端桡侧凹陷中。(图 2-59)

【层次解剖】有腕静脉网及尺神经手背支。

【主治病症】①目视不明。②肩、背、肘、臂痠痛,急性腰痛。

【针灸方法】向肘方向斜刺 0.5～0.8 寸。

7. 支正 Zhī zhèng (SI₇)

【类别】络穴。

【体表定位】在前臂背面尺侧,当阳谷与小海的连线上,腕背横纹上 5 寸。(图 2-59)

【层次解剖】有前臂骨间背侧动、静脉的末支及尺神经手背支。

【主治病症】①关节松弛无力,肘部酸痛不用。②皮肤赘生小疣。

【针灸方法】直刺或斜刺 0.5～0.8 寸。

8. 小海 Xiǎo hǎi (SI₈)

【类别】合穴。

【体表定位】在肘内侧,当尺骨鹰嘴与肱骨内上髁之间凹陷处。(图 2-59)

【层次解剖】有尺侧上、下副动、静脉及尺神经。

【主治病症】①肘臂疼痛。②癫痫。

【针灸方法】直刺 0.3～0.5 寸。

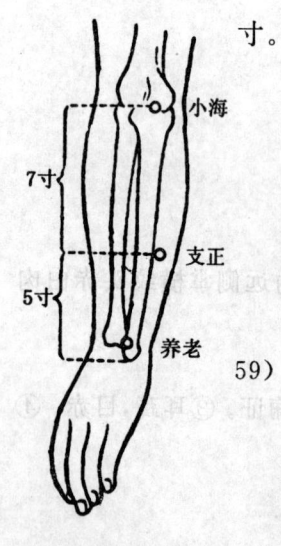

图 2-59

9. 肩贞 Jiān zhēn (SI₉)

【体表定位】在肩关节后下方,臂内收时,腋后纹头上1寸(指寸)。(图2-60)

【层次解剖】有旋肩胛动、静脉,深部上方为桡神经。

【主治病症】①肩臂疼痛,②瘰疬,耳鸣。

【针灸方法】直刺1～1.5寸。

10. 臑俞 Nào shū (SI₁₀)

【类别】手、足太阳、阳维脉、阳蹻脉交会穴。

【体表定位】在肩部,当腋后纹头直上,肩胛冈下缘凹陷中。(图2-60)

【层次解剖】有旋肱后动、静脉,腋神经。

【主治病症】①肩臂疼痛。②瘰疬。

【针灸方法】直刺0.5～1.5寸。

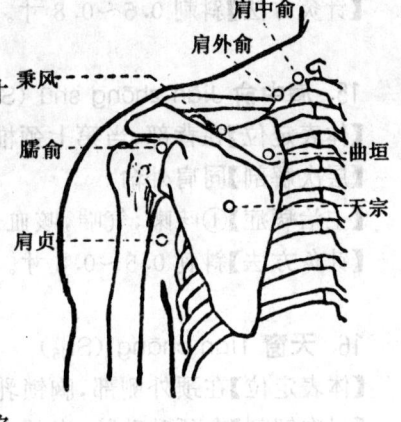

图2-60

11. 天宗 Tiān zōng (SI₁₁)

【体表定位】在肩胛部,当冈下窝中央凹陷处,与第四胸椎相平。(图2-60)

【层次解剖】有旋肩胛动、静脉肌支,分布着肩胛上神经。

【主治病症】①肩胛疼痛,②气喘,③乳痈。

【针灸方法】直刺或斜刺0.5～1寸。

12. 秉风 Bǐng fēng (SI₁₂)

【类别】手三阳与足少阳经交会穴。

【体表定位】在肩胛部,冈上窝中央,天宗直上,举臂有凹陷处。(图2-60)

【层次解剖】有肩胛上动、静脉,及为肩胛上神经。

【主治病症】肩胛疼痛,上肢痠麻。

【针灸方法】直刺或斜刺0.5～1寸。

13. 曲垣 Qǔyuán (SI₁₃)

【体表定位】在肩胛部,冈上窝内侧端,当臑俞与第二胸椎棘突连线的中点处。(图2-60)

【层次解剖】深层为肩胛上动、静脉肌支,及为肩胛上神经肌支。

【主治病症】肩胛疼痛。

【针灸方法】直刺或斜刺0.5～1寸。

14. 肩外俞 Jiān wài shū (SI₁₄)

【体表定位】在背部,当第一胸椎棘突下,旁开3寸。(图2-60)

【层次解剖】深层有颈横动、静脉,及为肩胛背神经。

【主治病症】肩背疼痛,颈项强急。

【针灸方法】斜刺 0.5～0.8 寸。

15. 肩中俞 Jiān zhōng shū (SI$_{15}$)
【体表定位】在背部,当第七颈椎棘突下,旁开 2 寸。(图 2-60)
【层次解剖】同肩外俞。
【主治病症】①咳嗽,气喘,咳血。②肩背疼痛。
【针灸方法】斜刺 0.5～0.8 寸。

16. 天窗 Tiān chāng (SI$_{16}$)
【体表定位】在颈外侧部,胸锁乳突肌的后缘,扶突后,与喉结相平。(图 2-61)
【层次解剖】有颈升动脉,当耳大神经丛的发出部。
【主治病症】①咽喉肿痛,暴喑,颈项强痛。②耳鸣,耳聋。
【针灸方法】直刺 0.5～1 寸。

17. 天容 Tiān róng (SI$_{17}$)
【体表定位】在颈外侧部,当下颌角的后方,胸锁乳突肌的前缘凹陷中。(图 2-61)
【层次解剖】深层为颈内动、静脉,分布着耳大神经的前支,深层有交感神经链通过。
【主治病症】耳鸣,耳聋,咽喉肿痛,颈项肿痛。
【针灸方法】直刺 0.5～1 寸。

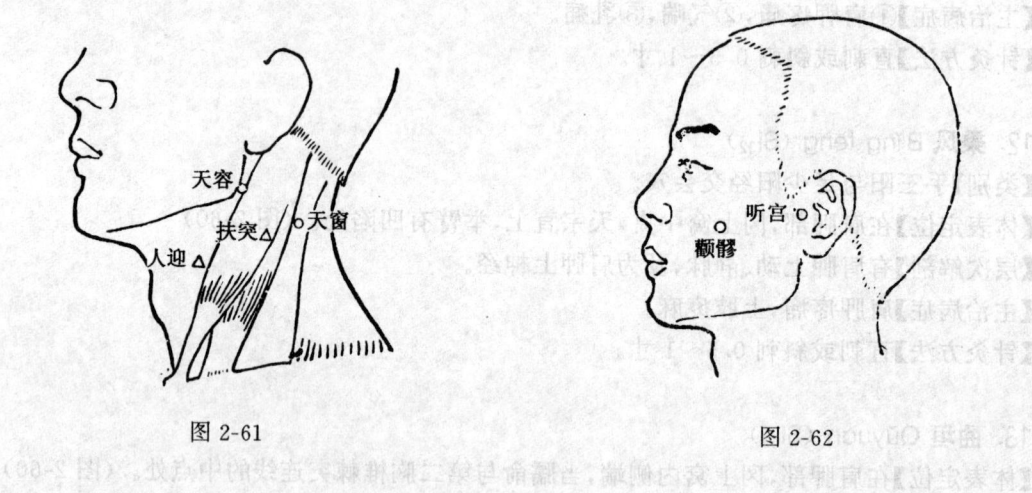

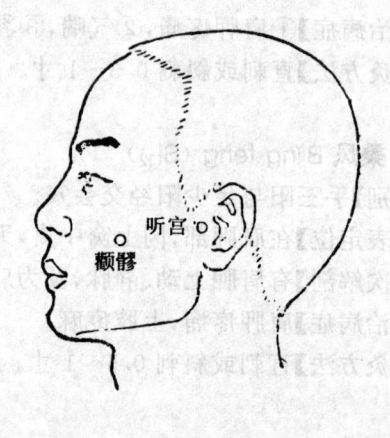

图 2-61

图 2-62

18. 颧髎 Quán liáo (SI$_{18}$)
【类别】手少阳、太阳经交会穴。
【体表定位】在面部,当目外眦直下,颧骨下缘凹陷处。(图 2-62)
【层次解剖】有面横动、静脉分支,分布着面神经及眶下神经。
【主治病症】①口眼歪斜,眼睑瞤动。②牙痛,颊肿。
【针灸方法】直刺 0.3～0.5 寸,斜刺或平刺 0.5～1 寸。《图翼》:禁灸。

19. 听宫 Tīng gōng (SI$_{19}$)

【类别】手、足少阳,手太阳经交会穴。

【体表定位】在面部,耳屏前,下颌骨髁状突的后方,张口时呈凹陷处。(图 2-62)

【层次解剖】有颞浅动、静脉的耳前支,分布着面神经分支及耳颞神经。

【主治病症】①耳鸣,耳聋,聤耳。②牙痛,牙关不利。

【针灸方法】张口,直刺 1～1.5 寸。

第七节　足太阳膀胱经穴

本经经穴起于睛明,止于至阴,左右各 67 穴。(图 2-63)

1. 睛明　Jīng míng (BL1)

【类别】手、足太阳、足阳明、阴跷、阳跷五脉之会穴。

【体表定位】在面部,目内眦角上方凹陷处。(图 2-64)

【层次解剖】有内眦动、静脉,分布着滑车上、下神经,深层为动眼神经和眼神经。

【主治病症】①视物不明,近视,夜盲,色盲。②胬肉攀睛,目翳,目赤肿痛,迎风流泪。③急性腰痛。

【针灸方法】嘱患者闭目,医者左手轻推眼球向外侧固定,右手缓慢进针,紧靠眶缘直刺 0.5～1 寸。不捻转,不提插(或只轻微地捻转)。出针后按压针孔片刻,以防出血。本穴禁灸。

2. 攒竹 Cuán zhú (BL2)

【体表定位】在面部,当眉头陷中,眶上切迹处。(图 2-64)

【层次解剖】有额动、静脉,分布着额神经内侧支。

【主治病症】①眉棱骨痛,目视不明,目赤肿痛。②呃逆。③腰痛。④膈肌痉挛。

【针灸方法】平刺 0.5～0.8 寸,或点刺放血。禁灸。

3. 眉冲　Méi chōng (BL$_3$)

【体表定位】在头部,当攒竹直上入发际 0.5 寸,神庭与曲差连线之间。(图 2-65)

【层次解剖】同攒竹穴。

【主治病症】①头痛,眩晕,鼻塞。②癫痫。

【针灸方法】平刺 0.3～0.5 寸。

4. 曲差　Qū chā (BL$_4$)

【体表定位】在头部,当前发际正中直上 0.5 寸,旁开 1.5 寸,即神庭与头维连线的内 1/3 与中 1/3 交点上。(图 2-65)

【层次解剖】有额动、静脉。分布着额神经外侧支。

【主治病症】①头痛,鼻塞,衄血。②目视不明。

【针灸方法】平刺 0.5～0.8 寸。

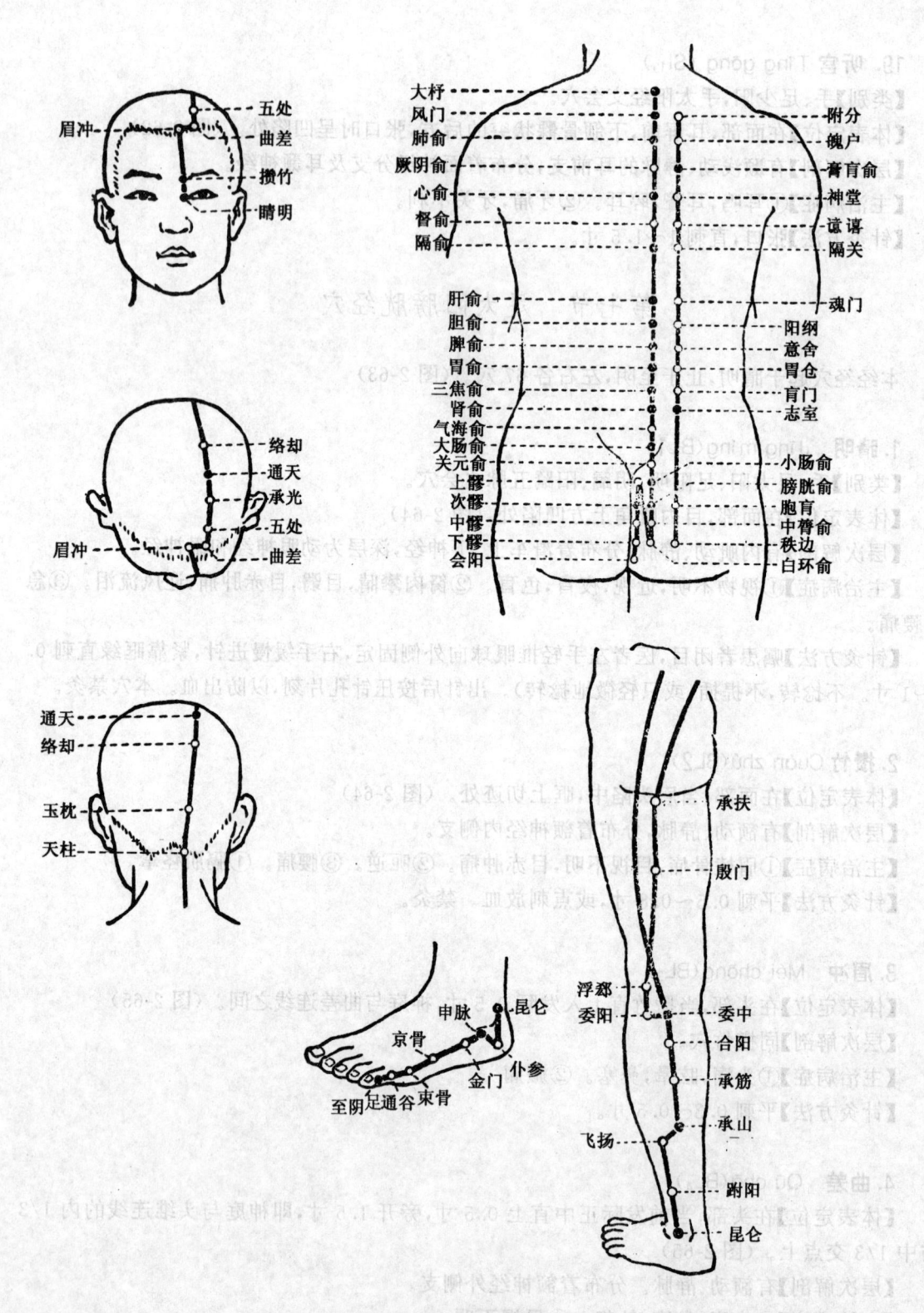

图 2-63 膀胱经经穴总图

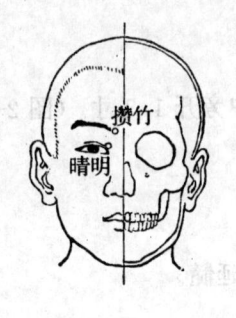

图 2-64 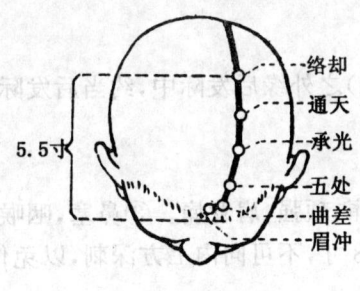　　　　　　　　　图 2-65 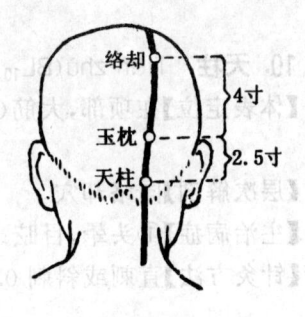　　　　　　　　　图 2-66

5. 五处　Wǔ chù(BL₅)

【体表定位】在头部,当前发际正中直上1寸,旁开1.5寸。(图2-65)

【层次解剖】同曲差穴。

【主治病症】①头痛,头晕。②中风偏瘫。③癫痫。

【针灸方法】平刺0.5～0.8寸。

6. 承光　Chéng guāng(BL₆)

【体表定位】在头部,当前发际正中直上2.5寸。旁开1.5寸。(图2-65)

【层次解剖】有额、颞、枕动、静脉的吻合网。当额神经外侧支和枕大神经吻合支处。

【主治病症】①目视不明。②中风偏瘫,癫痫。③头晕目眩。

【针灸方法】平刺0.3～0.5寸。

7. 通天　Tōng tiān(BL₇)

【体表定位】在头部,当前发际正中直上4寸,旁开1.5寸,(图2-65)

【层次解剖】有颞浅和枕动、静脉的吻合网,分布着枕大神经分支。

【主治病症】①鼻塞,鼻中瘜肉,鼻疮,鼻渊,鼻衄。②头痛,目眩。③中风偏瘫,癫痫。

【针灸方法】平刺0.3～0.5寸。

8. 络却　Luò què(BL₈)

【体表定位】在头部,当前发际正中直上5.5寸,旁开1.5寸。(图2-65)

【层次解剖】有枕动、静脉分支,分布着枕大神经分支。

【主治病症】①目视不明。②中风偏瘫,癫痫。③耳鸣。

【针灸方法】平刺0.3～0.5寸。

9. 玉枕　Yù zhěn(BL₉)

【体表定位】在后头部,当后发际正中直上2.5寸,旁开1.3寸,平枕外粗隆上缘的凹陷处。(图2-66)

【层次解剖】同络却穴。

【主治病症】①头项痛,目视不明。②鼻塞。③脚癣。

【针灸方法】平刺0.3～0.5寸。

10. 天柱　Tiān zhù（BL₁₀）

【体表定位】在项部，大筋（斜方肌）之外缘后发际中，约当后发际正中旁开1.3寸。（图2—66）

【层次解剖】同络却穴。

【主治病症】①头晕，目眩。②头痛，项强，肩背痛。③鼻塞，咽喉痛。

【针灸方法】直刺或斜刺0.5～0.8寸，不可向内上方深刺，以免伤及延髓。

11. 大杼　Dà zhù（BL₁₁）

【类别】八会穴（骨会），手、足太阳经交会穴。

【体表定位】在背部，当第一胸椎棘突下，旁开1.5寸。（图2-67）

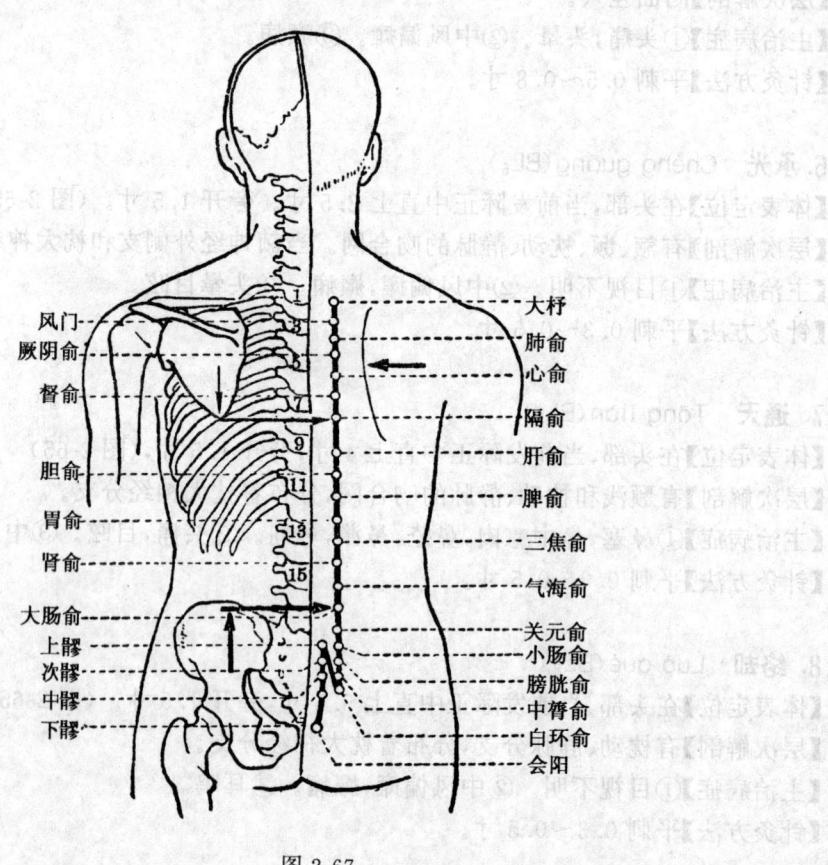

图2-67

【层次解剖】有肋间动、静脉后支的内侧支。分布着第一胸神经后支的内侧皮支，深层为外侧支。

【主治病症】①各种骨病（骨痛，肩、腰、骶、膝关节痛）。②发热，咳嗽，头痛鼻塞。

【针灸方法】斜刺0.5～0.8寸。

12. 风门 Fēng mén(BL₁₂)

【类别】足太阳经与督脉交会穴。
【体表定位】在背部,当第二胸椎棘突下,旁开1.5寸。(图2-67)
【层次解剖】血管分布同大杼。分布着第二、第三胸神经后支的内侧皮支,深层为外侧支。
【主治病症】①伤风,咳嗽。②发热,头痛,项强,胸背痛。
【针灸方法】斜刺0.5~0.8寸。

13. 肺俞 Fèi shū(BL₁₃)

【类别】肺的背俞穴。
【体表定位】在背部,当第三胸椎棘突下,旁开1.5寸。(图2-67)
【层次解剖】血管分布同大杼。分布着第三、四胸神经后支的内侧皮支,深层为外侧支。
【主治病症】①发热,咳嗽,咳血,盗汗,鼻塞。②毛发脱落,痘,疹,疮,癣。
【针灸方法】斜刺0.5~0.8寸。

14. 厥阴俞 Jué yīng shū(BL₁₄)

【类别】心包背俞穴。
【体表定位】在背部,当第四胸椎棘突下,旁开1.5寸。(图2-67)
【层次解剖】血管分布同大杼。分布着第四、五胸神经后支的内侧皮支,深层为外侧支。
【主治病症】①心痛,心悸。②咳嗽,胸闷。③牙痛。
【针灸方法】斜刺0.5~0.8寸。

15. 心俞 Xīn shū(BL₁₅)

【类别】心的背俞穴。
【体表定位】在背部,当第五胸椎棘突下,旁开1.5寸。(图2-67)
【层次解剖】血管分布同大杼。分布着第五、六胸神经后支的内侧皮支,深层为外侧支。
【主治病症】①心痛,心悸,胸闷,气短。②咳嗽,吐血。③失眠,健忘,癫痫。④梦遗,盗汗。
【针灸方法】斜刺0.5~0.8寸。

16. 督俞 Dū shū(BL₁₆)

【体表定位】在背部,当第六胸椎棘突下,旁开1.5寸。(图2-67)
【层次解剖】管分布同大杼。分布着第六、七胸神经后支的内侧皮支,深层为外侧支。
【主治病症】①心痛,胸闷。②胃痛,腹痛。③咳嗽,气喘。
【针灸方法】斜刺0.5~0.8寸。

17. 膈俞 Gé shū(BL₁₇)

【类别】八会穴(血会)。
【体表定位】在背部,第七胸椎棘突下,旁开1.5寸。(图2-67)
【层次解剖】血管分布同大杼。分布着第七、八胸神经后支的内侧支,深层为外侧支。

【主治病症】①急性胃脘痛,呃逆,噎膈,便血。②咳嗽,气喘,吐血,骨蒸盗汗。
【针灸方法】斜刺 0.5～0.8 寸。

18. 肝俞　Gān shū(BL$_{18}$)
【类别】肝的背俞穴。
【体表定位】在背部,当第九胸椎棘突下,旁开1.5寸。(图2-67)
【层次解剖】血管分布同大杼。分布着第九、十胸神经后支的内侧皮支,深层为外侧支。
【主治病症】①胁痛,黄疸。②目疾,吐,衄。③癫狂,脊背痛。
【针灸方法】斜刺 0.5～0.8 寸。

19. 胆俞　Dǎn shū(BL$_{19}$)
【类别】胆的背俞穴。
【体表定位】在背部,当第十胸椎棘突下,旁开1.5寸。(图2-67)
【层次解剖】血管分布同大杼。分布着第十、十一胸神经后支的内侧皮支,深层为外侧支。
【主治病症】①黄疸,口苦,胁痛。②肺痨,潮热。
【针灸方法】斜刺 0.5～0.8 寸。

20. 脾俞　Pǐ shū(BL$_{20}$)
【类别】脾的背俞穴。
【体表定位】在背部,当第十一胸椎棘突下,旁开1.5寸。(图2-67)
【层次解剖】血管分布同大杼。分布着第十一、十二胸神经后支的内侧皮支,深层为外侧支。
【主治病症】①腹胀,黄疸,呕吐,泄泻,痢疾,便血。②水肿。
【针灸方法】斜刺 0.5～0.8 寸。

21. 胃俞　Wèi shū(BL$_{21}$)
【类别】胃的背部穴。
【体表定位】在背部,当第十二胸椎棘突下,旁开1.5寸。(图2-67)
【层次解剖】有肋下动,静脉后支的内侧支。分布着第十二胸神经后支的内侧皮支,深层为外侧支。
【主治病症】①胃脘痛,呕吐。②腹胀,肠鸣。
【针灸方法】斜刺 0.5～0.8 寸。

22. 三焦俞　Sān jiāo shū(BL$_{22}$)
【类别】三焦背俞穴。
【体表定位】在腰部,当第一腰椎棘突下,旁开1.5寸。(图2-67)
【层次解剖】有第一、二腰动、静脉后支。布有第一、二腰神经后支。
【主治病症】①水肿,小便不利。②腹胀,肠鸣,泄泻,痢疾。③膝关节无力。
【针灸方法】直刺 0.5～1 寸。

23. 肾俞 Shèn shū(BL₂₃)
【类别】肾的背俞穴。
【体表定位】在腰部,当第二腰椎棘突下,旁开1.5寸。(图2-67)
【层次解剖】有第二、三腰动、静脉后支。分布着第二、三腰神经后支的肌支。
【主治病症】①遗尿,小便不利,水肿。②遗精,阳痿,月经不调,白带。③耳聋,耳鸣,咳嗽,气喘。④中风偏瘫,腰痛,骨病。
【针灸方法】直刺0.5～1寸。

24. 气海俞 Qì hǎi shū(BL₂₄)
【体表定位】在腰部,当第三腰椎棘突下,旁开1.5寸。(图2-67)
【层次解剖】有第三、四腰动、静脉后支。分布有第三、四腰神经后支的肌支。
【主治病症】①腹胀,肠鸣,痔漏。②痛经,腰痛。
【针灸方法】直刺0.5～1寸。

25. 大肠俞 Dà cháng shū(BL₂₅)
【类别】大肠背俞穴。
【体表定位】在腰部,当第四腰椎棘突下,旁开1.5寸。(图2-67)
【层次解剖】有第四、五腰动、静脉。分布有第四、五腰神经后支的肌支。
【主治病症】①腹胀,泄泻,便秘,痔疮出血。②腰痛。③荨麻疹。
【针灸方法】直刺0.8～1.2寸。

26. 关元俞 Guān yuán shū(BL₂₆)
【体表定位】在腰部,当第五腰椎棘突下,旁开1.5寸。(图2-67)
【层次解剖】有第五腰和第一骶动、静脉。布有第五腰神经后支的肌支。
【主治病症】①腰骶痛。②腹胀,泄泻。③小便频数或不利,遗尿。
【针灸方法】直刺0.8～1.2寸。

27. 小肠俞 Xiǎo cháng shū(BL₂₇)
【类别】小肠背俞穴。
【体表定位】在骶部,当骶正中嵴旁开1.5寸,平第一骶后孔。(图2-67)
【层次解剖】有骶外侧动、静脉后支。分布着第一骶神经后支的外侧支。
【主治病症】①腰骶痛,膝关节痛。②小腹胀痛,小便不利。③遗精,白带。
【针灸方法】直刺或斜刺0.8～1.2寸。

28. 膀胱俞 Páng Guāng shū(BL₂₈)
【类别】膀胱背俞穴。
【体表定位】在骶部,当骶正中嵴旁1.5寸,平第二骶后孔。(图2-67)
【层次解剖】血管分布同小肠俞。分布着第一、二骶神经后支的外侧支。

【主治病症】①小便不利,遗尿。②腰脊强痛,腿痛。③泄泻,便秘。
【针灸方法】直刺或斜刺 0.8～1.2 寸。

29. 中膂俞　Zhōng lǔ shū(BL₂₉)
【体表定位】在骶部,当骶正中嵴旁 1.5 寸,平第三骶后孔。(图 2-67)
【层次解剖】有骶外侧动、静脉后支,臀下动、静脉分支。分布着第三、四骶神经后支的外侧支。
【主治病症】①泄泻。②疝气,腰脊强痛。
【针灸方法】直刺 1～1.5 寸。

30. 白环俞　Bái huán shū(BL₃₀)
【体表定位】在骶部,当骶正中嵴旁 1.5 寸,平第四骶后孔。(图 2-67)
【层次解剖】有臀下动、静脉,深层为阴部内动、静脉。分布着第三、四骶神经后支的外侧支及臀下神经。
【主治病症】①遗精,白带,月经不调,遗尿。②腰骶疼痛,疝气。
【针灸方法】直刺 1～1.5 寸。

31. 上髎　Shàng liáo(BL₃₁)
【体表定位】在骶部,当髂后上嵴与后正中线之间,适对第一骶后孔处。(图 2-67)
【层次解剖】有骶外侧动、静脉后支,为第一骶神经后支通过处。
【主治病症】①月经不调,赤白带下,阴挺。②遗精,阳痿。③大、小便不利,腰骶痛。
【针灸方法】直刺 1～1.5 寸。

32. 次髎　Cì liáo(BL₃₂)
【体表定位】在骶部,当髂后上棘内下方,适第二骶后孔处。(图 2-67)
【层次解剖】血管分布同上髎。为第二骶神经后支通过处。
【主治病症】①遗精,阳痿。②月经不调,赤白带下。③腰骶痛,下肢痿痹。
【针灸方法】直刺 1～1.5 寸。

33. 中髎　Zhōng liáo(BL₃₃)
【体表定位】当次髎内下方,适对第三骶后孔处。(图 2-67)
【层次解剖】血管分布同上髎。为第三骶神经后支通过处。
【主治病症】①月经不调,白带,小便不利,便秘,泄泻。②腰骶疼痛。
【针灸方法】直刺 1～1.5 寸。

34. 下髎　Xià liáo(BL₃₄)
【体表定位】在骶部,当中髎内下方,适对第四骶后孔处。(图 2-67)
【层次解剖】有臀下动、静脉分支。为第四骶神经后支通过处。
【主治病症】①腰骶痛,小腹痛。②小便不利,带下。

【针灸方法】直刺 1~1.5 寸。

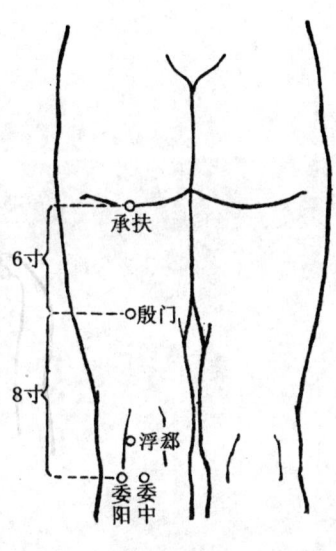

35. 会阳 Huì yáng(BL$_{35}$)
【体表定位】在骶部,尾骨端旁开 0.5 寸。(图 2-67)
【层次解剖】有臀下动、静脉分支。分布着尾神经。
【主治病症】①大便失禁,泄泻,便血,痔疾。②阳痿。③带下。
【针灸方法】直刺 1~1.5 寸。

36. 承扶 Chéng fú(BL$_{36}$)
【体表定位】在大腿后面,臀下横纹的中点。(图 2-68)
【层次解剖】有与坐骨神经并行的动、静脉。深层正当坐骨神经。
【主治病症】腰骶臀股部疼痛,痔疾。
【针灸方法】直刺 1~2 寸。

37. 殷门 Yīn mén(BL$_{37}$)
【体表定位】在大腿后面,当承扶与委中的连线上,承扶下 6 寸。(图 2-68)
【层次解剖】外侧为股深动、静脉第三穿支。深层正当坐骨神经。
【主治病症】腰痛,下肢痿痹。
【针灸方法】直刺 1~2 寸。

38. 浮郄 Fú xì(BL$_{38}$)
【体表定位】在腘横纹外侧端,委阳上 1 寸,股二头肌腱的内侧。(图 2-68)
【层次解剖】有膝上外侧动、静脉。分布着腓总神经。
【主治病症】腘窝部疼痛、麻木或挛急。
【针灸方法】直刺 1~1.5 寸。

39. 委阳 Wěi yáng(BL$_{39}$)
【类别】三焦下合穴。
【体表定位】在腘横纹外侧端,当股二头肌腱的内侧。(图 2-68)
【层次解剖】血管、神经分布同浮郄。
【主治病症】①腰脊强痛,小腹胀满,小便不利。②腿足拘挛疼痛,痿厥。
【针灸方法】直刺 1~1.5 寸。

40. 委中 Wěi zhōng(BL$_{40}$)
【类别】合穴。

图 2-68

【体表定位】在腘横纹中点,当股二头肌腱与半腱肌肌腱的中间。(图 2-68)
【层次解剖】有股腘静脉,深层为腘动脉。分布着胫神经。
【主治病症】①腰脊疼痛,腘筋挛急,半身不遂,下肢痿痹。②丹毒,皮疹,周身搔痒,疔疮,发背。③腹痛吐泻。④遗尿,小便不利。
【针灸方法】直刺 1～1.5 寸,或用三棱针点刺腘静脉出血。

41. 附分 Fù fēn (BL₄₁)

【类别】手、足太阳之会穴
【体表定位】在背部,当第二胸椎棘突下,旁开 3 寸。(图 2-69)

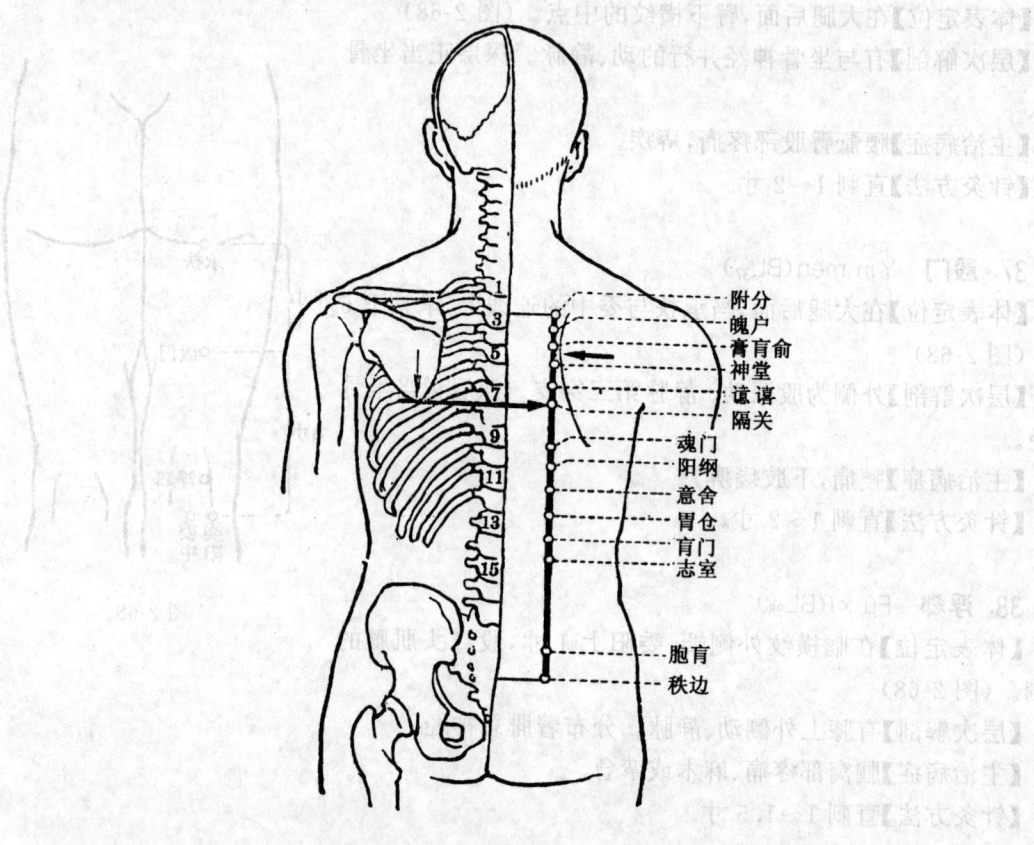

图 2-69

【层次解剖】有肋间动、静脉分支。分布着第一、二胸神经分支,深层为肩胛背神经。
【主治病症】颈项强痛,肩背拘急,肘臂麻木。
【针灸方法】斜刺 0.5～0.8 寸。

42. 魄户 Pò hù (BL₄₂)

【体表定位】在背部,当第三胸椎棘突下,旁开 3 寸。(图 2-69)
【层次解剖】血管分布同附分,分布着第二、三胸神经分支及肩胛背神经。
【主治病症】①咳嗽,气喘,肺痨。②项强,肩背痛。

【针灸方法】斜刺 0.5~0.8 寸。

43. 膏肓　Gāo huāng(BL₄₃)
【体表定位】在背部，当第四胸椎棘突下，旁开3寸。(图 2-69)
【层次解剖】血管分布同附分。分布着第三、四胸神经分支及肩胛背神经。
【主治病症】①肺痨咳嗽气喘，纳差，便溏，消瘦乏力。②遗精，盗汗，健忘。③肩背痠痛。
【针灸方法】斜刺 0.5~0.8 寸。

44. 神堂　shén táng(BL₄₄)
【体表定位】在背部，当第五胸椎棘突下，旁开3寸。(图 2-69)
【层次解剖】血管分布同附分，分布着第四、五、胸神经分支及肩胛背神经。
【主治病症】①心痛，心悸，失眠。②胸闷，咳嗽，气喘。③肩背痛。
【针灸方法】斜刺 0.5~0.8 寸。

45. 譩譆　Yì xǐ(BL₄₅)
【体表定位】在背部，当第六胸椎棘突下，旁开3寸。(图 2-69)
【层次解剖】有肋间动、静脉后支。分布着第五、六胸神经分支。
【主治病症】①咳嗽，气喘。②肩背痛。
【针灸方法】斜刺 0.5~0.8 寸。

46. 膈关　Gé guān(BL₄₆)
【体表定位】在背部，当第七胸椎棘突下，旁开3寸。(图 2-69)
【层次解剖】血管分布同诶诀穴。分布着第六、七胸神经后支的分支。
【主治病症】①饮食不下，呃逆，呕吐。②脊背强痛。
【针灸方法】斜刺 0.5~0.8 寸。

47. 魂门　Hún mén(BL₄₇)
【体表定位】在背部，当第九胸椎棘突下，旁开3寸。(图 2-69)
【层次解剖】血管分布同诶诀穴。分布着第八、九胸神经分支。
【主治病症】①胸胁胀满，呕吐，泄泻。②背痛。
【针灸方法】斜刺 0.5~0.8 寸。

48. 阳纲　Yáng gāng(BL₄₈)
【体表定位】在背部，当第十胸椎棘突下，旁开3寸。(图 2-69)
【层次解剖】血管分布同诶诀穴。分布着第九、十胸神经的分支。
【主治病症】①黄疸，腹痛，肠鸣，泄泻。②消渴。
【针灸方法】斜刺 0.5~0.8 寸。

49 意舍 Yì shè(BL₄₉)
【体表定位】在背部,当第十一胸椎棘突下,旁开3寸。(图2-69)
【层次解剖】血管分布同谚诀穴,分布着第十、十一胸神经分支。
【主治病症】腹胀,肠鸣,呕吐,泄泻。
【针灸方法】斜刺0.5~0.8寸。

50. 胃仓 Wèi cāng(BL₅₀)
【体表定位】在背部,当第十二胸椎棘突下,旁开3寸。(图2-69)
【层次解剖】有肋下动、静脉分支。分布着第十一胸神经分支。
【主治病症】①胃脘痛,腹胀。②小儿食积。③水肿。
【针灸方法】斜刺0.5~0.8寸。

51. 肓门 Huāng mén(BL₅₁)
【体表定位】在腰部,当第一腰椎棘突下,旁开3寸。(图2-69)
【层次解剖】有第一腰动、静脉后支。分布着第十二胸神经分支。
【主治病症】①腹痛,便秘。②痞块,乳疾。
【针灸方法】斜刺0.5~0.8寸。

52 志室 Zhì shì(BL₅₂)
【体表定位】在腰部,当第二腰椎棘突下,旁开3寸。(图2-69)
【层次解剖】有第二腰动、静脉的后支。分布着第十二胸神经及第一腰神经的分支。
【主治病症】①遗精,阳痿。②小便不利,水肿。③腰脊强痛。
【针灸方法】斜刺0.5~0.8寸。

53. 胞肓 Bāo huāng(BL₅₃)
【体表定位】在臀部,平第二骶后孔,骶正中嵴旁开3寸。(图2-69)
【层次解剖】有臀上动、静脉。分布着臀上皮神经,深层为臀上神经。
【主治病症】①尿闭,阴肿。②腰脊痛。③肠鸣腹胀。
【针灸方法】直刺1~1.5寸。

54. 秩边 Zhì biān(BL₅₄)
【体表定位】在臀部,平第四骶后孔,骶正中嵴旁开3寸。(图2-69)
【层次解剖】有臀下动、静脉。分布着臀下神经及坐骨神经。
【主治病症】①腰骶痛,下肢痿痹。②小便不利,便秘,痔疾。
【针灸方法】直刺1.5~2寸。

55. 合阳 Hé yáng(BL₅₅)
【体表定位】在小腿后面,当委中与承山的连线上,委中下2寸。(图2-70)

【层次解剖】有小隐静脉,深层为腘动、静脉。深层有胫神经。
【主治病症】①腰脊强痛,下肢痿痹。②疝气。③崩漏。
【针灸方法】直刺1～2寸。

56. 承筋 Chéng jīn(BL$_{56}$)

【体表定位】在小腿后面,当委中与承山的连线上,腓肠肌肌腹中央,委中下5寸。(图2-70)
【层次解剖】血管神经分布同合阳。
【主治病症】①痔疾。②腰腿拘急疼痛。
【针灸方法】直刺1～1.5寸。

57. 承山 Chéng shān(BL$_{57}$)

【体表定位】在小腿后面正中,委中与昆仑之间,当伸直小腿或足跟上提时,腓肠肌肌腹下出现尖角凹陷处。(图2-70)
【层次解剖】血管神经分布同合阳。
【主治病症】①痔疮,便秘。②腰腿拘急疼痛。③脚气。
【针灸方法】直刺1～2寸。

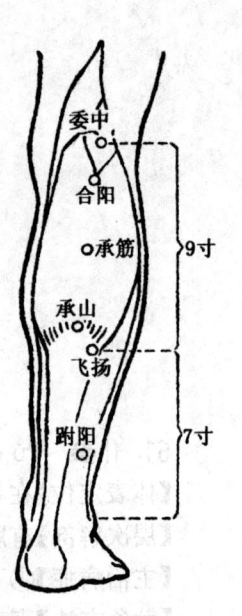

图2-70

58. 飞扬 Fēi yáng(BL$_{58}$)

【类别】络穴。
【体表定位】在小腿后面,当外踝后,昆仑穴直上7寸,承山外下方1寸处。(图2-70)
【层次解剖】有胫后动脉,分布着腓肠外侧皮神经。
【主治病症】①头痛,目眩,鼽衄。②腰腿疼痛无力。③痔疾。
【针灸方法】直刺0.7～1寸。

59. 跗阳 Fū yáng(BL$_{59}$)

【类别】阳跷脉郄穴。
【体表定位】在小腿后面,外踝后,昆仑穴直上3寸。(图2-70)
【层次解剖】有小隐静脉,深层为腓动脉末支。当腓肠神经分布处。
【主治病症】①头痛,头重。②腰骶疼痛,下肢痿痹,外踝肿痛。
【针灸方法】直刺0.8～1.2寸。

60. 昆仑 Kūn lún(BL$_{60}$)

【类别】经穴。
【体表定位】在足部外踝后方,当外踝尖与跟腱之间的凹陷处。(图2-71)
【层次解剖】有小隐静脉及外踝后动、静脉。分布着腓肠神经。
【主治病症】①急性腰痛,足跟肿痛。②难产。③头痛,项强,目眩,鼻衄。④小儿惊风。
【针灸方法】直刺0.5～1寸。

图 2-71

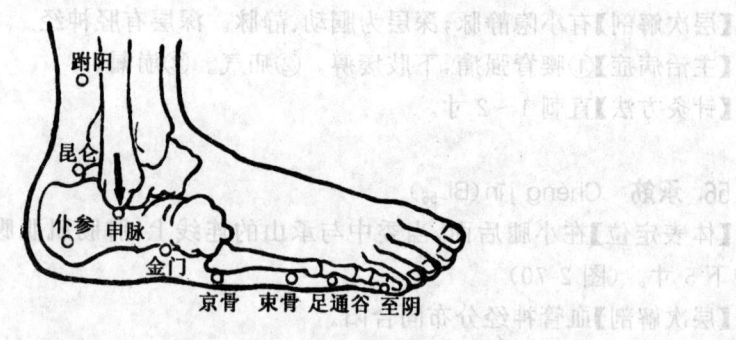

61. 仆参 Pú cān（BL₆₁）
【体表定位】在足外侧部,外踝后下方,昆仑直下,跟骨外侧,赤白肉际处。（图 2-71）
【层次解剖】有腓动、静脉分支。分布着腓肠神经分支。
【主治病症】①下肢痿痹,足跟痛。②癫痫。
【针灸方法】直刺 0.3～0.5 寸。

62. 申脉 Shēn mài（BL₆₂）
【类别】八脉交会穴通于阳蹻。
【体表定位】在足外侧部,外踝直下方凹陷处。（图 2-71）
【层次解剖】有外踝动脉网。分布着腓肠神经。
【主治病症】①痫症,癫狂。②失眠,足外翻。③头痛,项强,腰腿痛。④眼睑下垂。
【针灸方法】直刺 0.3～0.5 寸。

63. 金门 Jīn mén（BL₆₃）
【类别】郄穴。
【体表定位】在足外侧,当外踝前缘直下,骰骨下缘处。（图 2-71）
【层次解剖】有足底外侧动、静脉。分布着足背外侧皮神经,深层为足底外侧神经。
【主治病症】①癫狂,痫症,小儿惊风。②头痛,腰痛,下肢痿痹,外踝痛。
【针灸方法】直刺 0.3～0.5 寸。

64. 京骨 Jīng gǔ（BL₆₄）
【类别】原穴。
【体表定位】在足外侧,第五跖骨粗隆下方,赤白肉际处。（图 2-71）
【层次解剖】血管神经分布同金门。
【主治病症】①头痛,项强,目翳。②腰腿痛。③癫痫。
【针灸方法】直刺 0.3～0.5 寸。

65. 束骨 Shù gǔ（BL₆₅）
【类别】输穴。

【体表定位】在足外侧,足小趾本节(第五跖趾关节)的后方,赤白肉际处。(图2-71)
【层次解剖】有第四趾底总动、静脉。分布着第四趾跖侧总神经及足背外侧神经。
【主治病症】①癫狂,头痛项强。②腰腿痛,肛门痛。
【针灸方法】直刺0.3～0.5寸。

66. 足通谷 Zú tōng gǔ(BL$_{66}$)
【类别】荥穴。
【体表定位】在足外侧,足小趾本节(第五跖趾关节)的前方,赤白肉际处。(图2-71)
【层次解剖】有趾跖动、静脉,分布着趾跖固有神经,足背外侧皮神经。
【主治病症】①头痛,项强,目眩,鼻衄。②癫狂。
【针灸方法】直刺0.2～0.3寸。

67. 至阴 Zhì yīn(BL$_{67}$)
【类别】井穴。
【体表定位】在足小趾末节外侧,距趾甲角0.1寸(指寸)。(图2-71)
【层次解剖】有动脉网。神经分布同足通谷。
【主治病症】①胎位不正,难产。②头目痛,鼻塞,鼻衄。
【针灸方法】浅刺0.1寸,胎位不正用灸法。

第八节 足少阴肾经穴

本经经穴起于涌泉,止于俞府。左右各27穴。(图2-72)

1. 涌泉 Yǒng quán(KL$_1$)
【类别】井穴。
【体表定位】在足底部,卷足时足前部凹陷处,约当足底二、三趾趾缝纹头端与足跟连线的前1/3与后2/3交点上。(图2-73)
【层次解剖】深层有胫前动脉的足底弓,分布着第二趾足底总神经。
【主治病症】①昏厥,头顶痛,眩晕,小儿惊风,癫狂。②恶心,呕吐。③咽肿舌干,小便不利,大便难。④足心热。
【针灸方法】直刺0.5～1寸。
【参考资料】现代观察,涌泉穴有很好的降血压作用。艾灸涌泉穴有矫正胎位的作用。

2. 然谷 Rán gǔ(KL$_2$)
【类别】荥穴。
【体表定位】在足内侧,舟骨粗隆下方,赤白肉际。(图2-74)
【层次解剖】有足底内侧及跗内侧动脉分支。分布着小腿内侧皮神经末支及足底内侧神经。
【主治病症】①阴挺,阴痒,月经不调,带下病。②小儿脐风,口噤。③遗精,消渴,足背肿痛。

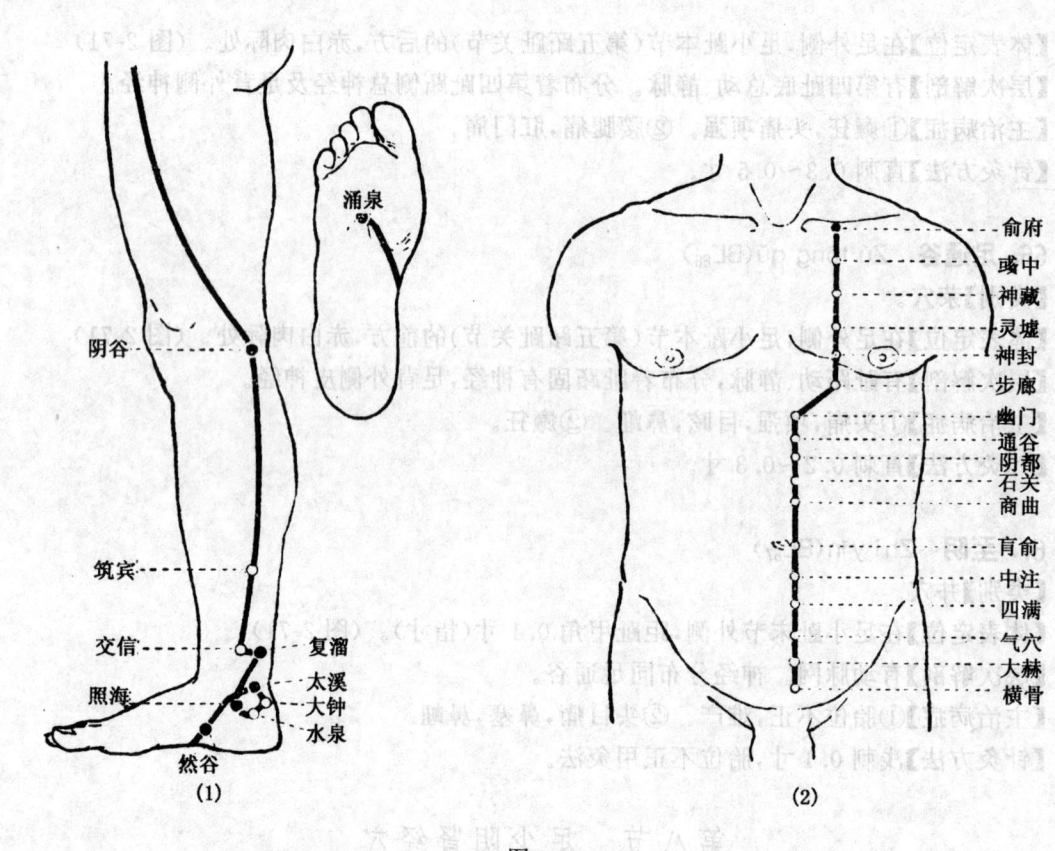

图 2-72

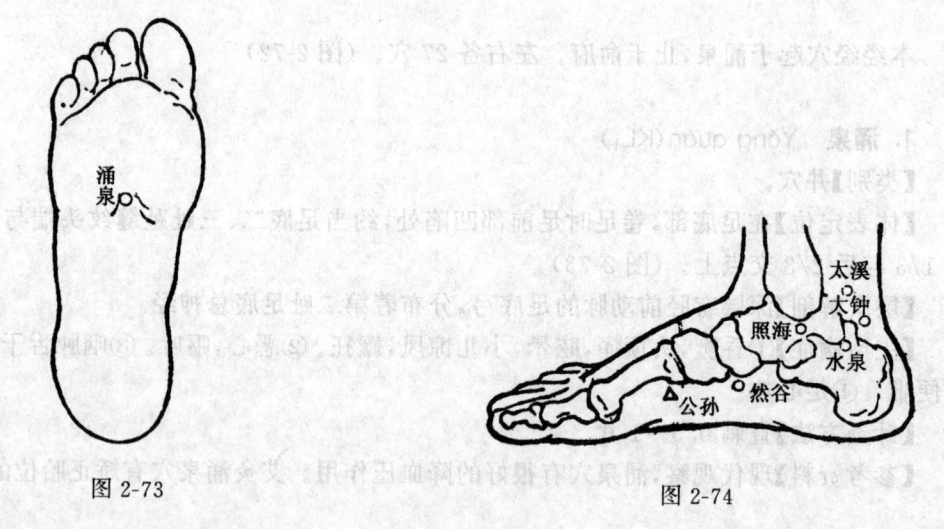

图 2-73

图 2-74

【针灸方法】直刺 0.5~1 寸。

3. **太溪** Tài xī(KL₃)

【类别】原穴，输穴。

【体表定位】在足内侧、内踝后方，当内踝尖与跟腱之间的凹陷处。（图 2-74）

542

【层次解剖】有胫后动、静脉。分布着胫神经的分支。
【主治病症】①阳痿，遗精，小便频数，耳聋，耳鸣，月经不调，腰疼。②头痛，头晕，目视不明，牙痛，咽肿。③咳嗽，气喘，消渴。④失眠。
【针灸方法】直刺0.5～1寸。

4. 大钟 Dà zhōng(KL₄)
【类别】络穴。
【体表定位】在足内侧、内踝后下方，当跟腱附着部的内侧前方凹陷处。((图2-74)
【层次解剖】有胫后动脉的跟骨内侧支，布有小腿内侧皮神经及胫神经的跟骨内侧支。
【主治病症】①癃闭，遗尿，便秘。②咳血，气喘。③痴呆，足跟痛。
【针灸方法】直刺0.3～0.5寸。

5. 水泉 Shuǐ quán(KL₅)
【类别】郄穴。
【体表定位】在足内侧，内踝后下方，当太溪穴直下1寸（指寸），跟骨结节的内侧凹陷处。(图2-74)
【层次解剖】血管，神经分布同大钟穴。
【主治病症】①月经不调，痛经，闭经，阴挺。②小便不利。
【针灸方法】直刺0.3～0.5寸。

6. 照海 Zhào hǎi(KL₆)
【类别】八脉交会穴通于阴跷脉。
【体表定位】在足内侧，内踝尖下方凹陷处。(图2-74)
【层次解剖】有胫后动、静脉。分布着小腿内侧皮神经，深部为胫神经本干。
【主治病症】①咽喉干痛，便秘，癃闭。②月经不调，赤白带下，阴挺，阴痒。③癫痫夜发。
【针灸方法】直刺0.3～0.5寸。

7. 复溜 Fù liū(KL₇)
【类别】经穴。
【体表定位】在小腿内侧，太溪直上2寸，跟腱的前方。(图2-75)
【层次解剖】深层前方有胫后动、静脉。深层为胫神经。
【主治病症】①水肿，腹胀，泄泻。②热病汗不出，或汗出不止，盗汗。③下肢痿痹。
【针灸方法】直刺0.6～1寸。

8. 交信 Jiāo xìn(KL₈)
【类别】阴跷脉郄穴。
【体表定位】在小腿内侧，当太溪直上2寸，复溜前0.5寸，胫骨内侧缘的后方。(图2-75)

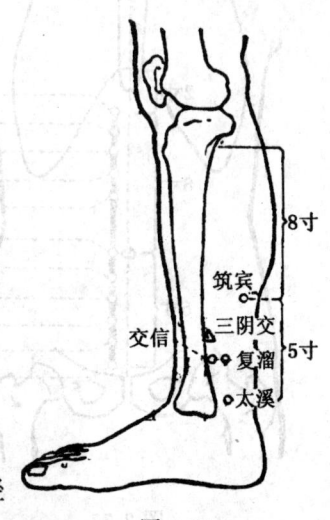

图2-75

【层次解剖】深层为胫后动、静脉。深部为胫神经本干。
【主治病症】①月经不调,崩漏,阴挺。②疝气。③泄泻,便秘。
【针灸方法】直刺 0.6～1.2 寸。

9. **筑宾** Zhù bīn(KL₉)

【类别】阴维脉郄穴。
【体表定位】在小腿内侧,当太溪与阴谷的连线上,太溪上 5 寸,腓肠肌肌腹的内下方。(图 2-75)
【层次解剖】深部有胫后动、静脉。深层为胫神经本干。
【主治病症】①癫狂。②疝气。③小腿疼痛。
【针灸方法】直刺 1～1.5 寸。

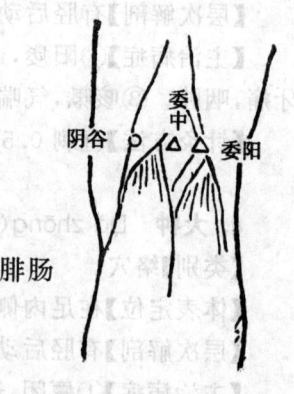

图 2-76

10. **阴谷** Yīn gǔ(KL₁₀)

【类别】合穴。
【体表定位】在腘窝内侧,屈膝时,当半腱肌肌腱与半膜肌肌腱之间。(图 2-76)
【层次解剖】有膝上内侧动、静脉。分布着股内侧皮神经。
【主治病症】①阳痿,疝气,崩漏。②小便不利。③膝腘痠痛。
【针灸方法】直刺 1～1.5 寸。

11. **横骨** Héng gǔ(KL₁₁)

【类别】足少阴与冲脉交会穴
【体表定位】在下腹部,当脐中下 5 寸,前正中线旁开 0.5 寸。(图 2-77)
【层次解剖】有腹壁下动、静脉,阴部外动脉,分布着髂腹下神经的分支。
【主治病症】①少腹胀痛,小便不利,遗尿。②遗精,阳痿。③疝气,阴部痛。
【针灸方法】直刺 1～1.5 寸。

12. **大赫** Dà hè(KL₁₂)

【类别】足少阴与冲脉交会穴。
【体表定位】在下腹部,当脐中下 4 寸,前正中线旁开 0.5 寸。(图 2-77)
【层次解剖】有腹壁下动、静脉的肌支,分布着髂腹下神经。
【主治病症】①遗精,阳痿。②阴挺,带下。
【针灸方法】直刺 1～1.5 寸。

13. **气穴** Qì xué(KL₁₃)

【类别】足少阴与冲脉交会穴。

图 2-77

【体表定位】在下腹部,当脐中下3寸,前正中线旁开0.5寸。(图2-77)
【层次解剖】血管分布同大赫。为十二肋间神经分布处。
【主治病症】①月经不调,带下。②小便不利。③泄泻。
【针灸方法】直刺1~1.5寸。

14. 四满 Sì mǎn(KL$_{14}$)
【类别】足少阴与冲脉的交会穴。
【体表定位】在下腹部,当脐中下2寸,前正中线旁开0.5寸。(图2-77)
【层次解剖】血管分布同大赫。当第十一肋间神经分布处。
【主治病症】①腹痛,腹胀,泄泻,水肿。②月经不调,痛经。
【针灸方法】直刺1~1.5寸。

15. 中注 Zhōng zhù(KL$_{15}$)
【类别】足少阴与冲脉交会穴。
【体表定位】在中腹部,当脐中下1寸,前正中线旁开0.5寸。(图2-77)
【层次解剖】血管分布同大赫。为第十肋间神经分布处。
【主治病症】①月经不调,痛经。②腹痛,便秘,泄泻。
【针灸方法】直刺1~1.5寸。

16. 肓俞 Huāng shū(KL$_{16}$)
【类别】足少阴与冲脉交会穴。
【体表定位】在中腹部,当脐中旁开0.5寸。(图2-77)
【层次解剖】血管、神经分布同中注。
【主治病症】腹痛,腹胀,呕吐,便秘,泄泻。
【针灸方法】直刺1~1.5寸。

17. 商曲 Shāng qū(KL$_{17}$)
【类别】足少阴与冲脉交会穴。
【体表定位】在上腹部,当脐中上2寸,前正中线旁开0.5寸。(图2-77)
【层次解剖】有腹壁上下动、静脉。分布着第九肋间神经。
【主治病症】腹痛,泄泻,便秘。
【针灸方法】直刺1~1.5寸。

18. 石关 Shí guān(KL$_{18}$)
【类别】足少阴与冲脉交会穴。
【体表定位】在上腹部,当脐中上3寸,前正中线旁开0.5寸。(图2-77)。
【层次解剖】血管分布同商曲,分布着第八肋间神经。
【主治病症】①呕吐,腹痛,便秘。②不孕。
【针灸方法】直刺1~1.5寸。

19. 阴都 Yīn dū(KL₁₉)

【类别】足少阴与冲脉交会穴。

【体表定位】在上腹部,当脐上4寸,前正中线旁开0.5寸。(图2-77)

【层次解剖】血管,神经分布同石关。

【主治病症】①腹痛,腹胀,便秘。②不孕。

【针灸方法】直刺1～1.5寸。

20. 腹通谷 Fù tōng gǔ(KL₂₀)

【类别】足少阴与冲脉交会穴。

【体表定位】在上腹部,当脐中上5寸,前正中线旁开0.5寸。(图2-77)

【层次解剖】血管,神经分布同石关。

【主治病症】腹胀,腹痛,呕吐。

【针灸方法】直刺0.5～1寸。

21. 幽门 Yōu mén(KL₂₁)

【类别】足少阴与冲脉交会穴。

【体表定位】在上腹部,当脐中上6寸,前正中线旁开0.5寸。(图2-77)

【层次解剖】血管分布同石关。为第七肋间神经分布处。

【主治病症】腹痛,腹胀,呕吐,泄泻。

【针灸方法】直刺0.5～1寸,不可深刺,以免伤及肝脏。

22. 步廊 Bù láng(KL₂₂)

【体表定位】在胸部、当第五肋间隙,前正中线旁开2寸。(图2-78)

【层次解剖】有第五肋间动、静脉。深部为第五肋间神经。

【主治病症】①咳嗽,气喘,胸胁胀满。②呕吐。

【针灸方法】斜刺或平刺0.5～0.8寸。本经胸部诸穴,不可深刺,以免伤及心、肺。

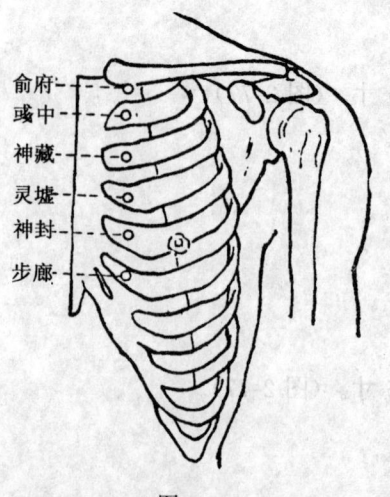

图2-78

23. 神封 Shén fēng(KL₂₃)

【体表定位】在胸部,当第四肋间隙,前正中线旁开2寸。(图2-78)

【层次解剖】有第四肋间动、静脉。深部为第四肋间神经。

【主治病症】①咳嗽,气喘,胸胁胀满。②乳痈。

【针灸方法】斜刺或平刺0.5～0.8寸。

24. 灵墟 Líng xū(KL₂₄)

【体表定位】在胸部,当第三肋间隙,前正中线旁开2寸。(图2-78)

【层次解剖】有第三肋间动、静脉。深层为第三肋间神经。
【主治病症】①咳嗽,气喘,胸胁胀满。②乳痈。
【针灸方法】斜刺或平刺 0.5～0.8 寸。

25. 神藏　Shén cáng(KL$_{25}$)
【体表定位】在胸部,当第二肋间隙,前正中线旁开 2 寸。(图 2-78)
【层次解剖】有第二肋间动、静脉。深层为第二肋间神经。
【主治病症】①咳嗽,气喘,胸痛。②呕吐。
【针灸方法】斜刺或平刺 0.5～0.8 寸。

26. 彧中　Yù zhōng(KL$_{26}$)
【体表定位】在胸部,当第一肋间隙,前正中线旁开 2 寸。(图 2-78)
【层次解剖】有第一肋间动、静脉。锁骨上神经前支,深层为第一肋间神经。
【主治病症】咳嗽,气喘,胸胁胀满。
【针灸方法】斜刺或平刺 0.5～0.8 寸。

27. 俞府　Shū fǔ(KL$_{27}$)
【体表定位】在胸部,当锁骨下缘,前正中线旁开 2 寸。(图 2-78)
【层次解剖】有乳房内动、静脉支。分布着锁骨上神经的前支。
【主治病症】①咳嗽,气喘,胸痛。②呕吐。
【针灸方法】斜刺或平刺 0.5～0.8 寸。

第九节　手厥阴心包经

本经经穴起于天池,止于中冲,左右各 9 穴。(图 2-79)

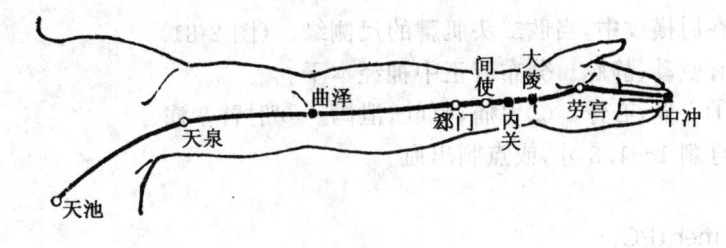

图 2-79

1. 天池　Tiān chí(PC$_1$)
【类别】手厥阴与足少阳经交会穴。
【体表定位】在胸部,当第四肋间隙,乳头外 1 寸,前正中线旁开 5 寸。(图 2-80)
【层次解剖】有胸外动、静脉分支。分布着第四肋间神经。
【主治病症】①乳痈,胁肋疼痛,瘰疬。②咳喘,胸闷。
【针灸方法】斜刺或平刺 0.3～0.5 寸,不可深刺,以免伤及肺脏。

图 2-80　　　　　　　　　图 2-81　　　　　　　　　图 2-82

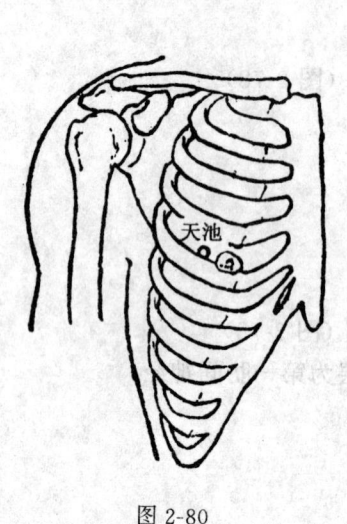

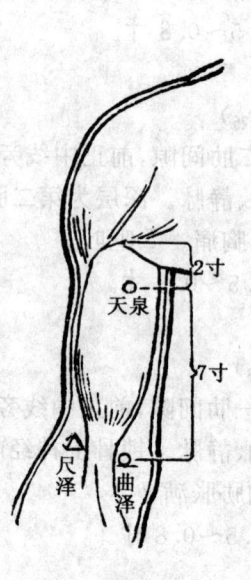

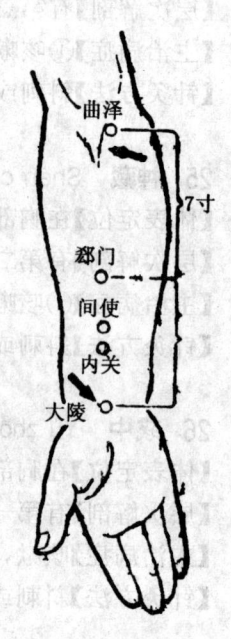

2. 天泉　Tiān quán（PC₂）
【体表定位】在臂内侧,当腋前纹头下2寸,肱二头肌的长、短头之间。（图2-81）
【层次解剖】有肱动、静脉肌支,为臂内侧皮神经。
【主治病症】①心痛,咳嗽,胸胁胀痛。②臂痛。
【针灸方法】直刺1～1.5寸。

3. 曲泽　Qū zé（PC₃）
【类别】合穴。
【体表定位】在肘横纹中,当肱二头肌腱的尺侧缘。（图2-81）
【层次解剖】有肱动、静脉。分布着正中神经本干。
【主治病症】①心痛,心悸。②胃痛,呕吐,泄泻。③肘臂挛痛。
【针灸方法】直刺1～1.5寸,或点刺出血。

4. 郄门　Xī mén（PC₄）
【类别】郄穴。
【体表定位】在前臂掌侧,当曲泽与大陵的连线上,腕横纹上5寸。（图2-82）
【层次解剖】有前臂正中动、静脉。深层为正中神经。
【主治病症】①心痛,心悸。②呕血,咳血。③疔疮。④癫痫。
【针灸方法】直刺0.5～1.0寸。

5. 间使　Jiān shǐ（PC₅）
【类别】经穴。

【体表定位】在前臂掌侧,当曲泽与大陵的连线上,腕横纹上3寸。掌长肌腱与桡侧腕屈肌腱之间。(图2-82)

【层次解剖】血管分布同郄门。分布着正中神经分支。

【主治病症】①心痛,心悸。②胃痛,呕吐。③热病,疟疾。④癫狂痫。

【针灸方法】直刺0.5~1.0寸。

6. **内关** Nèi guān(PC$_6$)

【类别】络穴,八脉交会穴通阴维脉。

【体表定位】在前臂掌侧,当曲泽与大陵的连线上,腕横纹上2寸,掌长肌腱与桡侧腕屈肌腱之间。(图2-82)

【层次解剖】血管、神经分布同间使。

【主治病症】①胸闷,胁痛,心痛,心悸。②癫痫,失眠,产后血晕。③胃脘痛,呕吐,呃逆。④郁症,眩晕,偏头痛,中风,偏瘫,上肢痹痛。⑤咳嗽,哮喘。⑥心烦,疟疾。

【针灸方法】直刺0.5~1.0寸。

7. **大陵** Dà líng(PC$_7$)

【类别】原穴。

【体表定位】在腕掌横纹的中点处,当掌长肌腱与桡侧腕屈肌腱之间。(图2-82)

【层次解剖】有腕掌侧动、静脉网。深层为正中神经本干。

【主治病症】①心痛,心悸,胸胁痛。②胃痛,呕吐。③癫狂。④足跟痛。

【针灸方法】直刺0.5~0.8寸。

8. **劳宫** Láo gōng(PC$_8$)

【类别】荥穴。

【体表定位】在手掌心,当第二、三掌骨之间偏于第三掌骨,握拳屈指时中指尖处。(图2-83)

【层次解剖】有指掌侧总动脉。分布着正中神经的第二掌侧总神经。

【主治病症】①口疮,口臭。②中风昏迷,鹅掌风。③心痛,呕吐。

【针灸方法】直刺0.3~0.5寸。

9. **中冲** Zhōng chōng(PC$_9$)

【类别】井穴。

【体表定位】在手中指末节尖端中央。(图2-83)

【层次解剖】有指掌侧固有动、静脉所形成的动、静脉网。分布着正中神经之指掌侧固有神经。

【主治病症】①中风昏迷,中暑昏厥。②心痛,心烦,舌强肿痛。

【针灸方法】浅刺0.1寸或点刺出血。

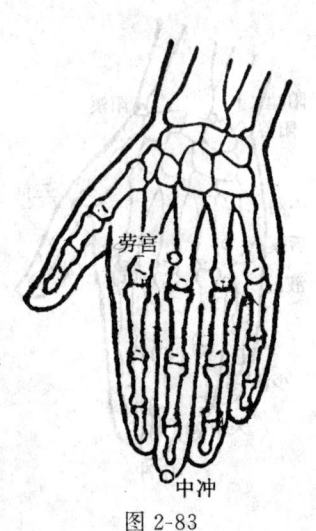

图2-83

第十节 手少阳三焦经穴

本经经穴起于关冲,止于丝竹空,左右各23穴。(图2-84)

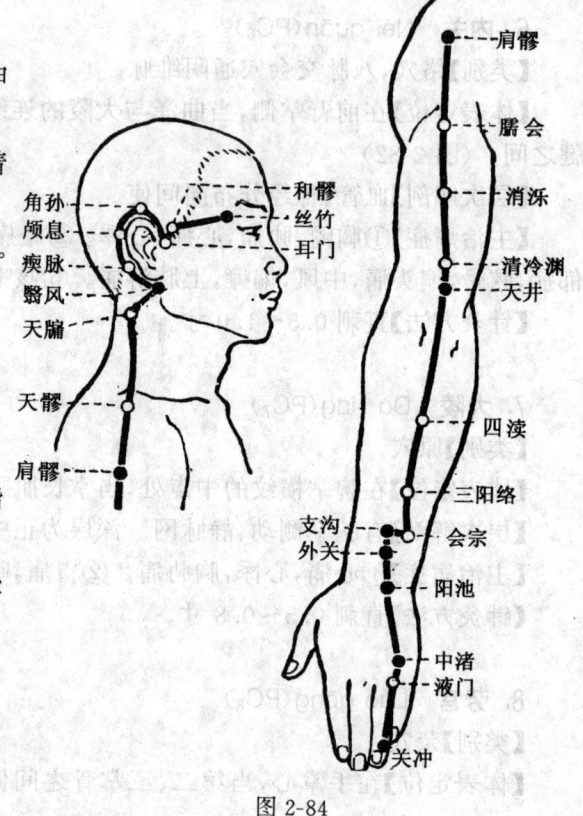

1. **关冲** Guān chōng(SJ₁)

【类别】井穴。

【体表定位】在手环指末节尺侧,距指甲角0.1寸(指寸)。(图2-85)

【层次解剖】有指掌侧动、静脉网。分布着尺神经的分支。

【主治病症】①热病,昏厥。②咽喉肿痛。③头痛,目赤,耳聋。

【针灸方法】浅刺0.1寸或点刺出血。

2. **液门** Yè mén(SJ₂)

【类别】荥穴。

【体表定位】在手背部,当第四、五指间指蹼缘后方赤白肉际处。(图2-85)

【层次解剖】有指背动脉。分布着尺神经手背支。

【主治病症】①疟疾。②咽喉肿痛。③头痛,目赤,耳聋。

【针灸方法】直刺0.3～0.5寸。

图 2-84

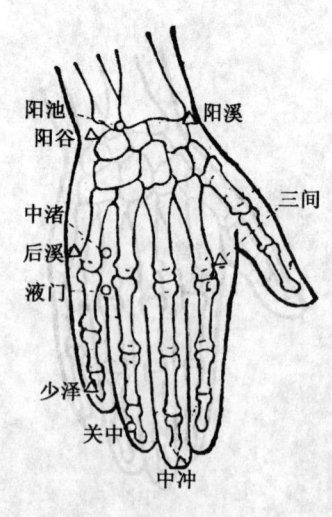

图 2-85

3. **中渚** Zhōng zhǔ(SJ₃)

【类别】输穴。

【体表定位】在手背部,当环指本节(掌指关节)的后方,第四、五掌骨间凹陷处。(图2-85)

【层次解剖】有手背静脉网及第四掌背动脉。分布着尺神经的手背支。

【主治病症】①头痛,目赤。②耳鸣,耳聋。③咽喉肿痛。④两肩胛之间痛,腿疼,手指不能屈伸。

【针灸方法】直刺0.3～0.5寸。

4. **阳池** Yáng chí(SJ₄)

【类别】原穴。

【体表定位】在腕背横纹中,当指伸肌腱的尺侧缘凹陷处。(图2-85)

【层次解剖】有腕背静脉网,腕背动脉。分布着尺神经手背支。
【主治病症】①消渴。②疟疾。③腕痛。④耳聋。
【针灸方法】直刺0.3～0.5寸。

5. **外关** Wài guān(SJ$_5$)
【类别】络穴,八脉交会穴通阳维脉。
【体表定位】在前臂背侧。当阳池与肘尖的连线上,腕背横纹上2寸,尺骨与桡骨之间。(图2-86)
【层次解剖】深层有前臂骨间背侧和掌侧动、静脉本干,桡神经分支和正中神经的分支。
【主治病症】①热病,头痛,目赤肿痛。②耳鸣,耳聋。③胁肋病,上肢痹痛。
【针灸方法】直刺0.5～1寸。

6. **支沟** Zhī gōu(SJ$_6$)
【类别】经穴。
【体表定位】在前臂背侧,当阳池与肘尖的连线上,腕背横纹上3寸,尺骨与桡骨之间。(图2-86)
【层次解剖】血管、神经分布同外关。
【主治病症】①便秘。②胁肋病。③耳聋耳鸣。
【针灸方法】直刺0.8～1.2寸。

图2-86

7. **会宗** Huì zōng(SJ$_7$)
【类别】郄穴。
【体表定位】在前臂背侧,当腕背横纹上3寸,支沟尺侧,尺骨的桡侧缘。(图2-86)
【层次解剖】有前臂骨间背侧动、静脉。分布着前臂背侧皮神经。
【主治病症】①耳聋。②癫痫。③上肢痹痛。
【针灸方法】直刺0.5～1寸。

8. **三阳络** Sān yáng luò(SJ$_8$)
【体表定位】在前臂背侧,腕背横纹上4寸,尺骨与桡骨之间。(图2-86)
【层次解剖】血管、神经分布同会宗穴。
【主治病症】①耳聋,暴喑。②齿痛。③上肢痹痛。
【针灸方法】直刺0.8～1.2寸

9. **四渎** Sì dú(SJ$_9$)
【体表定位】在前臂背侧,阳池与肘尖的连线上,肘尖下5寸,尺骨与桡骨之间。(图2-86)
【层次解剖】血管、神经分布同会宗穴。
【主治病症】①偏头痛。②耳聋。③暴喑,咽喉肿痛,④上肢痹痛。

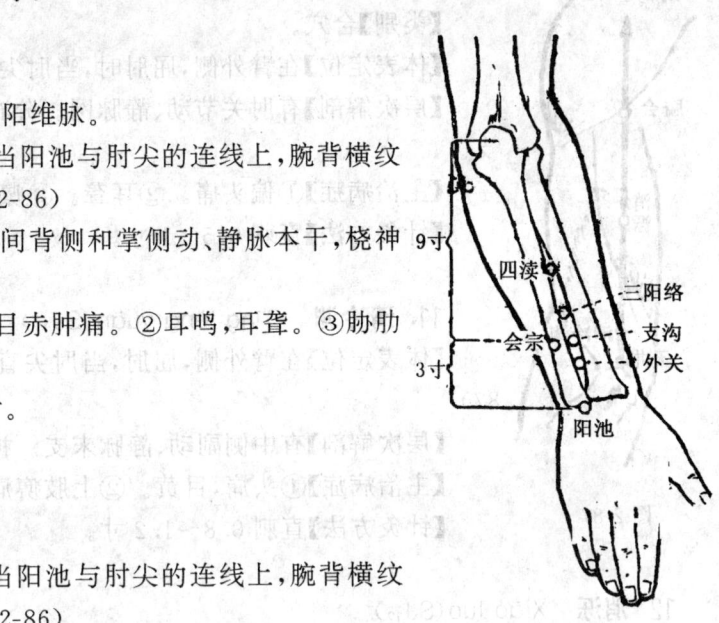

【针灸方法】直刺0.5～1寸。

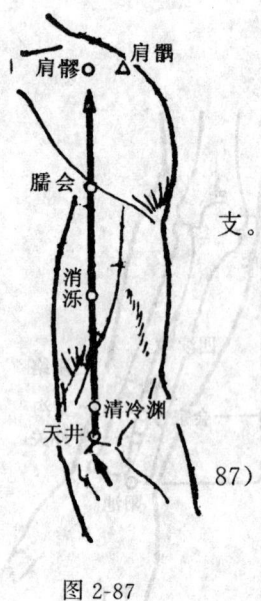

10. 天井 Tiān jǐng(SJ$_{10}$)

【类别】合穴。

【体表定位】在臂外侧,屈肘时,当肘尖直上1寸凹陷处。(图2-87)

【层次解剖】有肘关节动、静脉网。分布着臂背侧皮神经和桡神经的肌支。

【主治病症】①偏头痛。②耳聋。③瘰疬。④癫痫。

【针灸方法】直刺0.5～1寸。

11. 清冷渊 Qīng lěng yuān(SJ$_{11}$)

【体表定位】在臂外侧,屈肘,当肘尖直上2寸,即天井上1寸。(图2-87)

【层次解剖】有中侧副动、静脉末支。神经分布同天井。

【主治病症】①头痛,目黄。②上肢痹痛。

【针灸方法】直刺0.8～1.2寸。

图2-87

12. 消泺 Xiāo luò(SJ$_{12}$)

【体表定位】在臂外侧,当清冷渊与臑会连线的中点处。(图2-87)

【层次解剖】血管、神经分布同清冷渊。

【主治病症】头痛,项强,肩背痛。

【针灸方法】直刺1～1.5寸。

13. 臑会 Nào huì(SJ$_{13}$)

【体表定位】在臂外侧,当肘尖与肩髎的连线上,肩髎下3寸,三角肌的后下缘。(图2-87)

【层次解剖】血管神经分布除同清冷渊穴外,深层还分布桡神经。

【主治病症】①瘿气,瘰疬。②上肢痹痛。

【针灸方法】直刺1～1.5寸。

14. 肩髎 Jiān liáo(SJ$_{14}$)

【体表定位】在肩部,肩髃穴后方,当臂外展时,于肩峰后下方呈现凹陷处。(图2-87)

【层次解剖】有旋肱后动脉肌支。分布着腋神经肌支。

【主治病症】肩臂挛痛不遂。

【针灸方法】向肩关节直刺1～1.5寸。

15. 天髎 Tiān liáo(SJ$_{15}$)

【类别】手少阳与阳维脉交会穴。

【体表定位】在肩胛部,肩井与曲垣的中间,当肩胛骨上角处。(图2-88)

【层次解剖】有颈横动脉降支,分布着副神经、肩胛上神经分支。

图 2-88

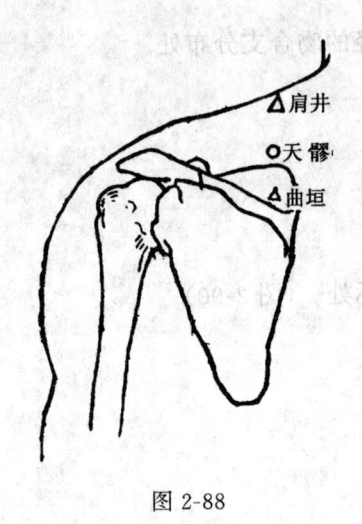

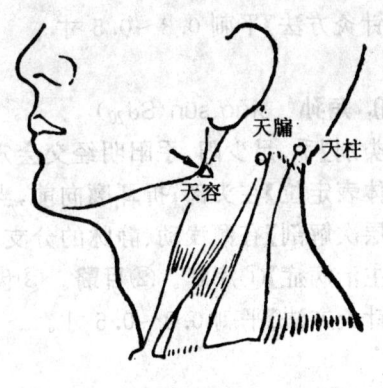

图 2-89

【主治病症】肩臂痛,颈项强急。
【针灸方法】直刺 0.5～0.8 寸。

16. 天牖 Tiān yǒu(SJ$_{16}$)
【体表定位】在颈侧部,当乳突的后方直下,平下颌角,胸锁乳突肌的后缘。(图 2-89)
【层次解剖】有耳后动脉及枕小神经。
【主治病症】①头痛,项强。②目痛,耳聋。③瘰疬。
【针灸方法】直刺 0.5～1 寸。

17. 翳风 Yì fēng(SJ$_{17}$)
【类别】手、足少阳经交会穴。
【体表定位】耳垂后方,下颌角与乳突间凹陷处。(图 2-90)
【层次解剖】有耳后动、静脉。分布着耳大神经,深层为面神经干从茎乳突孔穿出处。
【主治病症】①耳鸣,耳聋。②口眼㖞斜,颊肿。③牙痛。④瘰疬。
【针灸方法】直刺 0.8～1.2 寸。

18. 瘛脉 Chì mài(SJ$_{18}$)
【体表定位】在头部,耳后乳突中央,当角孙至翳风之间,沿耳轮连线的中、下 1/3 的交点处。(图 2-90)
【层次解剖】有耳后动、静脉。为耳大神经的耳后支。
【主治病症】①小儿惊风。②头痛,耳鸣,耳聋。
【针灸方法】平刺 0.3～0.5 寸或点刺出血。

19. 颅息 Lú xī(SJ$_{19}$)
【体表定位】在头部。当角孙与翳风之间沿耳轮连线的上、中 1/3 的交点处(图 2-90)

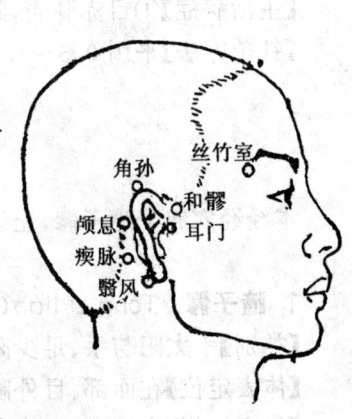

图 2-90

553

【层次解剖】有耳后动静脉。为耳大神经和枕大神经的吻合支分布处。
【主治病症】①头痛,耳鸣,耳聋。②小儿惊风。
【针灸方法】平刺0.3~0.5寸。

20. 角孙 Jiǎo sūn(SJ₂₀)
【类别】手、足少阳,手阳明经交会穴。
【体表定位】在头部,折耳廓向前,当耳尖直上入发际处。(图2-90)
【层次解剖】有颞浅动、静脉的分支及耳颞神经分支。
【主治病症】①痄腮。②目翳。③齿痛。④项强。
【针灸方法】平刺0.3~0.5寸。

21. 耳门 Er mén(SJ₂₁)
【体表定位】在面部,当耳屏上切迹的前方,下颌骨髁突后缘凹陷处。(图2-90)
【层次解剖】有颞浅动、静脉的分支,耳颞神经及面神经分支。
【主治病症】①耳鸣,耳聋,聤耳。②齿痛。
【针灸方法】张口,直刺0.5~1寸。

22. 耳和髎 Er hé liáo(SJ₂₂)
【类别】手、足少阳与手太阳交会穴。
【体表定位】在头侧部,当鬓发后缘,平耳廓根之前方,颞浅动脉的后缘。(图2-90)
【层次解剖】血管神经同耳门。
【主治病症】①头痛,耳鸣。②牙关紧闭,口㖞。
【针灸方法】避开动脉,斜刺或平刺0.3~0.5寸。

23. 丝竹空 Sī zhú kōng(SJ₂₃)
【体表定位】在面部,当眉梢凹陷处。(图2-90)
【层次解剖】有颞浅动、静脉。分布着面神经颧支及耳颞神经分支。
【主治病症】①目赤肿痛,眼睑瞤动。②头痛。③癫狂痫。
【针灸方法】平刺0.5~1.0寸。

第十一节 足少阳胆经穴

本经经穴起于瞳子髎,止于足窍阴,左右各44穴。(图2-91)

1. 瞳子髎 Tóng zi liáo(GB₁)
【类别】手太阳与手、足少阳经交会穴。
【体表定位】在面部、目外眦旁,当眶外侧缘处。(图2-92)
【层次解剖】有颧眶动、静脉及面神经的颧支。
【主治病症】头痛,目赤肿痛,目翳,青盲。

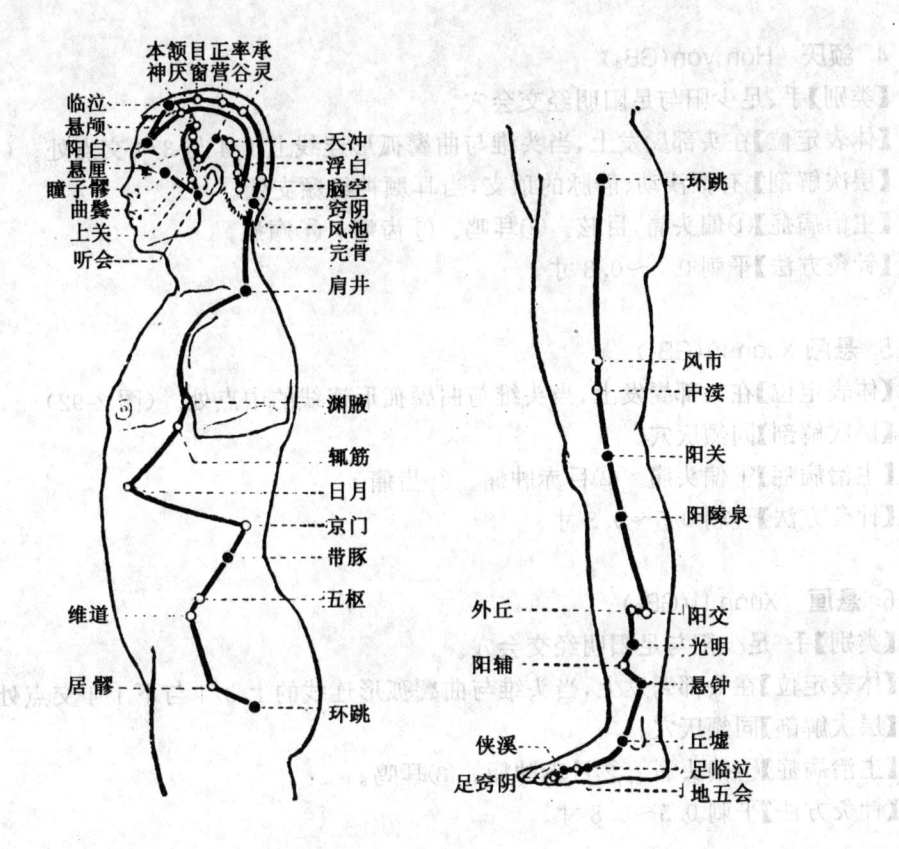

图 2-91　胆经经穴总图

【针灸方法】平刺 0.3～0.5 寸。

2. 听会　Tīng huì(GB₂)

【体表定位】在面部,当耳屏间切迹的前方,下颌骨髁突的后缘,张口有凹陷处。(图 2-92)
【层次解剖】有颞浅动脉,分布着耳大神经和面神经。
【主治病症】①耳鸣,耳聋。②齿痛。③口㖞。
【针灸方法】张口,直刺 0.5～1 寸。

3. 上关　Shàng guān　(GB₃)

【别名】客主人。
【类别】手、足少阳与足阳明经交会穴。
【体表定位】在耳前、下关直上,当颧弓的上缘凹陷处。(图 2-92)
【层次解剖】有颞眶动、静脉,分布着面神经的颧支。
【主治病症】①偏头痛。②耳鸣,耳聋。③口眼㖞斜。④齿痛,口噤。
【针灸方法】直刺 0.5～1 寸。

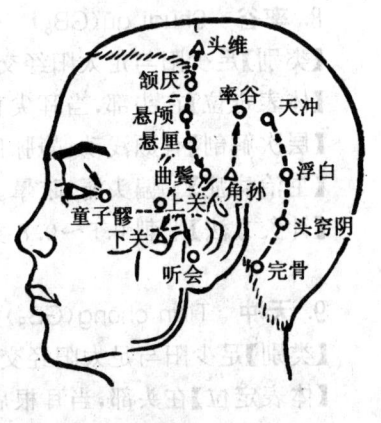

图 2-92

4. 颔厌　Hàn yàn（GB$_4$）
【类别】手、足少阳与足阳明经交会穴。
【体表定位】在头部鬓发上,当头维与曲鬓弧形连线上1/4与3/4交点处。（图2-92）
【层次解剖】有颞浅动、静脉的顶支,当耳颞神经颞支处。
【主治病症】①偏头痛,目眩。②耳鸣。③齿痛。④癫痫。
【针灸方法】平刺0.5~0.8寸。

5. 悬颅　Xuán lú（GB$_5$）
【体表定位】在头部鬓发上,当头维与曲鬓弧形连线的中点处。（图2-92）
【层次解剖】同颔厌穴。
【主治病症】①偏头痛。②目赤肿痛。③齿痛。
【针灸方法】直刺0.5~0.8寸。

6. 悬厘　Xuán lí（GB$_6$）
【类别】手、足少阳与足阳明经交会穴。
【体表定位】在头部鬓发上,当头维与曲鬓弧形连线的上3/4与下1/4交点处。（图2-92）
【层次解剖】同颔厌穴。
【主治病症】①偏头痛。②目赤肿痛。③耳鸣。
【针灸方法】平刺0.5~0.8寸。

7. 曲鬓　Qū bìn（GB$_7$）
【类别】足少阳与足太阳经交会穴。
【体表定位】在头部,当耳前鬓角发后缘的直上,平角孙穴处。（图2-92）
【层次解剖】血管、神经分布同颔厌穴。
【主治病症】①头痛。②牙痛,牙关紧闭,暴喑。
【针灸方法】平刺0.5~0.8寸。

8. 率谷　Shuài gǔ（GB$_8$）
【类别】足少阳与足太阳经交会穴。
【体表定位】在头部,当耳尖直上入发际1.5寸,角孙直上方。（图2-92）
【层次解剖】有颞浅动、静脉顶支,分布着耳颞神经和枕大神经的吻合支。
【主治病症】①偏头痛,眩晕。②小儿急、慢惊风。
【针灸方法】平刺0.5~0.8寸。

9. 天冲　Tiān chōng（GB$_9$）
【类别】足少阳与足太阳经交会穴。
【体表定位】在头部,当耳根后缘直上入发际2寸,率谷后0.5寸处。（图2-92）
【层次解剖】有耳后动、静脉。分布着枕大神经分支。

【主治病症】①头痛。②耳聋，耳鸣。③癫疾。④牙龈肿痛。
【针灸方法】平刺 0.5～0.8 寸。

10. 浮白 Fú bái（GB$_{10}$）
【类别】足少阳与足太阳经交会穴。
【体表定位】在头部，当耳后乳突的后上方，天冲与完骨的弧形连线的中 1/3 与上 1/3 交点处。（图 2-92）
【层次解剖】同天冲。
【主治病症】①头痛。②耳鸣，耳聋。③目痛。④瘿气。
【针灸方法】平刺 0.5～0.8 寸。

11. 头窍阴 Tóu qiào yīn（GB$_{11}$）
【类别】足少阳与足太阳经交会穴。
【体表定位】在头部，当耳后乳突的后上方，天冲与完骨的中 1/3 与下 1/3 交点处。（图 2-92）
【层次解剖】有耳后动、静脉分支。分布着枕大神经和枕小神经吻合支。
【主治病症】①头痛。②耳鸣，耳聋，耳痛。
【针灸方法】平刺 0.5～0.8 寸。

12. 完骨 Wán gǔ（GB$_{12}$）
【类别】足少阳与足太阳经交会穴。
【体表定位】在头部，当乳突的后下方凹陷处。（图 2-92）
【层次解剖】有耳后动、静脉。分布着枕小神经本干。
【主治病症】①头痛，颈项强痛。②齿痛，颊肿。③口眼歪斜。
【针灸方法】斜刺 0.5～0.8 寸。

13. 本神 Běn shén（GB$_{13}$）
【类别】足少阳与阳维脉交会穴。
【体表定位】在头部，当前发际上 0.5 寸，神庭旁开 3 寸，神庭与头维连线的内 2/3 与外 1/3 的交点处。（图 2-93）
【层次解剖】有颞浅动、静脉额支及额神经外侧支。
【主治病症】①头痛，目眩。②癫痫。③小儿惊风。
【针灸方法】平刺 0.5～0.8 寸。

14. 阳白 Yáng bái（GB$_{14}$）
【类别】足少阳与阳维脉交会穴。
【体表定位】在前额部，当瞳孔直上，眉上 1 寸。（图 2-93）

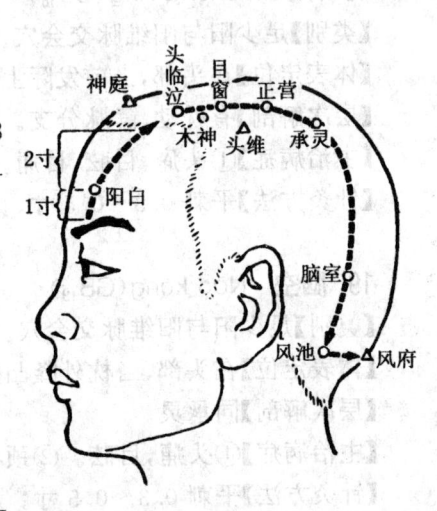

图 2-93

【层次解剖】有额动、静脉及额神经外侧支处。
【主治病症】①面瘫,眼睑下垂,闭眼困难。②视物模糊,眼痛。③前额痛,眩晕。
【针灸方法】平刺 0.3～0.5 寸。

15. 头临泣　Tóu lín qì(GB$_{15}$)
【类别】足少阳、太阳与阳维脉交会穴。
【体表定位】在头部,当瞳孔直上入前发际 0.5 寸,神庭与头维连线的中点处。(图 2-93)
【层次解剖】有额动、静脉。分布着额神经内、外侧支的吻合支。
【主治病症】①头痛,鼻塞。②目眩,流泪。③小儿惊痫。
【针灸方法】平刺 0.3～0.5 寸。

16. 目窗　Mù chuāng(GB$_{16}$)
【类别】足少阳与阳维脉交会穴。
【体表定位】在头部,当前发际上 1.5 寸,头正中线旁开 2.25 寸。(图 2-93)
【层次解剖】同头临泣穴。
【主治病症】①视物模糊,青盲,目赤肿痛。②头痛,鼻塞,面肿。③癫痫。
【针灸方法】平刺 0.3～0.5 寸。

17. 正营　Zhèng yíng(GB$_{17}$)
【类别】足少阳与阳维脉交会穴。
【体表定位】在头部,当前发际上 2.5 寸,头正中线旁开 2.25 寸。(图 2-93)
【层次解剖】有颞浅动、静脉顶支和枕动、静脉的吻合网及额神经和枕大神经吻合支。
【主治病症】①头痛,目眩,唇吻急强。②齿痛。
【针灸方法】平刺 0.3～0.5 寸。

18. 承灵　Chéng líng(GB$_{18}$)
【类别】足少阳与阳维脉交会穴。
【体表定位】在头部,当前发际上 4.0 寸,头正中线旁开 2.25 寸。(图 2-93)
【层次解剖】有枕动、静脉分支。分布着枕大神经分支。
【主治病症】①头痛,目眩,目痛。②鼻塞,衄血。
【针灸方法】平刺 0.3～0.5 寸。

19. 脑空　Nǎo kōng(GB$_{19}$)
【类别】足少阳与阳维脉交会穴。
【体表定位】在头部,当枕外隆凸的上缘外侧,头正中线旁开 2.25 寸,平脑户。(图 2-93)
【层次解剖】同承灵。
【主治病症】①头痛,目眩。②颈项强痛。③癫狂痫。
【针灸方法】平刺 0.3～0.5 寸。

20. 风池 Fēng chí(GB$_{20}$)

【类别】足少阳与阳维脉交会穴。

【体表定位】在项部,当枕骨之下,与风府相平,胸锁乳突肌与斜方肌上端之间的凹陷处。(图2-93)

【层次解剖】有枕动、静脉分支。分布着枕小神经分支。

【主治病症】①感冒,鼻塞,头痛,目赤肿痛,鼻渊,衄血,颈项强痛,肩痛不举。②头晕,目眩,中风偏瘫,癫痫。

【针灸方法】向鼻尖斜刺0.8～1.2寸,或平刺透风府穴。深部中间为延髓,必须严格掌握针刺的角度与深度。

21. 肩井 Jiān jǐng(GB$_{21}$)

【类别】手、足少阳、足阳明与阳维脉交会穴。

【体表定位】在肩上,前直乳中,当大椎与肩峰端连线的中点上。(图2-94)

【层次解剖】有颞横动、静脉。分布着锁骨上神经后支和副神经。

【主治病症】①乳痈,乳汁不下。②头晕,头痛,颈项强痛,上肢不遂。③难产,瘰疬。

【针灸方法】直刺0.5～0.8寸。内为肺尖,不可深刺。孕妇禁针。

图2-94

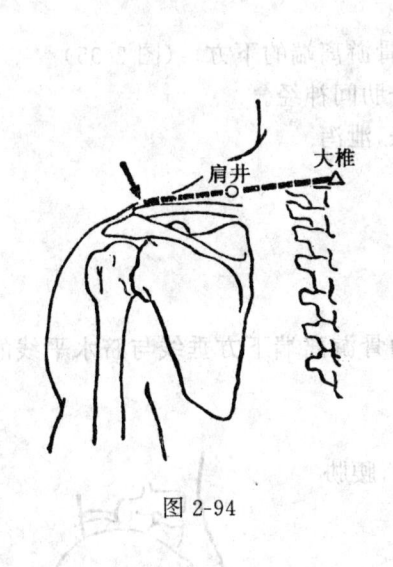

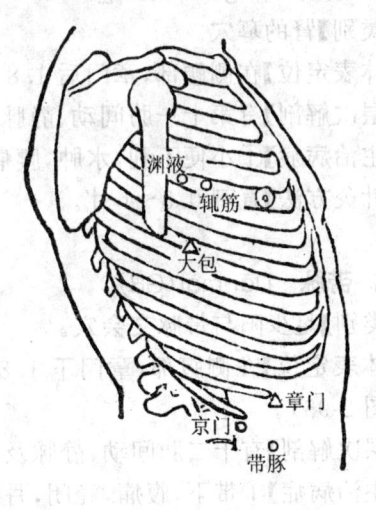

图2-95

22. 渊腋 Yuān yè(GB$_{22}$)

【体表定位】在胸部,举臂,当腋中线上,腋下3寸。第四肋间隙中。(图2-95)

【层次解剖】有第四肋间动、静脉及第四肋间神经的外侧皮支。

【主治病症】①胸满,胁痛。②上肢痹痛。

【针灸方法】斜刺或平刺0.5～0.8寸。本经渊腋至京门诸穴,不可深刺,以免伤及内部重要脏器。

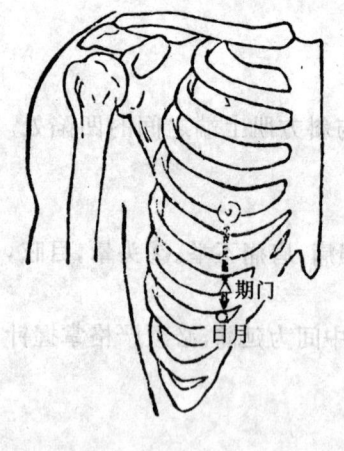

23. 辄筋 Zhé jīn (GB₂₃)

【体表定位】在侧胸部,渊腋前1寸,平乳头,第四肋间隙中。(图2-95)

【层次解剖】同渊腋穴。

【主治病症】①胸满,胁痛。②气喘。

【针灸方法】斜刺或平刺0.5～0.8寸。

24. 日月 Rì yuè (GB₂₄)

【类别】募穴,足少阳、足太阴经交会穴。

【体表定位】在上腹部,当乳头直下,第七肋隙,前正中线旁开4寸。(图2-96)

【层次解剖】有第七肋间动、静脉。分布着第七肋间神经。

【主治病症】①胁肋胀痛。②黄疸。③呕吐,呃逆,吞酸。

【针灸方法】斜刺或平刺0.5～0.8寸。

25. 京门 jīng mén (GB₂₅)

【类别】肾的募穴。

【体表定位】在侧腰部,章门后1.8寸,当第十二肋骨游离端的下方。(图2-95)

【层次解剖】有第十一肋间动、静脉。分布着第十一肋间神经。

【主治病症】①小便不利,水肿,腰痛。②胁痛,腹胀,泄泻。

【针灸方法】直刺0.5～1寸。

26. 带脉 Dài mài (GB₂₆)

【类别】足少阳与带脉交会穴。

【体表定位】在侧腹部,章门下1.8寸,当第十一肋骨游离端下方垂线与脐水平线的交点上。(图2-95)

【层次解剖】有十二肋间动、静脉及十二肋间神经。

【主治病症】①带下,腹痛,经闭,月经不调。②疝气,腰胁痛。

【针灸方法】直刺1～1.5寸。

27. 五枢 Wǔ shū (GB₂₇)

【类别】足少阳与带脉交会穴。

【体表定位】在侧腹部,当髂前上棘的前方,横平脐下3寸处。(图2-97)

【层次解剖】有旋髂浅深动、静脉。分布着髂腹下神经。

【主治病症】①腹痛,疝气。②便秘,阴挺,带下。

【针灸方法】直刺1～1.5寸。

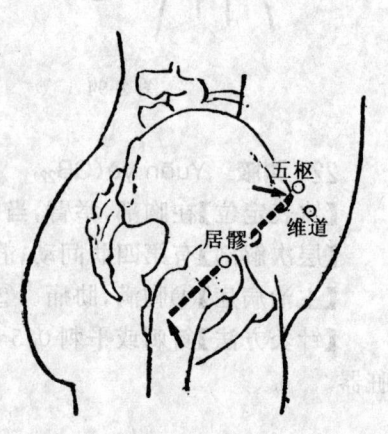

28. 维道 wéi dào（GB₂₈）

【类别】足少阳与带脉交会穴。

【体表定位】在侧腹部，当髂前上棘的前下方，五枢穴前下0.5寸（图2-97）。

【层次解剖】血管分布同五枢穴。分布着髂腹股沟神经。

【主治病症】①腹痛，疝气。②阴挺。③带下。

【针灸方法】直刺或向前下方斜刺1～1.5寸。

29. 居髎 Jū liáo（GB₂₉）

【类别】足少阳与阳蹻脉交会穴。

【体表定位】在髋部，当髂前上棘与股骨大转子最凸点与连线的中点处。（图2-97）

【层次解剖】有旋髂浅动、静脉分支及旋股外侧动、静脉升支。分布着股外侧皮神经。

【主治病症】腰痛，翻身困难，下肢痿痹。

【针灸方法】直刺1～1.5寸。

30. 环跳 Huán tiào（GB₃₀）

【类别】足少阳、太阳经交会穴。

【体表定位】在股外侧部，侧卧屈股，当股骨大转子最凸点与骶管裂孔连线的外1/3与中1/3交点处。（图2-98）

【层次解剖】分布着臀下皮神经，臀下神经，深部为坐骨神经。

【主治病症】下肢痿痹，腰腿痛，半身不遂。

【针灸方法】直刺2～3寸。

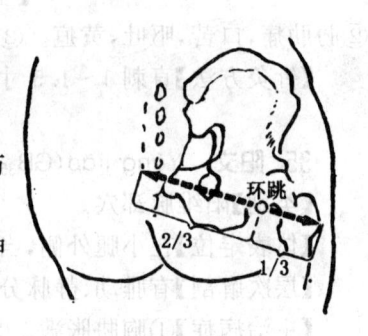

图2-98

31. 风市 Fēng shì（GB₃₁）

【体表定位】在大腿外侧部的中线上，当腘横纹上7寸。或直立垂手时，中指尖处。（图2-99）

【层次解剖】有股外侧皮神经及股神经肌支。

【主治病症】①下肢痿痹，脚气。②遍身瘙痒。③暴聋。

【针灸方法】直刺1～2寸。

32. 中渎 Zhōng dú（GB₃₂）

【体表定位】在大腿外侧，当风市下2寸，腘横纹上5寸，股外侧肌与股二头肌之间。（图2-99）

【层次解剖】同风市。

【主治病症】下肢痿痹，半身不遂。

【针灸方法】直刺1～2寸。

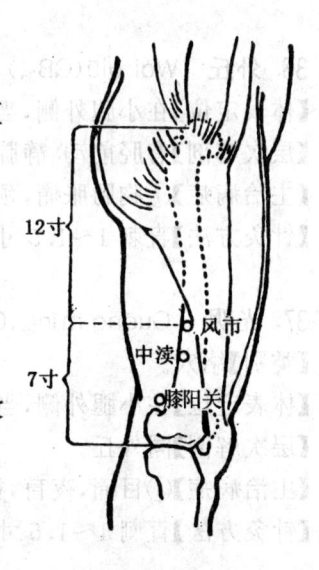

图2-99

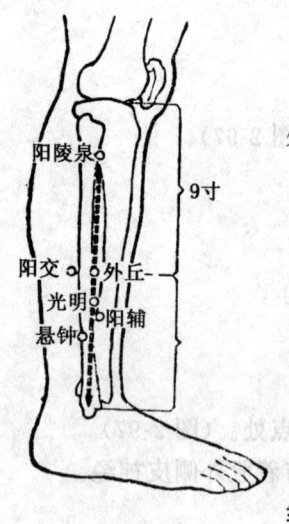

33. 膝阳关 Xī yáng guān (GB₃₃)

【体表定位】在膝外侧,当阳陵泉上3寸,股骨外上髁上方的凹陷处。(图2-99)
【层次解剖】同风市穴。
【主治病症】膝冷痛,腘筋挛急,小腿麻木。
【针灸方法】直刺1~1.5寸。

34. 阳陵泉 Yáng líng quán (GB₃₄)

【类别】合穴,八会穴(筋会)。
【体表定位】在小腿外侧,当腓骨小头前下方凹陷处。(图2-100)
【层次解剖】有膝下外侧动、静脉。当腓总神经分为腓浅及腓深神经处。
【主治病症】①半身不遂,肩痛,下肢痿痹,麻木,膝髌肿痛,脚气。②胁肋痛,口苦,呕吐,黄疸。③小儿惊风。
【针灸方法】直刺1~1.5寸。

35. 阳交 Yáng jiāo (GB₃₅)

【类别】阳维脉郄穴。
【体表定位】在小腿外侧,当外踝尖上7寸,腓骨后缘。(图2-100)
【层次解剖】有腓动、静脉分支。分布着腓肠外侧皮神经。
【主治病症】①胸胁胀满。②下肢痿痹。
【针灸方法】直刺1~1.5寸。

36. 外丘 Wài qiū (GB₃₆)

【体表定位】在小腿外侧,当外踝尖上7寸,腓骨前缘,平阳交。(图2-100)
【层次解剖】有胫前动、静脉肌支。分布着腓浅神经。
【主治病症】①胸胁胀痛,颈项痛。②下肢痿痹。③猘犬伤,毒不出。
【针灸方法】直刺1~1.5寸。

37. 光明 Guāng míng (GB₃₇)

【类别】络穴。
【体表定位】在小腿外侧,当外踝尖上5寸,腓骨前缘。(图2-100)
【层次解剖】同外丘。
【主治病症】①目痛,夜盲,视物模糊。②下肢痿痹。③乳房胀痛。
【针灸方法】直刺1~1.5寸。

38. 阳辅 Yáng fǔ (GB₃₈)

【类别】经穴。

【体表定位】在小腿外侧,当外踝尖上4寸,腓骨前缘稍前方。(图2-100)

【层次解剖】同外丘。

【主治病症】①偏头痛,目外眦痛。②腋下肿痛。③胸胁胀痛,下肢痿痹。

【针灸方法】直刺1～1.5寸。

39. 悬钟 Xuán zhōng(GB$_{39}$)

【别名】绝骨。

【类别】八会穴(髓会)。

【体表定位】在小腿外侧,当外踝尖上3寸,腓骨前缘。(图2-100)

【层次解剖】同外丘。

【主治病症】①中风偏瘫,颈项强痛,下肢痿痹,脚气。②胁肋痛。

【针灸方法】直刺1～1.5寸。

40. 丘墟 Qiū xū(GB$_{40}$)

【类别】原穴。

【体表定位】在足外踝前下方,当趾长伸肌腱的外侧凹陷处。(图2-101)

【层次解剖】有外踝前动、静脉分支及腓浅神经。

【主治病症】①胸胁胀痛。②下肢痿痹,外踝肿痛。③疟疾。

【针灸方法】直刺0.5～0.8寸。

41. 足临泣 Zú lín qì(GB$_{41}$)

【类别】输穴,八脉交会穴通于带脉。

【体表定位】在足背外侧,当足四趾本节(第四跖趾关节)的后方,小趾伸肌腱的外侧凹陷处。(图2-101)

【层次解剖】有足背动、静脉网及足背中间皮神经分支。

【主治病症】①偏头痛,目赤痛,胁肋痛,足跗肿痛,足趾挛痛。②乳痈,乳胀,月经不调。③瘰疬,疟疾。

【针灸方法】直刺0.3～0.5寸。

42. 地五会 Dì wǔ huì(GB$_{42}$)

【体表定位】在足背外侧,当足四趾本节(第四跖趾关节)的后方,第四、五跖骨之间,小趾伸肌的内侧缘。(图2-101)

【层次解剖】同足临泣穴。

【主治病症】①乳痈,乳胀。②头痛,目痛,耳鸣,耳聋。③胁肋痛,足跗肿痛。

【针灸方法】直刺0.3～0.5寸。

43. 侠溪 Xiá xī(GB$_{43}$)

【类别】荥穴。

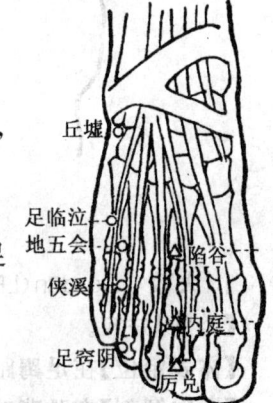

图2-101

【体表定位】在足背外侧,当第四、五趾间,趾蹼缘后方赤白肉际处。(图2-101)
【层次解剖】有足趾动、静脉。分布着趾背神经。
【主治病症】①头痛,目眩,目赤肿痛。②耳鸣,耳聋。③乳痈,胁肋疼痛。④热痛。
【针灸方法】直刺0.3~0.5寸。

44. 足窍阴 Zú qiào yīn(GB₄₄)
【类别】井穴。
【体表定位】在足第四趾末节外侧,距趾甲角0.1寸(指寸)。(图2-101)
【层次解剖】有动、静脉网和趾背神经。
【主治病症】①偏头痛,目赤痛,胸胁痛。②耳鸣、耳聋。③中风偏瘫。
【针灸方法】直刺0.1~0.3寸。

第十二节 足厥阴肝经穴

本经经穴起于大敦,止于期门,左右各14穴。(图2-102)

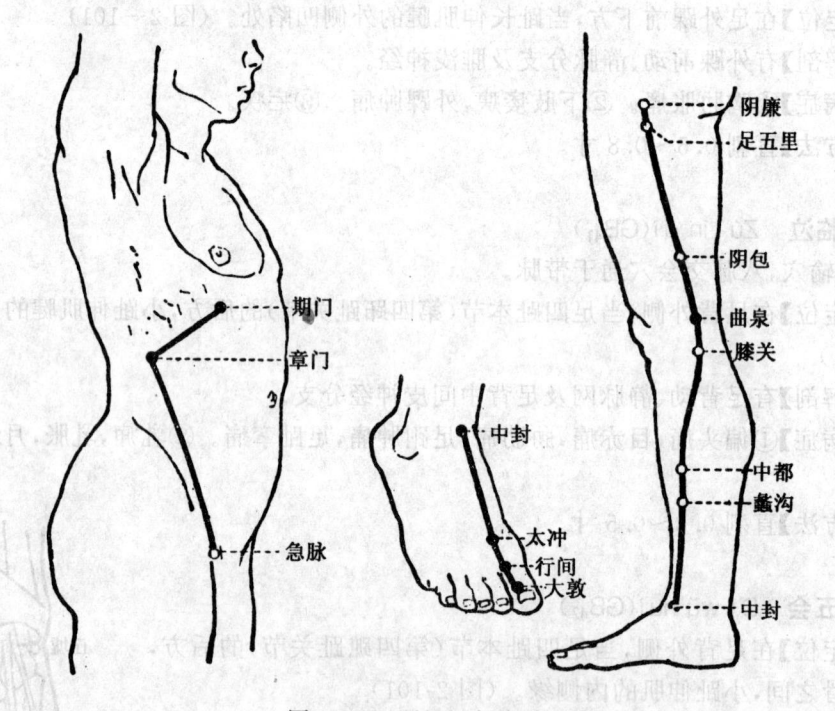

图2-102 肝经经穴总图

1. 大敦 Dà dūn(LR₁)
【类别】井穴。
【体表定位】在足蹞趾末节外侧,距趾甲角0.1寸(指寸)。(图2-103)
【层次解剖】有趾背动、静脉及趾背神经。
【主治病症】①疝气。②遗尿。③崩漏,阴挺,经闭。④癫痫。

【针灸方法】斜刺 0.1～0.2 寸或点刺出血。《图翼》：孕妇产前产后皆不宜灸。

2. 行间 Xíng jiān(LR$_2$)
【类别】荥穴。
【体表定位】在足背，当第一、二趾间，趾蹼缘的后方赤白肉际处。(图 2-103)
【层次解剖】有第一趾背动、静脉及趾背神经。
【主治病症】①目赤肿痛，青盲。②失眠，癫痫。③月经不调，痛经，崩漏，带下。④小便不利，尿痛。
【针灸方法】斜刺 0.5～0.8 寸。

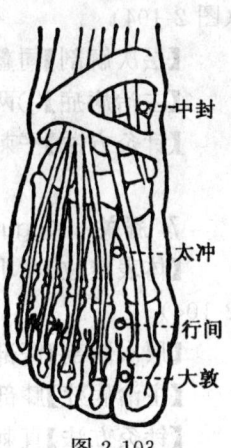

图 2-103

3. 太冲 Tài chōng(LR$_3$)
【类别】输穴。原穴。
【体表定位】在足背，当第一、二跖骨结合部前方凹陷处。(图 2-103)
【层次解剖】有足背静脉网，第一跖骨背动脉，分布着腓深神经的分支。
【主治病症】①头痛，眩晕，目赤肿痛，口眼歪斜。②郁证，胁痛，腹胀，呃逆。③下肢痿痹，行路困难。④月经不调，崩漏，疝气，遗尿。⑤癫痫，小儿惊风。
【针灸方法】直刺 0.5～0.8 寸。

4. 中封 Zhōng fēng(LR$_4$)
【类别】经穴。
【体表定位】在足背侧，商丘与解溪连线之间，胫骨前肌腱的内侧凹陷处。(图 2-103)
【层次解剖】有内踝前动脉及隐神经。
【主治病症】①疝气，腹痛。②遗精。③小便不利。
【针灸方法】直刺 0.5～0.8 寸。

5. 蠡沟 Lí gōu(LR$_5$)
【类别】络穴。
【体表定位】在小腿内侧，当足内踝尖上 5 寸，胫骨内侧面中央。(图 2-104)
【层次解剖】有隐神经的分支。
【主治病症】①外阴搔痒，阳强。②月经不调，带下。③小便不利，疝气，足肿疼痛。
【针灸方法】平刺 0.5～0.8 寸。

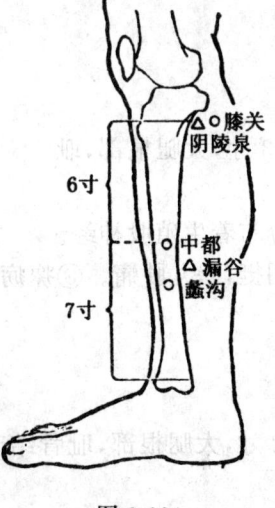

图 2-104

6. 中都 Zhōng dū(LR$_6$)
【类别】郄穴。
【体表定位】在小腿内侧，当内踝尖上 7 寸，胫骨内侧面的中央。

(图 2-104)

【层次解剖】同蠡沟穴。

【主治病症】①两胁痛,腹胀,腹痛,泄泻。②恶露不尽。③疝气。

【针灸方法】平刺 0.5～0.8 寸。

7. 膝关 Xī guān(LR₇)

【体表定位】在小腿内侧,当胫骨内髁的后下方,阴陵泉后 1 寸,腓肠肌内侧头的上部。(图 2-104)

【层次解剖】深部有胫后动脉及胫神经。

【主治病症】膝部肿痛。

【针灸方法】直刺 1～1.5 寸。

8. 曲泉 Qū quán(LR₈)

【类别】合穴。

【体表定位】在膝内侧,屈膝,当膝内侧横纹头上方凹陷中,股骨内上髁的后缘,半腱肌、半膜肌止端的前缘凹陷处。(图 2-105)

【层次解剖】有大隐静脉,膝最上动脉。分布着隐神经。

【主治病症】①小腹痛,小便不利。②遗精,阴挺,阴痒,外阴疼痛。③月经不调,赤白带下,痛经。④膝股内侧痛。

【针灸方法】直刺 1～1.5 寸。

9. 阴包 Yīn bāo(KR₉)

【体表定位】在大腿内侧,当股骨内上踝上 4 寸,股内肌与缝匠肌之间。(图 2-105)

【层次解剖】有旋股内侧动脉浅支及闭孔神经前支。

【主治病症】①腰骶引小腹痛,小便不利,遗尿。②月经不调。

【针灸方法】直刺 1～2 寸。

图 2-105

10. 足五里 Zú wǔ lǐ(LR₁₀)

【体表定位】在大腿内侧,当气冲穴直下 3 寸,大腿根部,耻骨结节的下方,长收肌的外缘。(图 2-106)

【层次解剖】有旋股内侧动、静脉浅支。分布着生殖股神经。

【主治病症】①小腹胀痛,小便不利。②阴挺,睾丸肿痛。③瘰疬。

【针灸方法】直刺 1～2 寸。

11. 阴廉 Yīn lián(LR₁₁)

【体表定位】在大腿内侧,当气冲穴直下 2 寸,大腿根部,耻骨结节的下方。长收肌的外缘。(图 2-106)

【层次解剖】有旋股内侧动、静脉的分支及生殖股神经。

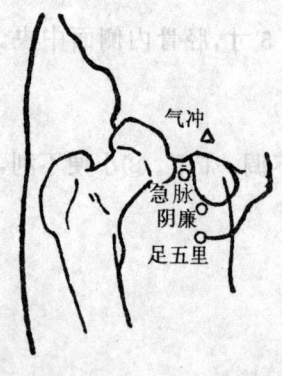

图 2-106

【主治病症】①月经不调,带下。②小腹胀痛。
【针灸方法】直刺1～2寸。

12. 急脉　Jí mài(LR$_{12}$)

【体表定位】在耻骨结节的外侧,当气冲穴外下方,腹股沟股动脉搏动处。前正中线旁开2.5寸。(图2-106)

【层次解剖】有阴部外动、静脉的分支。分布着髂腹股沟神经。

【主治病症】①疝气,腹痛。②外阴肿痛,阴茎痛,阴挺,阴痒。

【针灸方法】避开动脉,直刺0.5～0.8寸。

【附注】《素问》王注:可灸而不可刺。

13. 章门　Zhāng mén(LR$_{13}$)

【类别】脾募穴;八会穴(脏会),足厥阴、少阳经交会穴。

【体表定位】在侧腹部,当第十一肋游离端的下方。(图2-107)

【层次解剖】有第十肋间动脉末支。分布着第十、十一肋间神经。

【主治病症】①腹胀,泄泻。②胁痛,痞块。

【针灸方法】直刺0.8～1寸。

14. 期门　Qī mén(LR$_{14}$)

【类别】肝募穴,足厥阴、太阴与阴维脉交会穴。

【体表定位】在胸部,当乳头直下,第六肋间隙,前正中线旁开4寸。(图2-107)

【层次解剖】有第六肋间动、静脉。分布着第六肋间神经。

【主治病症】①郁证。②胸胁胀痛。③腹胀,呃逆,吞酸。

【针灸方法】斜刺或平刺0.5～0.8寸。

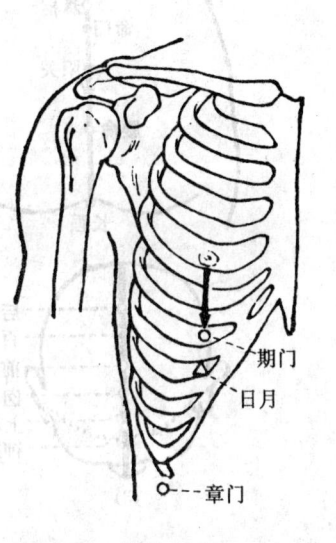

图2-107

第十三节　督脉穴

本经经穴起于长强,止于龈交。一名一穴,共28穴。(图2-108)

1. 长强　Cháng qiáng(Du$_1$)

【类别】督脉、足少阳、足太阴经交会穴,络穴。

【体表定位】在尾骨端下,当尾骨端与肛门连线的中点处。(图2-109)

【层次解剖】有肛门动、静脉分支。分布着尾神经后支及肛门神经。

【主治病症】①泄泻,便血,便秘,痔疾,脱肛。②癫狂痫。

【针灸方法】紧靠尾骨前面斜刺0.8～1寸。

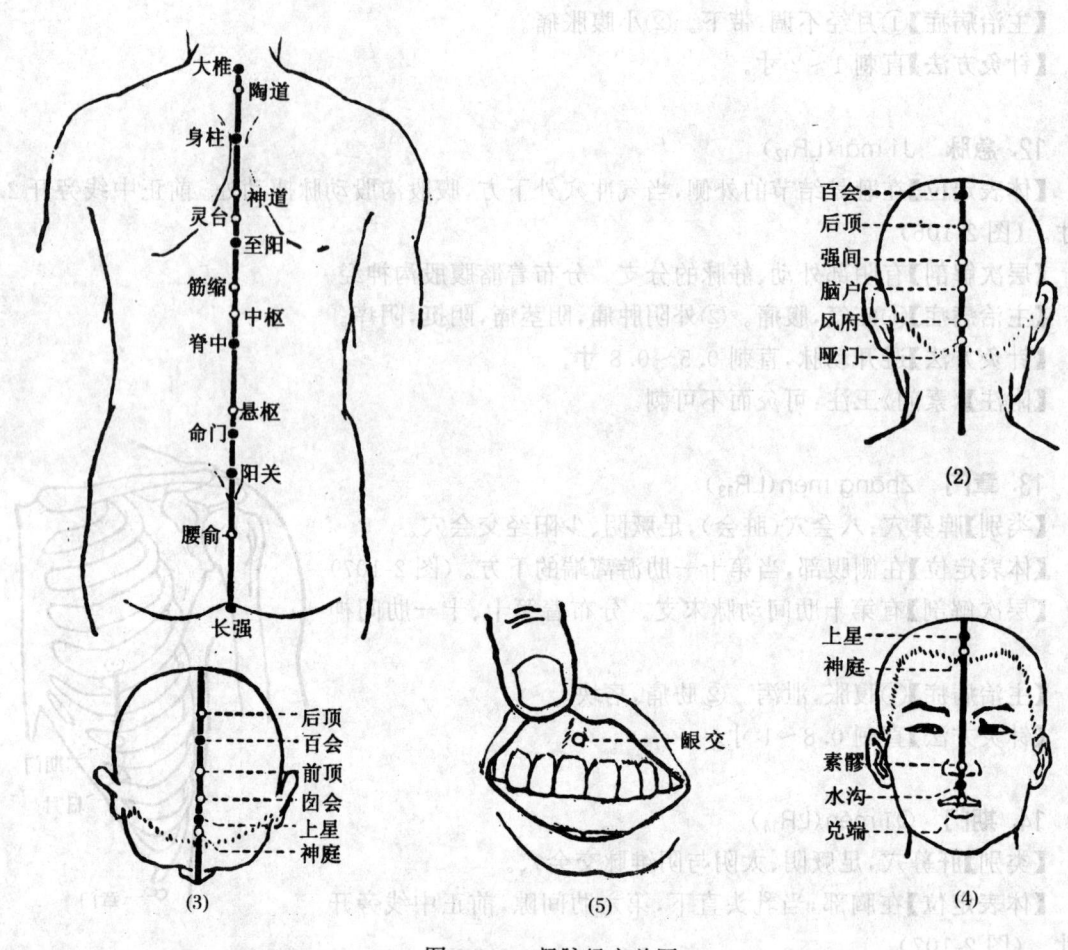

图 2-108　督脉经穴总图

2. 腰俞　Yāo shū(Du₂)

【体表定位】在骶部、当后正中线上,适对骶管裂孔。（图 2-109）
【层次解剖】有骶中动、静脉分支及尾神经分支。
【主治病症】①癫狂,癫痫。②痔疾。③腰脊强痛,下肢痿痹。④月经不调。
【针灸方法】向上斜刺 0.5～1 寸。

3. 腰阳关　Yāo Yáng guān(Du₃)

【体表定位】在腰部,当后正中线上,第四腰椎棘突下凹陷中。（图 2-109）
【层次解剖】有腰动脉后支及腰神经后支的内侧支。
【主治病症】①月经不调,遗精,阳痿。②腰骶痛,下肢痿痹。
【针灸方法】向上斜刺 0.5～1 寸。

4. 命门　Mìng mén(Du₄)

【体表定位】在腰部,当后正中线上,第二腰椎棘突下凹陷中。（图 2-109）
【层次解剖】同腰阳关穴。

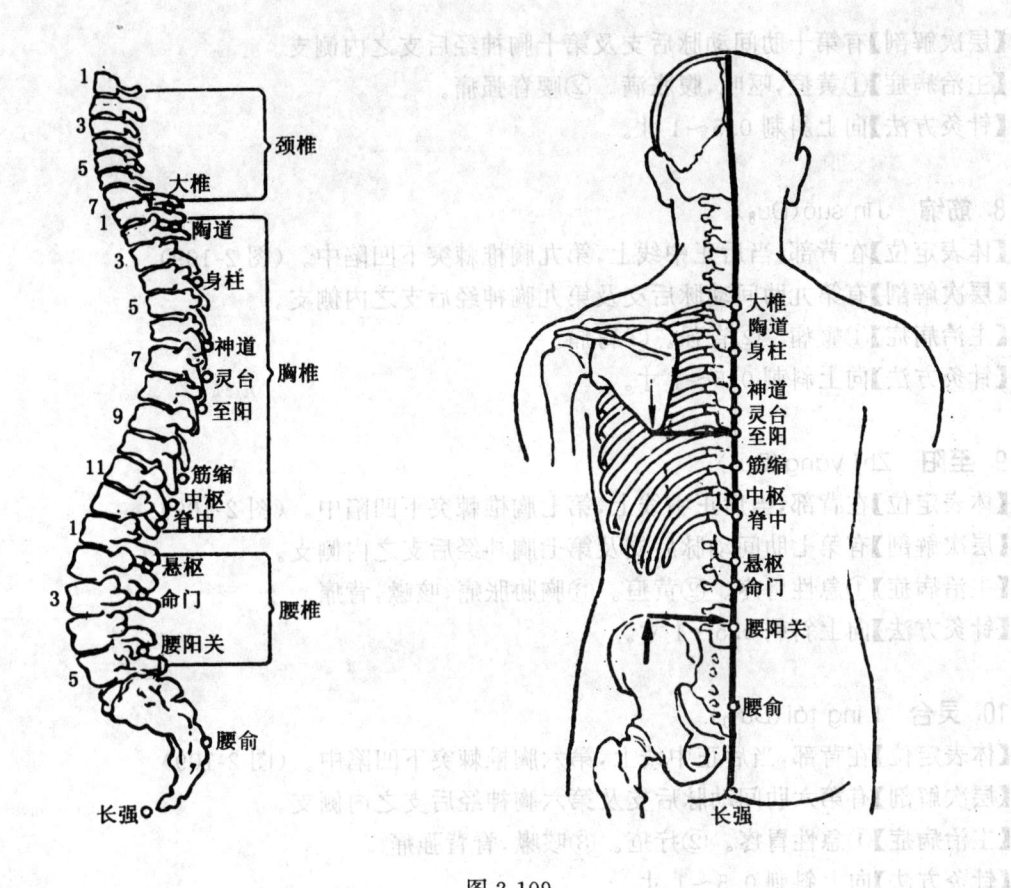

图 2-109

【主治病症】①遗精,阳痿。②月经不调,带下。③泄泻。④腰脊强痛。
【针灸方法】向上斜刺 0.5～1 寸。

5. **悬枢** Xuán shū(Du₅)
【体表定位】在腰部,当后正中线上,第一腰椎棘突下凹陷中。(图 2-109)
【层次解剖】同腰阳关穴。
【主治病症】①腰脊强痛。②泄泻,腹痛。
【针灸方法】向上斜刺 0.5～1 寸。

6. **脊中** Jǐ zhōng(Du₆)
【体表定位】有背部,当后正中线上,第十一胸椎棘突下凹陷中。(图 2-109)
【层次解剖】同腰阳关穴。
【主治病症】①泄泻。②黄疸。③痔疾。④癫痫。
【针灸方法】向上斜刺 0.5～1 寸。

7. **中枢** Zhōng shū(Du₇)
【体表定位】在背部,当后正中线上,第十胸椎棘突下凹陷中。(图 2-109)

569

【层次解剖】有第十肋间动脉后支及第十胸神经后支之内侧支。
【主治病症】①黄疸,呕吐,腹胀满。②腰脊强痛。
【针灸方法】向上斜刺 0.5～1 寸。

8. **筋缩** Jīn suō(Du$_8$)
【体表定位】在背部,当后正中线上,第九胸椎棘突下凹陷中。(图 2-109)
【层次解剖】有第九肋间动脉后支及第九胸神经后支之内侧支。
【主治病症】①癫痫。②脊强。③胃痛。
【针灸方法】向上斜刺 0.5～1 寸。

9. **至阳** Zhì yáng(Du$_9$)
【体表定位】在背部,当后正中线上,第七胸椎棘突下凹陷中。(图 2-109)
【层次解剖】有第七肋间动脉后支及第七胸神经后支之内侧支。
【主治病症】①急性胃疼。②黄疸。③胸胁胀痛,咳嗽,背痛。
【针灸方法】向上斜刺 0.5～1 寸。

10. **灵台** Líng tái(Du$_{10}$)
【体表定位】在背部,当后正中线上,第六胸椎棘突下凹陷中。(图 2-109)
【层次解剖】有第六肋间动脉后支及第六胸神经后支之内侧支。
【主治病症】①急性胃疼。②疔疮。③咳嗽,脊背强痛。
【针灸方法】向上斜刺 0.5～1 寸。

11. **神道** Shén dào(Du$_{11}$)
【体表定位】在背部、当后正中线上,第五胸椎棘突下凹陷中。(图 2-109)
【层次解剖】有第五肋间动脉后支及第五胸神经后支之内侧支。
【主治病症】①心悸,心痛,失眠,健忘。②咳嗽,喧膈。③脊背强痛。
【针灸方法】向上斜刺 0.5～1 寸。

12. **身柱** Shēn zhù(Du$_{12}$)
【体表定位】在背部,当后正中线上,第三胸椎棘突下凹陷中。(图 2-109)
【层次解剖】有第三肋间动脉后支及第三胸神经后支内侧支。
【主治病症】①咳嗽,气喘。②癫痫。③脊背强痛。
【针灸方法】向上斜刺 0.5～1 寸。

13. **陶道** Táo dào(Du$_{13}$)
【类别】督脉与足太阳经交会穴。
【体表定位】在背部,当后正中线上,第一胸椎棘突下凹陷中。(图 2-109)
【层次解剖】有第一肋间动脉的后支及第一胸神经后支之内侧支。
【主治病症】①热病,疟疾。②头痛,脊强。

【针灸方法】向上斜刺 0.5～1 寸。

14. 大椎　Dà zhuī(Du₁₄)
【类别】督脉、手、足三阳脉交会穴。
【体表定位】在后正中线上,第七颈椎棘突下凹陷中。(图 2-109)
【层次解剖】有颈横动脉分支及第八颈神经后支。
【主治病症】①热病,疟疾,骨蒸盗汗。②周身畏寒,感冒,目赤肿痛,头项强痛。③癫痫。④咳喘。
【针灸方法】向上斜刺 0.5～1 寸。

15. 哑门　Yǎ mén(Du₁₅)
【类别】督脉与阳维脉交会穴。
【体表定位】在项部,当后发际正中直上 0.5 寸,第二颈椎棘突下缘。(图 2-110)
【层次解剖】有枕动、静脉分支及第三枕神经。
【主治病症】①情志变化引起的精神障碍、乏力。②聋哑。③中风,舌强不语,暴瘖。④癫狂痫。⑤后头痛,项强。⑥鼻衄。
【针灸方法】直刺或向下斜刺 0.5～1 寸,不可向上斜刺或深刺。深部接近延髓,必须严格掌握针刺的角度和深度。

16. 风府　Fēng fǔ(Du₁₆)
【类别】督脉与阳维脉交会穴。
【体表定位】在项部,当后发际正中直上 1 寸,枕外隆凸直下,两侧斜方肌之间凹陷中。(图 2-110)
【层次解剖】同哑门穴。
【主治病症】①中风不语,半身不遂,癫狂。②颈痛项强,眩晕,咽痛。
【针灸方法】直刺或向下斜刺 0.5～1 寸,不可深刺。深部为延髓,针刺注意安全。

17. 脑户　Nǎo hù(Du₁₇)
【类别】督脉与足太阳经交会穴。
【体表定位】在头部,后发际正中直上 2.5 寸,风府上 1.5 寸,枕外隆凸的上缘凹陷处。(图 2-110)
【层次解剖】有左右枕动、静脉分支及枕大神经分支。
【主治病症】①头晕,项强。②癫痫。
【针灸方法】平刺 0.5～0.8 寸。

18. 强间　Qiáng jiān(Du₁₈)
【体表定位】在头部,当后发际正中直上 4

图 2-110

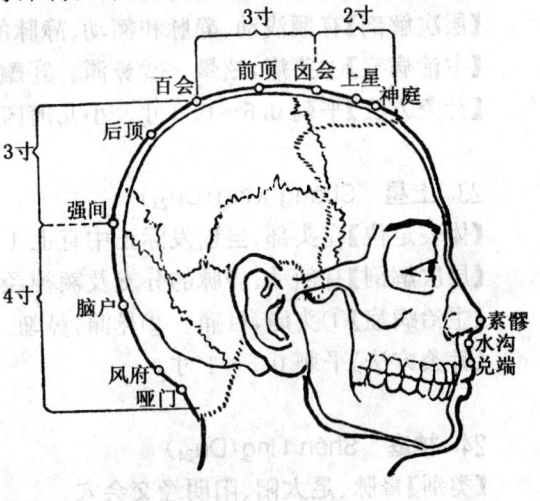

寸(脑户上1.5寸)。(图2-110)
【层次解剖】同脑户穴。
【主治病症】①头痛,眩晕。②癫狂痫。③中风偏瘫。
【针灸方法】平刺0.5～0.8寸。

19. 后顶 Hòu dǐng(Du₁₉)
【体表定位】头部,后发际正中直上5.5寸(脑户上3寸)。(图2-110)
【层次解剖】同脑户穴。
【主治病症】①头痛,眩晕。②癫狂痫症。③中风偏瘫。
【针灸方法】平刺0.5～0.8寸。

20. 百会 Bǎi huì(Du₂₀)
【类别】督脉、足太阳经交会穴。
【体表定位】在头部,当前发际正中直上5寸,或两耳尖连线的中点处。(图2-110)
【层次解剖】有左右颞浅动、静脉,左右枕动、静脉的吻合网及枕大神经分支。
【主治病症】①眩晕,头痛。②昏厥,中风偏瘫,不语。③脱肛,阴挺。④癫狂不寐。
【针灸方法】平刺0.5～0.8寸。

21. 前顶 Qián dǐng(Du₂₁)
【体表定位】在头部,当前发际正中直上3.5寸(百会前1.5寸)。(图2-110)
【层次解剖】同百会穴。
【主治病症】①头痛,眩晕。②鼻渊。③中风偏瘫,癫痫。
【针灸方法】平刺0.5～0.8寸。

22. 囟会 Xìn huì(Du₂₂)
【体表定位】在头部,当前发际正中直上2寸(百会前3寸)。(图2-110)
【层次解剖】有颞浅动、静脉和额动、静脉的吻合网。分布着额神经分支。
【主治病症】①头痛,眩晕。②鼻渊。③癫痫。④小儿惊痫。
【针灸方法】平刺0.5～0.8寸。小儿前囟未闭者禁针。

23. 上星 Shàng xīng(Du₂₃)
【体表定位】在头部,当前发际正中直上1寸。(图2-110)
【层次解剖】有额动、静脉的分支及额神经分支。
【主治病症】①头痛,目痛。②鼻渊,鼻衄。③癫狂。④中风偏瘫。
【针灸方法】平刺0.5～1寸。

24. 神庭 Shén tíng(Du₂₄)
【类别】督脉、足太阳、阳明经交会穴。
【体表定位】在头部、当前发际正中直上0.5寸。(图2-110)

【层次解剖】同上星穴。
【主治病症】①失眠,惊悸,癎症。②头痛,眩晕。③鼻渊。
【针灸方法】平刺0.5～0.8寸。《甲乙》:禁不可刺,令人癫疾。

25. **素髎** Sù liáo (Du$_{25}$)
【体表定位】在面部,当鼻尖的正中央。(图2-110)
【层次解剖】有面动、静脉鼻背支及眼神经支。
【主治病症】①昏迷,昏厥,新生儿窒息。②鼻塞、鼻衄、鼻渊、酒皶鼻。③目胀痛,视物不清。④足跟痛。
【针灸方法】向上斜刺0.3～0.5寸。

26. **水沟** Shuǐ gōu (Du$_{26}$)
【类别】督脉与手足阳明之会。
【体表定位】在面部、当人中沟的上1/3与中1/3交点处。(图2-110)
【层次解剖】有上唇动、静脉及面神经颊支、眶下神经分支。
【主治病症】①晕厥,中暑,中风昏迷,精神障碍,牙关紧闭。为急救要穴。②癫狂、癎症。③急性腰痛。④胃疼不止,口㖞面肿。
【针灸方法】向上斜刺0.3～0.5寸。

27. **兑端** Duì duān (Du$_{27}$)
【体表定位】在面部,当上唇的尖端,人中沟下端的皮肤与唇的移行部。(图2-110)
【层次解剖】同水沟穴。
【主治病症】①癫狂。②牙龈肿痛,口㖞。
【针灸方法】向上斜刺0.2～0.3寸。

28. **龈交** Yín jiāo (Du$_{28}$)
【体表定位】在上唇内,唇系带与上齿龈的相接处。(图2-111)
【层次解剖】有上唇动、静脉及上齿槽神经分支。
【主治病症】①急性腰痛。②痔疮出血、痔疾疼痛。③齿龈肿痛。④鼻渊。⑤癫狂。
【针灸方法】向上斜刺0.2～0.3寸。或点刺出血。

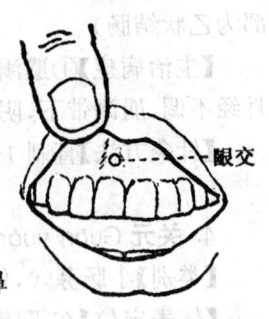

图2-111

第十四节 任脉穴

本经经穴起于会阴,止于承浆,一名一穴,共24穴。(图2-112)

1. **会阴** Huì yīn (RN$_1$)
【类别】任脉、督脉、冲脉交会穴。
【体表定位】在会阴穴,男性当阴囊根部与肛门连线的中点。女性当大阴唇后联合与肛门连

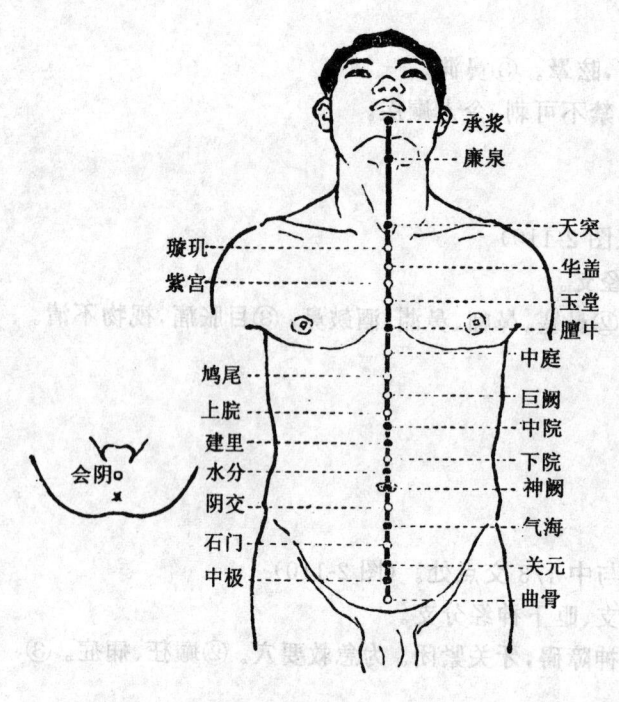

图 2-112 任脉经穴总图

线的中点。(图 2-112)

【层次解剖】有会阴动、静分支及会阴神经分支。

【主治病症】①二便不利或失禁,痔疾,脱肛。②遗精,阳痿,阴部痒。③溺水窒息,昏迷,癫狂。

【针灸方法】直刺 0.5~1 寸。

2. **曲骨** Qū gǔ(RN₂)

【类别】任脉、足厥阴交会穴。

【体表定位】在下腹部,当前正中线上,耻骨联合上缘的中点处。(图 2-113)

【层次解剖】有腹壁下动脉分支及髂腹下神经分支。

【主治病症】①小便不利,遗溺。②遗精,阳痿。③月经不调,带下。

【针灸方法】直刺 1~1.5 寸。

3. **中极** zhōng jí(RN₃)

【类别】膀胱募穴,任脉、足三阴经交会穴。

【体表定位】在下腹部,前正中线上,当脐中下 4 寸。(图 2-113)

【层次解剖】有腹壁浅动、静脉分支及腹壁下动、静脉分支,分布着髂腹下神经的分支。(内部为乙状结肠)

【主治病症】①遗溺、小便不利。②遗精,阳痿。③月经不调,崩漏带下,阴挺,不孕。④疝气。

【针灸方法】直刺 1—1.5 寸。

4. **关元** Guān yuán(RN₄)

【类别】小肠募穴,任脉与足三阴经交会穴。

【体表定位】在下腹,前正中线上,当脐中下 3 寸。(图 113)

【层次解剖】血管同中极,分布着十二肋间神经的前皮支的内侧支。(内部为小肠)

【主治病症】①阳痿,遗精,遗溺,小便频数,小便不通。②月经不调,崩漏,带下,痛经,阴挺,阴痒,不孕,产后出血。③中风脱症,虚劳体弱,本穴有强壮作用,为保健要穴。④泄泻,脱肛,完谷不化。

【针灸方法】直刺 1~2 寸。

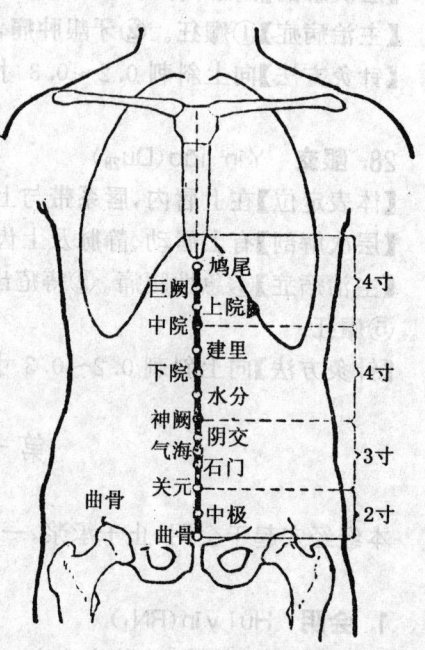

图 2-113

5. 石门 Shí mén(RN5)
【类别】三焦募穴。
【体表定位】在下腹部,前正中线上,当脐中下2寸。(图2-113)
【层次解剖】血管同中极穴,分布着第十一肋间神经的前皮支。
【主治病症】①小便不利,水肿。②疝气,腹痛,泄泻。③经闭,带下,崩漏。
【针灸方法】直刺1~2寸。

6. 气海 Qì hǎi(RN6)
【体表定位】在下腹部,前正中线上,当脐中下1.5寸。(图2-113)
【层次解剖】血管、神经分布同石门穴。
【主治病症】①腹痛,泄泻,便秘。②遗溺。③疝气。④遗精,阳痿。⑤月经不调,经闭。⑥虚劳体弱,本穴有强壮作用,为保健要穴。
【针灸方法】直刺1~2寸。

7. 阴交 Yīn jiāo(RN7)
【类别】任脉与冲脉交会穴。
【体表定位】在下腹部,前正中线上,当脐中下1寸。(图2-113)
【层次解剖】同石门穴。
【主治病症】①小便不利,水肿。②疝气腹痛。③月经不调,带下,崩漏,阴痒,产后出血。
【针灸方法】直刺1~2寸。

8. 神阙 Shén què(RN8)
【体表定位】在腹中部,脐中央。(图2-113)
【层次解剖】有腹壁下动、静脉。分布着第十肋间神经的前皮支。
【主治病症】①中风脱证,四肢厥冷。②泄泻,偏身出汗。③水肿。
【针灸方法】艾条悬灸或隔物灸(盐、姜等)。

9. 水分 Shuǐ fēn(RN9)
【体表定位】在上腹部,前正中线上,当脐中上1寸。(图2-113)
【层次解剖】血管分布同神阙。当第八肋及第九肋间神经前皮支分布处。
【主治病症】①水肿,小便不通。②腹痛,泄泻,翻胃吐食。
【针灸方法】直刺0.5~1寸。《铜人》:水病灸之大良,禁不可针。

10. 下脘 Xià wǎn(RN10)
【类别】任脉与足太阴交会穴。
【体表定位】在上腹部,前正中线上,当脐中上2寸。(图2-113)
【层次解剖】血管同神阙穴。分布着第八肋间神经前皮支。
【主治病症】胃脘痛,腹胀泄泻,呕吐,呃逆。

575

【针灸方法】直刺1～2寸。

11. 建里 Jiàn lǐ(RN₁₁)
【体表定位】在上腹部，前正中线上，当脐中上3寸。(图2-113)
【层次解剖】有腹壁上、下动脉交界处的分支。分布着第八肋间神经的前皮支。
【主治病症】①胃痛，呕吐。②食欲不振。③腹胀肠鸣。
【针灸方法】直刺1—2寸。

12. 中脘 Zhōng wǎn(RN₁₂)
【类别】胃募穴，八会穴(腑会)，任脉、手太阳、少阳与足阳明经交会穴。
【体表定位】在上腹部，前正中线上，当脐中上4寸。(图2-113)
【层次解剖】有腹壁上动、静脉，分布着第七肋间神经的前皮支。
【主治病症】①胃脘痛，呕吐，呃逆，吞酸。②腹胀，泄泻，饮食不化。③咳喘痰多。④黄疸。⑤失眠。

13. 上脘 Shàng wǎn(RN₁₃)
【类别】任脉、足阳明与手太阳经交会穴。
【体表定位】在上腹部，前正中线上，当脐中上5寸。(内为肝下缘及胃幽门部)(图2-113)
【层次解剖】同中脘。
【主治病症】①胃痛，呕吐，腹胀。②癫痫。
【针灸方法】直刺1—1.5寸。不可深刺，以免伤及肝脏。

14. 巨阙 Jù què(RN₁₄)
【类别】心募穴。
【体表定位】在上腹部，前正中线上，当脐中上6寸。(图2-113)
【层次解剖】内部为肝上缘及幽门部。血管、神经同中脘穴。
【主治病症】①心胸痛，心悸。②癫狂痫。③胃痛，呕吐。
【针灸方法】向下斜刺0.5～1寸。不可深刺，以免伤及肝脏。

15. 鸠尾 Jiū wěi(RN₁₅)
【类别】任脉络穴。
【体表定位】在上腹部，前正中线上，当胸剑结合部下1寸。(图2-113)
【层次解剖】同中脘。
【主治病症】①癫狂痫。②胸痛，心悸，腹胀。
【针灸方法】向下斜刺0.4～0.6寸。

16. 中庭 Zhōng tíng(RN₁₆)
【体表定位】在胸部，当前正中线上，平第五肋间，即胸剑结合处。(图2-114)
【层次解剖】有乳房内动、静脉的前穿支。分布着第六肋间神经的前皮支。

【主治病症】①胸胁胀满,心痛。②呕吐,小儿吐乳。
【针灸方法】平刺 0.3～0.5 寸。

17. 膻中 Dàn zhōng(RN$_{17}$)
【类别】心包募穴,八会穴(气会)。
【体表定位】在胸部,当前正中线上,平第四肋间,两乳头连线的中点。(图 2-114)
【层次解剖】血管同中庭穴,分布着第四肋间神经的前皮支。
【主治病症】①气喘,胸痛,胸闷。②心痛,心悸。③乳汁少,呃逆,噎膈。
【针灸方法】平刺 0.3～0.5 寸。

图 2-114

18. 玉堂 Yù táng(RN$_{18}$)
【体表定位】在胸部,当前正中线上,平第三肋间。(图 2-114)
【层次解剖】血管同中庭,分布着第三肋间神经前皮支。
【主治病症】①咳嗽,气喘。②胸痛,乳痛。
【针灸方法】平刺 0.3～0.5 寸。

19. 紫宫 zǐ gōng(RN$_{19}$)
【体表定位】在胸部,当前正中线上,平第二肋间。(图 2-114)
【层次解剖】血管同中庭,分布着第二肋间神经的前皮支。
【主治病症】咳嗽,气喘,胸痛。
【针灸方法】平刺 0.3～0.5 寸。

20. 华盖 Huá gài(RN$_{20}$)
【体表定位】在胸部,当前正中线上,平第一肋间。(图 2-114)
【层次解剖】血管同中庭。分布着第一肋间神经的前皮支。
【主治病症】咳嗽,气喘,胸胁胀痛。
【针灸方法】平刺 0.3～0.5 寸。

21. 璇玑 Xuán jī(RN$_{21}$)
【体表定位】在胸部,当前正中线上,天突下 1 寸。(图 2-114)
【层次解剖】血管同中庭穴,当锁骨上神经前支处。
【主治病症】①咳嗽,气喘。②胸痛,咽喉肿痛。
【针灸方法】平刺 0.3～0.5 寸。

22. 天突 Tiān tū(RN$_{22}$)
【类别】任脉、阴维脉交会穴。

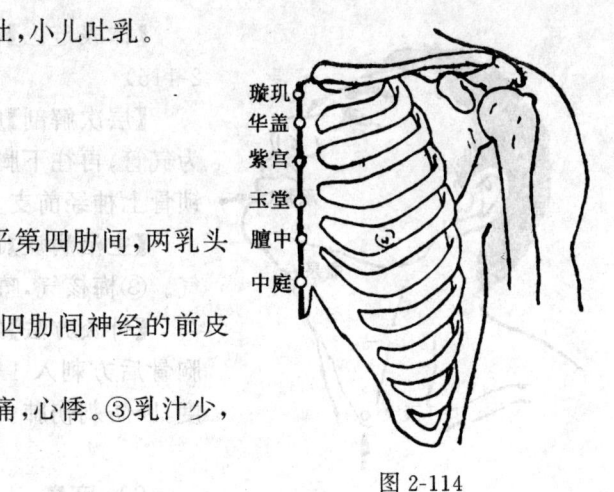

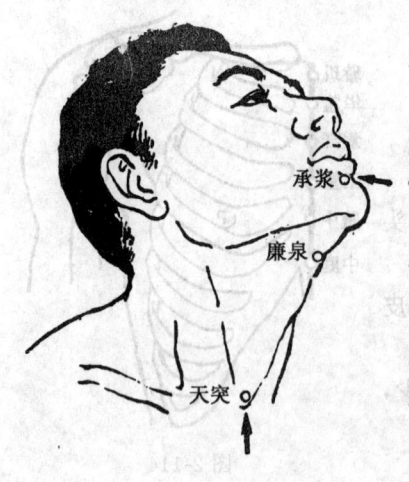

【体表定位】在颈部,当前正中线上,胸骨上窝中央。(图2-115)

【层次解剖】皮下有颈静脉弓,甲状腺下动脉分支,深部为气管,再往下胸骨柄后方为无名静脉及主动脉弓。分布着锁骨上神经前支。

【主治病症】①咳嗽,气喘,胸痛。②咽喉肿痛,暴喑,瘿气。③梅核气,噎膈。

【针灸方法】先直刺0.2寸,然后将针尖转向下方,紧靠胸骨后方刺入1—1.5寸。必须严格掌握针刺的角度和深度,以防刺伤肺。

图 2-115

23. 廉泉 Lián quán(RN₂₃)

【类别】任脉、阴维脉交会穴。

【体表定位】在颈部,当前正中线上,结喉上方,舌骨上缘凹陷处。(图2-115)

【层次解剖】有颈前静脉及舌下神经和舌咽神经的分支。

【主治病症】舌下肿痛,舌缓流涎,舌强不语,暴喑,吞咽困难。

【针灸方法】向舌根斜刺0.5～0.8寸。

24. 承浆 Chéng jiāng(RN₂₄)

【类别】任脉、足阳明经交会穴。

【体表定位】在面部,当颏唇沟的正中凹陷处。(图2-115)

【层次解剖】有唇下动、静脉的分支。当面神经分布处。

【主治病症】①口眼歪斜,牙龈肿痛,流涎。②癫狂。③遗溺。

【针灸方法】斜刺0.3～0.5寸。

第四章 经外奇穴

第一节 头颈部

1. 四神聪 Sì shén cōng(EX—HN₁)

【体表定位】在头顶部,当百会前后左右各1寸,共四穴。(图2-116)

【层次解剖】有枕动、静脉,颞浅动、静脉顶支和眶上动、静脉的吻合网。分布着枕大神经、耳颞神经和眶上神经分支。

【主治病症】①头痛,眩晕。②失眠,健忘。③癫痫。

【针灸方法】平刺0.5～0.8寸。

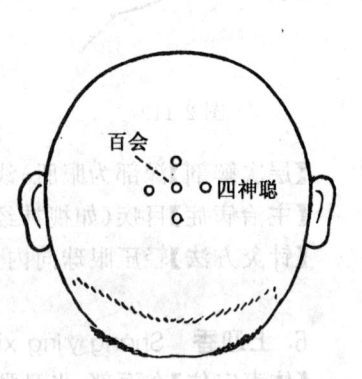

图 2-116

2. 印堂 Yìn táng(EX—HN₃)

【体表定位】在额部,当两眉头之中间。(图2-117)

【层次解剖】有额内动、静脉分支及滑车上神经。

【主治病症】①头痛,头重,眩晕。②鼻渊,鼻衄。③小儿惊风。④失眠。

【针灸方法】平刺0.3～0.5寸。

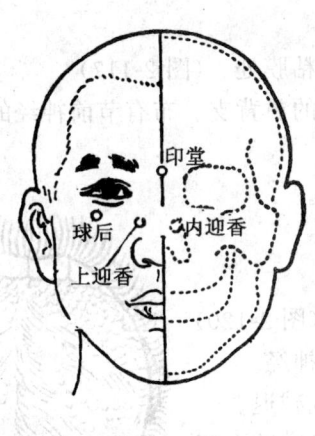

图 2-117 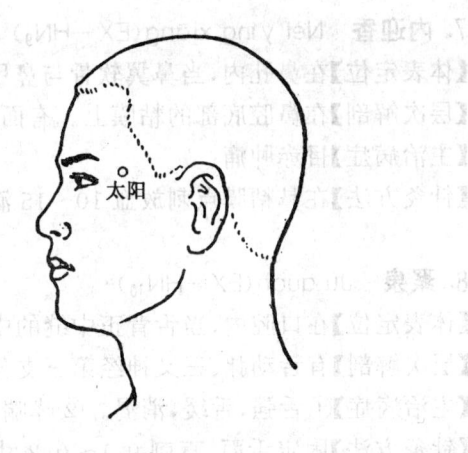   图 2-118

3. 太阳 Tài yáng(EX—HN₅)

【体表定位】在颞部,当眉梢与目外眦之间,向后约一横指的凹陷处。(图2-118)

【层次解剖】有颞浅动、静脉。分布着三叉神经第二、三支分支,面神经颞支。

【主治病症】①头痛,目赤肿痛。②牙痛,面痛。

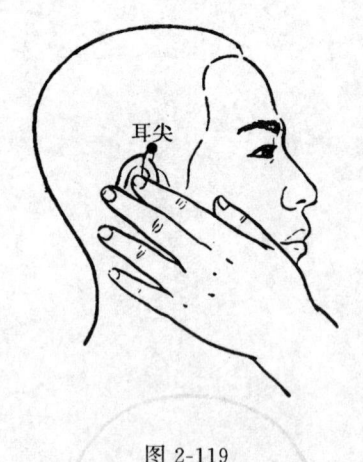

【针灸方法】直刺或斜刺0.5～0.8寸，或点刺出血。

4. 耳尖 Ěr jiān(EX—HN₆)

【体表定位】在耳廓的上方,当折耳向前,耳廓上方的尖端处。(图2-119)

【层次解剖】有耳后动、静脉；布有耳颞神经。

【主治病症】①目赤肿痛,目翳,视物模糊。②自汗,心悸。

【针灸方法】点刺放血。

5. 球后 Qiú hòu(EX—HN₇)

【体表定位】在面部,当眶下缘外1/4与内3/4交界处。(图2-117)

图2-119

【层次解剖】深部为眼肌,浅层有面动、静脉,深层有动眼神经和视神经。

【主治病症】目疾(如视神经炎,视神经萎缩,视网膜色素变性,青光眼,早期白内障,近视)。

【针灸方法】轻压眼球向内上,沿眶缘缓慢直刺0.5～1.5寸,不提插。不灸。

6. 上迎香 Shàng yíng xiāng(EX—HN₈)

【体表定位】在面部,当鼻翼软骨与鼻甲的交界处,近鼻唇沟上端。(图2-117)

【层次解剖】有面动、静脉分支。布有节前神经。

【主治病症】鼻渊,鼻部疮疖。

【针灸方法】向内上方平刺0.3～0.5寸。

7. 内迎香 Nèi yíng xiāng(EX—HN₉)

【体表定位】在鼻孔内,当鼻翼软骨与鼻甲交界的粘膜处。(图2-117)

【层次解剖】在鼻腔底部的粘膜上。有面动、静脉的鼻背支。布有节前神经的鼻外支。

【主治病症】目赤肿痛。

【针灸方法】在鼻粘膜点刺放血10～15滴。不灸。

8. 聚泉 Jù quán(EX—HN₁₀)

【体表定位】在口腔内,当舌背正中缝的中点处。(图2-120)

【层次解剖】有舌动脉、三叉神经第三支分支及舌神经。

【主治病症】①舌强,舌缓,消渴。②哮喘。③味觉减退。

【针灸方法】固定舌面,直刺0.1～0.2寸；或用三棱针点刺出血。《针灸大成》:"若灸,则不过七壮。灸法:用生姜切片如钱厚,搭于舌上穴中,然后灸之。灸毕,以清茶连生姜细嚼咽下,又治舌苔,舌强,用小针出血"。

9. 金津 Jīn jīn(EX—HN₁₂)

【体表定位】在口腔内,当舌下系带左侧的静脉上。(图

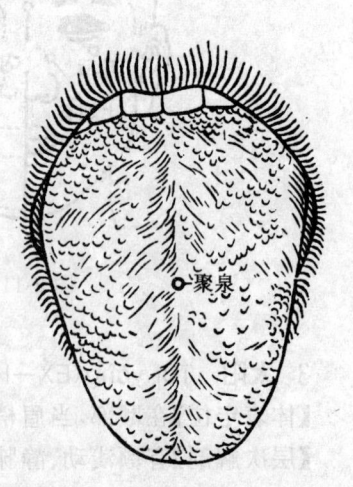

图2-120

2-121)

【层次解剖】有舌下静脉。分布着舌神经，舌下神经。

【主治病症】①口舌生疮，舌肿。②呕吐，消渴。

【针灸方法】固定舌体，点刺出血。不灸。

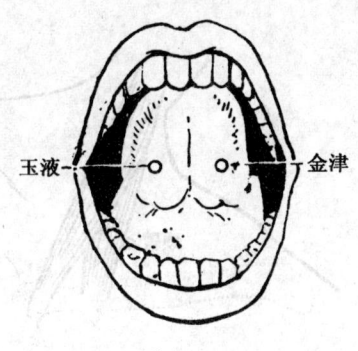

10. 玉液 Yù yè(EX—HN₁₃)

【体表定位】在口腔内，当舌下系带右侧的静脉上。（图2-121）

层次解剖，主治病症，针灸方法，同金津穴。

图 2-121

11. 翳明 Yì míng(EX—HN₁₄)

【体表定位】在项部，当翳风后1寸。（图2-122）

【层次解剖】有耳后动、静脉。布有耳大神经和枕小神经。

【主治病症】①目疾（近视，远视，雀目，青盲，早期白内障。）②耳鸣，耳聋。③失眠。

【针灸方法】直刺0.5～1寸。

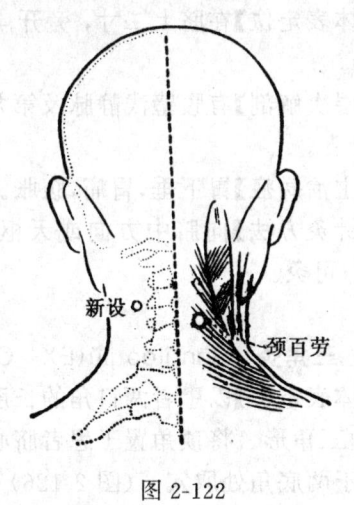

图 2-122 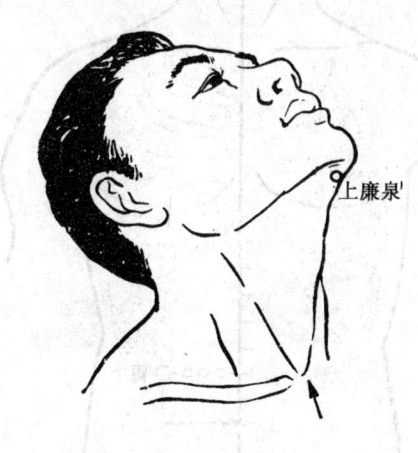　　　图 2-123

12. 颈百劳 Jǐng bǎi láo(EX—HN₁₅)

【体表定位】在项部，当大椎直上2寸，后正中线旁开1寸。（图2-122）

【层次解剖】有枕动、静脉和椎动、静脉。分布着枕大神经、枕小神经分支。

【主治病症】①骨蒸潮热，盗汗，自汗。②瘰疬。③咽肿，咳喘。④颈项强痛。

【针灸方法】直刺0.5～1寸。

13. 上廉泉 Shàng lián quán(EX—HN)

【体表定位】正坐仰靠，在颈上部正中，下颌下缘与舌骨体之间的凹陷处。（图2-123）

【层次解剖】有舌动、静脉及舌下神经。

【主治病症】舌强，喑哑，语言不清，失语，流涎，咽喉疼痛，舌面溃疡。

【针灸方法】向舌根方向斜刺0.5～0.8寸。

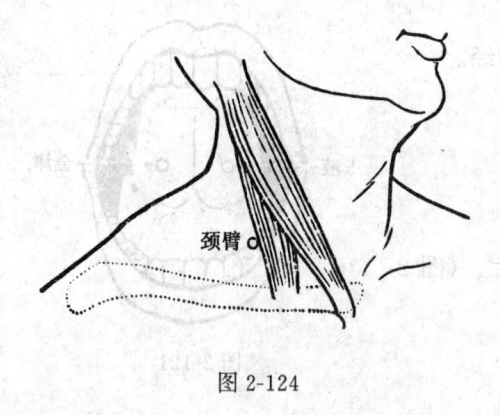

14. 颈臂 Jǐng bì(EX—HN)

【体表定位】仰卧去枕、头转向对侧,于锁骨内1/3与外2/3交点处直上一寸,胸锁乳突肌胸骨头后缘处。(图2-124)

【层次解剖】颈外侧动,静脉之分支。分布有臂丛神经。

【主治病症】肩、臂、手指麻木或疼痛,上肢痿痹。

【针灸方法】直刺0.3～0.5寸,不宜深刺,免伤肺尖。

图2-124

第二节 胸腹部

1. 胃上 Wèi shàng(EX—CA)

【体表定位】在脐上二寸,旁开4寸处。(图2-125)

【层次解剖】有腹壁浅静脉及第九、十肋间神经外侧支。

【主治病症】胃下垂,胃痛,腹胀。

【针灸方法】向脐中方向或天枢方向斜刺2～3寸;可灸。

2. 三角灸 Sān jiǎo jiǔ(EX—CA)

【体表定位】以患者两口角的长度为一边,作一等边三角形。将顶角置于患者脐心,底边呈水平线,于两底角处取穴。(图2-126)

【层次解剖】有腹壁下动、静脉肌支及第十肋间神经。

【主治病症】疝气奔豚。绕脐疼痛,妇人不孕。

【刺灸方法】艾炷灸5～7壮。

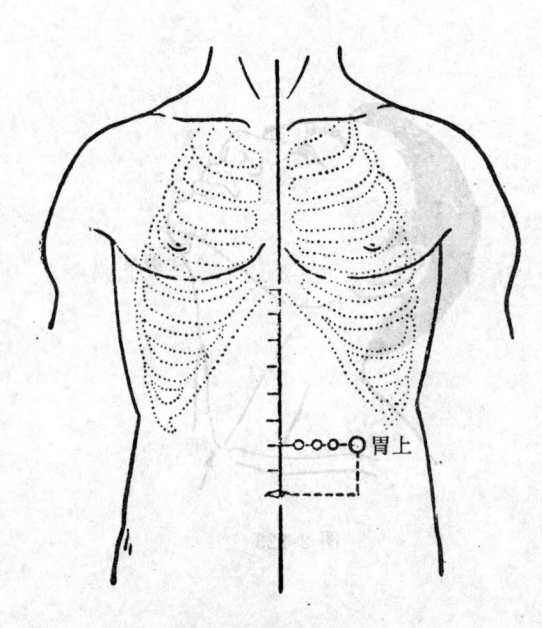

图2-125

3. 利尿穴 Lì niào xué(EX—CA)

【体表定位】神阙穴与耻骨联合上缘连线的中点取穴。(图2-127)

【层次解剖】有腹壁下动、静脉分支及第十二肋间神经前皮支的内侧支。

【主治病症】癃闭,淋沥,血尿,腹痛,泄泻,子宫下垂,胃下垂。

【刺灸方法】直刺0.5～1寸;可灸;或用手指按压。

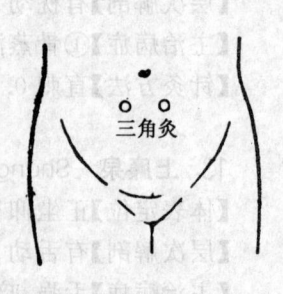

图2-126

4. 气门 Qì mén(EX—CA)

【体表定位】关元穴旁开 3 寸处。(图 2-127)

【层次解剖】同利尿穴。

【主治病症】妇人不孕,产后恶露不止,崩漏,癃闭,淋症,少腹疼。

【刺灸方法】直刺 0.5～1 寸;可灸。

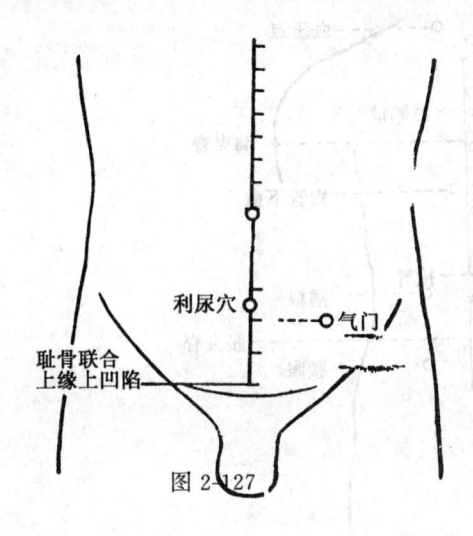

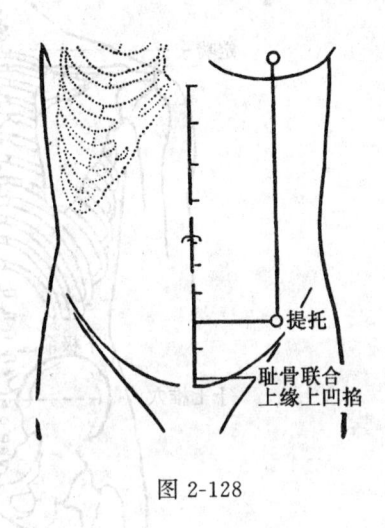

图 2-127

图 2-128

5. 提托 Tí tuō(EX—CA)

【体表定位】关元穴旁开 4 寸处。(图 2-128)

【层次解剖】有旋髂浅动、静脉;布有髂腹下神经。

【主治病症】子宫下垂,痛经,腹胀,疝气,肾下垂。

【刺灸方法】向阴部平刺 3～4 寸或直刺 0.5～1 寸;可灸。

6. 子宫穴 Zǐ gōng xúe(EX—CA$_1$)

【体表定位】在下腹部,当脐中下 4 寸,中极旁开 3 寸。(图 2-127)

【层次解剖】有腹壁浅动、静脉及髂腹下神经。

【主治病症】①子宫脱垂,月经不调,崩漏,痛经,经闭,不孕。②疝气,腰疼。

【针灸方法】直刺 0.8～1.2 寸。

第三节 背腰部

1. 定喘 Dìng chuǎn(EX—B$_1$)

【体表定位】在背部,当第七颈椎棘突下,旁开 0.5 寸。(图 2-129)

【层次解剖】有颈横动脉和颈深动脉分支,分布着第七、八颈神经后支。

【主治病症】①气喘,咳嗽,胸闷,气短。②咽喉肿痛。

【针灸方法】直刺 0.5～0.8 寸。

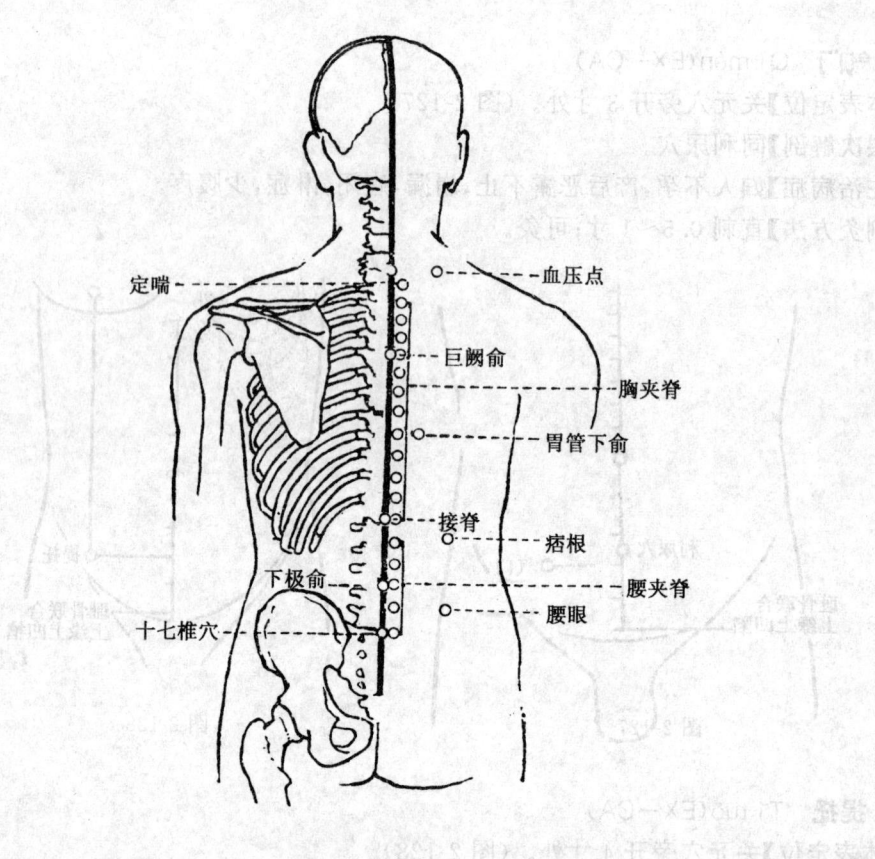

图 2-129

2. 夹脊 Jiá jí(EX—B₂)

【体表定位】在背腰部,当第一胸椎至第五腰椎棘突下两侧,后正中线旁0.5寸。一侧17穴。左右共34穴。(图2-129)

【层次解剖】在横突间的韧带和肌肉中。每穴都有相应椎骨下方发出的脊神经后支及其伴行的动脉和静脉分布。

【主治病症】①上胸部穴位治疗咽喉、心、肺、上肢部病。②下胸部穴位治疗肝、胆、脾、胃疾病。③腰部穴位治疗泌尿,生殖,肠腑,腰骶及下肢部病症。

【针灸方法】直刺0.3～0.5寸,或用梅花针叩刺。

3. 胃脘下俞 Wèi wǎn xià shū(EX—B₃)

别名:八俞、胰俞。

【体表定位】在背部,当第八胸椎棘突下,旁开1.5寸。(图2-129)

【层次解剖】有第八肋间动、静脉背侧支的内侧支。布有第八胸神经后支内侧皮支。深层为外侧支。

【主治病症】①消渴,咽干。②胃痛,胁痛。

【针灸方法】斜刺0.3～0.5寸。

4. 痞根 Pǐ gēn(EX—B₄)
【体表定位】在腰部,当第一腰椎棘突下,旁开3.5寸。(图2-129)
【层次解剖】有第一腰动、静脉背侧支,深层为第一腰神经后支。
【主治病症】①痞块,肝脾肿大。②腰痛,疝气。
【针灸方法】每次灸10~20壮,日一次。或直刺0.5~1寸。

5. 下极俞 Xià jí shū(EX—B₅)
【体表定位】在腰部,当后正中线上,第三腰椎棘突下。(图2-129)
【层次解剖】有棘间皮下静脉网。分布有腰神经后支内侧支。
【主治病症】①腰痛。②腹痛,泄泻。
【针灸方法】直刺0.5~1寸。

6. 腰眼 Yāo yǎn(EX—B₇)
【体表定位】在腰部,当第四腰椎棘突下,旁开约3.5寸凹陷中。(图2-129)
【层次解剖】有第二腰动、静脉背侧支。分布有第一腰神经外侧支。
【主治病症】①腰痛,尿频。②肺痨羸瘦。③月经不调,带下。
【针灸方法】直刺1.5寸。

7. 十七椎 Shí qī Zhuī(EX—B₈)
【体表定位】在腰部,当后正中线上,第五腰椎棘突下。(图2-129)
【层次解剖】有腰动脉后支,棘间皮下静脉网。分布有腰神经后支内侧支。
【主治病症】①腰腿痛,下肢瘫痪。②崩漏,月经不调。
【针灸方法】向上斜刺1—1.5寸。

8. 血压点 Xuè Yā diǎn(EX—B)
【体表定位】俯伏,于后正中线,第六、七颈椎棘突之间左右各开2寸处。(图2-129)
【层次解剖】有颈横动脉及颈深动脉分支,分布有第七颈神经后支。
【主治病症】高血压、低血压。
【针灸方法】直刺0.5~1寸;可灸。

9. 巨阙俞 Jù què shū(EX—B)
【体表定位】俯伏,于背部中线第四、五胸椎棘突之间凹陷处。(图2-129)
【层次解剖】有第四肋间动脉后支及第四肋间神经后支内侧支。
【主治病症】①心痛,失眠。②咳嗽,气喘,胸胁痛。③肩背痛。
【针灸方法】斜刺0.5~1寸;可灸。

10. 接脊 Jiē jǐ(EX—B)
【体表定位】俯伏,于背部中线,第十二胸椎棘突与第一腰椎棘突之间凹陷处。(图2-129)

【层次解剖】有第十二肋间动脉后支及十二肋间神经后支内侧支。
【主治病症】①小儿赤白痢疾,脱肛,腹痛,腹泻,消化不良。②癫痫。③疝气。
【针灸方法】斜刺 0.5～1 寸;可灸。

第四节 四肢部

1. 肘尖 Zhǒu jiān(EX—UE₁)

【体表定位】在肘后部,屈肘,当尺骨鹰嘴的尖端。(图 2-130)

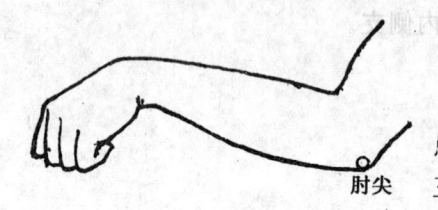

【层次解剖】有肘关节动脉网。布有前臂背侧皮神经。
【主治病症】①瘰疬,痈疽,疔疮,肠痈。③霍乱。
【针灸方法】瘰疬:如患左灸右肘,患右灸左肘,左右俱患,两肘皆灸,以三、四十壮为期,更服补剂。一年灸一次,三次其疮自除。

图 2-130

2. 二白 Èr bái(EX—UE₂)

【体表定位】在前臂掌侧,腕横纹上 4 寸,桡侧腕屈肌腱的两侧,一侧各一穴,一臂二穴,左右两臂共四穴。(图 2-131)
【层次解剖】有骨间掌侧动,静脉及正中神经和桡神经。
【主治病症】①痔疮,脱肛。②前臂痛,胸胁痛。
【针灸方法】直刺 0.5～0.8 寸。

3. 中泉 Zhōng quán(EX—UE₃)

【体表定位】在腕背侧横纹中,当指总伸肌腱桡侧的凹陷中。(图 2-132)
【层次解剖】有桡动脉腕背支,腕背静脉网。布有桡神经浅支。
【主治病症】①胸胁胀满。②胃脘疼痛,腹胀。③心痛。
【针灸方法】直刺 0.3～0.5 寸。

4. 中魁 Zhōng kuí(EX—UE₄)

【体表定位】在中指背侧近端,指骨关节横纹中点处。(图 2-133)
【层次解剖】有指背动脉和神经。
【主治病症】①噎膈,翻胃。②白癜风。
【针灸方法】灸。

5. 大骨空 Dà gǔ kōng(EX—UE₅)

【体表定位】在拇指背侧,指间关节的中点处。(图 2-133)
【层次解剖】有指背动脉和神经。
【主治病症】①目痛,目翳,内障。②吐、衄血。

图 2-131

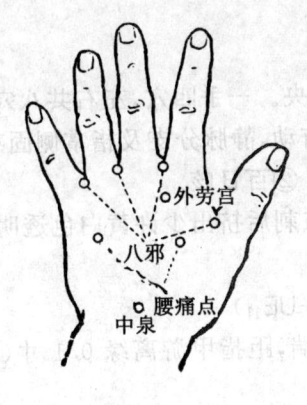

图 2-132 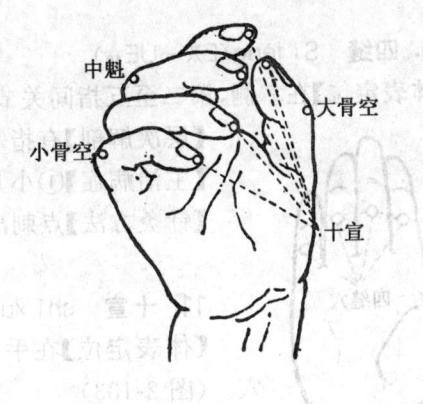　　　　　　　　图 2-133

【针灸方法】灸。

6. 小骨空　Xiǎo gǔ kōng (EX－UE₆)

【体表定位】在小指背侧近端,指间关节的中点处。(2-133)

【层次解剖】有指背动脉和神经。

【主治病症】目翳,目赤肿痛。

【针灸方法】灸。

7. 腰痛点　yāo tòng diǎn (EX－UE₇)

【体表定位】在手背侧,当第二、三掌骨及第四、五掌骨之间,腕横纹与掌指关节中点处。一侧二穴,左右共四穴。(图 2-132)

【层次解剖】有掌背动脉,布有掌背神经,指掌侧总神经。

【主治病症】急性腰扭伤。

【针灸方法】由两侧向掌中斜刺 0.5～0.8 寸。

8. 外劳宫　wài láo gōng (EX－UE₈)

【体表定位】在手背侧,第二、三掌骨之间,掌指关节后 0.5 寸(指寸)。(图 2-132)

【层次解剖】有掌背动脉,手背静脉网。布有桡神经分支。

【主治病症】①落枕,手臂痛。②胃痛。

【针灸方法】直刺或斜刺 0.5～0.8 寸。

9. 八邪　Bā xié (EX－UE₉)

【体表定位】在手背侧,微握拳,第一至五指的指蹼缘后方赤白肉际处,左右共八穴。(图 2-132)

【层次解剖】有掌背动脉,手背静脉网及尺、桡神经的手背支。

【主治病症】①毒蛇咬伤手背肿痛。②烦热,目痛。

【针灸方法】向上斜刺 0.5～0.8 寸;或点刺出血。

10. 四缝 Sì fèng(EX—UE₁₀)

【体表定位】在掌侧,第二至五指间关节近端中央。一手四穴,左右共八穴。(图 2-134)

【层次解剖】有指掌侧固有动、静脉分支及指掌侧固有神经。

【主治病症】①小儿疳积。②百日咳。

【针灸方法】点刺出血或点刺后挤出少许黄白色透明粘液。

11. 十宣 shí xuān(EX—UE₁₁)

【体表定位】在手十指尖端,距指甲游离缘0.1寸(指寸),左右共十穴。(图 2-133)

【层次解剖】有指掌侧动、静脉网及丰富的痛觉感受器。

【主治病症】①昏迷,癫痫。②高热、咽喉肿痛。

【针灸方法】浅刺0.1~0.2寸;或用三棱针点刺出血。

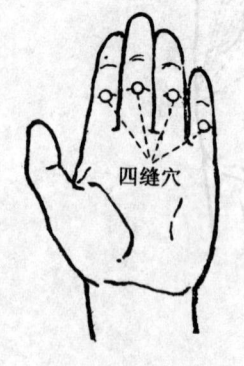

图 2-134

12. 五虎 Wǔ hǔ (EX—UE)

【体表定位】握拳、于手背第二、四掌骨小头高点处。(图 2-135)

【层次解剖】有指背动、静脉;分布有尺、桡神经的手背支。

【主治病症】手指拘挛。

【针灸方法】灸。

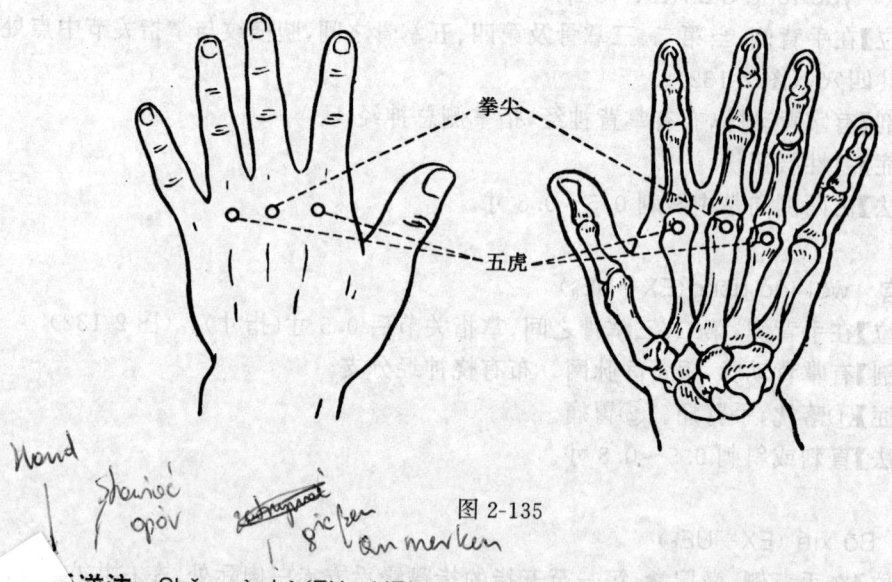

图 2-135

手逆注 Shǒu nì zhù(EX—UE)

【体表定位】伸臂仰掌,于掌长肌腱与桡侧腕屈肌腱之间,腕横纹与肘横纹连线的中点处。

【层次解剖】有前臂正中动、静脉及前臂掌侧骨间神经。

【主治病症】①前臂疼痛,上肢麻痹或痉挛。②乳腺炎、胸胁痛。③小腿痠痛。④癔病。

【针灸方法】0.5~0.8寸;可灸。

14. 肩前 Jiān qián (EX—UE)

【体表定位】于腋前皱襞尽端与肩髃穴连线的中点处(图2-131)

【层次解剖】有胸肩峰动、静脉,深部为腋神经。

【主治病症】肩痛不举,上肢瘫痪,肩关节及周围软组织疾患。

【针灸方法】直刺0.5～1寸;可灸。

15. 鹤顶 Hè dǐng (EX—LE$_2$)

【体表定位】在膝上部,髌底的中点上方凹陷处。(图2-136)

【层次解剖】有膝关节动脉网。布有股神经前皮支及肌支。

【主治病症】膝关节痠痛,腿足无力,鹤膝风,脚气。

【针灸方法】直刺0.5～0.8寸。

16. 百虫窝 Bǎi chōng wō (EX—LE$_3$)

【体表定位】屈膝,在大腿内侧,髌底内侧端上3寸,即血海上1寸。(2-136)

【层次解剖】有股动、静脉。布有股神经。

【主治病症】①皮肤瘙痒,风疹块,下部生疮。②蛔虫病。

【针灸方法】直刺0.5～1寸。

17. 内膝眼 Nèi xī yǎn (EX—LE$_4$)

【体表定位】屈膝,在髌韧带内侧凹陷处。(图2-136)

【层次解剖】有膝关节动、静脉网。及隐神经分支。

【主治病症】膝关节肿痛。

【针灸方法】向外上方斜刺0.5～1寸。

18. 胆囊 Dǎn náng (EX—LE$_6$)

【体表定位】在小腿外侧上部,当腓骨小头前下方凹陷处(阳陵泉)直下2寸。(图2-136)

【层次解剖】有胫前动、静脉分支。布有腓肠外侧皮神经,腓浅神经。

【主治病症】①急慢性胆囊炎,胆石症,胆道蛔虫症 ②下肢痿痹。

【针灸方法】直刺1—2寸。

19. 阑尾 Lán wěi (EX-LE$_7$)

【体表定位】在小腿前侧上部,当犊鼻下5寸,胫骨前缘旁开一横指。(图2-136)

【层次解剖】有胫前动、静脉,布有腓肠外侧皮神经、腓深神经。

【主治病症】①急、慢性阑尾炎。②消化不良。③下肢瘫痪。

【针灸方法】直刺1.5～2寸。

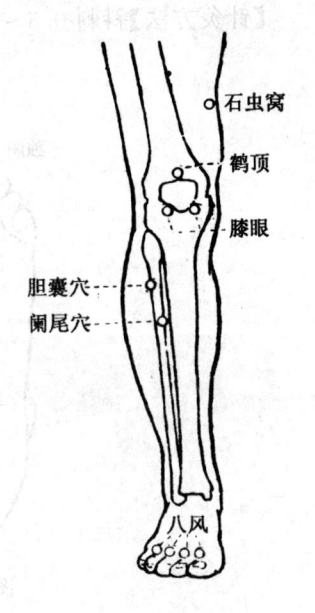

图 2-136

20. **八风** Bā fēng(EX-LE₁₀)

【体表定位】在两足背侧,第一至五趾间,趾蹼缘后方赤白肉际处。一足四穴,左右共八穴。(图2-138)

【层次解剖】有趾背动、静脉。布有腓浅、深神经。

【主治病症】①脚气,趾痛。②毒蛇咬伤,足跗肿痛。

【针灸方法】斜刺0.5～0.8寸,或点刺出血。

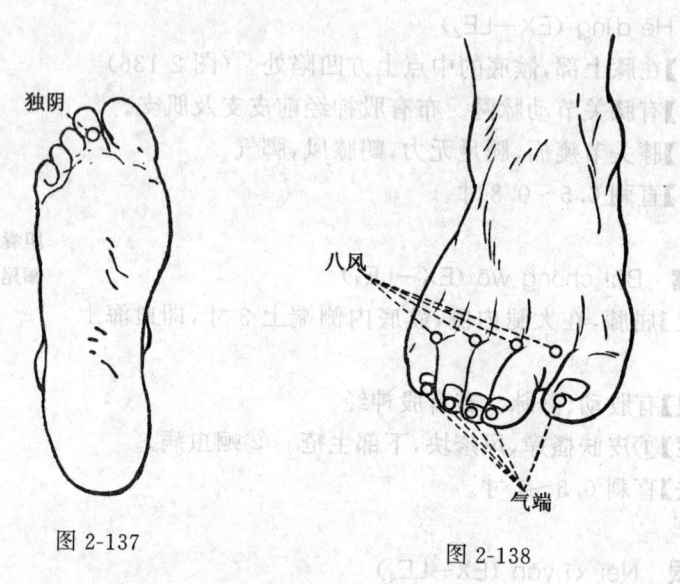

图 2-137

图 2-138

21. **独阴** Dú yīn(EX-LE₁₁)

【体表定位】在足第二趾的跖侧远端,趾间关节的中点。(图2-137)

【层次解剖】有趾底固有动、静脉,布有趾足底固有神经。

【主治病症】①卒心痛,胸胁痛。②月经不调,胎衣不下,死胎。③疝气。

【针灸方法】直刺0.1～0.2寸。

22. **气端** Qì duān(EX-LE₁₂)

【体表定位】在足十趾尖端,距趾甲游离缘0.1寸(指寸),左右共十穴。(图2-138)

【层次解剖】有趾背动脉及神经。

【主治病症】①中风急救,足趾麻木。②脚背红肿疼痛。

【针灸方法】直刺0.1～0.2寸;可灸。

中篇 刺灸方法

刺法和灸法是两种不同的治病方法。刺法亦称针法,是用针具刺入腧穴运用不同的手法以防治疾病的一种方法。临床常用的针具有毫针、皮肤针、皮内针、三棱针等,其中以毫针最为常用。灸法,是用艾绒为主要材料制成的艾炷或艾条,点燃后熏灼腧穴来防治疾病的一种方法。针和灸在临床上常相互配合应用,故合称为针灸。

第一章 毫针刺法

第一节 毫针的构造、规格

毫针是现在临床应用最广泛的一种针具,现多采用不锈钢针。毫针的结构共分五个部分:针柄、针尾、针尖、针身、针根。(图 2-139)

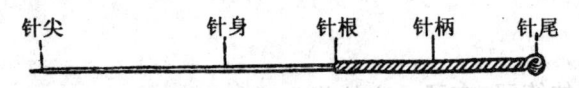

针尖　　针身　　针根　针柄　针尾

图 2-139

毫针的规格,主要是指针身的粗细和长短。常用毫针的长短、粗细规格分别如下表:

表 2-12　毫针的长短规格

寸	0.5	1.0	1.5	2.0	2.5	3.0	3.5	4	4.5	5
毫米	15	25	40	50	65	75	90	100	115	125

表 2-13　毫针的粗细规格

号数	26	28	30	32	34
直径(毫米)	0.45	0.38	0.32	0.28	0.22

临床上以 28～32 号、1.0～3 寸长的毫针最为常用。

第二节 针刺练习

由于毫针针身细软,如果没有一定的能力,很难进针和随意进行各种手法的操作。练习指力是学习针刺的基础,是进针顺利、减少疼痛、提高疗效的基本保证。

1. 纸垫练针法

用松软的纸,折迭成 5×8 厘米大小,厚约 2 厘米的纸块,用线如"#"字形扎紧,做成纸垫。练针时,以左手平执纸垫,右手执针,在纸块上反复进行捻进、捻出的练习,使指力运用自如,然后反复练习左右捻转,上下提插等基本手法。(图 2-140)

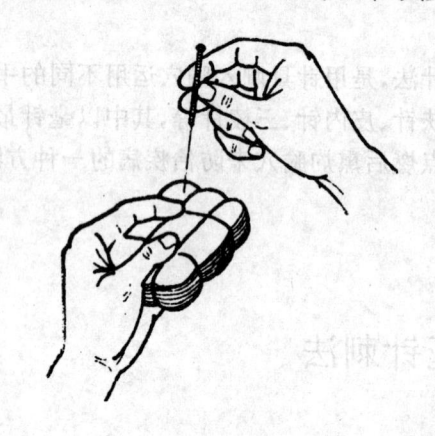

图 2-140 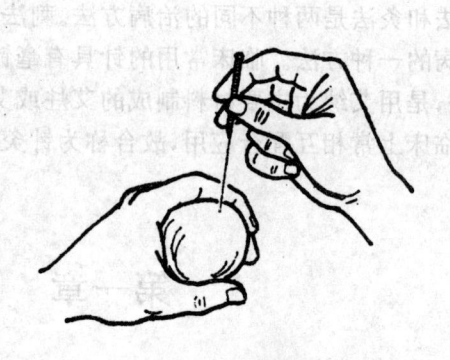　　　　　　　　　　　　　图 2-141

2. 棉球练习法

用棉花做成一个 6～7 厘米直径的棉团,外用纱布包裹,用线将口扎紧。练针方法同纸垫练针法,所不同的是棉团松软,可做提插捻转和补泻等多种基本手法的练习。(图 2-141)

3. 自身试针

通过以上两种方法的练习,有了一定的指力和行针基本手法后,就要在自己身上试针,或学员之间互相试针,细心体会进针手法以及针感情况,要求做到进针无痛,操作时针身不弯,刺入后针感强,并使针感向一定方向扩散。在针刺技术达到一定熟练程度后,才能在患者身上进行操作治疗。

第三节　针刺前的准备

1. 检查用具

在施行针刺操作以前,必先检查所用的各种针具器械,例如毫针、针盘、镊子、艾绒、火罐、消毒棉球、75%酒精或 1.5%碘酊、2%龙胆紫等是否准备齐全。

2. 选择体位

病人的体位是否合适,对于正确取穴和顺利进行针刺操作、持久留针、防止晕针、弯针、滞针、断针等都有很大影响。因此,选择体位应以医者能正确取穴,操作方便,病人肢体舒适并能持久留针为原则。临床常用的体位有以下几种:

仰卧位:适用于取头面、胸腹部的腧穴,以及四肢的部分腧穴。(图 2-142)

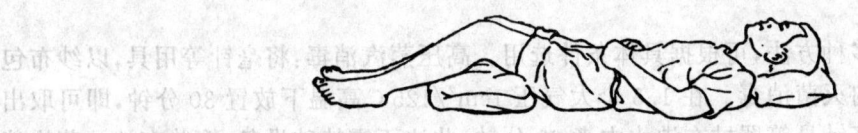

图 2-142

侧卧位:适用于身体侧面的腧穴。(图 2-143)

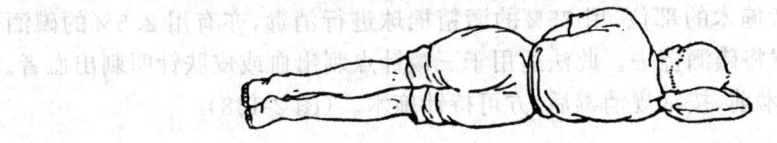

图 2-143

伏卧位:适用于头项、背、腰、臀部以及下肢后面的腧穴。(图 2-144)

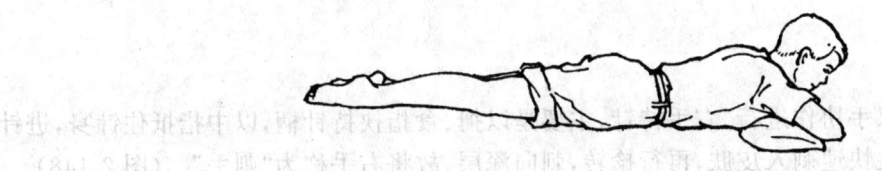

图 2-144

仰靠坐位:适用于头面、颈部、胸部以及四肢部位腧穴。(图 2-145)

俯伏坐位:适用于取头项、背部腧穴。(图 2-146)

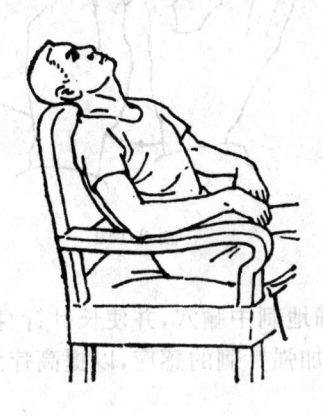

图 2-145　　　　　　　　图 2-146

侧伏坐位:适用于一侧取、耳颊部腧穴。(图 2-147)

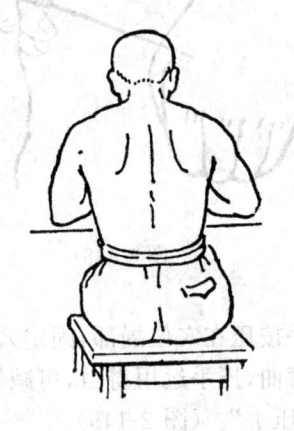

图 2-147

3. 消毒

①针具消毒：有多种方法，可根据具体条件选用。高压蒸汽消毒：将毫针等用具，以纱布包扎，放在高压蒸汽锅内灭菌消毒。在1.5个大气压1cm²/125℃高温下放置30分钟，即可取出使用。煮沸消毒：即将针具等器械在沸水中煮30分钟，此法不需特殊设备，简单有效。药物消毒：将针具放在75%酒精内浸泡30分钟至1小时，取出擦干应用。与毫针直接接触的针盘、镊子等也应进行消毒。此外，曾用于治疗某些传染病患者的针具，必须另外放置，严格消毒。

②皮肤消毒：患者施术的部位，用75%的酒精棉球进行消毒，亦有用2.5%的碘酒先给皮肤消毒，再用酒精棉球将碘酒擦去。此法适用于三棱针点刺出血或皮肤针叩刺出血者。

医生的两手在施术前，按常规消毒后，方可持针施术。（图2-148）

第四节 操 作

1. 进针法

针刺操作，需双手协作进行。右手持针，主要是以拇、食指挟持针柄，以中指抵住针身，进针时运用指力，使针尖快速刺入皮肤，再行捻转，刺向深层，故将右手称为"刺手"。（图2-148）

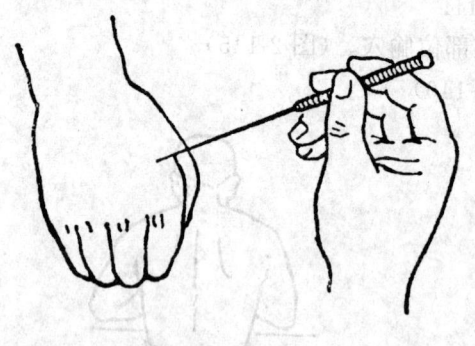

图2-148 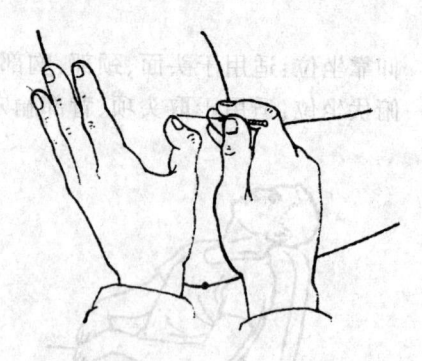　　　　　图2-149

左手按压在穴位局部，固定穴位的皮肤，使针能准确地刺中腧穴，并使长针针身有所依靠，不摇晃弯曲，压手运用得当，可减轻针刺的疼痛，调整和加强针刺的感应，以提高疗效。故将左手称为"压手"。（图2-149）

《灵枢·九针十二原》说："右主推之，左持而御之"。《难经·七十八难》说："知为针者，信其左；不知为针者，信其右。"《标幽赋》中进一步阐明了"左手重而多按，欲令气散；右手轻而徐入，不痛之因。"都说明了针时左右手互相配合的重要性。临床上常用的进针法有如下几种：

①指切进针法：左手拇指端或食指尖切按在穴位旁边，右手持针，针尖紧靠指甲刺入腧穴。此法多适用于短针的进针。（图2-149）

②夹持进针法：左手拇、食两指夹捏棉球，裹住针身，露出针尖，直对腧穴，下按，右手捻动针柄，将针刺入。此法多适用于长针的进针。（图2-150）

③舒张进针法：左手拇、食二指将腧穴的皮肤向两侧撑开，使皮肤绷紧，易于进针。此法多适用于皮肤松弛的部位，如腹部的进针。（图2-151）

图 2-150　　　　　　　　　　　　　　　图 2-151

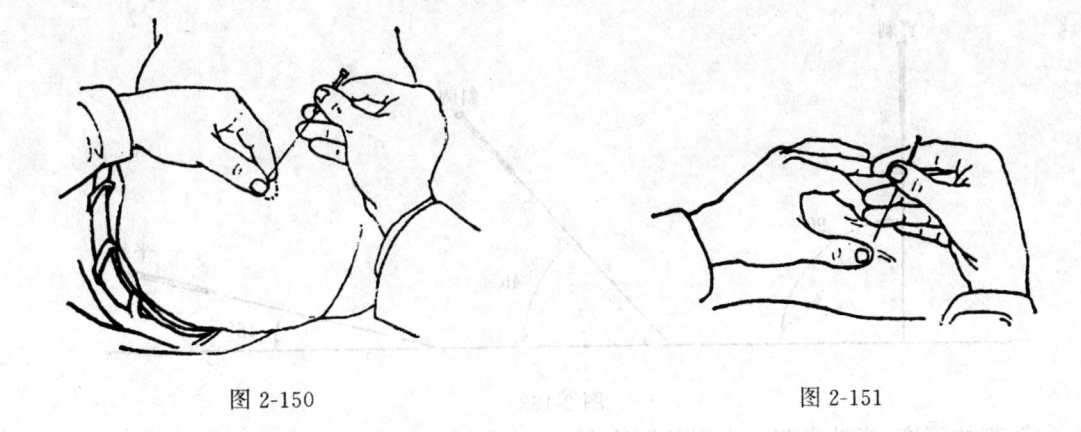

④提捏进针法：以左手拇、食二指将针刺部位的皮肤捏起，右手持针从捏起的上端刺入腧穴，此法多适用于皮肉浅薄的部位。如面部腧穴的进针。（图 2-152）

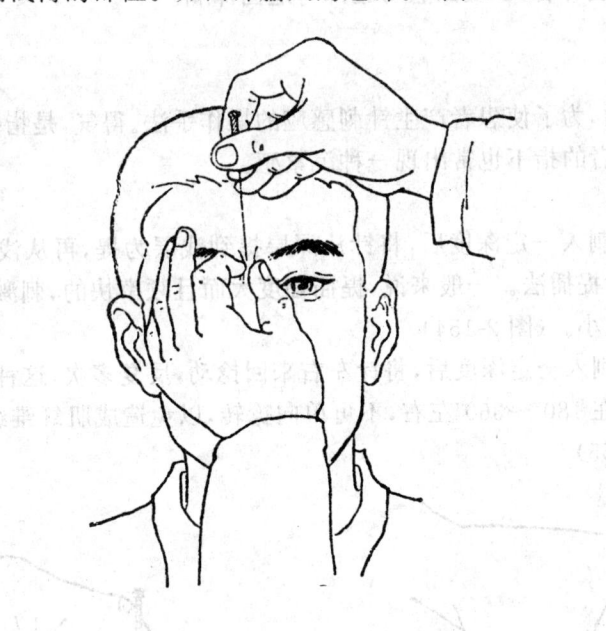

图 2-152

2. 针刺的角度和深度

临床上对所针腧穴的角度和深度，主要根据施术部位，病情需要以及患者的体质强弱、形体胖瘦等具体情况而定。

①针刺的角度：指进针时针身与皮肤表面所构成的夹角。有直刺、斜刺和横刺三种。

直刺：将针体垂直，与腧穴的皮肤表面呈90°角刺入，全身的腧穴大多可以直刺。（图2-153）

斜刺：针身与腧穴的皮肤表面呈45°角左右倾斜刺入，适用于肌肉较薄或穴下有重要脏器不宜深刺的部位。如胸、背部。（图 2-153）

横刺：又称平刺。针身与腧穴皮肤表面呈15°角左右沿皮刺入，适用于肌肉浅薄处。（图2-153）

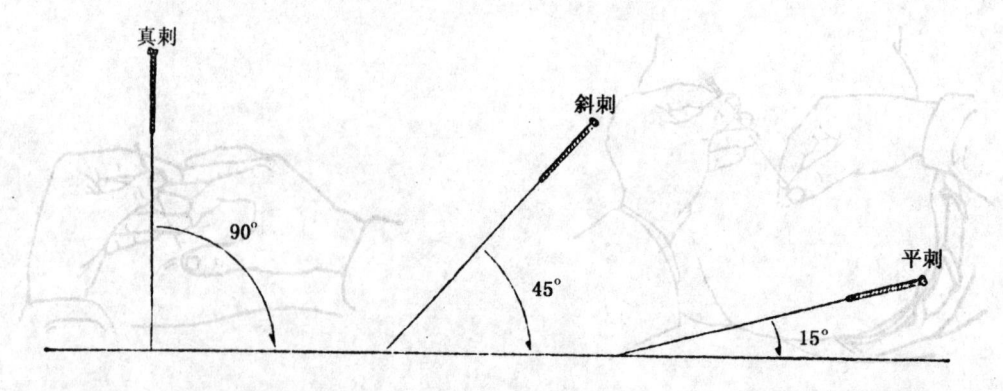

图 2-153

②针刺的深度:指针身刺入皮肉的深浅。以既有针感又不伤及重要脏器为原则。多根据体质、部位、病情而决定。如年老气血虚弱、小儿娇嫩之体、形体瘦弱以及头面、背部等宜浅刺;青壮年体质强壮或形体肥胖者,以及四肢臀腹部可适当深刺。

3. 行针与得气

行针,是指进针后,为了使患者产生针刺感应的操作手法。得气,是指针刺后患者有痠、麻、胀、重等感觉,同时医者的指下也常出现一种沉紧感。

①行针基本手法:

(1)提插法:针尖刺入一定深度后,将针从深层提到浅层为提,再从浅层插向深层为插,如此反复上下提插,称为提插法。一般来说,提插幅度大而且频率快的,刺激量就大,提插幅度小而频率慢的,刺激量就小。(图 2-154)

(2)捻转法:针尖刺入一定深度后,将针左右来回捻动,反复多次,这种行针手法,称为捻转法。捻转的幅度一般在 180°～360°左右,不可单向捻转,以免造成肌纤维缠住针身而产生疼痛和行针困难。(图 2-155)

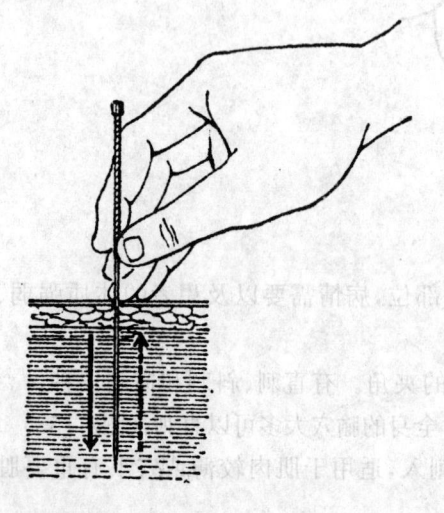

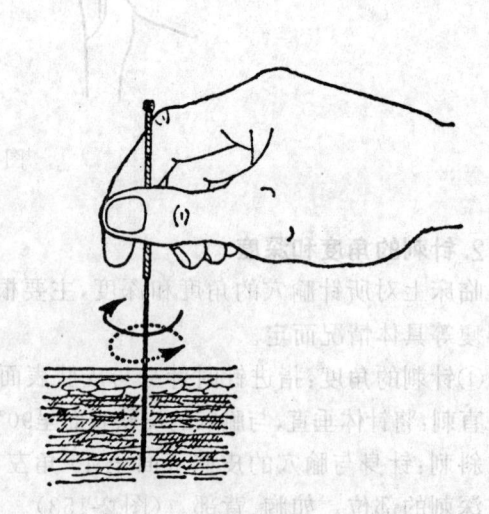

图 2-154 图 2-155

②辅助手法：在针刺过程中，不论用何种手法，都必须达到得气。《灵枢·九针十二原》说："刺之要，气至而有效……"。《金针赋》还说："气速效速，气迟效迟"。都说明了针刺的得气与否以及得气快慢与治疗效果均有密切关系。故历代针灸家对此都十分重视，并总结出了多种催气手法（又称辅助手法）。当针刺后，毫无得气现象或得气不明显，应施以催气手法使之得气。临床常用的催气辅助手法有如下六种：

（1）循法：用手指沿着经脉的循行路径，在针刺腧穴的所属经脉的上下部轻轻地循按。目的是激发经气的运行，容易得气，适用于经气阻滞，气至迟缓的病证。（图2-156）

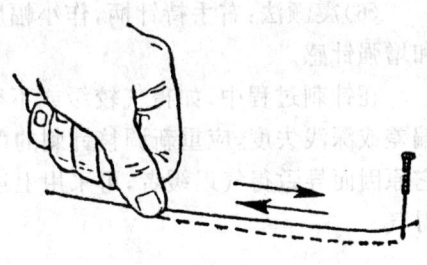

（2）飞法：操作时以捻转为主，连续捻转3次，然后拇食指立即张开，如飞鸟展翼之状，反复数次，可催气，并使针感增强。（图2-157）

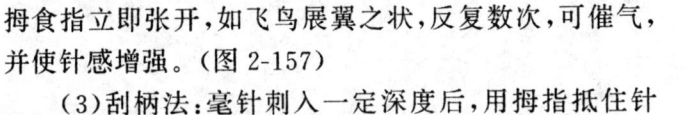

图 2-156

（3）刮柄法：毫针刺入一定深度后，用拇指抵住针尾，以食指或中指的指甲刮动针柄；或用食、中指抵住针尾，以指甲刮动针柄，以加强针感和促进针感的扩散。（图2-158）

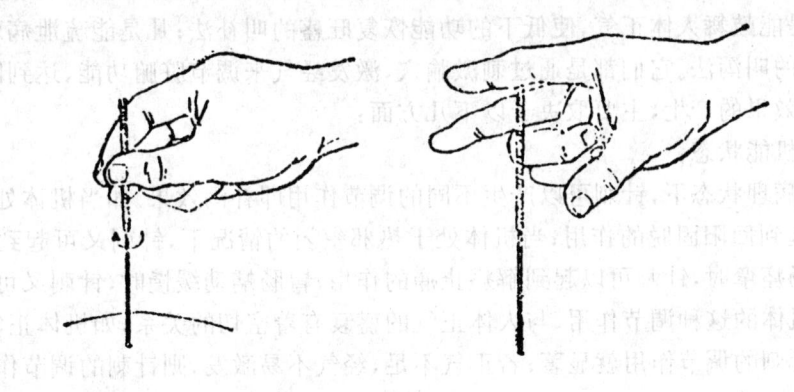

图 2-157

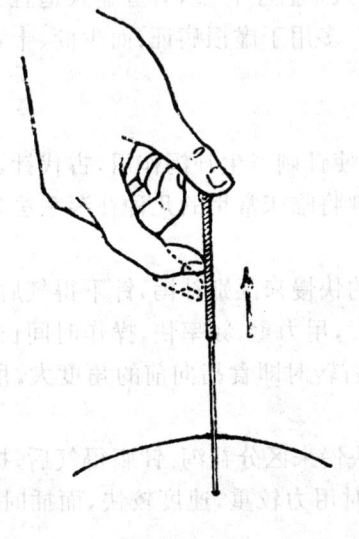

图 2-158 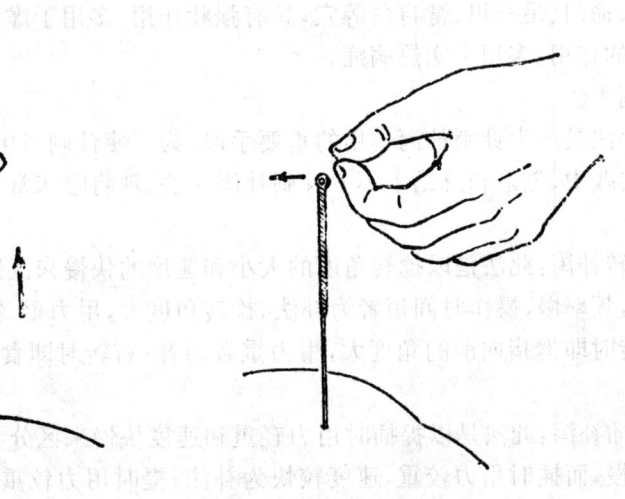　　　　　图 2-159

(4)弹柄法：用手指轻弹针尾，使针体微微震动以增强针感。用于留针过程中需稍加刺激者。（图2-159）

(5)摇柄法：手持针柄进行摇动如摇橹或摇辘轳之状。若直立针身而摇，多自深而浅，随摇随提，用以出针泻邪。若卧针斜刺或平刺而摇，一左一右，不进不退，如青龙摆尾，可以促使针感向一定方向传导。

(6)震颤法：右手持针柄，作小幅度快速的提插或捻转，使针身产生轻微震颤，以促使得气和增强针感。

在针刺过程中，如得气较缓或不得气，就要分析其原因，如属取穴不准，针刺角度、方向有偏差或深浅失度，应重新调整针刺的部位、角度、方向和深度。如患者病久体虚，经气不足，或其它原因而导致得气迟缓者，可采用上述一些辅导手法催气，或加艾灸，亦可留针候气，促使针下得气。

4. 针刺补泻

针刺补泻是根据《内经》"实则泻之，虚则补之"的治疗原则而确立的两类相对应的治疗方法。依据患者的体质、病情、功能状态、腧穴的特性而运用不同的操作方法，以促进机体内在因素的转化。凡是能鼓舞人体正气，使低下的功能恢复旺盛的叫补法；凡是能疏泄病邪，使亢进的功能恢复正常的叫泻法。它们都是通过刺激腧穴，激发经气来调节脏腑功能，达到阴阳平衡的。

针刺补泻效果的产生，主要取决于以下几方面：

①机体的机能状态：

在不同的病理状态下，针刺可以产生不同的调节作用即补泻效果。如当机体处于虚脱状态时，针刺可以起到回阳固脱的作用；当机体处于热邪壅闭的情况下，针刺又可起到泄热启闭的效果。又如胃肠痉挛时，针刺可以起到解痉止痛的作用；胃肠蠕动缓慢时，针刺又可使胃肠蠕动增强。针刺对机体的这种调节作用，与人体正气的盛衰有着密切的关系，如机体正气充盛，则经气易于激发，针刺的调节作用就显著；若正气不足，经气不易激发，则针刺的调节作用就较差。

②腧穴特性：

不同的腧穴在功能上具有相对的特异性，有些腧穴适宜于补虚，有些腧穴适宜于泻实。如气海、关元、命门、足三里、膏肓俞等穴，具有强壮作用，多用于虚损病证；而少商、十宣等穴具有清热、启闭的作用，多用于实热病症。

③针刺手法：

针刺手法是产生针刺补泻作用的重要手段。为了使针刺产生补泻作用，古代针灸医家在长期的医疗实践中，创造和总结了不少针刺补泻手法。现将临床常用的几种补泻手法分别介绍如下：

(1)捻转补泻：此法是以捻转角度的大小和速度的快慢来区别补泻。针下得气后，捻转角度小，用力轻，频率慢，操作时间短者为补法。捻转角度大，用力重，频率快，操作时间长者为泻法。也有以左转时即拇指向前的角度大，用力重者为补；右转时即食指向前的角度大，用力重者为泻。

(2)提插补泻：此法是以提插时用力轻重和速度快慢来区分补泻。针刺得气后，提时用力较轻，速度较慢，而插时用力较重，速度较快为补法；提时用力较重，速度较快，而插时用力较轻，速度较慢为泻法。

(3)徐疾补泻：此法是以进针、退针过程的快慢来区分补泻。行补法时，进针要慢，逐步进针达到一定的深度，出针要快，迅速提至皮下，稍停片刻出针；行泻法时，进针要快，一次就插到所需的深度，出针要慢，逐步分层退出。

(4)开合补泻：此法是以出针时是否按闭针孔来区分补泻。补法时，出针较快，出针后立即按闭针孔，意在使真气留存；行泻法时，出针时右手持针摇大针孔，一面摇一面退出，出针后不闭针孔。

(5)迎随补泻：此法是以经脉循行的顺逆来定补泻，行补法，将针尖顺经而刺；行泻法时，针尖要逆经而刺。

(6)呼吸补泻：当病人呼气时进针，吸气时出针为补法；吸气时进针，呼气时出针为泻法。

(7)平补平泻：进针得气后均匀地提插，捻转后即可出针。

以上各种手法，临床上可以单独应用，亦可以相互配合应用。此外尚有如下复式手法：(1)烧山火：将针刺入腧穴应刺深度的上1/3(天部)，得气后将针紧按慢提(即重插轻提)九次，再将针刺入中1/3(人部)，再紧按慢提九次，然后将针刺入下1/3(地部)，紧按慢提九次，然后将针慢慢提至上1/3(天部)，即三进一退，此为一度。如未出现热感再依前法反复操作二次，使之产生温热感，即将针紧按至地部留针。在操作过程中，可配合呼吸补泻法的补法。此法多用于治疗冷痹顽麻，虚寒性疾病等。

透天凉：将针刺入腧穴应刺深度的下1/3(地部)，得气后将针紧提慢按六次，再将针提至中1/3(人部)，再紧提慢按六次，然后将针提至上1/3(天部)，再紧提慢按六次，即一进三退，此为一度，如未出现凉感，再将针插至下1/3处，如前法反复操作二次，使之产生凉感。在操作过程中，可配合呼吸补泻法中的泻法。此法多用于热痹、急性痈肿等热性疾病。

5. 留针与出针

①留针：留针是指将针刺入腧穴行针施术后，将针留置穴内。留针的目的是为了加强针感和便于继续行针施术。留针与否和留针时间的长短，主要依病情而定。一般病症，针下得气后留针15—20分钟；但对某些慢性顽固性疼痛、痉挛性病证，可适当延长留针时间，有的病证留针可达数小时之久，在留针过程中作间歇行针，以增强疗效。对针感较差患者，留针还可以起到候气的作用。

②出针：出针时先以左手拇、食两指按住针孔周围皮肤，右手持针轻微捻转并慢慢将针提至皮下，然后将针起出，并用消毒棉球轻揉针孔，以防出血。最后检查针数，以防遗漏。

第五节 异常情况处理及预防

针刺治病，虽然比较安全，但如操作不慎，疏忽大意，或犯刺禁，或针刺手法不当，或对人体解剖部位缺乏全面的了解，在临床上也会出现一些异常情况，常见的有以下几种：

1. 晕针

原因：由于患者精神紧张、体质虚弱、疲劳、饥饿，或因体位不适，或医者操作不当，手法过重等因素造成。

症状：患者在针刺过程，突然感觉心慌、头晕目眩，或恶心欲吐，出冷汗，面色苍白，脉象微弱;严重者出现肢体厥冷,血压下降,二便失禁,不省人事等。

处理:立即停止针刺,将已经针刺的毫针取出,令患者平卧,头部稍低,注意保暖。轻者静卧片刻,喝点温开水或热水,即可恢复。重者以指掐或针刺人中、合谷、内关、足三里,或艾灸百会、气海、关元、涌泉等穴,如仍不缓解时,可配合其它急救措施。

预防:对于初次接受针刺治疗和精神紧张者,应先做好解释工作,消除顾虑。手法不宜过重,尽量采取卧位,少留针或留针时间不宜过长;对于过度劳累、饥饿者不宜针刺;医者在针刺过程中,发现患者面色苍白,出汗或诉说头晕等晕针先兆时,应及时采取处理措施。

2. 滞针

原因:患者精神紧张,针刺入后,局部肌肉强烈收缩;或行针时向同一方向连续捻转,而致肌纤维缠绕针身;或因针身刺入肌腱;或针刺后体位改变,都可引起滞针。

现象:进针后针下异常紧涩,出现提插、捻转及出针困难。

处理:嘱患者消除紧张情绪,使局部肌肉放松,因单向捻转而致者,则须反向捻转。如属肌肉一时性紧张,可留针一段时间,然后再行捻转出针,也可轻轻按揉针刺周围的皮肤肌肉,或在附近部位加刺一针,以宣散气血,缓解痉挛,因体位改变者,应恢复体位后随之将针取出。

预防:对精神紧张者,先作好解释工作,消除紧张心理,行针时不可用力过猛,避免单向捻针及将针刺入肌腱,留针过程中不宜随意改变体位。

3. 弯针

原因:医者手法不熟练,进针时用力过猛,或针下碰到坚硬组织;或留针时患者体位移动;针柄受到外物的压迫和碰撞;以及滞针没有及时处理。

现象:针身弯曲,针柄改变了进针时刺入的方向,提插、捻转及出针均感困难,患者感觉疼痛。

处理:发现弯针后,不可再行提插、捻转等手法。应顺势慢慢将针退出;如因患者体位改变所致,应使患者慢慢恢复体位,使局部肌肉放松后,再将针慢慢退出,切忌强行拔针,以免将针断入体内。

预防:医者进针手法要熟练,指力要均匀轻巧;针刺前应选择舒适的体位,留针期间不能随意变动体位;针刺部位和针柄应避免被外物碰撞和压迫。

4. 断针

原因:针具质量欠佳,针根或针身有剥蚀损坏;行针时手法过重,肌肉强烈收缩;或患者体位改变,滞针和弯针现象未能及时正确处理等,均可造成断针。

现象:针身折断,或部分针身尚露于皮肤之外,或针身残端全部没入皮肤之下。

处理:嘱患者不要紧张、乱动,以防断针继续向肌肉深层陷入,如残端部分针身尚露于体外,可立即用手指或镊子取出;如残端与皮肤相平,可按压针孔两旁,使断端暴露于体外,用镊子取出;如断针完全深入皮下或肌肉时,应在X线下定位,手术取出。

预防:认真检查针具,对不符合质量要求的针具应剔出不用。针刺不要将针身全部刺入,应留一小部分在体外。进针过程中,如发生弯针时,应立即出针,切不可强行刺入。当发生滞针、弯针时应及时正确处理,不可强行拔出。

5. 血肿

原因:针刺时误伤血管,起针时没有及时按压。

现象:出针后,局部肿胀疼痛,皮肤呈青紫色。

处理:轻度血肿,一般不必处理,可自行消退。若局部疼痛较剧,肿胀明显者,先作冷敷或加压止血,血止后再作热敷以促使局部瘀血消散。

预防:避开血管针刺,出针时立即用消毒干棉球揉按压迫针孔。

第六节 针刺注意事项

(1)过饥、过饱、醉酒、劳累过度时,不宜立即进行针刺,身体过于虚弱的患者,手法不宜过强,并尽量选用卧位。

(2)孕妇腹部、腰骶部和一些能引起子宫收缩的腧穴,如合谷、三阴交、昆仑、至阴等,不宜针刺;月经期间如不是为了调经,也不宜针刺。

(3)小儿囟门未闭合时,头顶部腧穴一般不宜针刺。此外,小儿不能合作,一般采用速刺不留针。

(4)避开血管针刺,防止出血,有自发性出血倾向或损伤后出血不止的患者,不宜针刺。

(5)皮肤有感染、溃疡、瘢痕的部位,不宜针刺。

(6)眼区、项部、胸背部、胁肋部等部位,应掌握好针刺的角度、方向和深度,严格按要求操作,以免发生事故。

第二章 灸法(附:拔罐)

灸法是以艾绒作为主要原料,制成艾炷或艾条,或将艾绒置于特制的容器中,点燃后,在体表一定的穴位上熏灼、温熨,借助灸火的温和热力的刺激,并通过经络的传导,腧穴的功用,起到温通经络,行气活血,扶正祛邪的作用,从而达到治疗疾病和防病保健目的的一种疗法。

艾叶性温而气味芳香,用作灸料,具有易燃,热力温和,能穿透皮肤,直达病部等优点。据《本草从新》记载艾叶有"理气血、逐寒湿、温经、止血、安胎等作用,故可用于风寒湿痹、气血虚弱、阳气虚脱、痈疽等诸种疾病,常灸关元、气海、足三里等强壮腧穴,尚可鼓舞人体正气,增强抗病能力,起到防病保健的作用。

第一节 常用灸法

常用灸法的种类如下:

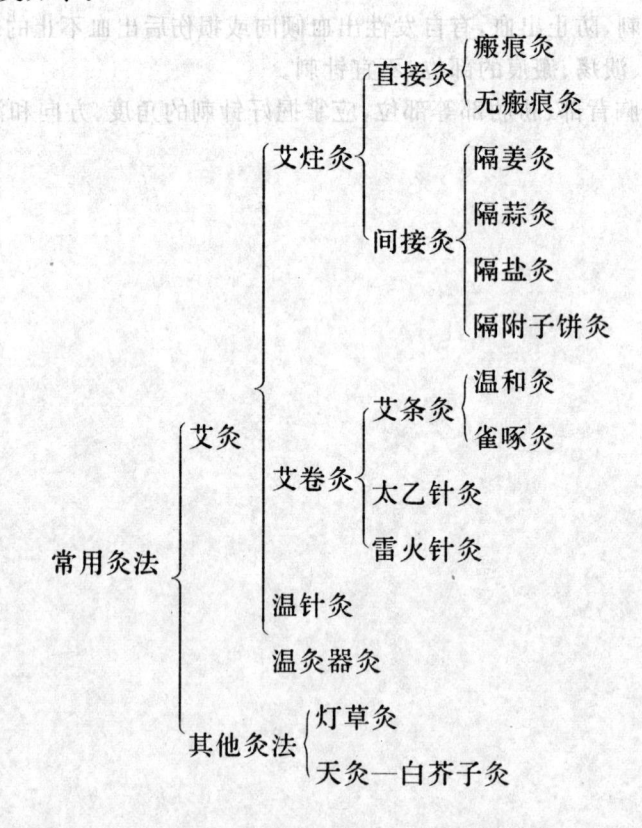

```
                    ┌ 直接灸 ┬ 瘢痕灸
                    │        └ 无瘢痕灸
            ┌ 艾炷灸┤
            │       │        ┌ 隔姜灸
            │       │        │ 隔蒜灸
            │       └ 间接灸 ┤
            │                │ 隔盐灸
            │                └ 隔附子饼灸
            │
            │       ┌ 艾条灸 ┬ 温和灸
    ┌ 艾灸 ┤       │        └ 雀啄灸
    │       │ 艾卷灸┤
常用│       │       │ 太乙针灸
灸法┤       │       └ 雷火针灸
    │       │
    │       │ 温针灸
    │       │
    │       └ 温灸器灸
    │
    │       ┌ 灯草灸
    └ 其他灸法┤
            └ 天灸—白芥子灸
```

1. 艾炷灸

是将纯净的艾绒,放在平板上,用手搓捏成圆锥形的艾炷,常用的艾炷或如麦粒,或如苍耳子,或如莲子,或如半截橄榄等大小不一。(图2-161)

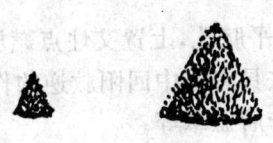

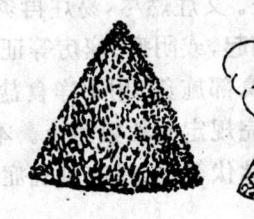

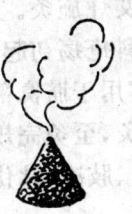

图 2-161

艾炷灸分直接灸和间接灸两类:
①直接灸:是将艾炷直接放在穴位皮肤上施灸的一种方法。若施灸时需将局部组织烫伤、化脓、愈后保留有瘢痕者,称为瘢痕灸;若不使皮肤烧伤化脓,不留瘢痕者,称为无瘢痕灸。(图2-162)

(1)瘢痕灸:又称"化脓灸"。施灸前用大蒜汁涂敷施灸部位,以增加粘附和刺激作用,然后将大小适宜的艾炷置于腧穴上,用火点燃艾炷施灸。每壮艾炷必须燃尽,除去灰烬后,方可易炷再灸,待规定壮数灸完为止,一般灸5～7壮。燃烧过程中,患者感觉灼痛时,可用手在施灸部位的周围轻轻拍打,以减轻疼痛。在正常情况下,灸后一周左右,施灸部位化脓形成灸疮,5～6周左右,灸疮自行痊愈,结痂脱落后留下瘢痕。此法适应于某些慢性疾患如哮喘、肺痨、顽固性痹症等。

灸疮要注意清洁,避免继发感染。

(2)无瘢痕灸:将艾炷放在腧穴上点燃,待其烧到三分之二左右,患者感到灼痛时,即将烧剩的艾炷去掉,另换一炷继续再灸。连续灸3～17壮,以局部皮肤产生红晕,而不起水泡为度。此法适应范围较广,多用于虚寒性疾患,如哮喘、慢性腹泻、消化不良等。

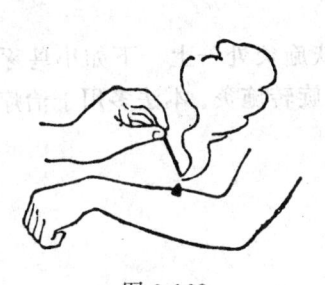

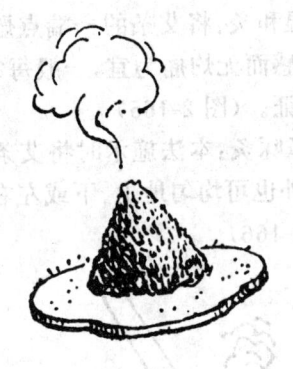

图 2-162 图 2-163

②间接灸:亦称隔物(药)灸,是用药物将艾炷与施灸部位的腧穴皮肤隔开,进行施灸的方法。临床常用的有:隔姜灸,隔盐灸,隔蒜灸、隔附子饼灸等。

(1)隔姜灸:用鲜姜切成直径大约2～3厘米直径,厚约0.2～0.3厘米,中间以针刺数孔,置于施灸部位,再将艾炷放在姜片上点燃施灸。(图2-163)当艾炷燃尽或患者感觉灼痛,易炷再灸,灸完规定的壮数,以局部皮肤潮红为度。本法具有温中散寒的作用,多用于脾胃虚寒、腹痛、泄泻、痹证及属于阳虚一类的病证。

(2)隔蒜灸:用大蒜(独头大蒜更好)切成0.2～0.3厘米厚的薄片,中间以针刺数孔,置于施灸部位,再加上艾炷施灸。艾炷燃尽,易炷再灸,至规定的数目灸完为止。本法具有消肿止痛的作用,多用于外科疮疡初起,或阴疽、瘰疬等证。

(3)隔盐灸:多用于脐窝部施灸。用干净食盐填平脐孔,上置艾炷点燃施灸。(图2-164)。待艾炷燃尽,易炷再灸,至灸完规定的壮数为止。本法具有温中回阳救逆的作用。多用于治疗急性吐泻所致的汗出、肢冷、脉伏等症,或中风脱症、产后血晕等。

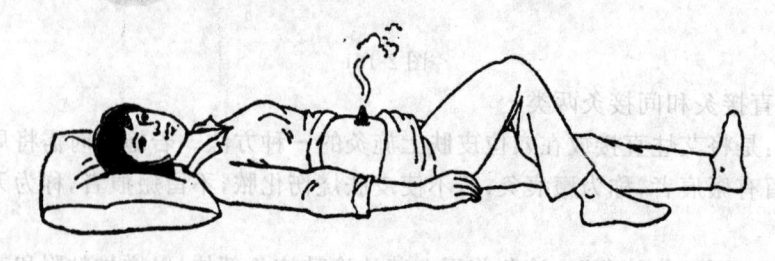

图 2-164

(4)隔附子饼灸:将附子研成粉末,用酒调和做成直径约3厘米,厚约0.3厘米的薄饼,中间以针刺数孔,置于施灸部位,上面放艾炷灸之。本法有温壮肾阳的作用,多用于治疗阳痿遗精、早泄、不孕或疮疡久溃不敛等症。

2. 艾卷灸
包括艾条灸、太乙针灸和雷火针灸。

①艾条灸:艾条灸是将艾绒卷成艾条,一端点燃,在离开穴位皮肤一定距离进行熏灸。根据操作方法分为温和灸和雀啄灸。

(1)温和灸:将艾条的一端点燃后,距施灸部位皮肤约2~3厘米处进行熏灸,使患者局部产生温热感而无灼痛为宜,一般每穴施灸15分钟左右,以皮肤潮红为度。本法适用于一切需要艾灸的病证。(图2-165)

(2)雀啄灸:本法施术时将艾条燃着的一端,对准皮肤施灸处一上一下如小鸟啄食一样地施灸。另外也可均匀地上、下或左右方向移动或作反复地旋转施灸。本法多用于治疗肢体麻痛者。(图2-166)

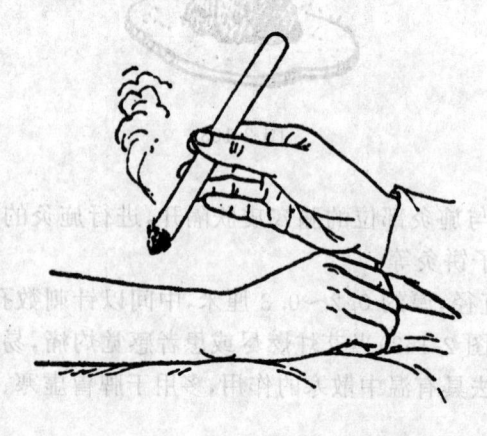

图 2-165 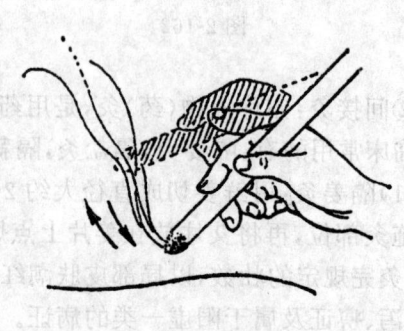　　　　　　　　　　图 2-166

②太乙针灸：是用纯净细软的艾绒150克，平铺在40厘米见方的桑皮纸上，将人参125克、穿山甲250克、山羊血90克、千年健500克、钻地风300克、肉桂500克、小茴香500克、苍术500克、甘草1000克、防风2000克、麝香少许，共为细末，取药末24克掺入艾绒内，紧卷成爆竹状，外用鸡蛋清封固，阴干后备用。

施灸时，将太乙针的一端烧着，用布七层包裹其烧着的一端，立即紧按于应灸的腧穴或患处，进行灸熨，冷则再燃再灸。如此反复灸熨7～10次为度。此法治疗风寒湿痹、顽麻、瘦弱无力、半身不遂等均有效。

③雷火针灸：其制做方法与"太乙针"相同，惟药物处方有异。方用纯净细软的艾绒125克，沉香、木香、乳香、羌活、干姜、穿山甲各9克，共为细末、麝香少许。

施灸方法及主治与"太乙针"基本相同。

3. 温针灸

是针刺与艾灸结合使用的一种方法，适用于既需要留针，又需要施灸的患者。操作方法是在针刺得气的基础上，将毫针留在适当的深度，用一小段艾条（约2厘米左右）套在针柄上，从下端点燃，直至燃尽为止。其作用是在针刺的基础上，借助艾火的热力以温通经脉，宣行气血，用以治疗寒湿痹痛、痿痹等症。（图2-167）

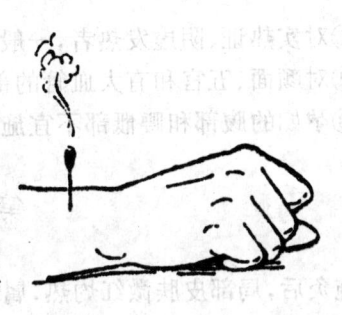

图2-167

4. 温灸器灸

温灸器又名灸疗器，是用金属特制的一种圆筒灸具，分为二层，内层是四周带有十孔的小筒，为放置艾绒的容器；外层为有均匀的小孔的圆柱状筒或锥状筒，附有持柄和支架。目前临床上使用的温灸器式样较多，但基本结构相似。

操作方法：将艾绒放置内筒点燃，然后用温灸器在施灸的腧穴或部位来回熨灸。或固定在施灸部位一定距离处温灸，以局部皮肤红润为度。本法用于需要艾灸及施灸范围较大的病症，对妇、儿及惧怕其它灸法者尤宜。

第二节 其它灸法

1. 灯草灸

又名十三元宵火，方法是用灯芯草一根，蘸麻油点燃后，于应灸的腧穴上迅速点灸。本法具有疏风解表，行气化痰，醒神定搐的作用。多用于治疗儿科疾患，如小儿惊风，胃痛，腹胀及腮腺炎等症。

2. 白芥子灸

用白芥子研末，用水或姜汁调和敷患处，使局部发泡，以此治疗阴疽、痰核及膝关节肿痛、口眼歪斜等。

第三节 注意事项

①施灸的先后顺序：一般先灸上部，后灸下部，先灸背部，后灸腹部；先灸头部，后灸四肢。临床上，可根据情况灵活运用。

②施灸的补泻方法：以灸补之者，灸时不吹其火，使其自然燃尽熄灭；以火泻之者，吹其火，使其旺。此法载于《灵枢·背腧》。

第四节 施灸的禁忌

①对实热证、阴虚发热者，一般不宜灸。
②对颜面、五官和有大血管的部位、关节部，不宜采用瘢痕灸。
③孕妇的腹部和腰骶部不宜施灸。

第五节 灸后的处理

施灸后，局部皮肤微红灼热，属正常现象，无需处理，如施灸过量，时间过长，局部出现小水泡，注意不要擦破，可自然吸收。如水泡较大，可用消毒针刺破，放出水液，再涂以龙胆紫，并以纱布包敷。如用化脓灸者，在灸疱化脓期间，要注意适当休息和加强营养，并保持局部清洁，以防污染，如灸疱感染，脓液呈黄绿色，或有渗血现象，可用消炎药膏或玉红膏涂敷。

〔附〕**拔罐法**：

拔罐法又称拔火罐，古称"角法"。是以罐子为工具，和用火燃烧排出罐内空气，造成相对负压，使罐子吸附于施术部位，产生温热刺激及局部皮肤充血、瘀血，以达到治疗疾病目的的一种疗法。多用于痹证，刺血拔罐运用于急性扭伤有瘀血者，疮疡、部分皮肤病，如丹毒、神经性皮炎等。

1. 罐的种类：

临床上常用罐有三种：玻璃罐、竹罐、陶罐。（图2-168）

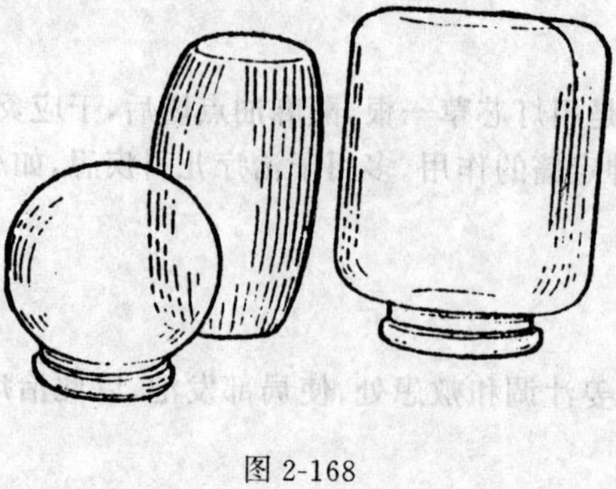

图 2-168

2. 拔罐的方法：

①火罐：是用火在罐内燃烧，形成负压，使罐吸附在皮肤上，具体操作方法有以下几种。

(1)闪火法：用镊子或止血钳夹住燃烧的酒精棉球，在火罐内绕一圈后，迅速退出，快速地将罐扣在施术部位。此法简便安全，不受体位限制，为目前临床常用的方法。(图2-169)

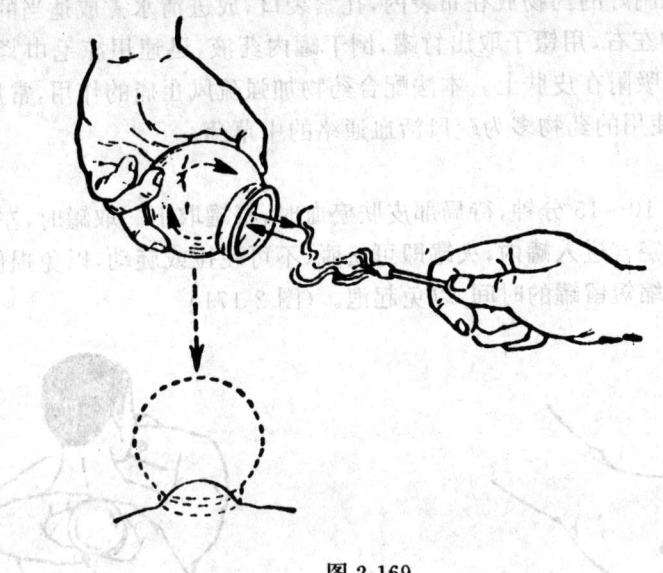

图 2-169

(2)投火法：将纸片或酒精棉球点燃后，投入罐内，然后迅速将火罐扣于施术部位。(图2-170)

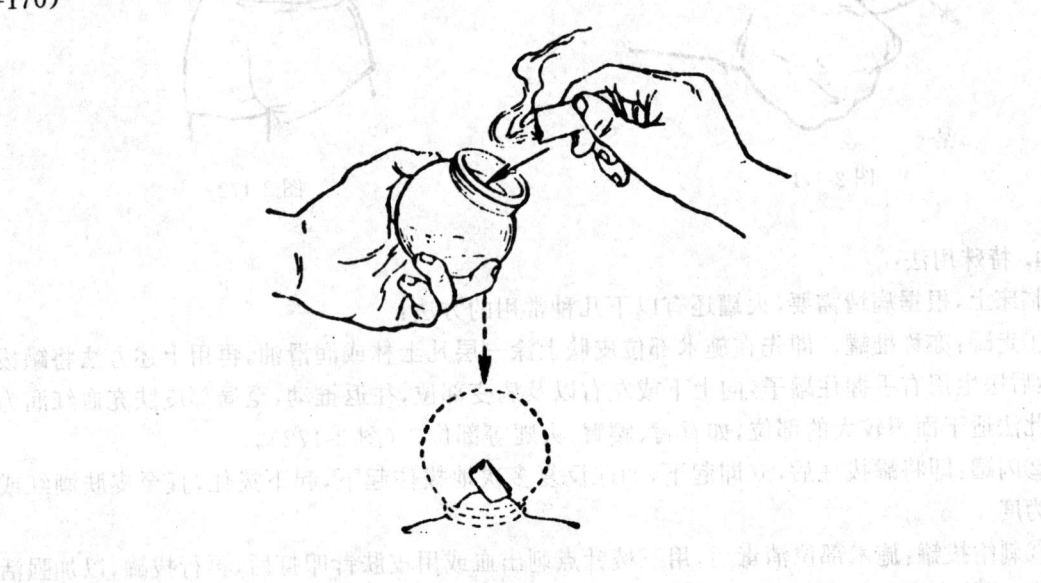

图 2-170

(3)滴酒法：是用95%酒精或白酒，滴入罐内1~3滴(切勿滴酒过多，以免拔罐时流出烧伤皮肤)，沿罐内壁摇匀，用火点燃后，迅速将罐扣在应拔的部位。

(4)贴棉法：是用大小适宜的酒精棉一块，贴在罐内壁的下1/3处，用火将酒精棉点燃后，迅速将罐扣在应拔的部位。

(5)架火法：即用不易燃烧、传热的物体，如瓶盖，小酒盅等，将95%酒精数滴或酒精棉球置其内，置于应拔部位，用火点燃，将罐迅速扣下。

②水煮法：先将配制好的药物放在布袋内，扎紧袋口，放进清水煮成适当的浓度，再把竹罐投入药液内煮15分钟左右，用镊子取出竹罐，倒干罐内药液，迅速用凉毛巾紧扣罐口，立即将罐扣在应拔部位，即能吸附在皮肤上。本法配合药物加强疏风止痛的作用，常用于风湿痹痛和某些软组织病证。所使用的药物多为疏风活血通络的中草药。

3．起罐：

拔罐时，一般留罐10～15分钟，待局部皮肤瘀血时，将罐取下。取罐时，左手扶住罐身，右手按压罐口的皮肤，使空气进入罐内，火罐即可松脱，不可硬拉或旋动，以免损伤皮肤。若罐大而吸附力强时，可适当缩短留罐的时间，以免起泡。(图2-171)

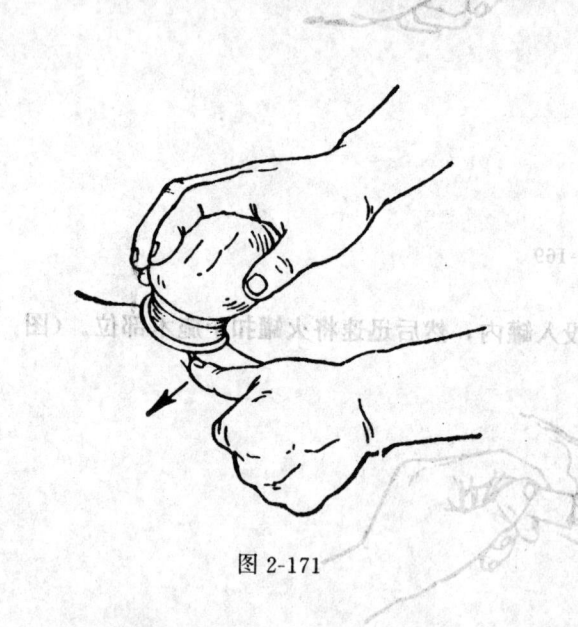

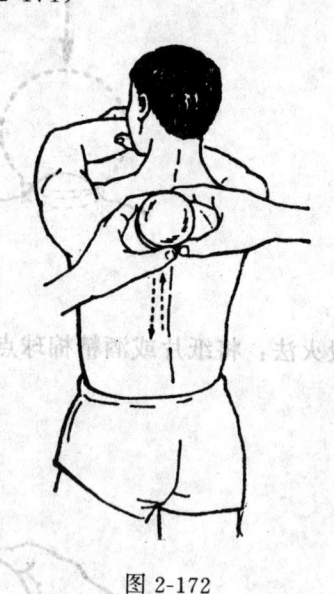

图2-171　　　　　　　　　　图2-172

4．特殊用法：

临床上，根据病情需要，火罐还有以下几种常用的方法：

①走罐：亦称推罐。即先在施术部位皮肤上涂一层凡士林或润滑油，再用上述方法将罐拔住，然后医生用右手握住罐子，向上下或左右以及病变部位，往返推动，至局部皮肤充血红润为度。此法适于面积较大的部位，如脊背、腰臀、大腿等部位。(图2-172)。

②闪罐：即将罐拔住后，立即起下，如此反复多次地拔住起下，起下拔住，直至皮肤潮红或充血为度。

③刺络拔罐：施术部位消毒后，用三棱针点刺出血或用皮肤针叩打后，再行拔罐，以加强活血祛瘀，消肿止痛的作用。

5．适应范围：

拔罐具有温通经络，行气活血，祛湿逐寒，散瘀消肿止痛的作用，常用于痹证(如腰腿痛、肩背痛)，胃肠道疾患(如胃痛、腹痛)，肺部疾患(如咳嗽、哮喘)。

刺络拔罐法适用于急性扭伤有瘀血者，疮疡、某些皮肤病，如丹毒、神经性皮炎、牛皮癣等。

6. 注意事项：

①患者体位要舒适，根据部位选用大小不同口径的火罐，注意选择肌肉较丰满，没有毛发和骨骼凹凸的部位，以防火罐脱落。

②拔罐时火力要足，罐口靠近拔罐的部位，操作要迅速轻巧，做到稳、准、快，才能将火罐拔紧，否则影响疗效。

③皮肤有溃疡、水肿及大血管的部位，不宜拔罐；高热抽搐者，以及孕妇的腹部和腰骶部也不宜拔罐。

④有自发性出血和损伤后出血不止的患者，不宜使用拔罐法。

⑤用火罐时注意勿灼伤或烫伤皮肤。若烫伤或留罐时间太长而皮肤起水泡时，小的勿须处理，水泡较大时，用消毒针将水放出，涂以龙胆紫药水后，覆盖敷料，以防感染。

第三章 其它针法

第一节 三棱针

三棱针是点刺放血的针具,目前所用的三棱针多为不锈钢制成,针长约2寸,针柄较粗呈圆柱形,针身呈三棱形,针尖锋利,三边有刃。(图 2-173)

图 2-173

1. 操作方法

右手拇、食指持针柄,中指扶住针尖部露出针尖 1—2 分许,以控制针刺深浅度,(图 2-174),针刺时左手捏住指(趾)部,或夹持、舒张皮肤,常用的刺法有四种。

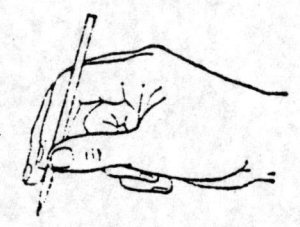

图 2-174

①腧穴点刺

先在腧穴部位上下推按,使血聚集穴部,右手持针对准消毒好的穴位迅速刺入 1—2 分,立即出针。轻轻挤压针孔周围,使血出数滴,然后用消毒干棉球按压针孔止血。如咽喉肿痛刺少商,目赤肿痛刺耳尖等。

②刺络

又称"络刺"。消毒后用三棱针刺入浅静脉,使之少量出血,然后用消毒干棉球按压针孔止血。如中暑时在肘窝、腘窝浅静脉刺络出血,急性淋巴管炎在红丝上多针刺血。

③散刺:

又称"豹纹刺"。即在患处局部或红肿部位的周围刺数针,然后用手轻轻挤压或用火罐吸拔,使恶血出尽,消肿止痛。如顽癣、疖肿、丹毒、扭、挫伤均可在局部散刺出血。

④挑刺

左手按压或捏住消毒后的皮肤,右手持针,将腧穴或反应点的表皮挑破,使出血或流出粘液;或再刺入半分许,挑断部分纤维组织,然后覆盖消毒敷料。如多发性毛囊炎、颈部瘰疬,在背部脊柱两侧的反应点挑刺。痔疾,在腰骶部或"八髎"的反应点挑刺。

2. 适应范围

三棱针刺法具有消肿散瘀、开窍泄热、通经活络的作用。适用于实证、热证、或寒实证,如高热、昏厥、中风闭证、咽喉肿痛、疖肿痔疾、顽固性痹证、扭挫伤、局部皮肤充血、肿胀、麻木等。

3. 注意事项

①三棱针刺激较强,注意防止晕针。

②注意无菌操作,以防感染。
③点刺时应轻、浅、快,出血不宜过多,切勿刺动脉。
④凡体弱、孕妇及有出血倾向的患者,均不宜刺血。
⑤每日或隔日针一次,3—5次为一疗程,急症可每日两次,刺血量多者,每周刺1—2次。挑刺多3—7日一次,3—5次为一疗程,10—14天后,可进行第二疗程。

第二节 皮 肤 针

皮肤针又叫"梅花针"、"七星针"。是用5—7枚不锈钢针集束固定在针柄的一端而成。(图2-175)

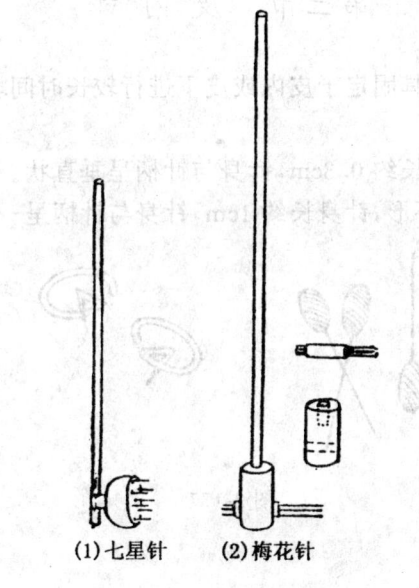

(1)七星针　(2)梅花针

图 2-175

1. 操作方法

常规消毒后,手握针柄的后部,食指压在针柄上,用手腕之力进行叩刺。针尖垂直叩打在皮肤上,并立即提起,反复进行。(图2-176)。叩刺的强度根据病人体质、年令、病情及部位的不同,有轻、中、重之分。轻叩用力稍小,使局部皮肤潮红即可,用于老弱妇儿、头面五官、肌肉浅薄处;重叩用力较大,使皮肤微出血,有痛感为度,用于强壮、实证、肌肉丰厚处;中等叩刺用力介于轻重二者之间,使皮肤潮红,但无渗血,稍痛,用于多数患者,一般病症及一般部位。叩刺部位分为循经、穴位、局部三种。

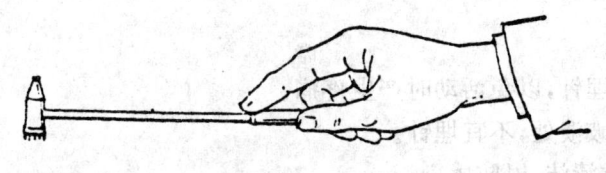

图 2-176

2. 适应范围

皮肤针多用于神经系统、皮肤等疾患。如头痛、胁痛、眩晕、不寐、近视、痿痹、胃肠病、妇科病及多种皮肤病等。

3. 注意事项

①针尖必须平齐无钩,叩刺时针尖须垂直而下,以减少疼痛。
②针具及叩刺部位皮肤必须消毒,以防感染。
③局部皮肤有外伤及溃疡者,不宜使用。

第三节 皮内针

皮内针是以特制的小型针具固定于皮内或皮下进行较长时间埋藏的一种方法。其针型有两种:图钉型和麦粒型。

图钉型:针柄呈环形,针身长约0.3cm,针身与针柄呈垂直状。
麦粒型:针柄呈麦粒形或环形,针身长约1cm,针身与针柄呈一直线。(图2-177)

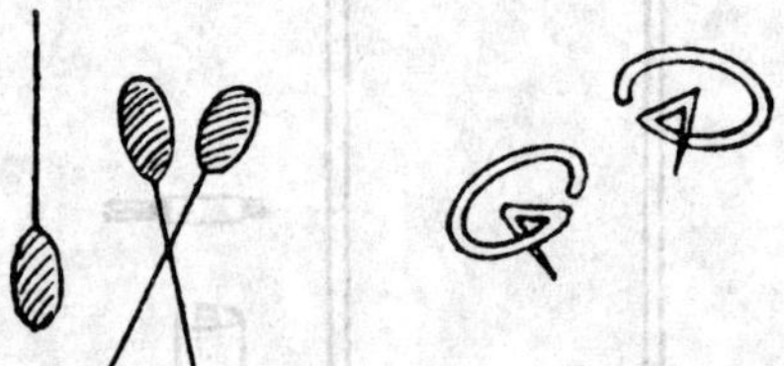

图 2-177

1. 操作方法

①图钉型皮内针:用镊子夹住针柄,针尖对准消毒好的穴位垂直刺入,使环状的针柄平整地留在皮肤上,用胶布固定。多用于面部和耳部腧穴。
②麦粒型皮内针:用镊子夹住针身,对准消毒好的穴位沿皮刺入0.5-1cm左右,用胶布将留于皮肤外的针身和针柄固定。适用于各部腧穴或压痛点。

2. 适应范围

常用于需要久留针的慢性顽固性或疼痛性疾病。如头痛、胃痛、胆绞痛、不寐、高血压、月经不调、遗尿、咳喘等。

3. 注意事项

①关节附近不宜埋针,以免活动时产生疼痛。
②皮肤有炎症及破溃处,不宜埋针。
③埋针期间,注意清洁,以防感染。
④留针时间,根据病情及季节的不同而定,夏季出汗多,留针部位易发生感染,一般留针1

~2天；秋冬季可留针3～7天。留针期间，每隔4小时左右按压埋针处1～2分钟，以加强刺激，增强疗效。

第四节 电　针

电针是针刺腧穴"得气"后，联接电针器，利用脉冲电流加强刺激，以防治疾病的一种方法。

电针器的种类很多，但主要区别在于输出波型和频率的选择。都是采用振荡发生器输出脉冲电流，要求输出电压（峰值）在40～80伏之间，输出电流小于1毫安。它的特点是：刺激量大，安全，可代替手法运针，节省人力。

1. 操作方法：

一般选取同侧肢体1—3对腧穴，毫针刺入腧穴得气补泻后，将电针器上的输出电位器调到"0"值，把一对输出导线分别连接在两根针的针柄上，打开电源开关，选择需要的波型和频率，逐步调高输出电流至所需的电流量，使病人出现能耐受的痠麻感。通电时间一般为10～20分钟左右，针麻时间可更长。如刺激感减弱时，可适当加大刺激量，或断电1～2分钟后再通电，或改变频率，以保持恒定的刺激作用。治疗完毕，把电位器调至"0"值，关闭电源，撤去导线，起出毫针。

2. 脉冲电流作用和电针的适应症

①脉冲电流作用：

低频脉冲电流通过毫针刺激腧穴，具有调整人体功能、肌肉张力、加强止痛、镇静、促进血循环等作用。由于脉冲电流的波形、频率不同，其作用亦不同。频率快的叫密波（高频），一般在50～100次/秒，频率慢的叫疏波（低频），一般在2～5次/秒。有的电针器有密波、疏波、疏密波、断续波等数种波形，用时可根据病情选择，以提高疗效。

密波：对感觉神经和运动神经产生抑制作用。常用于止痛、镇痛、缓解肌肉和血管痉挛，针刺麻醉等。

疏波：刺激作用较强，能引起肌肉收缩，提高肌肉韧带的张力。对感觉和运动神经的抑制发生较迟。常用于治疗痿症、肌肉、关节、韧带、肌腱的损伤等。

疏密波：是疏波、密波自动交替出现的一种波形。交替持续的时间约各1.5秒，能克服单一波形易产生适应的缺点。能促进代谢、气血循环，改善组织营养，消炎性水肿。常用于止痛，如扭挫伤、关节周围炎、气血运行障碍、坐骨神经痛、面瘫、肌无力、局部冻伤等。

断续波：是有节律地时断时续自动出现的一种疏波。断时，在1.5秒时间内无脉冲电输出，续时，是密波连续工作1.5秒。此波不易产生适应，能提高肌肉组织的兴奋性，对横纹肌有良好的刺激收缩作用。常用于治疗痿症、瘫痪等。（图2-178）

锯齿波：是脉冲波幅按锯齿形自动改变的起伏波，每分钟16～25次，其频率接近人体的呼吸规律，适用于刺激膈神经（相当于天鼎穴部）作人工电动呼吸，抢救呼吸衰竭，故又称呼吸波。并有提高神经肌肉兴奋性，调整经络的功能，改善气血循环等作用。

②电针的适应症：

凡毫针治疗有效的病症，均可适用。其中以癫狂、神经衰弱、神经痛、脑血管意外后遗症、脊

连续波

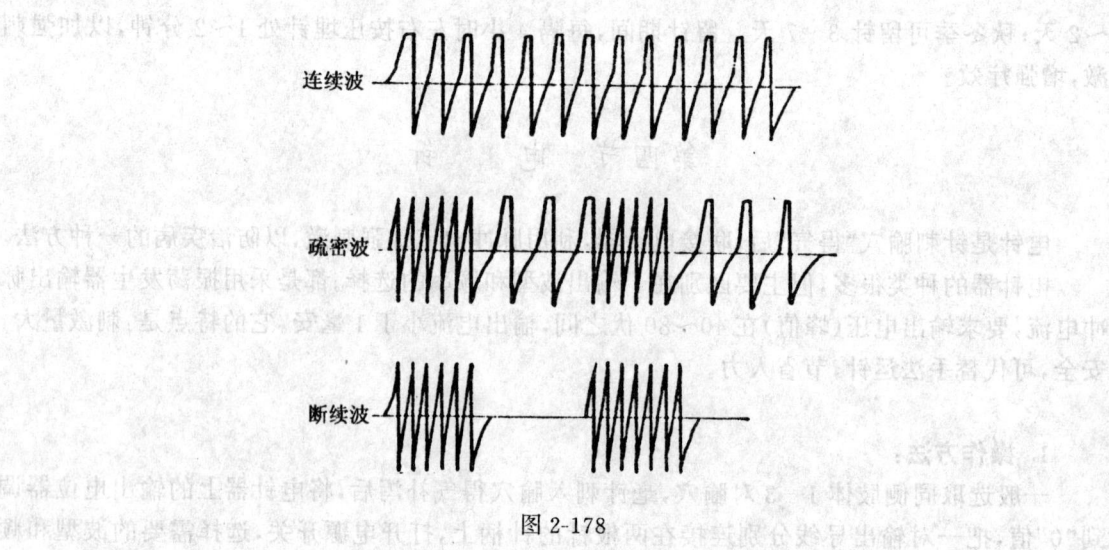

疏密波

断续波

图 2-178

髓灰质炎后遗症、痿症、胃肠道疾病、痹证等效果好,也可用于针刺麻醉。

3. 注意事项

①治疗前,检查电针机输出是否正常,治疗后应将输出调节电钮等全部退至"0"位,随后关闭电源,撤去导线。

②电针刺激量较大,需防止晕针。调节电流量时,应逐渐从小到大,不能突然增强,防止引起肌肉强烈收缩,造成弯针、断针。

③有心脏病者,避免电流回路通过心脏;在邻近延髓、脊髓等部位使用电针时,电流的强度要小一些,以免意外,孕妇慎用。

④温针灸用过的毫针,针柄表面因氧化不导电;有的针柄是因铝丝绕成,经过氧化处理镀成金黄色,氧化铝不导电,不宜使用。若使用,输出线应夹持在针身上。

⑤如果电流输出时断时续,可能是导线接触不良引起,应检查修理后再使用。

第五节 水 针

水针又称"穴位注射",是在穴位或相应部位进行药物注射,通过针刺和药液对穴位的刺激及药理作用,调整机体功能,改善病理状态的一种疗法。对某些疾病能提高疗效,是近代发展起来的针头。

根据使用药物的剂量大小及针刺部位选择不同型号的注射器及针头。常用的为1、2、5、10、20毫升注射器及5—6号普通注射针头。或牙科5号针头,或封闭用9号长针头。

1. 常用药物

凡是可供肌肉注射的药物,均可用于水针。如当归、红花、复方当归、复方丹参、川芎、板兰根、柴胡、鱼腥草、威灵仙、徐长卿等中药注射液,及维生素B_1、B_{12}、C,5—10%葡萄糖,0.25～2%盐酸普鲁卡因,25%硫酸镁、生理盐水、阿托品、利血平、安络血、麻黄素、抗生素、胎盘组织液等西药注射液。

2. 治疗方法
①选穴处方：

根据辨证论治，选择相应的腧穴，或阿是穴，或阳性反应物，2～4穴（处）作为注射部位。

②注射剂量：

水针注射的药物剂量取决于注射部位及药物性质和浓度。一般成人，中药制剂、维生素类每穴一次可注射1～2毫升；抗生素等药物每次可按原药物剂量的1/10～1/2注射；5～10%葡萄糖每次可注射5～20毫升。注射部位以四肢、腰、臀部肌肉较丰厚处，注射量可多一些，头面耳部皮肉较薄，注射量每穴不超过0.1～0.5毫升药液。

③操作方法：

病人取适宜的体位，选择所需的注射器和针头，抽好药液，穴位局部消毒，右手持注射器，对准腧穴（或阳性反应物），快速刺入，缓慢进针，得气后回抽无血，即可将药液注入。一般疾病用中等速度注入，急症、实热证注入宜速；慢性病、虚寒证注入宜缓。如药液多，可由深到浅，边退针边推药，或将针更换几个方向推药。

④注射疗程：

急症每日1—2次；慢性病一般每日或隔日一次，穴位可左右交替使用。6—10次为一疗程，一疗程后，休息一周再继续第二疗程。

适应证

凡是针灸的适应证，大部分都可以用水针注射治疗。多用于咳嗽、哮喘、胃腹痛、神经痛、痹症、痿证、腰腿痛、扭挫伤、皮肤病等。

3. 注意事项

①必须注意药物的性能、药理作用、剂量、质量、有效期、禁忌、副作用和过敏反应。凡是能引起过敏反应的药物（如青霉素等）必须先作皮试，副作用较强的药物应慎用。

②一般药液不宜注射到关节腔、脊髓腔和血管内。药液误入关节腔，可引起关节红肿、发热、疼痛，误入脊髓腔，有损害脊髓的可能。

③颈项、胸背部注射时，切勿过深，控制剂量。在主要神经干旁注射时应避开神经干，若针尖触及神经干，患者有触电感，要稍退针，然后注入药物，以免损伤神经。

④孕妇的下腹部、腰骶部及合谷、三阴交等穴，一般不宜做穴位注射，以防引起流产。

⑤严格遵守无菌操作，防止感染。

第四章　古代九针和《内经》刺法

第一节　九针

九针的记载首见于《内经》，书中有多篇论及了九针的形状、长短和用途。九针的出现，对于针刺方法的发展起了重要的作用。（图 2-179）

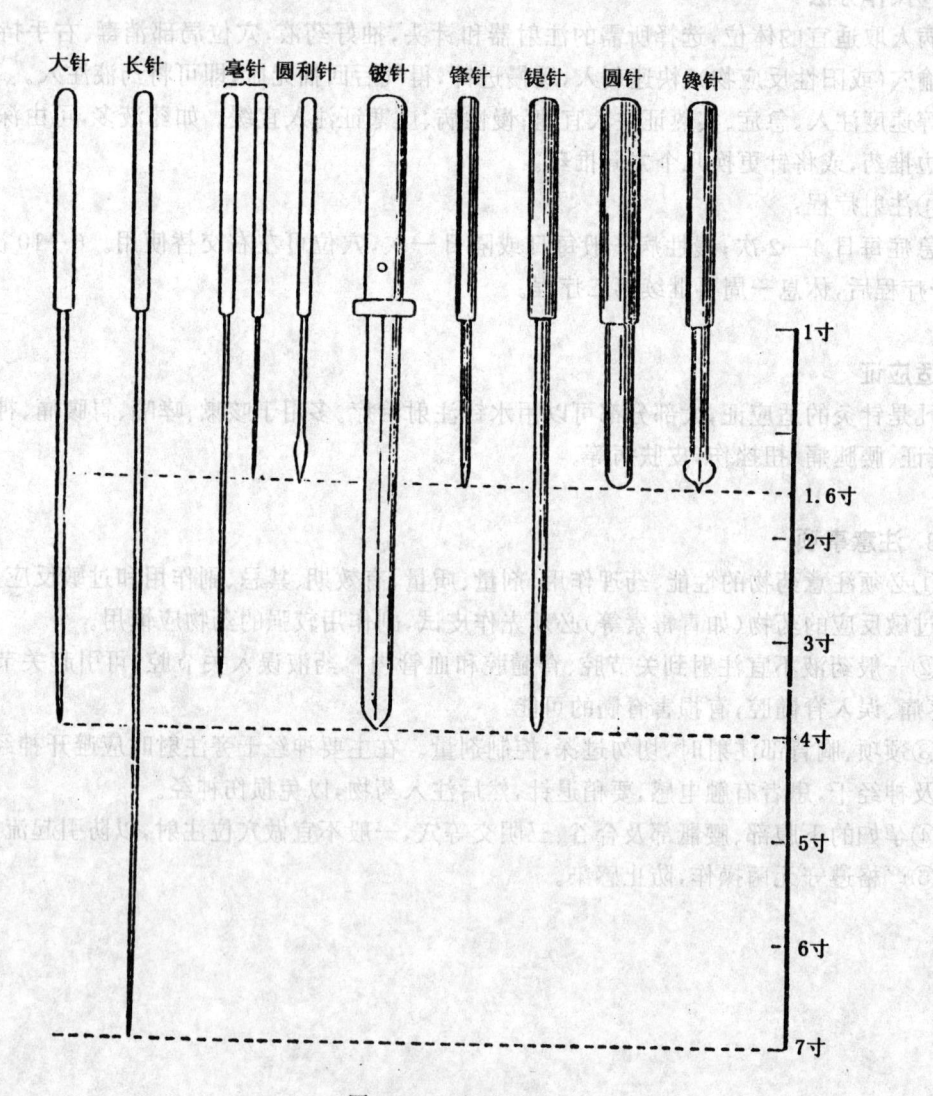

图 2-179　九针图

(1)镵针

形状:长一寸六分,形似箭头,末端十分尖锐。近人在此基础上发展为皮肤针。

用途:浅刺皮肤泻血,治头身热症等。

(2)圆针

形状:长一寸六分,针身圆柱形,针头卵圆。

用途:按摩体表,治分肉间气滞,不伤肌肉。为按摩用具。

(3)锟针

形状:长三寸半,针头如黍粟状,圆而微尖。

用途:按压经脉,不能深入,为按压穴位的用具。

(4)锋针

形状:长一寸六分,针身圆柱形,针头锋利,呈三棱锥形。后人称为"三棱针"。

用途:点刺泻血,治痈肿、热病等。

(5)铍针

形状:长四寸,宽二分半,形如剑。

用途:痈脓外症割治用。为外科用具。

(6)圆利针

形状:长一寸六分,针头微大,针身反细小,圆而且利,使能深刺。

用途:痈肿、痹症、深刺。

(7)毫针

形状:长三寸六分,针身细如毫(豪)毛,为常用针具。

用途:通调经络,治寒热,痛痹等。

(8)长针

形状:长七寸,针身细长锋利。近人又发展为芒针。

用途:深刺,治"深邪远痹"。

(9)大针

形状:长四寸,针身粗圆。

用途:泻水,治关节积液等。后人用作火针等。(图 2-179)

《内经》记载的针刺方法很多,其中最多的是《灵枢·官针》篇,其所论针法范围较广,简述如下:

第二节 九刺

《灵枢·官针》篇云:"凡刺有九,以应九变"。即指九种刺法适应九类不同的病变。

(1)输刺:是对五脏疾病的针治方法,五脏有病,可取该经脉的荥穴,输穴及背俞穴。

(2)远道刺:"病在上,取之下"为循经远取穴的一种刺法。适宜于治疗六腑的疾病。可取用足三阳经上的六腑下合穴。

(3)经刺:"刺大经之结络经分"。即刺经脉的瘀滞不通处,与络刺相对,主治经脉病。

(4)络刺:"刺小络之血脉"。即浅刺皮下浮络以泻除瘀血的方法。主治络脉病。

(5)分刺:"刺分肉之间"。是刺深部的肌肉以治疗肌肉的痹痛、痿证或陈伤的方法。

(6)大泻刺："刺大脓以铍针"。即用铍针切开引流，排脓放血、泻水的方法，多用于外科的疾病。

(7)毛刺："刺浮痹皮肤"。为浮浅刺法，治浅部的病证。现在的皮肤针刺法，是由此演进而来。

(8)巨刺："左取右，右取左"。是一种左病取右，右病取左，在健侧交叉取穴施治的一种方法。《素问》又分交叉取经穴为"巨刺"，交叉泻络为"缪刺"。

(9)焠刺："刺燔针以取痹"。燔针即火针，是将针烧红后刺入皮肤，多用于治疗瘰疬，阴疽等阴证。

第三节　十二刺

《灵枢·官针》篇云："凡刺有十二节，以应十二经。"即针刺有十二种方法，以应合十二经。

(1)偶刺："一刺前，一刺后，以治心痹。"这种前胸一针，后背一针，一前一后阴阳对偶的针法，称为偶刺。以治疗心气窒塞不通的心痹等证。

(2)报刺："刺痛无常处也。上下行者，直内无拔针，以左手随病所按之，乃出针复针也"即针刺后采用留针法，并以左手按压寻找痛处，然后出针再行针刺。这种刺而再刺的方法，称为报刺。以治疗游走不定的疼痛等症。

(3)恢刺："直刺傍之，举之前后，恢筋急，以治筋痹也。""恢"有恢复之意。即在筋肉拘挛的旁边垂直进针，得气后，令患者活动患处，以疏通经气，舒缓筋急，以治疗筋痹症。

(4)齐刺："直入一，傍入二，以治寒气小深者"。即正中先刺一针，并于两旁各刺一针，三针齐用，故名齐刺。以治疗寒邪所中病变范围小而部位较深的痹证。(图2-180)

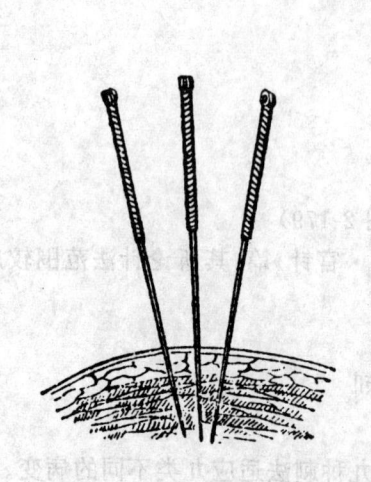

图2-180 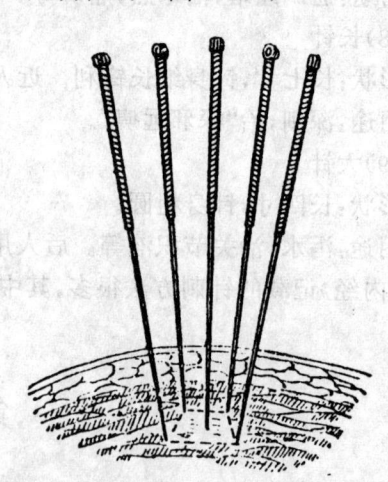　　　　　　　　　　　　　　　图2-181

(5)扬刺："正内一，傍内四而浮之，以治寒气之博大者也"。即中间刺入一针，周围刺入四针的浅刺法。适宜治疗寒气浅而面积较大的痹证。(图2-181)

(6)直针刺："引皮乃刺之，以治寒气之浅也"。即先挟持捏起穴位皮肤，然后将针沿皮卧刺，直对病所，称为直针刺。现称沿皮刺或横刺。适用于寒气较浅毋须深刺的疾病。

(7)输刺："直入直出，稀发针而深之，以治气盛而热者也。"即垂直刺之，垂直提出，针入较深,以输通经气,清泻热邪,治疗气盛而热的病症。

(8)短刺:"刺骨痹,稍摇而深之,致针骨所,以上下摩骨也。""短"是接近之意。即进针时稍摇动,将针刺入深部,使其接近于骨,上下轻轻提插捻转。以治骨痹等深部病痛。

(9)浮刺:"傍入而浮之,以治肌急而寒者也。"这是斜刺浅刺的一种方法。近代的皮内针法,就是从本法演变而来。以治疗因寒邪所致的肌肉拘急的疾病。

(10)阴刺:"左右率刺之,以治寒厥,中寒厥,足踝后少阴也"。即刺足少阴在足踝后的太溪穴,左右同刺的一种方法。适用于治疗少阴病手足逆冷,脉不至的寒厥证。

(11)傍针刺:"直刺、傍刺各一,以治留痹久居者也。"即正中直刺一针,旁边斜刺一针的方法。以治疗病程久远的留痹。(图2-182)

(12)赞刺:"直入直出,数发针而浅之出血,是谓治痈肿也。""赞"是赞助之意,其能帮助消散,故称赞刺。即直入直出,刺入浅而快出针,连续浅刺出血的刺法。多用于痈肿、丹毒等疾患。

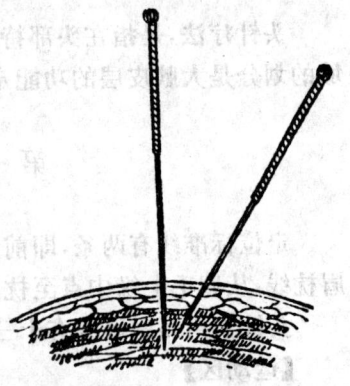

图2-182 傍针刺

第四节 五刺

《灵枢·官针》篇云:"凡刺有五,以应五脏"。这是指从五脏与皮脉筋肉骨的相应关系而分成的五种刺法。

(1)半刺:"浅内而疾发针,无针伤肉,如拔毛状,以取皮气,此肺之应也。"也是一种浅刺方法,刺得浅,出针快,刺不到半分,似拔毛状,故名半刺。主要用于宣泄在表之邪,因肺主皮毛,故与肺脏相应。适应于风寒束表、发热、咳嗽、喘息等与肺脏有关的疾病和皮肤病。

(2)豹文刺:"左右前后针之,中脉为故,以取经络之血,此心之应也。"即刺病变部位的前后左右使之出血,因针刺点如豹的斑纹一样,故名豹纹刺。因心主血脉、故本法与心气相应。治疗红肿热痛等症。

(3)关刺:"直刺左右尽筋止,以取筋痹,慎无出血,此肝之应也。"此法多刺在四肢关节附近的肌腱上,左右均刺。因筋会于节,四肢筋肉的尽端都在关节附近,故名关刺。由于针刺较深,不可伤脉出血。因肝主筋,故与肝脏相应。治疗筋痹。

(4)合谷刺:"左右鸡足,针于分肉之间,以取肌痹,此脾之应也。"即刺在肌肉丰厚之处,先将针刺入分肉之间,后退至浅层,再向左右各斜刺一针,形如鸡爪。因脾主肌肉,故与脾脏相应,可治疗肌痹。(图2-183)

(5)输刺:"直入直出,深内之至骨",以此肾骨痹,此肾之应也"。即直入直出,深刺至骨的一种刺法。因肾主骨,故与肾脏相应,治疗骨痹。

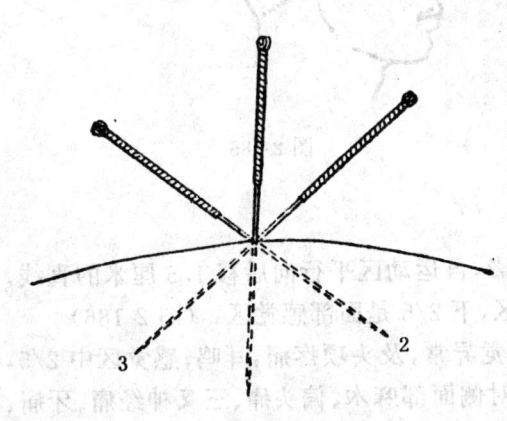

图2-183 合谷刺

第五章　头针疗法

头针疗法,是指在头部特定的区域针刺以治疗疾病的方法,多用于脑源性疾病。其刺激区域的划分是大脑皮层的功能定位在头皮上的投影。

第一节　刺激区线的定位及主治

定位标准线有两条,即前后正中线和眉枕线。前后正中线:从眉心至枕外粗隆下缘的连线;眉枕线:从眉毛上缘中点至枕外粗隆尖端的连线。(图 2-184)

头针常用刺激区线有十三条

【运动区】

部位及取法:运动区相当于大脑皮层中央前回在头皮上的投影。上点在前后正中线的中点向后移 0.5 厘米处,下点在眉枕线和鬓角发际前缘相交处。(若鬓角不明显者,可从颧弓中点向上引一垂直线,将此线与眉枕线交点前 0.5 厘米处作为下点),上下两点之间的连线即运动区。将运动区划分为五等分,上 1/5 为下肢、躯干运动区,中 2/5 为上肢运动区,下 2/5 为面部运动区。(图 2-185)

主治:运动区上 1/5 治疗对侧下肢瘫痪;运动区中 2/5,治疗对侧上肢瘫痪;运动区下 2/5,治疗对侧中枢性面瘫,运动性失语,流涎,发音障碍。

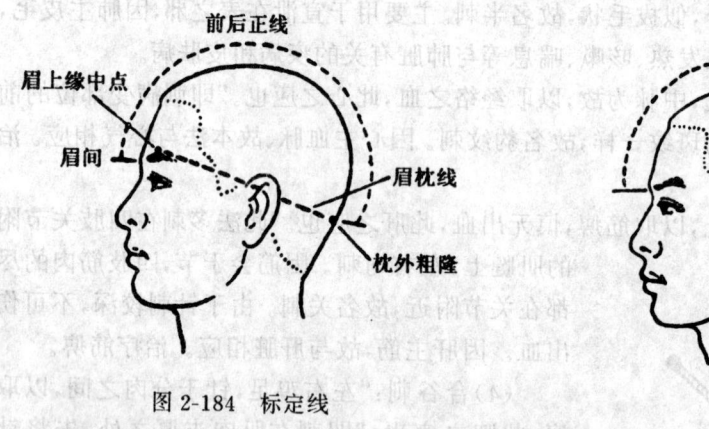

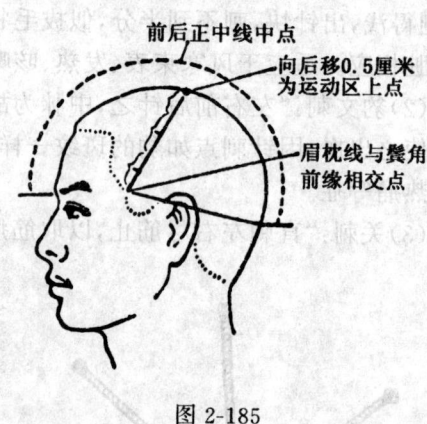

图 2-184　标定线

图 2-185

【感觉区】

部位:相当于大脑皮层中央后回在头皮上的投影,自运动区平行向后移 1.5 厘米的直线。上 1/5 是下肢、头、躯干感觉区;中 2/5 是上肢感觉区,下 2/5 是面部感觉区。(图 2-186)

主治:感觉区上 1/5,治疗对侧腰腿痛、麻木、感觉异常,及头项疼痛,耳鸣;感觉区中 2/5,治对侧上肢疼痛、麻木、感觉异常;感觉区下 2/5 治对侧面部麻木、偏头痛、三叉神经痛、牙痛、下颌关节炎。

感觉区配合相应的内脏区(胸腔区、胃区、生殖区),可用于有关部位手术的头针麻醉。

【舞蹈震颤控制区】

部位:自运动区向前平移 1.5 厘米的直线。(图 2-186)

主治:舞蹈病,震颤麻痹综合征(一侧病变针对侧,两侧病变针双侧)。

【晕听区】

部位:从耳尖直上 1.5 厘米处向前及后各引 2 厘米的平行线,共长 4 厘米。(图 2-186)

主治:眩晕、耳鸣、听力减退等。

【语言二区】

部位:相当于大脑顶叶的角回部。以顶骨结节下方 2 厘米处为起点,向后引平行于前后正中线的 3 厘米长的直线。(图 2-186)

主治:命名性失语

【语言三区】

部位:晕听区中点向后引 4 厘米长的水平线。(2-186)

主治:感觉性失语。

【运用区】

部位:从顶骨结节起向下引一长 3 厘米的垂线,再引与该线夹角为 40 度的前后两线,三条为运用区。(图 2-186)

主治:失用症。

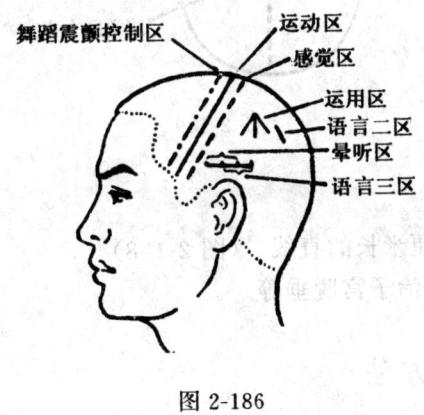

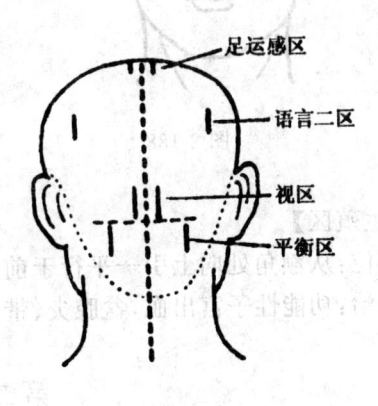

图 2-186

图 2-187

【足运感区】

部位:在前后正中线的中点旁开左右各 1 厘米处为起点,由此点向后引平行于前后正中线 3 厘米长的直线。(图 2-187,2-189)

主治:对侧下肢疼痛、麻木、瘫痪,急性腰扭伤,皮层性多尿、夜尿、子宫脱垂等。

【视区】

部位从枕外粗隆顶端旁开 1 厘米处向上引一平行于前后正中线的 4 厘米长的直线。(图 2-187)

主治:皮层性视力障碍。

【平衡区】

部位：相当于小脑半球在头皮上的投影。从枕外粗隆顶端，旁开3.5厘米处，向下引平行于前后正中线的4厘米长的直线。（图2-187）

主治：小脑平衡障碍。

【胃区】

部位：从瞳孔直上的发际处为起点，向上引一平行于前后正中线的2厘米长的直线。（图2-189）

主治：胃疼、上腹部不适等。

【胸腔区】

部位：在胃区与前后正中线之间，从发际向上下各引2厘米长的平行于前后正中线的直线。（图2-188）

主治：胸痛、胸闷、心悸、冠状动脉供血不足，哮喘、呃逆等。

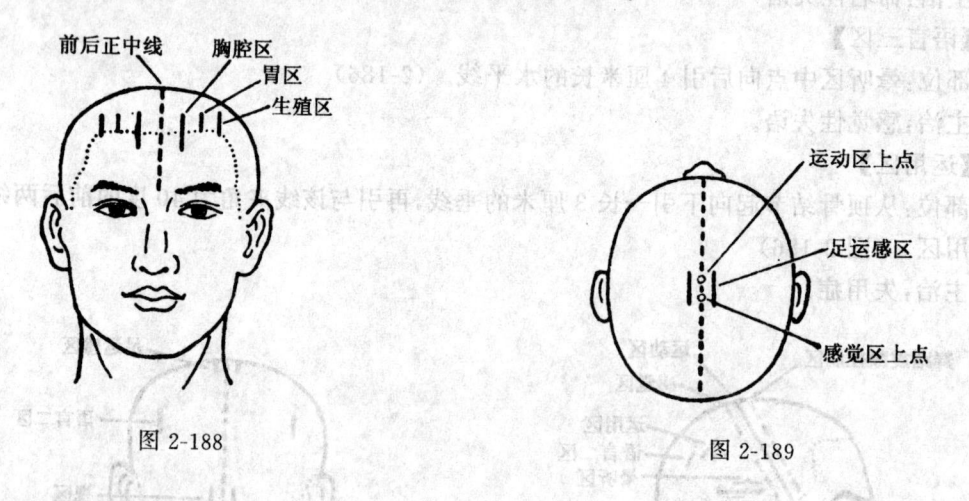

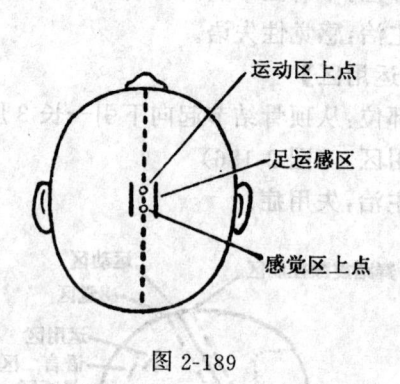

图2-188

图2-189

【生殖区】

部位：从额角处向上引一平行于前后正中线的2厘米长的直线。（图2-188）

主治：功能性子宫出血，盆腔炎、带下、配足运感区治子宫脱垂等。

第二节 操作方法

患者取坐位或卧位，依不同疾病选定刺激区后，局部常规消毒。

①进针：选28～30号1.5～2寸毫针，与头皮呈30度角快速将刺入皮下，针达帽状腱膜下层时，指下感到阻力减少，然后使针与头皮平行继续捻转推进，深达骨膜，根据不同穴区可刺入0.5～1.5寸，然后运针。（图2-190）

②运针：头针之运针只捻转，不提插，要保持针身的深度不变，每分钟130～200次左右，持续捻2～3分钟，留针5～10分钟。如此，反复操作2～3次后起针，偏瘫患者留针及运针期间，应积极配合肢体的活动。（重症患者可被动活动）以提高治疗效果。（图2-191）

③电针刺激：亦可用电针器在主要区线上通电，以代替手捻，以高频弱刺激为好。

④疗程：每日或隔日针1次，一般10次为一疗程，休息5～7天，再作下一疗程治疗。

图 2-190 头针持针式　　　　　　　　图 2-191 头针捻式

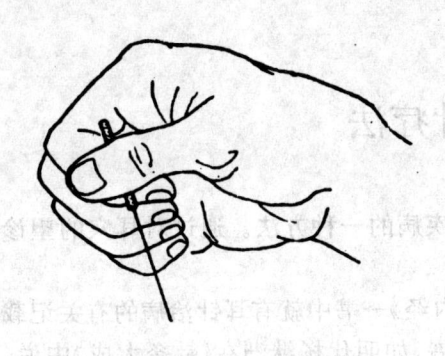

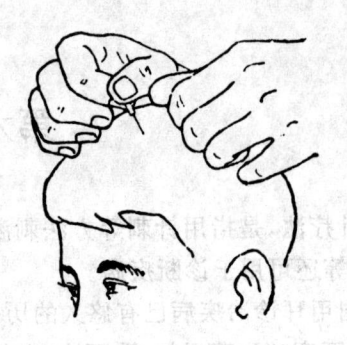

第三节　适应范围

头针主要用于治疗脑源性疾病，如偏瘫、麻木、失语、眩晕、耳鸣、舞蹈病等。此外，也可用于治疗头痛、腰腿疼、夜尿、三叉神经痛、肩周炎、各种神经系统疾病等。

第四节　注意事项

①头针刺激强度大，应注意防止晕针，观察患者面色，适当掌握刺激量。

②中风由脑出血引起者，在急性期有昏迷、发热、血压过高等，暂不用头针治疗。应待病情稳定时针治。对急性炎症、高热，及心力衰竭的病人，一般慎用头针治疗。

第六章 耳针疗法

耳针疗法,是指用针刺等方法刺激耳穴,以防治疾病的一种方法。通过对耳穴的望诊,压诊,电测等还可用于诊断疾病。

我国用耳诊治疾病已有悠久的历史。早在《黄帝内经》一书中就有耳针治病的有关记载。如《灵枢·厥病》"耳聋无闻,取耳中。"以后历代均有发展,如明代杨继洲在《针灸大成》中说:"耳尖二穴,在耳尖上,卷耳取尖上是穴,治眼生翳膜"。《证治准绳》有关于耳穴诊断的记述:"耳大则肾大,耳黑则肾败。"近几十年,在利用耳壳诊断治疗疾病方面又有新的突破,成为应用较广的一种针灸方法。

第一节 耳与脏腑经络的关系

耳与脏腑的关系:中医学认为人体虽可分为脏腑、经络、五官九窍、四肢百骸等组织和器官,但它们都是有机整体的一部分。耳并不单纯是一个孤立的听觉器官,它和脏腑有着密切的关系。如《灵枢·脉度》"肾气通于耳,肾和则耳能闻五音矣。"《证治准绳》有"肾为耳窍之主,心为耳窍之客"的论述。《厘定按摩要术》中进一步将耳朵分为心、肝、脾、肺、肾五部。即"耳珠属肾,耳轮属脾,耳上轮属心,耳皮肉属肺,耳背玉楼属肝"。此外,古今医家还通过观察耳廓的形态和色泽、压痛、敏感、皮肤电阻的改变等,来判断脏腑疾病的变化,说明耳与脏腑之间的密切关系。

耳与经络的关系:成书于两千多年前的《阴阳十一脉灸经》中就有"耳脉"之记载,至《内经》把耳脉发展为手少阳三焦经,而且对耳与经脉、经别、经筋的关系都作了比较详细的记载。

在十二经循行中,小肠经、三焦经、胆经、大肠经各经脉或经别分别入耳中,胃经过耳前,膀胱经至耳上角,六阴经虽然不入耳,但却通过经别与阳经相合。因此,十二经脉都直接或间接地上达于耳。正如《灵枢·邪气脏腑病形》篇所说:"十二经脉,三百六十五络,其血气皆上于面而走空窍,其精阳气上走于目而为睛,其别气走于耳而为听。"阐明了耳与经脉的密切关系。

第二节 耳廓表面的解剖名称(图 2-192)

①耳轮:耳廓外缘向前卷起的部分。
②耳轮结节:耳轮后上方一个不太明显的小结节。
③耳轮脚:指耳轮深入到耳腔的横行突起。
④对耳轮:指与耳轮相对的上部有分叉的隆起部分。上突起叫对耳轮上脚,下突起叫对耳轮下脚。
⑤三角窝:由对耳轮上、下脚之间构成的三角形凹窝。

⑥耳舟：对耳轮与耳轮之间的凹沟。
⑦耳屏：又称耳珠，指耳廓前面的瓣状突起。
⑧屏上切迹：耳屏上缘与耳轮脚之间的凹陷。
⑨对耳屏：耳垂上部，与耳屏相对的隆起部。
⑩屏间切迹：指耳屏与对耳屏之间的凹陷。
⑪轮屏切迹：指对耳轮与对耳屏之间的凹陷。
⑫耳甲艇：指耳轮脚与耳轮之间的凹窝。
⑬耳甲腔：指耳轮脚以下的凹窝。
⑭外耳道口：即耳甲腔中的孔窍。
⑮上耳根：即耳廓上缘与头皮附着处。
⑯下耳根：指耳廓根下缘处。

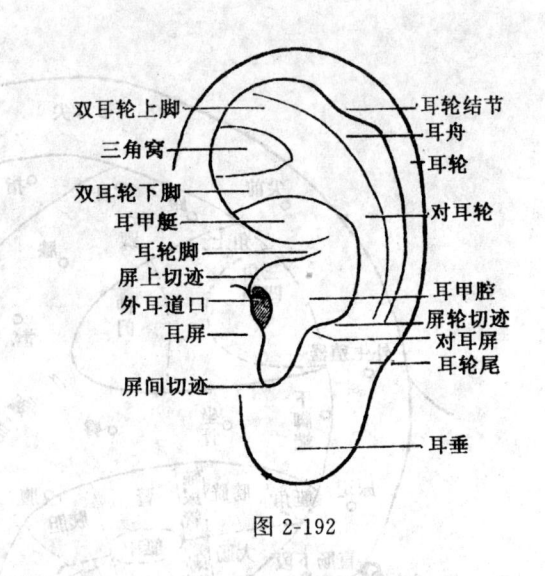

图 2-192

第三节 耳针穴位

耳穴是指耳廓上一些特定的刺激点或刺激部位。其在耳廓上的分布似一个倒置的胎儿（图 1-193）头部朝下，臀部朝上，其耳穴的分布是：头面部相应的穴位在耳垂及其邻近处；与上肢相应的穴位在耳舟；与躯干和下肢相应的穴位在对耳轮和对耳轮上、下脚；与内脏相应的穴位多集中在耳甲艇和耳甲腔；消化道在耳轮脚周围环形排列。

常用耳穴的定位及主治。（图 2-194）（表 2-14）

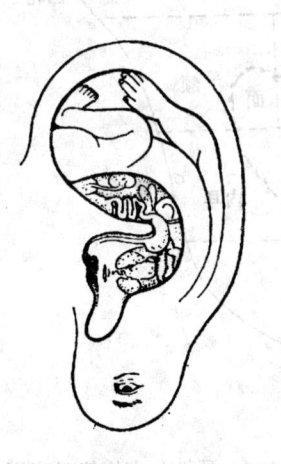

图 2-193 耳穴形象分布示意图

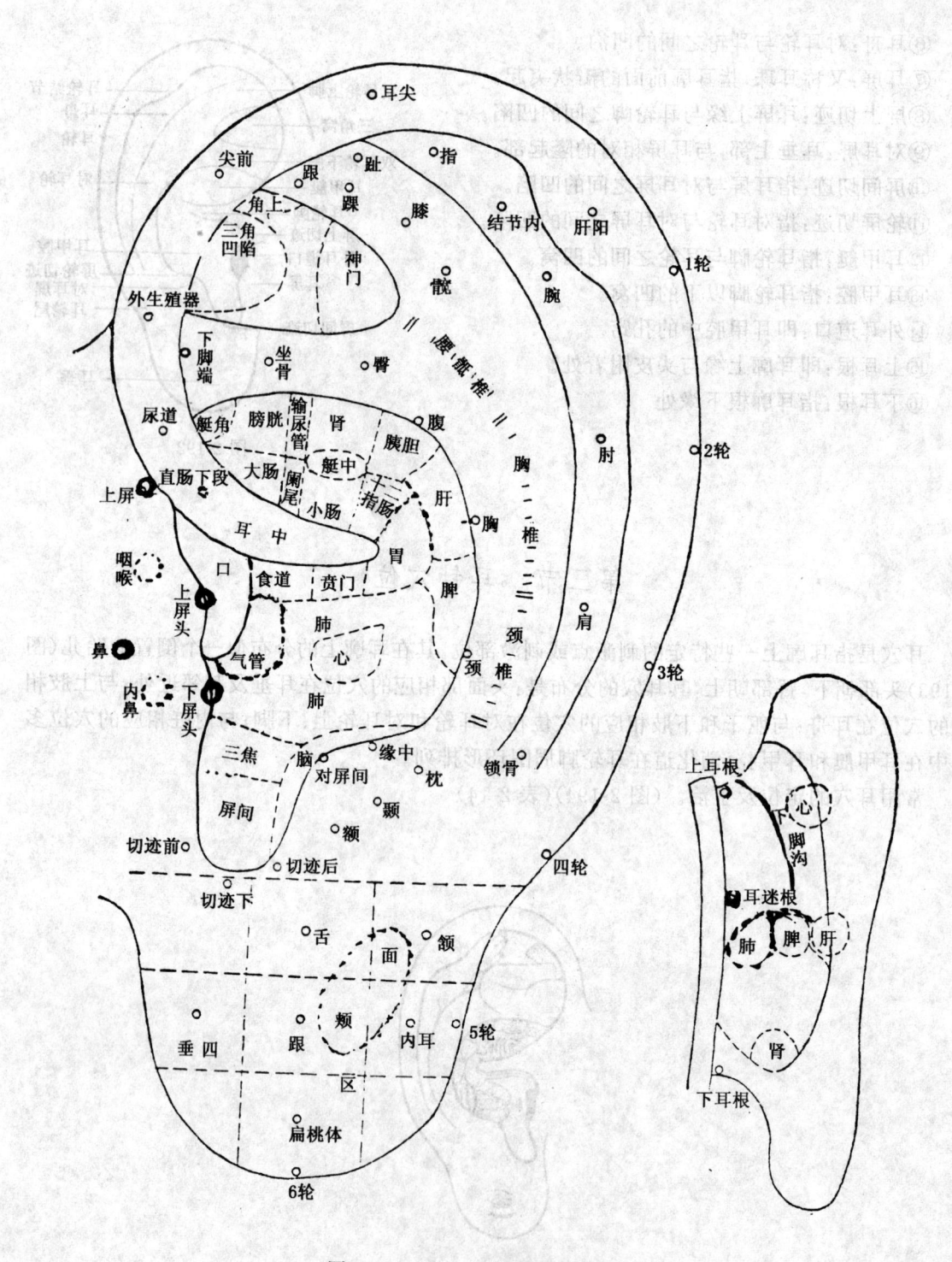

图 2-194 耳针分布规律示意图

表 2-14 耳穴定位、功能与主治表

解剖分部	穴名	原名	定位	功能与主治
	耳中	膈	即耳轮脚	降逆和胃,祛风利膈。主治:呃逆,黄疸等消化病症,皮肤病。
耳轮角及耳轮部	直肠下段		耳轮起点,近屏上切迹处	便秘、脱肛、内外痔、里急后重
	尿道		与对耳轮下脚下缘相平的耳轮处	遗尿、尿频、尿急、尿痛、尿潴留
	外生殖器		与对耳轮下脚上缘相平的耳轮处	外生殖器炎症及会阴部皮肤病、阳萎
	尖前	痔核点	耳尖穴与上耳根穴之间	内外痔(对痔疾有一定辅助诊断意义)
	肝阳		耳轮结节处	肝气郁结、肝阳上亢
	轮₁至轮₆		自耳轮结节下缘至耳垂正中下缘划为五等分共六点,自上而下依次为轮1、2、3、4、5、6	清热止痛,平肝熄风。主治:发热,扁桃体炎、高血压。
耳舟部	指		耳舟的顶端	手指麻木疼痛及功能障碍
	结节内	荨麻疹点过敏区	指、腕两穴之中点	祛风止痒。主治:荨麻疹,皮肤瘙痒症,哮喘
	腕		肘、指两穴之中点	腕部扭伤、肿痛及功能障碍
	肘		指、锁骨两穴之中点	相应部位疼痛及功能障碍
	肩		肘、锁骨两穴之中点	相应部位疼痛及功能障碍
	锁骨		与轮屏切迹同水平的耳舟部	相应部位疼痛,肩周炎,无脉症
对耳轮上脚部	趾		对耳轮上脚的外上角	足趾麻木疼痛及功能障碍
	跟		对耳轮上脚的内上角	足跟痛
	踝		跟、膝两穴之中点	踝关节扭伤等相应部位疼痛及功能障碍
	膝		对耳轮上脚的中部	相应部位疼痛及功能障碍(如膝关节扭伤,关节炎等)
	髋		对耳轮上脚的下 1/3 处	相应部疼痛
对耳轮下脚部	臀		对耳轮下脚外 1/3 处	相应部位疼痛,坐骨神经痛
	坐骨	坐骨神经	对耳轮下脚内 2/3 处	坐骨神经痛
	下脚端	交感	对耳轮下脚的末端	解痉镇痛,滋阴扶阳。主治:内脏疼痛、心悸、自汗、盗汗等,植物神经功能紊乱
对耳轮部	颈椎胸椎腰骶椎		自轮屏切迹至对耳轮上、下脚分叉处分为三等分。下 1/3 为颈椎。中 1/3 为胸椎,上 1/3 为腰骶椎	强脊益髓;主治相应部位疼痛
	颈		颈椎的耳腔缘	落枕、斜颈等相应部位病症
	胸		胸椎的耳腔缘	胸闷、胸痛、乳腺炎等相应部位病症
	腹		腰骶椎的耳腔缘	腹部及妇科病症、腰痛

续表 2-14

解剖分部	穴 名	原 名	定 位	功能与主治
三角窝	神门		对耳轮上、下脚分叉处,三角窝的外1/3处	镇静、安神、止痛、消炎、清热
	三角凹陷	天癸、子宫、精宫	三角窝内,近耳轮中点的凹陷处	扶阴益精,调和经血。主治:妇产科病症,阳痿,前列腺炎等
三角窝部	角上	降压点	三角窝外上	平肝熄风。主治:高血压
耳屏部	屏上	外耳	屏上切迹近耳轮部	滋肾水、潜肝阳。主治:眩晕、耳聋、耳鸣
	鼻	外鼻	耳屏外侧面的中央	疏通鼻部经络。主治:鼻尖鼻疖,鼻塞等鼻部病症
	上屏尖	屏尖	耳屏上部隆起的尖端	清热、止痛
	下屏尖	肾上腺	耳屏下部隆起的尖端	清热止痛,解痉,祛风。主治:低血压、昏厥、无脉症、咳喘、感冒、中暑、疟疾、乳腺炎
	咽喉		耳屏内侧面的上1/2处	清利咽喉。主治:急慢性咽炎,扁桃体炎
	内鼻		耳屏内侧面的下1/2处	疏利鼻窍。主治:过敏性鼻炎等鼻部病症
对耳屏部	对屏尖	平喘、腮腺	对耳屏的尖端	利肺定喘、清热解毒、祛风邪。主治:哮喘、气管炎、腮腺炎、皮肤瘙痒
	缘中	脑点	对屏尖与轮屏切迹间的中点	益脑安神。主治:智能发育不全,遗尿等
	枕		对耳屏外侧面的后上方	镇静止痛,安神熄风。主治:头昏、头痛、失眠等。
	颞	太阳	枕、额两穴之中点	镇静止痛。主治:少阳头痛
	额		对耳屏外侧面前下方	镇静止痛。主治:阳明头痛
	脑	皮质下	对耳屏内侧面	补髓益脑,止痛安神。主治:智能发育不全,失眠多梦,肾虚耳鸣等
耳轮角周围	口		外耳道口的上缘和后缘	清心火,除风邪。主治:面瘫、口腔炎等。
	食道		耳轮脚下方内2/3处	利膈和胃。主治:吞咽困难,食道炎等
	贲门		耳轮脚下方的外1/3处	利膈降逆。主治:贲门痉挛,神经性呕吐等
	胃		耳轮角消失处	和胃益脾,补中安神。主治:胃炎、胃溃疡等胃部病症及失眠

续表 2-14

解剖分部	穴 名	原 名	定 位	功能与主治
耳轮角周围	十二指肠		耳轮脚上方的1/3处	温中和胃。 主治:十二指肠溃疡,幽门痉挛等
	小肠		耳轮脚上方中1/3处	补脾和中,养心生血。 主治:消化不良,心悸等
	阑尾		大小肠两穴之间	清利下焦湿热。 主治:阑尾炎,腹泻等
耳轮脚周围	大肠		耳轮脚上方之内1/3处	清下焦、利肺气。 主治:腹泻,便秘
耳甲艇部	肝		胃和十二指肠穴的后方	清肝明目,舒筋活血。 主治:肝部气滞、眼病及少腹部病症
	胰胆		肝、肾两穴之间	利胆健胃疏肝除风。 主治:胆道病症,胰腺炎,偏头痛等
	肾		对耳轮下脚的下缘,小肠穴直上方	补肾聪耳、强骨填髓。 主治:肾炎,腰痛,耳鸣重听,遗精、阳萎等
	输尿管		肾与膀胱穴之间	输尿管结石绞痛
	膀胱		对耳轮下脚的下缘,大肠穴的直上方	利下焦,补下元。 主治:腰痛,坐骨神经痛,膀胱炎,遗尿,尿潴留等
	艇角		耳甲艇的内上角	清下焦、利前阴。 主治:前列腺炎
	艇中	脐周	耳甲艇中央	理中和脾。 主治:低热,腹胀,胆道蛔虫症,听力减退,腮腺炎等
耳中腔部	心		耳甲腔中心凹陷处	宁心安神,调和营血,止痛止痒。 主治:失眠,心悸,癔病,盗汗,心绞痛等
	肺		心穴的周围	推动气血运行,通利小便,补虚清热、利皮毛。 主治:咳喘、皮肤病,声嘶,又为针麻常用穴。
	气管		在肺区内,位于心口两穴之间	止咳祛痰。 主治:咳喘
	脾		肝穴下方,耳甲腔的外上方	化五谷,生营血,营养肌肉,健脾补气。 主治:腹胀,慢性腹泻,消化不良,口腔炎,功能性子宫出血等
	三焦		屏间穴的上方	通利水道,清热止痛。 主治:便秘,浮肿腹胀,手臂外侧疼痛等
	屏间	内分泌	耳甲腔底部,屏间切迹内	舒肝理气,通经活血,祛风邪,补下元。 主治:皮肤病,阳萎,月经不调,更年期综合症等内分泌功能紊乱病症

续表 2-14

解剖分部	穴 名	原 名	定 位	功能与主治
耳垂部	切迹前	目₁	屏间切迹外前下方	清肝明目。 主治:青光眼,假性近视等眼病。
	切迹下	升压点	屏间切迹下方	补气举阳。 主治:低血压
	切迹后	目₂	屏间切迹处后下方	清肝火明目。 主治:屈光不正,外眼炎症等
	面颊区		耳垂部眼穴的后上方	疏通面部经络。 主治:面瘫、痤疮等面部病症。
	舌		在2区	清心火。 主治:舌炎等
	颌		在3区	牙痛,下颌关节炎等
	垂四	神经衰弱点	在4区	交济水火,宁心安神。 主治:牙痛,神经衰弱
	眼		在5区	明目。 主治:急性结膜炎,电光性眼炎,近视等眼病
	内耳		在6区	除眩聪耳。 主治:耳鸣,听力减退,耳源性眩晕等
	扁桃体		在8区	清利咽喉。 主治:急性扁桃体炎等
	上耳根	郁中脊髓	在耳根的最上缘	止痛定喘。 主治:头痛,腹痛,哮喘
	下耳根	郁中脊髓	耳垂与面颊相交的下缘	止痛定喘。 主治:头痛,腹痛,哮喘
耳背部	耳迷根		耳背、乳突交界的根部,与耳轮脚同水平	通窍止痛,安脏腑。 主治:头痛,鼻塞,胆道蛔虫症等
	下脚沟	降压沟	在对耳轮上、下脚的耳廓背面呈"Y"形的凹沟中	平肝降逆,利皮肤。 主治:高血压、皮肤病
	心		耳背上部	清泻心火,宁心安神,止痛止痒。 主治:疖肿、失眠、多梦、高血压、头痛等
	脾		耳背中部	健脾和胃,生营血,养肌肉。 主治:腹胀、腹泻、消化不良等
	肝		耳背脾区外侧	舒肝和胃,利筋活血。 主治:胸胁胀满,急性阑尾炎,腰疲背痛等
	肺		耳背脾区内侧	补肺定喘、清热、利皮毛。 主治:哮喘、发热、消化系病症等
	肾		耳背下部	滋肾水、聪耳、强骨、填髓。 主治:头痛失眠,眩晕,月经不调

第四节 耳穴的应用

1. 探查耳穴诊病

当人体内脏或躯体某部位发生病变时,往往会在耳壳的相应区域出现各种反应,表现为变形、变色、脱屑、丘疹、压痛点、皮肤电阻低等。利用这些现象,可以帮助诊断,一般探查方法有三种。

①直接观察法:就是用肉眼或借助于放大镜在自然光线下,对照耳廓由上而下,从内至外,直接观察有无变形、变色等征象,如脱屑、水泡、丘疹、充血、硬结、疣赘、软骨增生,色素沉着以及血管的形状,颜色的变异等。

②压痛法:是利用按压寻找痛点。先通过初步诊断、有目的的在某区或全耳进行轻、慢、均匀地按压,压到痛点时,病人出现皱眉,眨眼,呼痛或躲闪等反应。依此协助诊断和进行治疗。

③电测法:是用特制的电子仪器测定耳穴皮肤电阻、电位的变化,以协助诊断的方法。病人一手握电极棒,医生手持探头,在耳廓上探查,当探头触及敏感点时,指示信号或音响或仪表则显示。

2. 耳针的选穴与操作

①耳针选穴有四种方法:

(1)辨证选穴:根据中医脏腑经络学说辨证选穴。如皮肤病可选肺穴,因肺主皮毛。

(2)经验选穴:如耳中穴治血液病、皮肤病;胃穴治消化系统病,神门穴、镇静安神;耳尖穴消炎退热等。

(3)根据现代医学的生理病理知识选穴:如月经病选内分泌;神经衰弱选皮质下等。

(4)按病变部位选穴:如眼病选眼、胃病选胃穴,妇科病选内生殖器、盆腔等。

②操作方法:耳针治病首先依病处方,在即定的穴区找最痛点。如反应点不明显即按耳穴治疗。刺激点选定后,要严格消毒,一般先用2%碘酒消毒,然后再用75%酒精脱碘并消毒。如消毒不严格,容易感染而致耳翼软骨膜炎,造成不良后果。其刺激方法有:

(1)毫针刺法:进针时,术者用左手拇、食指固定耳廓,中指托着针刺部的耳背,然后右手持针刺入穴位,以病人大痛为准。如针下无反应,应调换针刺方向,深度视耳壳厚薄灵活掌握,留针20~30分钟。慢性病、疼痛性疾病留针时间宜长,儿童与老年人留针时间宜短,刺激要轻。起针时左手托住耳背,右手拔针,马上用消毒干棉球压迫针眼片刻,以防出血,再用酒精棉球涂擦一次。

(2)电针:电针法适用于神经系统疾病、内脏痉挛痛、哮喘等病症。

(3)埋针:埋入耳穴后,需每天自行按压3次,留针3~5天。

(4)压迫法:是在耳穴表面贴敷小颗粒状药物的一种简易刺激方法。此法安全、无痛、副作用少,不易引起耳翼软骨膜炎,适用于老年及儿童、怕针的患者。其材料可就地选用,如菜籽、绿豆、莱菔子、王不留行籽、磁珠等。

第五节 注意事项

1. 严密消毒，防止感染。如针后针眼有红肿出现，需用2%碘酒涂擦，或用艾悬灸。
2. 一般应用毫针、电针刺，可隔日一次；激光照射耳穴，可每天1次；如用压籽压磁可5～7天换1次，可轮换使用耳穴，5—10次为一疗程。
3. 有习惯性流产的孕女，不宜应用耳穴，年老体弱的高血压及动脉硬化的患者，针刺前后要适应休息，手法要轻，以防发生意外。
4. 对肢体功能活动障碍及扭伤的患者，留针时可配合肢体活动，以提高疗效。

第六节 常见病症处方举例

1. 头痛：额、枕、脑、缘中、耳尖。
2. 落枕：额、颈椎的压痛敏感点。
3. 感冒：肺、内鼻、下屏尖。
4. 中暑：心、枕、脑。
5. 咳嗽：气管、肺、神门。
6. 哮喘：平喘、肺、下脚端、下屏尖。
7. 眩晕：肾、神门、内耳。
8. 胃痛：胃、神门、脑、下脚端。
9. 遗尿：肾、膀胱、缘中、脑。
10. 手术后切口痛：手术切口相应部位耳穴、脑、神门、肺。
11. 手术后腹胀：大肠、小肠穴压痛点。胃、下脚端、脾。
12. 癌肿疼痛：脑、心、耳尖、病变相应部位耳穴、下脚端、肝、神门。
13. 输尿管结石绞痛：肾、腹、下脚端、脑。
14. 痢疾：大肠、小肠、直肠下段。
15. 疟疾：下屏尖、脑、屏间。
16. 高血压：下屏尖、下脚端、心、神门。
17. 呃逆：耳中或耳迷根穴找压痛点针刺。
18. 呕吐：胃、肝、脾、神门。
19. 泻泄：大肠、胃。
20. 癔病：心、脑、枕、缘中、神门。

下篇 针灸治疗

第一章 治疗总论

第一节 针灸辨证

针灸治病,必须辨证论治,即根据脏腑经络学说及四诊八纲的理论,将临床上各种不同的病候进行分析、归纳、以明确病位(在经、在络、在脏、在腑、在表、在里)、病性(阴、阳、寒、热、虚、实),再依病因病机找出标本、缓急,这个过程就是辨证的过程;然后,根据辨证,进行相应的立法、处方,再依方取穴,依法施术,以通其经脉,调其气血,平其阴阳,和其脏腑,达到"阴平阳秘,精神乃治"的目的。这一过程叫论治。

针灸辨证:针灸是中医宝库中的一颗明珠,中医的辨证方法很多,有八纲辨证,脏腑经络辨证,气血辨证,六经辨证,卫气营血辨证,三焦辨证,病因辨证等等。这些辨证方法,各有其特点和侧重,而针灸临床最常用的是经络辨证,因为经络内属于脏腑,外络于肢节的原因,所以当经脉的运行发生异常时,就会在本经所循行络属的脏腑经络、五官九窍、皮肉筋骨等处有所反应。即十二经脉病候(见经络部分);奇经八脉病候(见经络部分);十五络脉病候(见经络部分),这是针灸临床诊断和治疗的基础。

第二节 针灸立法

针灸的立法包括两个内容,一是依据病位,确定选取的经穴;一是依据病性,制定治疗大法:即《灵枢·九针十二原》指出的"凡用针者,虚则实之,满则泻之,菀陈则除之"和《灵枢·经脉》所说的"热则疾之,寒则留之,陷下则灸之,不盛不虚,以经取之"等。"虚则实之"是指正气不足的人针时要用补法以恢复人体的正气,扶正而祛邪;"满则泻之"是指邪气盛满的病人要用泻的方法施术;"菀陈则除之"是指经脉瘀阻的病人用放血法以消除瘀滞;"热则疾之"是指治热性病要疾刺疾出,以退其热邪;"寒则留之"是指寒邪较重的病人应留针;"陷下则灸之"是指元阳暴脱,汗出不止,子宫下垂,脱肛等病人,要用灸法以升阳固脱;"不盛不虚,以经取之"是指病的虚实表现不明显时,可用平补平泻的方法取本经腧穴进行治疗。

随着针灸医学的发展,治疗方法及手段也越来越多,如皮下埋针,穴位注射,电针,激光,微波照射等等,为针灸学增添了新的内容。

第三节　针灸处方

针灸处方是把针灸立法所确定的经穴具体化。即针对主病取主穴，兼证配对症穴，使主穴、配穴协同作用，加强疗效。因疾病轻重不同，所涉及的经也不同，所以，处方就有大小之分。有时主病只用一穴，亦不配穴，即一方一穴为小方，但如病变涉及到几条经脉时，则必须用多个穴位组成大方才能生效。这就是《素问·至真要大论》所说："病有盛衰，治有缓急，方有大小"。及《灵枢·卫气失常》所说"间者少之，甚者众之，随变而调气"。的道理。

为了施术准确，书写病历方便，特规定了针灸施术的符号，即：T或十代表补法；⊥或—代表泻法；｜或±代表平补平泻法；∷代表皮肤针；↓代表三棱针刺血；—代表皮内埋针；∥代表电针；△代表艾灸；○代表拔罐等等。

组成针灸处方的方法很多，主要有近部取穴，远部取穴，对症取穴，对应取穴和特定穴的应用等。但是，不论哪种取穴方法，都必须以经络学说为基础，即"经脉所过，主治可及"的原则，具体说明如下：

1. 近部取穴法

此法是指在病变的局部和邻近选穴。是所有穴位都能主治穴位所在的局部病和邻近病的具体运用，如眼病取睛明穴，鼻病取迎香穴，耳病取听宫穴，胃病取中脘穴等，是局部取穴，多用于慢性病；如病变局部穴位有溃烂，创伤，瘢痕等，不宜针灸时，可选邻近穴位。邻近选穴，即在病位的邻近取穴，如鼻病取印堂、上星，胃病取天枢、气海等，此法多用于治疗脏腑、五官疾病。

2. 远部取穴

是指在离病位较远的部位取穴，通常以四肢肘膝以下的穴位为主。

《素问·五常正大论》说："病在上，取之下；病在下，取之上；病在中，傍取之"。如胃肠病取足三里，腰背病取委中，面口病取合谷，胸胁病取内关等等。临症时，近部取穴和远部取穴可以结合应用，以加强疗效，列表如下：

表 2-15　局部、邻近、远道选穴举例表

病位	局部	邻近	远道
前额	阳白	百会	合谷、内庭
侧头	太阳、率谷	风池	足临泣、环跳、足窍阴
后头	哑门	大椎	后溪、腰阳关 Z
眼	睛明	风池	合谷、光明
鼻	迎香	通天、巨髎	足三里
口	地仓	颊车	合谷、太冲
耳	听宫	风池	中渚、风市
喉	人迎	天容、大杼	少商、照海、列缺

续表 2-15

病位	局部	邻近	远道
胸	膻中	肺俞	内关、丘墟
胁	大包	肝俞	支沟
上腹	中脘	梁门	足三里、内关
下腹	关元	天枢	三阴交
腰	肾俞	居髎	委中、养老
肛门	长强	大肠俞	承山、二白

3. 对症选穴

依据某些穴位对某些病症具有相对特异性的特点取穴。

临床上某些病症可取相应的穴组，单穴的应用则是其最精华者，列表举例如下：

表 2-16 对症选穴举例

病症	选穴
发热	大椎 曲池 外关 合谷 十宣
昏迷	水沟 十宣 十二井 神阙
盗汗	阴郄 后溪
牙关紧闭	颊车 下关 合谷
咳喘	定喘 鱼际 天突 列缺
胸闷	膻中 内关 极泉
心区痛	膻中 内关 心俞 郄门
胃痛	足三里 梁丘 内关
便秘	支沟 照海
胎位不正	至阴
虚弱	足三里 关元 大椎
小儿疳积	四缝
痔疮出血	二白

对应选穴：依据经脉的上下相通，表里相合，同经相应的特点，在病位比较局限或急性疼痛时，可以取健侧的对应穴治疗，如左肘痛取右曲池穴，外踝下扭伤取养老，足跟痛取大陵等等。

4. 补母泻子法

此法是根据《难经》"虚者补其母，实者泻其子"的理论而定的取穴方法。

它是将五输穴的主治性能与木、火、土、金、水五行相配合，并结合脏腑的五行属性取穴。如肺在五行属金，实证，可取肺经五输穴中属"水"的合穴尺泽，因"金"生"水"，"水"为"金"之子，取尺泽即所谓"实者泻其子"。虚症，可取肺经五输穴中属"土"的输穴太渊，因"土"生"金"，"土"为"金"之母，取太渊即所谓"虚者补其母"。余可类推，详如下表：

表 2-17 补母泻子法取穴表

五行	金		水		木		火				土	
							君		相			
脏腑	肺	大肠	肾	膀胱	肝	胆	心	小肠	心包	三焦	脾	胃
母穴	太渊	曲池	复溜	至阴	曲泉	侠溪	少冲	后溪	中冲	中渚	大都	解溪
子穴	尺泽	二间	涌泉	束骨	行间	阳辅	神门	小海	大陵	天井	商丘	厉兑

5. 子午流注纳子法取穴

纳子法又叫纳支法,是将一天的十二个时辰配属脏腑和地支,结合病候和气血流注时间而行补母泻子的按时取穴方法。具体应用是,当本脏(或腑)有实邪时,就在本脏腑气血充盛时泻其子穴,如本脏腑虚时,则在气血方衰(即流注本脏腑的下一个时辰补其母穴;如果补泻时间已过,或病症的虚实不明显时,则取本经的原穴或与本经同一属性的穴(本经本穴)进行治疗,用平补平泻法。(见下表)

表 2-18 子午流注纳子法取穴表

脏腑	肺	大肠	胃	脾	心	小肠	膀胱	肾	心包	三焦	胆	肝
流注时间	3~5	5~7	7~9	9~11	11~13	13~15	15~17	17~19	19~21	21~23	23~1	1~3
地支	寅	卯	辰	巳	午	未	申	酉	戌	亥	子	丑
实泻时间及穴位	3~5 尺泽	5~7 二间	7~9 厉兑	9~11 商丘	11~13 神门	13~15 小海	15~17 束骨	17~19 涌泉	19~21 大陵	21~23 天井	23~1 阳辅	1~3 行间
虚补时间及穴位	5~7 太渊	7~9 曲池	9~11 解溪	11~13 大都	13~15 少冲	15~17 后溪	17~19 至阴	19~21 复溜	21~23 中冲	23~1 中渚	1~3 侠溪	3~5 曲泉
原穴	太渊	合谷	冲阳	太白	神门	腕骨	京骨	太溪	大陵	阳池	丘墟	太冲
本经本穴	经渠	商阳	足三里	太白	少府	阳谷	足通谷	阴谷	劳宫	支沟	足临泣	大敦

第二章 治疗各论

第一节 内科病证

一、中风

【概说】

中风是指突然昏倒,不省人事,口眼歪斜,语言不利,半身不遂或不经昏倒而见口眼歪斜,语言不利,半身不遂的疾病。因本病起病急,证候多,变化快,颇与自然界中"风"性善行数变相似,故名"中风";又因发病突然,又称"卒中"。因发病轻重不一,故有中脏腑(闭证、脱症)和中经络之不同。

本病相当于现代医学的脑出血、脑血栓形成、蛛网膜下腔出血、脑血管痉挛、病毒性脑炎、中枢性面神经瘫痪等病。

【病因病机】

中风多发生于中老年人,由于身体素虚,加之将息失宜,而使肝、肾、心、脾的功能失调,肝肾阴亏则肝阳偏亢,心阴不足则心火偏亢,脾阳不足则痰湿内生,如遇忧思恼怒,饮酒暴食,劳累过度,风寒外袭等诱因,即可肝阳暴张,引动肝风,心火暴盛,风火相煽,气血并走于上,挟痰浊,蒙闭清窍,发为闭证;如真元衰微,阴阳离绝则复生脱证;痰浊流窜经脉,则发为偏瘫。

【辨证治疗】

(一)中脏腑

1. 闭证

主证:突然昏倒,不省人事,两手握固,牙关紧闭,面赤气粗,喉中痰鸣,二便闭塞,舌赤红苔黄厚或灰黑,脉弦滑有力。

治法:取督脉、足厥阴经及十二井穴为主。毫针泻法,或点刺出血,以开窍醒神,平肝熄风,清化痰火。

处方:水沟 十二井穴 劳宫 丰隆 百会 太冲 涌泉

随证配穴:牙关紧闭:下关、颊车、合谷;舌强不语:哑门、廉泉、通里。

方义:水沟醒神清脑;十二井开窍、清热,点刺出血可交通十二经气;劳宫泄心火;丰隆为胃经络穴,针之以宣通脾胃气机,健脾胃以化痰浊;百会、太冲平肝熄风;涌泉滋肾水以平肝潜阳,诸穴共奏开窍醒神,平肝熄风,清化痰火之效;下关、颊车、合谷,疏调上下牙关以开闭;哑门醒脑开窍,配廉泉、通里利舌窍以治不语。

2. 脱证

主证:突然昏倒,不省人事,目合口开,鼻鼾息微,手撒遗尿,四肢厥冷,如面赤如妆,脉微欲绝或浮大无根。为真阳外越之危候。

治法:取任脉经穴为主,重用灸法,以回阳固脱。

处方:神阙 关元 气海 百会

方义:神阙位于脐中,为生命之根蒂,真气所系,关元、气海为任脉、足三阴经交会穴,位居小腹,关元为三焦元气所出,系命门真阳,气海为元气之海,故隔盐灸神阙,并灸关元、气海可大补元阳,回阳以固脱,灸百会以通督脉,醒脑开窍。

(二)中经络

风痰阻于经脉,未及脏腑,或中脏腑后,脏腑功能逐渐恢复,而经脉仍为风痰阻隔者。

主证:半身不遂,肌肤不仁,手足麻木,口角㖞斜,语言不利,或兼见头痛眩晕,手足抽动,面红目赤,咽干口渴,烦躁等症,脉多弦滑。

治法:取手足阳明,手足少阳、太阳经穴为主。针刺平补平泻法,以祛风痰、通经脉、调气血、平阴阳。

处方:

上肢:肩髃　曲池　手三里　支沟　合谷　后溪

下肢:肾俞　环跳　阳陵泉　足三里　太冲

头面:百会　风池　地仓　颊车　哑门　廉泉

方义:阳明为多气多血之经,气血旺盛,疾病易于恢复,故取肩髃、曲池、手三里、合谷、足三里、地仓、颊车,以通调上肢、下肢及头面之气血,祛风化痰;少阳为枢,主持全身之运动,取支沟、风池、环跳、阳陵泉各穴以舒筋通络,恢复肢体的运动功能;百会、风池、太冲,平肝熄风以治兼证;地仓、颊车治口角㖞斜;哑门、廉泉以通舌窍;后溪强刺激可通督脉以解痉挛,为治上肢不遂,手握不开之经验效穴。

【其它疗法】

1. 头针

取穴:对侧运动区,感觉区,足运感区,舞蹈震颤控制区。

方法:常规消毒后,依次针入各有关穴线,要深达骨膜后,进行捻转手法,每分钟140—160次左右,连续捻转2min,边捻针边叫患者活动肢体,停针5min,再捻转2min,如此操作,留针30—40min,每天或隔天一次,10次为一疗程,此法对大脑中动脉和前动脉分支的血栓形成效果好。

2. 耳针

取穴:脑、缘中、肝、三焦、瘫痪部位相应的耳穴。失语加心、脾;吞咽困难加口、耳迷根、咽喉。

方法:隔日一次,15—20次为一疗程。耳针适用于脑血管意外后遗症(中经络),宜在病情稳定,神志清醒后进行。

3. 电针

每次上下肢各选1—2穴,进针出现针感后,接通电疗机,逐渐加大电流,使有关肌群出现节律收缩,以患者能耐受的最大量为准,每次通电20min,隔日一次,10次为一疗程。电针适用于风中经络。

4. 穴位注射

选穴:上肢:曲池;下肢:阳陵泉。

方法:选用5%当归注射液,每穴注入1ml左右,隔日一次,10次为一疗程。此法适于中经络。

5. 皮肤针

轻刺头部督脉,膀胱经线,重刺胆经线,背腰部轻刺,骶部重刺,上肢内侧手三阴经轻刺,手三阳及手指端穴重刺,下肢膝以下足三阴经线轻刺,下肢足三阳及趾端穴重刺。每日一次,10

次为一疗程。适于中经络较轻的患者。

【附注】

预防中风：凡年高形盛气虚，痰多，并有眩晕，心悸等肝阳上亢的患者，若出现舌强，语言不利，嗜睡腿软，性格改变，指端麻木等现象，这是中风的先兆症状，宜注意饮食起居，避免劳累，并常灸足三里、悬钟，以预防中风的发生。

二、中暑

【概说】

中暑是以壮热，烦闷恶心，甚则卒然昏倒，不省人事为主证的夏季急病。多由于夏季酷热或长时间处在高温环境或烈日下所致。本病包括热射病、热痉挛、日射病等。

【病因病机】

夏季暑气当令，气候炎热，人若长时间在烈日下或高温中劳作，劳则伤气，暑热之邪乘机侵入而发病。依临床表现可分为轻证和重证两类。

【辨证治疗】

（一）轻证

主证：头痛头晕，汗多，皮肤灼热，气粗，舌燥，口干烦渴，脉浮大而数。

治法：取督脉、手厥阴、阳明经穴为主。针刺用泻法，以泄热祛暑。

处方：大椎　内关　曲池　委中

方义：大椎泻全身之热；委中又名血郄，放血以清血分热；曲池清热要穴；内关清热泄三焦火。

（二）重证

主证：先头痛，烦渴，呼吸喘息，继则突然昏倒，不省人事，汗出，脉沉而无力。

治法：取督脉经穴为主。针刺用泻法，以开窍、泄热、祛暑。

处方：水沟　百会　十宣　曲泽　委中

方义：神志昏迷，取水沟、百会以开窍醒神；曲泽为心包经合穴，配委中刺血以清血热；十宣放血以开窍苏厥。

【其它疗法】

刮痧疗法：适用于中暑轻证，用光滑平整的汤匙蘸食油或清水，刮背脊两侧，颈部，胸肋间隙，肩臂，胸窝及腘窝等处，刮至皮肤出现紫红色为度。

三、昏厥

【概说】

昏厥是指突然昏倒，不省人事，四肢厥冷为主症的一种病证。一般昏厥时间短暂，醒后无后遗症，也有一厥不复而死亡者。可见于单纯性晕厥，体位性低血压，低血糖，休克，癔病发作等。

【病因病机】

（一）虚证：元气素弱，每于过度疲劳，悲恐，剧烈疼痛时，气虚下陷，清阳不升，突发昏厥。或因失血过多，以致气随血脱，阴阳离绝，发生昏厥。

（二）实证：惊恐恼怒，气机逆乱，上壅心胸，痞塞气道，蒙闭窍隧，发为昏厥；或肝阳素旺，暴怒后血随气逆，气血上壅，清窍不利，则昏倒无知。

【辨证治疗】

(一)虚证

主证：突然昏倒,气息微弱,张口合眼,面色苍白,肢冷汗出,脉象沉细。

治法：取督脉、心包经穴为主。针刺用补法,并可加灸,以醒脑苏厥,益气升阳。

处方：水沟　百会　内关　关元　足三里。

方义：水沟醒神清脑开窍;百会升举元阳;内关宽胸理气;关元固本培元;足三里补益气血,五穴共奏醒脑苏厥,益气升阳之效。

(三)实证

主证：突然昏倒,呼吸气粗,四肢僵直,牙关紧闭,脉多沉实。

治法：取督脉、心包经穴为主。针刺用泻法,以醒脑开窍,调气苏厥。

处方：水沟　中冲　劳宫　合谷　太冲　涌泉

方义：水沟、中冲醒脑开窍;合谷、太冲通调气血;劳宫、涌泉清心降逆。

【其它疗法】

耳针

取穴：心　皮质下　神门　缘中　下脚端

方法：每次取2~3穴,留针30min,实证用强刺激,虚证用弱刺激,每5分钟捻转1次。

四、感冒

【概说】

感冒是以头痛,鼻塞,流涕,恶风寒,发热为主症的一种外感病。四季均可发生,尤以冬春两季为多。根据感邪性质和临床表现的不同,分为风寒、风热两大类。一般病轻者称"伤风",在一个时期内引起广泛流行者,为时行感冒,多见于上呼吸道感染,流行性感冒等疾病。

【病因病机】

本病的发生主要是由于体虚抗病能力减弱,当气候急剧变化时,人体卫外功能不能适应,于是邪气从皮毛、口鼻而入,引起一系列肺经症状。

(一)风寒束表,肺气不宣,阳气郁阻,毛窍闭塞而为风寒感冒。

(二)感受风热,则风热犯肺,肺失清肃,皮毛疏泄失常而为风热感冒。

【辨证治疗】

(一)风寒

主证：恶寒发热,无汗,头痛,四肢酸痛,鼻塞,流涕,喉痒,咳嗽声重,痰多清稀,舌苔薄白,脉浮紧。

治法：取手阳明、太阴和足太阳经穴为主。针用泻法,以祛风散寒,宣肺解表。

处方：列缺　合谷　风池　风门

随证配穴：挟湿加中脘、内关、足三里。

方义：风寒外束,毛窍闭塞,肺气失宣,故取手太阴络穴列缺宣肺利窍,以治鼻塞,喉痒,咳嗽;太阳主表,外感风寒,先犯太阳,故取风门以疏调太阳经气,祛风散寒,以治恶寒,发热,头痛等症;太阴、阳明互为表里,取手阳明经原穴合谷以宣肺解表,更用阳维脉与足少阳之会穴风池祛风解表,四穴相配,以达祛风散寒,宣肺解表的功效。挟湿针中脘、内关、足三里以健脾胃,化湿浊,理气降逆。

(二)风热

主证:发热,汗出,微恶风,头胀痛,咳嗽,吐黄稠痰,咽部红肿疼痛,口渴欲饮,苔薄白或微黄,脉浮数。

夏令感冒,多挟暑湿,症见发热较高,有汗而热不解,身重倦怠,口渴,小便黄赤,舌红苔黄,脉濡数。

治法:取督脉、手阳明、少阳、太阴经穴为主。针刺用泻法,以疏风清热,清肃肺气。

处方:大椎　尺泽　外关　合谷　鱼际　少商

随证配穴:挟暑湿加中脘、足三里。

方义:大椎为诸阳之会,功善表散阳邪而退热;尺泽为肺之合穴,鱼际为肺经荥穴,少商为肺经井穴,三穴合用可泄肺热、利咽喉;外关为手少阳络穴,又通阳维脉,阳维主表而维系诸阳经,故外关可解表热;挟暑湿加中脘、足三里以健脾胃,祛湿邪。

【其它疗法】

1. 耳针

取穴:肺　气管　耳尖

方法:针双耳,强刺激,留针10—20min。

2. 皮肤针

对发热汗不出及项背疼痛者,沿背部督脉、膀胱经用皮肤针叩打,之后再拔火罐。

【附注】

预防感冒法:在流行季节中,灸风门,或针足三里,可预防感冒。

五、疟疾

【概说】

疟疾,是指寒战,高热,汗出并周期性发作为特征的一种传染病。多发于夏秋之间,其它季节也可散在发病,主要是由于感受疟邪及瘴毒疫疠之气所致,有一日一发称日疟,二日一发为间日疟,三日一发为三日疟之不同,如久疟不愈,在胁下形成积块,称为疟母。

【病因病机】

(一)感受疟邪及风寒、暑湿之气,邪毒侵入人体,伏于半表半里,出入营卫之间,邪入则与阴争而寒;出则与阳争则热,邪正交争而发疟疾;如邪正相离,邪气伏藏,不与营卫相搏,则寒热休止。

(二)饮食不节,脾胃受损,气血生化不足,致气血虚弱,正气不足,或劳倦太过,体质虚弱,疟邪乘虚而入。张景岳说:"疟疾本由外感,……惟禀赋怯弱,劳倦过度者尤易感邪"。

【辨证治疗】

主证:寒热往来,先寒后热,汗出而息,发作有时。发病之初,呵欠乏力,毛孔粟起,旋即寒战鼓颔,寒去则内外皆热、体若燔炭,头痛如裂,面赤唇红,烦渴引饮,口苦而干,胸胁痞满,终则遍身汗出,热退身凉。舌苔白腻或黄腻。脉弦紧或弦数。如疟久不愈,则胁下结块而成疟母。

治法:取督脉、少阳经穴为主。毫针刺用泻法,以通调督脉,和解少阳。在发作前二小时针之为宜。发作时寒多热少的,针灸并用;热重寒轻的只针不灸。

处方:大椎　陶道　后溪　间使　液门　足临泣

随证配穴:热重加曲池,毫针泻法。疟母加章门,灸痞根。高热神昏谵语者,点刺十二井穴出血。

方义:大椎是手足三阳经与督脉之会,可宣通诸阳之气而祛邪,配陶道,退邪热,调阴阳,为治疟要穴;液门、足临泣和解少阳经气;后溪通督脉,为小肠经输穴,功可宣发太阳与督脉阳气,祛邪外出;间使为心包经经穴,厥阴、少阳相表里,故间使可调气机,引邪外出,为治疟之要穴,诸穴合用,能通阳祛邪,表里双解,调和营卫,使疟疾止而病痊愈;曲池配大椎以增退热之效;章门为脏会,可调脏气;痞根为治痞块奇穴。

【其它疗法】

1. 耳针

取穴:肾上腺　皮质下　内分泌　肝　脾

方法:在发作前1—2h针刺,强刺激,留针1h,连续针3天。

2. 穴位敷药

(1)取大椎穴,在发作前2h,用胡椒或朝天椒1—2个捣烂,外敷3—4h。

(2)取内关穴,用烟丝两份,生姜1份,共捣烂,取如硬币大小一块敷穴位上。

(3)取内关,用鲜毛茛或野薄荷或独头蒜适量,捣烂、在发作前1—2h敷穴上,外用胶布固定3—4h。

【附注】

针灸治疗疟疾,以间日疟效果较好。

六、咳嗽

【概说】

咳嗽为肺系疾患的主要证候。其发病原因,有外邪侵袭,肺气不得宣畅而咳嗽;也可由肺脏的病变,或其它脏腑有病,影响肺脏所致咳嗽。常见于上呼吸道感染,急、慢性支气管炎,支气管扩张,肺结核等疾患。

【病因病机】

(一)外感:肺主气,为五脏之华盖,上连喉咙,开窍于鼻,外合皮毛,职司呼吸,一旦遭受外邪侵袭,肺卫受邪,肺气壅遏不宣,肺气失其清肃,因而引起咳嗽。

由于四时气候变化不同,人体所受外邪各异,因而临床上分为风寒咳嗽和风热咳嗽两类。

(二)内伤:由于肺脏功能失调,或他脏有病,累及肺脏而致的咳嗽为内伤咳嗽。常见的有肺燥阴虚,肺失清肃之咳嗽;脾阳不振,聚湿为痰,痰浊上渍于肺,影响气机出入所致之咳嗽;肝气郁滞,日久化火,木火灼金伤肺之咳嗽;有肺肾阴虚,肺失宣降,清肃无权,而导致咳嗽。

【辨证治疗】

(一)外感咳嗽

1. 风寒

主证:咳嗽喉痒,痰液稀白,恶寒发热,无汗,头痛,鼻塞流涕,舌苔薄白,脉浮。

2. 风热

主证:咳痰黄稠,咳而不爽,口渴咽痛,身热,或见头痛,恶风,有汗等表证,苔薄黄,脉浮数。

治法:取手太阴、阳明经穴为主。风寒咳嗽针灸并用;风热证只针不灸,以宣肺解表。

处方:列缺　合谷　肺俞

随证配穴:咳嗽伴咽喉肿痛:少商;发热恶寒:大椎、外关。

方义：肺主皮毛，与大肠相表里，取肺之络穴列缺，大肠之原穴合谷，以散风祛邪，宣肺解表；肺俞为肺之背俞穴，功可通调肺气，加强宣肺解表之效；咽喉肿痛，少商放血以泄肺热；发热恶寒用大椎、外关以退热解表。

(二)内伤咳嗽

1. 痰浊阻肺

主证：咳嗽痰多，色白而粘，胸脘痞闷，胃纳减少，舌苔白腻，脉滑。

治法：取背俞和足阳明经穴为主。针刺补泻兼施，并可加灸，以健脾化痰。

处方：肺俞　脾俞　中脘　足三里　尺泽　丰隆

方义：肺俞、脾俞补益肺脾之气，以增强肺之宣降，脾之运化功能；中脘、足三里健脾胃以化痰浊；尺泽泻肺以止咳，丰隆化痰以降气。诸穴共收健脾化痰止咳之效。

2. 肺燥阴虚

主证：干咳无痰，或痰少不易咳出，鼻燥咽干或咽痛，或痰中有血丝，甚则咳血，潮热，颧红，舌红苔薄，脉象细数。

治法：取肺之俞、募穴为主。针刺平补平泻法，以益阴润燥，清肃肺气。

处方：肺俞　中府　列缺　照海

随证配穴：咯血加孔最、膈俞。

方义：肺俞、中府，俞募穴相配，以润肺调气；列缺为肺经络穴，通于任脉，以清肃润燥止咳，配照海养阴生津以清利咽喉；孔最为肺之郄穴，主治急症；膈俞血会，功专止血，两穴相配，以止咳血。诸穴共奏益阴润燥，清肃肺气，止咳止血之效。

【其它疗法】

1. 耳针

取穴：肺　气管　神门　脾

方法：取双侧，中等刺激，留针10～20min，隔日一次，10次为一疗程；并可用王不留行贴压耳穴。

2. 皮肤针

取穴：颈背部督脉、膀胱经、喉两侧。

方法：轻或中度叩刺，每日一次，10次为一疗程。

七、哮喘

【概说】

哮喘是一种常见的反复发作性疾病，哮是以喉间有声为主症，喘是以呼吸困难为主症。两者常同时发作，病因病机相似，故合并叙述。其发病的根本原因是气机升降失度所致，一般可分虚、实两类。常见于支气管哮喘、喘息性支气管炎、阻塞性肺气肿等病。

【病因病机】

导致哮喘的病因甚多，但不外乎外感与内伤两途，明代医家张景岳认为："实喘者有邪，邪气实也；虚喘者无邪，元气虚也。"外感多为实证，内伤多为虚证。

(一)实证

1. 风寒：重感风寒，侵袭于肺，内则壅阻肺气，外则郁遏肌表，肺卫为邪所伤，以致肺气壅盛，不得宣降，因发哮喘。

2. 痰热：饮食不节，脾失健运，积湿生痰；或素体湿痰内蕴，久郁化热；或肺火素盛，蒸液成痰，则痰火交阻于肺，宣发肃降功能失常，而成哮喘。

(二)虚证

1. 肺虚：久病体弱，咳伤肺气，或劳倦内伤，均可导致肺气不足，而发为气短喘促。

2. 肾虚：房劳伤肾，或大病久病之后，正气亏损，精气内伤；或喘促日久，累及肾脏，均可导致肾气受损，不能纳气，气逆而喘。

【辨证治疗】

(一)实证

1. 风寒

主证：哮喘而咳痰，痰液清稀，兼恶寒发热，头痛，无汗，口不渴，舌苔白，脉浮紧。

治法：取督脉、手太阴、手阳明经穴为主。毫针刺用泻法，并可用灸法，以解表散寒，宣肺平喘。

处方：大椎　合谷　列缺　肺俞　风门

方义：大椎温阳解表，合谷理气解表，列缺宣肺解表，肺俞调理肺气，风门祛风解表，诸穴共奏解表散寒，宣肺平喘之效。

2. 痰热

主证：哮喘声高气粗，胸闷烦热，口干，咳吐黄痰，舌苔黄厚而腻，脉滑数。

治法：取手太阴、足阳明经穴为主。毫针刺用泻法，以清化痰热，宣肺定喘。

处方：鱼际　尺泽　定喘　丰隆

方义：鱼际为肺经荥火穴，清泄肺火以止喘；尺泽为肺经合水穴，合主逆气而泄，水能制火，故尺泽泄肺清热以止喘；定喘为治喘之奇穴；丰隆为胃经络穴，健脾和胃，清化痰热，宣肺定喘。

(二)虚证

1. 肺虚

主证：喘促气短，语言无力，咳声低弱，自汗，舌质淡，脉虚弱。

治法：取手太阴、足阳明经穴为主。毫针刺，用补法，酌用灸法，以补肺定喘。

处方：肺俞　中府　太渊　太白　足三里

方义：肺俞、中府二穴为俞募穴相配，再加太渊，肺之原穴，二穴相配，补肺定喘；足三里胃经合穴，太白脾经原穴，二穴相配补土生金，乃"虚则补其母"之义。脾气健，肺气足则喘自平。

2. 肾虚

主证：喘促日久，动则喘甚，张口抬肩，气不接续，神疲体倦，汗出肢冷，舌质淡，脉沉细。

治法：取足少阴、任脉经穴为主。毫针用补法，酌用灸法，以补肾纳气定喘。

处方：肾俞　太溪　肺俞　膏肓俞　膻中　关元　脾俞　中脘

方义：久喘伤肾，太溪、肾俞补益肾气以纳气定喘；肺俞、膻中理气宽胸；脾俞、中脘健脾胃以益肾气；关元培元固本，益肾定喘；膏肓俞为人之大补穴，功可补益一身之气。诸穴共收补肾纳气，培元固本止喘之效。

【其它疗法】

1. 耳针

取穴：平喘　肺　下脚端　下屏尖。

方法：轻刺激，留针 20min。

2. 灸法

取穴：肺俞　膏肓俞　脾俞　肾俞

方法：艾炷如枣核大，隔姜灸，每穴3～5壮，以皮肤微红不起泡为度。每日1次，在三伏天施灸。

3. 皮肤针

取穴：手太阴肺经循行部位，两侧胸锁乳突肌部。

方法：依顺序轻叩15min左右，以皮肤微红为度。用于哮喘发作期，有缓解作用。

4. 穴位注射

取穴：夹脊穴胸1—6。

方法：用胎盘组织液，每次取一对穴，每穴注射0.5～1ml，由上而下，逐日更换。常用于哮喘缓解期。

5. 药物敷穴

取穴：肺俞　定喘　膻中　尺泽　足三里

方法：每次选3～4穴，用消喘膏(白芥子21g，元胡21g，细辛15g，甘遂12g)共研细末，用姜汁调成糊状，取少许敷穴上，胶布固定，持续敷30～60min，擦掉药膏。每10天治疗一次。

八、胃痛

【概说】

胃痛，又称胃脘痛。因疼痛在上腹胃脘及近心窝附近，故古代又有"心痛"、"心腹痛"之名称。胃痛常见于急、慢性胃炎，胃或十二指肠溃疡及胃神经官能症等病。

【病因病机】

(一)饮食不节，嗜食生冷，饥饱无常，损伤脾胃，以致脾不运化，胃失和降，饮食停滞而疼痛。

(二)忧思恼怒，气郁伤肝，肝失疏泄，横逆犯胃，气机阻滞，发生疼痛。

(三)脾胃素虚，感受寒邪，凝滞胃脘，发生疼痛。

【辨证治疗】

(一)饮食积滞

主证：胃脘胀痛，拒按，嗳气有腐臭味，不思饮食，食则痛甚，舌苔厚腻，脉沉实而滑。

治法：取胃之募穴、足阳明经穴为主。针刺用泻法。以消食化滞，和胃止痛。

处方：中脘　内关　足三里　里内庭　天枢

方义：中脘为胃之募穴，又为八会穴之腑会，六腑病之要穴；足三里为胃之下合穴，"合治内腑"，亦为治胃病之主穴；内关穴理气宽胸和胃止痛，为治胃痛胸痛之主穴，三穴合用可消食化滞，和胃止痛；里内庭为治食积胃痛的经验穴；天枢为大肠募穴，取"和胃必通肠"之意。

(二)肝气犯胃

主证：胃脘胀痛，攻及两胁，嗳气频频，恶心，吐酸，腹胀，食少，苔薄白，脉沉弦。

治法：取手足厥阴、足阳明经穴为主。针刺用泻法，以疏肝理气，和胃止痛。

处方：内关　期门　太冲　中脘　足三里

方义：期门为肺之募穴，太冲为肝之原穴二穴合用可疏肝理气，消胀止痛；足三里、内关、中脘，和胃止痛，降气止呕。

(三)脾胃虚寒

主证：胃脘隐痛，喜按，喜暖，得热痛减，泛吐清水，四肢倦怠，舌苔薄白，脉象沉迟。

治法：取背俞、任脉经穴为主。针灸并用，以温中散寒，行气止痛。

处方：中脘　气海　脾俞　内关　公孙　足三里

方义：寒者温之，虚则补之，针灸中脘、足三里，以温胃散寒，行气止痛；公孙配内关为八脉交会穴，既可健脾和胃，又能行气止痛；隔姜灸气海穴，是取以生姜之温中散寒，艾绒之通经活络止痛作用，最适用于脾胃虚寒之久病患者。

【其它疗法】

1. 拔罐疗法：拔罐部位以上腹部及背部腧穴为主，可用大型和中型火罐，时间约10～15min左右。适用于虚寒性胃痛。

2. 耳针

取穴：胃　神门　脑　下脚端

方法：轻刺激留针20min。

3. 穴位注射

取穴：足三里　中脘　内关

方法：选用1%普鲁卡因注射液或阿托品注射液0.5mg，或当归注射液，红花注射液注于上述穴位，每次1～2穴，每穴1～2ml。

九、呕吐

【概述】

呕吐是由于胃失和降，气逆于上所引起的病证。有物有声为呕，有物无声为吐，无物有声为干呕，因呕与吐常同时发生，病因病机相似，故一并叙述。

呕吐可见于现代医学的神经性呕吐，急、慢性胃炎，胃扩张，贲门痉挛，幽门痉挛或梗阻，胆囊炎等。

【病因病机】

(一)外邪犯胃：外感风寒暑湿之邪，循经犯胃，胃失和降，上逆则呕吐。

(二)食伤胃腑：过食生冷，肥甘以及误食腐败不洁之物，胃腑受伤，胃气不能下降，上逆而为呕吐。

(三)脾胃虚弱：运化无力，水谷难以消磨，水津不布，痰饮内生，积于胃脘，上逆而为呕吐。

(四)肝气犯胃：情志失调，肝气郁结，木旺尅土致胃气上逆而发生呕吐。

【辨证治疗】

(一)外邪犯胃

主证：时呕清水或稀涎，喜暖畏寒，大便溏薄，或呕吐频繁，食入即吐，口渴喜冷饮，大便秘结，脉迟或数。

(二)食伤胃腑

主证：呕吐酸腐，脘腹胀满，嗳气厌食，舌苔厚腻，脉多滑实。

(三)脾胃虚弱

主证：饮食稍多即胃脘不适，甚则呕吐，或劳累之后，眩晕作呕，食不甘味，倦怠乏力，大便微溏，舌质淡，苔薄白，脉细弱。

(四)肝气犯胃

主证:呕吐吞酸,嗳气频繁,胸胁胀痛,烦闷不舒,舌苔白腻,脉弦。
治法:取胃之募穴和下合穴为主。实证用泻法,虚证用补法以和胃降逆止呕。
处方:中脘　内关　足三里　涌泉(男左女右)
随证配穴:外邪犯胃:大椎、至阳;食伤胃脘:建里、天枢;脾胃虚弱:脾俞、三阴交;肝气犯胃:太冲、阳陵泉。
方义:中脘是胃之募穴,腑之会穴,用以和胃理气;足三里为胃之下合穴,用以降逆止呕;内关为心包经络穴,与三焦经相表里,故可通调三焦,为降逆止呕吐的效穴;肾为胃之关,涌泉穴可导胃气下行,为止呕吐的经验效穴。寒邪犯胃灸至阳以温胃散寒止呕吐;热蕴胃腑泻大椎以泻胃降逆止呕吐;建里健胃腑以助消化,天枢通肠腑以降胃气。二穴共奏和胃止呕吐之效,为治伤食之有效穴组;脾俞、三阴交健脾以升清降浊;太冲、阳陵泉疏肝以降冲逆。

【其它疗法】
1. 耳针
取穴:胃　肝　脾　神门
方法:轻刺激,留针20min。
2. 穴位敷药
寒性呕吐取涌泉穴,以吴茱萸研细末,用醋或开水调成膏状,敷穴上。本法对小儿因消化不良引起的呕吐效果好,一般敷药1~4h见效。

十、呃逆

【概说】
呃逆俗称"打呃",古代称"哕",是指胸膈气逆上冲,喉间呃呃连声,令人不能自止,甚则妨碍谈话、进食、呼吸和睡眠的病证。如偶然发作者,大都轻微而自愈;如持续不止,则需要治疗。
本证常见于胃肠神经官能症引起的膈肌痉挛;其它如胃、肠、纵膈、食道等疾病引起的膈肌痉挛亦可发生呃逆之证。

【病因病机】
(一)暴饮暴食,至中焦阻滞不通,胃气不得下降,上逆为呃逆。
(二)情志不畅,郁怒气滞,上逆为呃逆。
(三)过食生冷及寒凉药物,寒气留于中焦,胃阳被遏,气不顺利,上逆而为呃逆。
(四)久病不愈,胃气衰败,气竭而逆。

【辨证治疗】
(一)食积
主证:呃声洪亮,脘腹胀满,厌食,舌苔厚腻,脉滑实。
(二)气滞
主证:呃呃连声,常因情志改变发病或加重,胸胁胀痛,烦闷不舒,苔薄,脉弦有力。
(三)胃寒
主证:呃逆得热则减轻,遇寒则甚,脘痛喜温,舌苔白润,脉迟缓。
(四)胃气衰败
主证:呃声低而无力,神疲气怯,形体消瘦,舌质淡,体胖有齿痕,苔白,脉细弱或结代。
治法:取胃经及有关腧穴为主。食积气滞者,针刺用泻法;胃寒则针灸并施;胃气衰败则用重灸,以和胃,降逆,平呃。

处方:中脘　足三里　膈俞　内关　太渊　攒竹

随证取穴:食滞:梁门、天枢;气滞:膻中、太冲;胃寒:上脘;胃气衰败:关元。

方义:中脘、足三里募合相配,和胃降逆;膈俞血会,位近胸膈,功可补血益气止呃;内关调气止呃;太渊为输土穴,降胃气以止呃逆;攒竹为治呃逆之经验穴。食滞加梁门、天枢以和胃通肠,降逆止呃;气滞加膻中、太冲,理气疏肝止呃;胃寒加灸上脘以温胃;胃气衰败加灸关元以大补元阳。

【其它疗法】

1. 耳针

取穴:耳中或在耳迷根找压痛点针刺。

方法:轻刺激,留针20min。

2. 拨罐

取穴:膈俞　膈关　肝俞　中脘　乳根

方法:留罐5～10min,以皮肤红润,皮下瘀血为度。

十一、泄泻

【概说】

泄泻,是指排便次数增多,粪便稀薄,甚至泻出如水样的一种疾病。其病变主要在脾、胃与大、小肠,临床上根据发病情况及病程长短,有急性、慢性之分。急性泄泻多因内伤饮食,外受寒湿,以致传导功能失调;或因夏秋感受湿热所致。慢性泄泻多因脾肾阳虚,运化失常所致。

泄泻多见于急、慢性肠炎、消化不良、肠功能紊乱、过敏性结肠炎、肠结核、神经官能性腹泻等疾病。

【病因病机】

(一)急性泄泻

1. 寒湿:寒湿侵及肠胃,脾胃升降失司,水湿下注大肠而泄泻。

2. 湿热:夏秋季节伤于暑热,留于肠胃,传导失常而泄泻。

3. 伤食:暴饮暴食,或食不洁之物,或过食生冷,肥甘,致食滞中焦,损伤脾胃,运化失司而致泄泻。

(二)慢性泄泻

1. 脾虚:脾阳不足,运化无力,水湿内停,留于肠胃而成泄泻。

2. 肾虚:肾阳不足,无以温化,水湿内停而作泄泻。

【辨证治疗】

(一)急性泄泻

1. 寒湿

主证:泄泻清稀,腹痛肠鸣,喜温畏冷,口不渴,舌淡苔白,脉多沉迟。

2. 湿热

主证:腹痛即泻,泻下黄糜热臭,肛门灼热,小便短赤,或兼身热,口渴等症,舌苔黄腻,脉象滑数。

3. 饮食所伤

主证:泻下粪便臭如败卵,腹痛肠鸣,泻后痛减,脘腹痞满,嗳气不欲食,舌苔垢浊,脉象滑数或弦。

治法:取足阳明经穴为主。寒湿证针灸并用(或隔姜灸)以温中利湿;湿热证针刺用泻法,以清热利湿;饮食所伤,针刺用泻法,以调中消导。

处方:天枢　足三里

随证配穴:寒湿:加中脘、关元;湿热:曲池、阴陵泉;饮食所伤:内关、梁门。

方义:天枢为大肠募穴,可调整大肠的传导功能;足三里为胃经合穴,可通调胃腑气机;针灸中脘、关元可温中散寒祛湿浊以止泻;曲池清阳明之热,阳陵泉利小便以除湿,二穴合用以清肠胃之热治湿热之泄泻;饮食所伤针内关通调三焦气机,梁门以消食导滞,二穴共收调中消导之效。

(二)慢性泄泻

1.脾虚

主证:大便溏薄,甚则完谷不化,不思饮食,食后脘闷不舒,面色萎黄,神疲倦怠,舌淡苔白,脉弱无力。

2.肾虚

主证:每天黎明之前即泻,肠鸣腹痛,泻后则安,腹部凉,时有腹胀,下肢不温,舌淡苔白,脉沉细无力。

治法:取任脉、及脾胃经穴为主。针用补法及灸法,以温补脾肾,固肠止泻。

处方:中脘　天枢　关元　足三里　地机

随证配穴:脾虚:脾俞、太白;肾虚:肾俞、太溪。

方义:中脘腑会,又为胃之募穴,健胃调肠止泻;天枢大肠募穴,调肠以止泻;关元温肾,足三里健胃,地机健脾,三穴共收温中散寒止泻之效;脾阳虚加灸脾俞、太白以健脾温阳,肾虚加肾俞、太溪以温肾止泻。

【其它疗法】

1.耳针

取穴:大肠　胃

方法:轻刺激留针20min。

2.拨火罐

取穴:天枢　关元　大肠俞　小肠俞

方法:留罐10min,日二次。

十二、便秘

【概说】

便秘是指大肠秘结,排便困难,两天以上不能自解者。主要由大肠的传导功能失常所致。并与脾胃及肾脏有关。依发病特点可分虚实两类。现代医学之习惯性便秘可依此治疗。

【病因病机】

(一)实秘

1.阳盛嗜食:素体阳盛,又嗜食辛辣厚味,致肠腑积热,灼伤津液,肠枯便秘。

2.情志不畅:忧愁思虑,情志不舒,致气机郁滞,津液不布,肠腑传导失常而便秘。

(二)虚秘

1. 气血两亏：病后，产后气血未复，年迈体衰，致气血两虚，气虚则大肠传导无力；血虚则津液不足，不能滋润大肠，而成便秘。

2. 下焦虚寒：下焦阳气不足，阴寒凝结，肠道腑气受阻导致便秘。

【辨证治疗】

(一)实秘

主证：大便坚涩难下，经常三、五日或更长时间一次。或身热，烦渴，口臭，脉数，苔黄燥；或胁腹胀满疼痛，嗳气频作，纳食减少，苔厚腻，脉弦。

(二)虚秘

主证：便秘而排便无力，或见面色口唇㿠白无华，头晕心悸，神疲气怯，舌淡苔薄，脉象虚细；或见腹中冷痛，喜热畏寒，舌淡，苔白润，脉沉迟。

治法：取大肠俞、募穴及三焦、肾经穴为主。实秘用泻法，以清热润肠，疏肝理气；虚秘用补法，以补益气血，润肠通便；寒秘：加灸以温下焦通便秘。

处方：大肠俞　天枢　支沟　照海　左水道

随证配穴：热盛，加曲池、合谷；气滞：加中脘、太冲；气血两亏：加脾俞、胃俞、足三里；下焦虚寒：灸神阙，气海。

方义：便秘病因不同，但其本质是津液不能濡润大肠，使大肠的传导功能失调所致。大肠俞为大肠背俞穴，天枢为大肠募穴，俞募相配，以疏通大肠腑气，腑气通则传导功能复常，便秘可止；支沟为三焦经火穴，可宣泄三焦之火以通便；照海穴滋肾水以增液润肠；曲池、合谷泻大肠腑气以泄热通便；中脘疏通三焦，太冲疏肝理气以通肠腑；补脾俞、胃俞、足三里，扶助中气，脾胃气旺，则能生化气血，为虚秘治本之法；灸神阙、气海，温下焦理气滞以通便；左水道是治疗便秘的经验穴。

【其它疗法】

1. 耳针

选穴：直肠下段　大肠　脑

方法：捻转中、强刺激，留针20～30min。

【附注】

针灸治疗便秘，效果较好，如经多次治疗而无效者，应采用多种方法治疗，并进一步查明病因，以防延误病情，平时宜坚持体育锻炼，多食蔬菜，逐步养成定时排便的习惯。

十三、腹胀

【概说】

腹胀是指腹部发生胀满，叩之如鼓的一种病证。可见于上腹和小腹，脾胃居上腹，大肠，小肠位居小腹，四者的功能失常即可造成腹胀。本证可见于胃下垂，急性胃扩张，肠麻痹，肠梗阻，胃肠神经官能症等病。

【病因病机】

(一)饮食过量，或暴饮暴食，损伤脾胃，运化功能失调，宿食积滞，气机阻滞而腹胀。

(二)脾胃素虚，年高，久病体虚，均可使脾胃失于健运，使胃肠气机不利而腹胀。

(三)腹部手术，胃肠气机紊乱，亦可致腹胀。

【辨证治疗】

(一)实性腹胀

主证:腹胀拒按,甚则胀痛,嗳气,口臭,小便黄,大便秘结;或有发热,呕吐,舌苔黄厚,脉滑数有力。

(二)虚性腹胀

主证:腹胀,时轻时重,喜按,肠鸣便溏,食少神疲,精神不振,小便清长,舌质淡,苔白,脉弱无力。

治法:取足太阴、足阳明及任脉经穴为主。实证针刺用泻法,以通调腑气;虚证用补法并配合灸,以健脾和胃,理气消胀。

处方:公孙 中脘 天枢 气海 足三里

随证配穴:实胀加商丘、厉兑;虚胀加关元、大都、解溪。

方义:公孙为脾经络穴,功可健脾益胃;中脘腑会以和胃气;天枢大肠之募以通肠导滞;气海理气消胀;足三里通降胃气;五穴共奏健脾和胃,通肠导滞,理气和胃之效。实胀加商丘、厉兑泻脾胃为实则泻其子;虚胀加大都、解溪补益脾胃,为虚则补其母。

十四、痢疾

【概说】

痢疾是指以腹痛,里急后重,痢下赤白脓血为主证的一种肠道传染性疾病。多发生于夏、秋季节。本病《内经》称为"肠澼",《金匮》名为"下利"。《诸病源候论》又有"赤白痢"、"血痢"、"脓血痢"、"热痢"等名称。以病程长短分,则病程较久的称"久痢",时作时止的为"休息痢"。临床常见的有湿热痢、寒湿痢、噤口痢、休息痢四种。本病多由外受湿热疫毒之气,内伤生冷不洁之物,邪积交阻,损伤肠胃而成。本病包括现代医学之急、慢性菌痢和阿米巴痢疾。

【病因病机】

(一)感受暑湿:感受暑湿之邪,暑湿热毒侵于肠胃,湿热郁蒸,肠胃气血与暑湿热毒搏结,化为脓血,而成痢疾。湿胜于热则为白痢;热胜于湿则为赤痢;湿热俱盛,则为赤白痢。

(二)嗜食肥甘:素有湿热内结,复加嗜食肥甘,或食不洁之物,致使腑气阻滞,湿热蕴结,气血凝滞,化为脓血而为痢疾。

(三)恣食生冷:寒湿内蕴,再加恣食生冷,或食不洁之物,致寒湿伤于肠胃,气机阻滞,损及营血,而成寒湿痢。

上述病因,虽有外邪与饮食之分,但二者实是互相影响,往往是内外交感发病。痢疾的病位在肠,但与胃关系密切,如疫毒湿热之气上攻于胃,则胃不纳食,成为噤口痢;如痢疾迁延,邪恋正衰,则可成为久痢或休息痢。

【辨证治疗】

(一)湿热痢

主证:腹痛,里急后重,下痢赤白粘冻,肛门灼热,小便短赤,或有恶寒发热,心烦口渴,苔多黄腻,脉象滑数或濡数。

(二)寒湿痢

主证:下痢白腻粘冻,喜暖畏寒,腹中隐痛,胸脘痞闷,口淡不渴,舌苔白腻,脉沉迟。

(三)噤口痢

主证：痢下赤白，饮食不进，恶心呕吐，舌苔黄腻，脉濡数。
（四）休息痢
主证：下痢时作时止，日久难愈，倦怠怯冷，嗜卧，食欲不振，舌淡苔腻，脉濡。
治法：取手阳明及大肠募穴、下合穴为主。以通肠导滞。湿热痢针刺用泻法；寒湿痢针灸并用；久痢针灸补泻兼施。
处方：天枢　上巨虚
随证配穴：发热：大椎；脱肛：灸百会，针长强。湿热痢加曲池、合谷；寒湿痢加中脘、阴陵泉，灸气海；噤口痢：加中脘，内关；休息痢：加脾俞、胃俞、关元、足三里。
方义：天枢为大肠募穴，上巨虚为大肠下合穴，"合治内腑"，痢疾病在大肠，故取大肠之募穴下合穴为主，以通调大肠腑气，使气调而湿化滞行；曲池、合谷清泻肠胃湿热以止痢；灸中脘、气海能温中、下焦，调气行滞，阴陵泉健脾利湿，三穴合用以治寒湿痢疾；噤口痢用中脘开胃进食，内关通利三焦，二穴可和胃气化湿降浊；休息痢灸脾俞、胃俞，针足三里，既能温补脾胃，又可消除肠中积滞；关元为小肠募穴，取之分利清浊，益气助阳。

【其它疗法】
1. 耳针
取穴：大肠　小肠　直肠下段
方法：轻刺激，留针20min。
2. 穴位注射
取穴：天枢　足三里
方法：用10%葡萄糖水或维生素B_1注射液，每穴注入0.5～1ml；每日一次。

十五、脱肛

【概说】
脱肛，又称直肠脱垂，是指直肠下段和直肠粘膜脱出肛门之外的一种疾病。
【病因病机】
本病多由久痢久泄，及病后体弱，元气未复，中气下陷，收摄无力所致；亦有因长期便秘，肛门怒张，失于约束能力而成。
【辨证治疗】
主证：发病缓慢，始则仅在大便时感肛门胀坠，时或脱出，便后能自行回纳，经久失治，则稍有劳累即发，脱垂后收摄无力，须以手助其回纳。或伴有神疲肢软，心悸气短，面色萎黄等症，舌质淡，苔薄白，脉多细弱。
治法：取督脉、足太阳、阳明经穴为主。针用补法并灸。
处方：百会　长强　大肠俞　承山
方义：大肠下连肛门，补大肠俞充养大肠腑气；长强为督脉别络，位近肛门，刺入可增加肛门的约束能力；承山属足太阳膀胱经，其经别别入于肛，其经筋结于臀，与长强相配可增强直肠的回收之力；百会位于巅顶，灸之可使阳气旺盛，有升提收摄之力。数穴同用，则陷者能举，脱肛自收。

【其它疗法】
1. 耳针

取穴：直肠下段　皮质下　神门
方法：取双侧，用中等刺激，留针30min，每日一次。

十六、黄疸

【概说】

黄疸以目黄、肤黄、尿黄为主要症状，其中尤以目睛黄染为主要特征。依临床表现分为阳黄和阴黄两大类。乃由脾胃湿热，蕴伏中焦，胆液不循常道，溢于肌肤，眼目所致。

本病可见于急性黄疸性肝炎，阻塞性黄疸和溶血性黄疸等病。

【病因病机】

(一)时疫病毒，结于脾胃，致湿热内生，湿热蕴蒸，伤及肝胆，胆汁外溢肌肤，发为黄疸。

(二)饮食不节，损伤脾胃，运化失常，湿浊内生，郁而化热，湿热交蒸，熏染肌肤，发为黄疸。

(三)素体脾胃气弱，或过于劳伤，均能导致中阳不振，运化失常，寒湿内阻，发为阴黄。如《临证指南》说："阴黄之作，湿以寒化，脾阳不能化湿，胆液为湿所阻，渍于脾，浸淫肌肉，溢于肌肤，色如熏黄。"

(四)阳黄迁延失治，阳气受损，脾阳不振，寒湿内阻，亦可转为阴黄。

【辨证治疗】

(一)阳黄

主证：身目俱黄，黄色鲜明，发热口渴，小便黄赤短少，身重腹满，胸闷呕恶，舌苔黄腻，脉弦数。

治法：取足少阳、督脉、足太阳经穴为主。针刺用泻法，以疏肝利胆，清热利湿。

处方：至阳　胆俞　阳陵泉　阴陵泉　太冲

随证配穴：热重：大椎、曲池；湿重：足三里、三阴交；便秘：支沟。

方义：至阳为督脉经穴，泻之可清热，为治黄疸之要穴；胆俞为胆之背俞穴，阳陵泉为胆之下合穴，太冲为肝之原穴，泻三穴以疏肝利胆；阴陵泉为脾之合穴，泻之可清利湿热，五穴合用，可使热退湿除，胆汁循于常道，黄疸消退。热重加大椎、曲池以泻热；湿重加足三里、三阴交以健脾和胃化湿浊；便秘加支沟泻三焦之火以通便。

(二)阴黄

主证：黄色晦暗，身重倦怠，纳少脘闷，神疲畏寒，口不渴，舌质淡，苔白腻，脉沉迟。

治法：取足阳明、太阴经穴为主。针刺用补法，并灸。以健脾疏肝利胆，温化寒湿。

处方：脾俞　胆俞　足三里　三阴交　阴陵泉。

随证配穴：神疲肢倦加关元、命门；脘腹胀满加气海；大便溏加天枢；痞块加痞根。

方义：阴黄由寒湿为患，脾胃虚寒为其主因；灸脾俞、足三里、三阴交以温补脾胃，运化寒湿；针胆俞、阳陵泉，俞合相配以利胆退黄；神疲者元气不足，灸关元、命门大补元气；腹胀满乃气滞之象针气海以理气消胀；大便溏灸天枢以止溏泄；痞块加灸痞根以软坚消痞。

【其它疗法】

1. 耳针

取穴：胆　肝　脾　胃　耳迷根　膈

方法：每次取2~3穴，中等刺激，每日一次，10次为一疗程。

2. 穴位注射

取穴：肝俞　胆俞　期门　日月　中都

方法：板兰根注射液，维生素 B_1 注射液。每次选 2～3 穴，每穴注入药物 0.5～1ml，每日一次，10 次为一疗程。

十七、水肿

【概说】

水肿，是指体内水液潴留，泛溢肌肤引起头面、眼睑、四肢、腹背，甚至全身浮肿而言。水肿是全身气化功能障碍的一种表现，与肺、脾、肾、三焦各脏腑密切相关。依据症状表现不同而分为阳水、阴水二类，常见于肾炎、肺心病、肝硬化、营养障碍及内分泌失调等疾病。

【病因病机】

（一）风湿外袭，内舍于肺，肺失宣降，则水道不通，水液溢于肌肤，发为水肿。

（二）饮食劳倦，伤及脾胃，运化失司，水湿停聚，横溢肌肤，发为水肿。

（三）房劳过度，内伤肾元，不能化气行水，水湿内停，溢于肌肤而水肿。

【辨证治疗】

（一）阳水

主证：发病急，初起面目微肿，继之则遍及全身，腰以上肿甚，皮肤光亮，阴囊肿亮，胸中烦闷，呼吸急促。或形寒无汗，苔白滑，脉浮紧；或咽喉肿痛，苔薄黄，脉浮数。

治法：取肺、脾经穴为主。针用平补平泻法，以宣肺、解表、利水；表邪退后，宜参用阴水治法。

处方：列缺　合谷　偏历　阴陵泉　委阳

方义：阳水为病，系肺气失宣，水湿内停所致，腰以上肿宜发汗，故取列缺、合谷发汗解肌，通利肺气；腰以下肿宜利小便，故取偏历、阴陵泉利小便以消水肿；委阳为三焦下合穴，功可调三焦气化功能以消水肿。

（二）阴水

主证：发病较缓，足跗水肿，渐及周身，身肿以腰以下为甚，按之凹陷，复平较慢，皮肤晦暗，小便短少。或兼脘闷腹胀，纳减便溏，四肢倦怠，舌苔白腻，脉象濡缓；或兼腰痛腿酸，畏寒肢冷，神疲乏力，舌淡苔白，脉沉细无力。

治法：取足太阴、少阴经穴为主。针刺用补法，并用灸法，以温补脾肾，利水消肿。

处方：脾俞　肾俞　水分　复溜　关元　三阴交

方义：阴水病因脾肾阳虚，针灸脾俞、肾俞、复溜可温脾肾元阳，促三焦气化；灸水分利水以消水肿；灸关元培补元气以温下焦；补三阴交健脾利湿，通利小便。

【其它疗法】

耳针

取穴：肺　脾　肾　三焦　膀胱　皮质下

方法：每次取 2～3 穴，中等刺激，隔日一次。也可用耳穴埋豆法。

十八、遗尿

【概说】

遗尿是指睡梦中小便自遗的病证。多发生于三岁以上之儿童和少数成年人。本病由肾气不足,膀胱不能制约所致。

【病因病机】

肾气不足,下元不能固摄,每致膀胱约束无权,膀胱失约而遗尿。

【辨证治疗】

主证:夜间睡梦中排尿,或在遗尿后立即惊醒发觉,轻者数日一次,重者一夜数次。如迁延日久,可见面色萎黄,食欲不振,肢体乏力等全身症状,舌淡苔白,脉细尺弱。

治法:取任脉及膀胱经穴为主。针刺用补法或灸法,以补益肾气,约束膀胱。

处方:肾俞　膀胱俞　中极　三阴交　大敦

随证配穴:梦遗加神门;食欲不振加脾俞、足三里。

方义:肾与膀胱相表里,取肾俞、膀胱俞及膀胱之募穴中极,三穴合用以补益肾气,固摄下元;三阴交以调理肝、脾、肾之经气,健脾补肝益肾;大敦为肝之井穴,灸之可温经壮阳,以固下元。

【其它疗法】

耳针

取穴:肾　膀胱　皮质下　尿道

方法:毫针中等刺激,每次选用2~3穴,每日1次,每次留针20min,亦可用贴压法。

【附注】

针灸对大脑排尿中枢发育不全所致遗尿效果较好。对器质性病变,如尿道畸形,隐性脊柱裂,大脑器质性病变或蛲虫病引起的遗尿,应治疗其原发病。

十九、癃闭

【概说】

癃闭是指排尿困难,少腹胀痛,甚则小便闭塞不通的病证。癃证病势较缓,小便不畅,点滴而出;闭指小便闭塞不通,病势较急。因二者病位同在膀胱,病机上可相互转化,故合称癃闭。

本病的发生,主要是各种原因引起的膀胱气化不利,即《内经》所说的"膀胱不利为癃"。多见于各种原因引起的尿潴留。

【病因病机】

(一)热结膀胱:下焦有热,积于膀胱,或肾热移于膀胱,致膀胱气化失司而小便癃闭。

(二)命门火衰:肾与膀胱互为表里,膀胱的气化有赖于肾阳的温煦,今肾阳不足,命门火衰,膀胱气化不利,而成癃闭。

(三)外伤:跌扑损伤,外科手术,均可导致经络瘀阻,膀胱受损,而成癃闭。

【辨证治疗】

(一)热结膀胱

主证:点滴而下,尿道热痛,小便黄少或闭塞,小腹胀满,口渴不欲饮,舌质红,苔黄,脉数。

治法:取膀胱俞募穴为主。针用泻法,以清热利尿。

处方:膀胱俞 中极 三阴交 委阳 束骨

方义:热结膀胱,小便癃闭,取膀胱俞、中极,俞募相配,以清膀胱积热,助膀胱气化,三阴交健脾利湿,清热利尿;委阳为三焦下合穴,针之以促三焦气化,通利下焦;束骨为膀胱经输穴,五行属木,乃实则泻其子之义。

(二)命门火衰

主证:尿液清少,排出无力,小腹胀满,面色㿠白,手足不温,舌质淡,脉沉细尺弱。

治法:取督、任脉及膀胱经穴为主。针用补法或用灸法,以温补肾阳,促进膀胱气化。

处方:命门 肾俞 关元 阴谷 三阴交

方义:命门火衰,膀胱气化不利,取命门、肾俞、阴谷温肾阳以补命门之火;关元温下焦以培元固本促膀胱气化;三阴交利小便以通癃闭。

(三)外伤

主证:小便闭塞,小腹膨隆,甚则胀痛。

治法:取膀胱募穴及肾、脾经穴为主。针用平补平泻法。以通经活络,恢复膀胱气化。

处方:利尿穴 中极 三阴交 照海

方义:利尿穴位于膀胱,指压可促进膀胱气化,通利小便;中极为膀胱募穴,配三阴交疏调膀胱经气;照海补肾气,利小便。诸穴共奏通经活络,恢复膀胱气机以利小便之效。

【其它疗法】

1. 耳针

取穴:膀胱 肾 尿道 三焦

方法:中等刺激,每次选1~2穴,留针40~60min,每10~15min捻转一次。

2. 穴位注射

取穴:足三里 关元 三阴交

方法:用维生素B_1注射液,每穴注入0.2~0.3ml。

3. 电针

取穴:水道。

方法:沿皮向曲骨透刺2~3寸,通电15~30min。

4. 穴位贴敷

(1)大葱,剥去老皮切碎,捣烂,敷神阙穴。一般于敷后24~48h,小便可通畅,初为点滴而下,逐渐转为正常。

(2)大蒜2枚,蝼蛄2个,共捣烂,纱布包,敷神阙穴。

二十、淋证

【概说】

淋证是指小便频数,淋沥刺痛,溲之不尽的一种病证。多由于热炽膀胱引起,亦有因七情及肾虚而发病。前人依临床证候,将淋证分为五种,即:气淋、石淋、血淋、膏淋、劳淋,合称"五淋"。

本病多见于泌尿系感染和泌尿系结石等病。

【病因病机】

(一)石淋:多食肥甘酒热之品,致湿热蕴积下焦,尿液受其煎熬,日久结为砂石,小者如砂,大者如石,或在于肾,或在膀胱,或在尿道,故名石淋。

(二)血淋:湿热聚于膀胱,或心火下移膀胱,热伤血络,迫血妄行,小便涩痛有血,则为血淋。

(三)膏淋:湿热蕴结于下,以致气化不利,不能制约脂液,则小便粘稠,如脂如膏,而为膏淋。

(四)气淋:忿怒伤肝,气郁化火,或气滞火郁下焦,膀胱气化失司,则小便艰涩而痛,余沥不尽,成为气淋。

(五)劳淋:房室劳伤,致肾虚不固,或脾虚气陷,因而小便艰涩疼痛,遇劳即发,成为劳淋。

【辨证治疗】

(一)石淋

主证:尿中有时挟有砂石,小便难,色黄赤而混浊,时或突然阻塞,尿来中断,或小便刺痛窘迫难忍,或觉腰痛腹痛难忍,甚或尿中带血,舌色如常。

(二)气淋

主证:小便涩滞,少腹满痛,舌苔薄白,脉多沉弦。

(三)血淋

主证:尿血红紫,疼痛满紧,小便时热涩刺痛,舌苔薄黄,脉数有力。

(四)膏淋

主证:小便混浊如米泔,或有粘腻之物,尿时尿道热涩疼痛,舌质红苔腻,脉细数。

(五)劳淋

主证:小便涩而淋沥不已,时作时止,遇劳则发,缠绵难愈,脉多虚弱。

治法:取膀胱俞募穴为主。针用泻法或补泻兼施。以疏利膀胱气机。

处方:膀胱俞　中极　阴陵泉

随证配穴:石淋:委阳;气淋:行间;血淋:血海、三阴交;膏淋:肾俞、照海;劳淋:百会、气海、足三里。

方义:淋证以膀胱病变为主,故取膀胱俞和膀胱募穴中极,以疏理膀胱气机;配脾经合穴阴陵泉以利小便,使气化复常,小便通利,含通则不痛之意;石淋为湿热蕴结于下焦,煎熬尿液而成,故取足太阳膀胱经之委阳,又系三焦下合穴,能清下焦,除湿热,利膀胱;行间为肝经荥穴,故气淋取之以泻肝火,理气通淋;血海、三阴交清下焦热而止血;膏淋日久则肾虚不能制约脂液而下流,故取肾俞、照海,可益肾气;劳淋乃脾肾俱虚,取百会为诸阳之会,配气海、足三里,可补益脾、肾之气。

二十一、阳痿

【概说】

阳痿是指阳事不举,或临房举而不坚的一种病证。《内经》又称"阴痿",张景岳说:"阴痿者,阳不举也"。由各种原因造成宗筋弛纵而发病。多见于性神经衰弱,及某些慢性虚弱性疾病。

【病因病机】

(一)命门火衰:恣情纵欲,或少年误犯手淫,损伤肾气,命门火衰,宗筋失养;或惊恐,伤肾,思虑太过,相火妄动,耗损肾精,宗筋失养而成阳痿。即《类证治裁》所说:"伤于内则不起,故阳之痿,多由色欲泻精,斫丧太过,或思虑伤神,或恐惧伤肾"。从而导致阳萎。

(二)湿热下注:饮酒厚味,脾胃受伤,运化失常,湿浊内生,郁而化热,湿浊下注,宗筋弛纵而发阳痿,但此类阳痿较少见,如张景岳曾说:"火衰者十居七八,火盛者只有之耳"。

【辨证治疗】

(一)命门火衰

主证:阳事不举,或举而不坚,面色㿠白,形寒肢冷,头晕目眩,精神不振,腰腿痠软,舌淡苔白,脉沉细,若兼心脾损伤者,则有心悸胆怯,失眠等证。

治法:取任脉、足少阴经穴为主。针用补法,并用灸法,以补肾壮阳。

处方:命门　关元　肾俞　太溪

随证配穴:心脾亏损加心俞、神门、三阴交。

方义:命门火衰,肾阳不足之阳痿,取命门、肾俞、太溪补肾壮阳;关元为足三阴与任脉之会穴,补之能壮人身之元气,培元固本壮阳;心俞、神门、三阴交补益心脾。

(二)湿热下注

主证:阴茎萎弱不能勃起,兼见口苦或渴,小便热赤,下肢痠困,苔黄腻,脉濡数。

治法:取任脉、足太阴经穴为主。针用泻法,以清利湿热。

处方:中极　三阴交　阴陵泉　足三里。

方义:湿热下注所致阳痿,病由脾被湿困,郁久化热,故取三阴交、阴陵泉,健脾利湿;中极清下焦之湿热;足三里以助脾利湿。

【其它疗法】

耳针

取穴:外生殖器　睾丸　内分泌

方法:中等刺激,每10分钟捻转一次,留针30min。

二十二、遗精

【概说】

遗精是指梦遗和滑精两个病证。有梦而遗的,名为梦遗;不因梦交或见色而精自滑出者,名为滑精。其病因主要是各种原因引起的精关不固。多见于性神经衰弱、精囊炎、睾丸炎,以及某些慢性疾病。

【病因病机】

(一)心肾不交:思虑过度,或恣情纵欲,心火不能下交于肾,肾水不能上济于心,心肾不交,水亏而心火独亢,扰动精室,多梦有感而遗。

(二)肾虚失藏:房室不节,或久病伤肾,封藏失司,精关不固,而滑精。
(三)湿热下注:湿热内蕴,流注于下,扰动精室,精关不固,而致遗精。

【辨证治疗】
(一)心肾不交
主证:梦中遗精,头晕心悸,心烦,腰疲耳鸣,小便黄,舌质红,脉细数。
治法:取手少阴经穴,针用泻法;足少阴经穴,针用补法。以交通心肾,固精止遗。
处方:神门　心俞　太溪　志室
方义:神门、心俞,降心火以交通心肾;太溪益肾气,配志室以固精关。

(二)肾虚失藏
主证:遗精频作,不拘昼夜,动念,见色则常有精液滑出,神疲体瘦,面色㿠白,舌质淡,脉沉细弱。
治法:取足太阳、足太阴及任脉经穴为主。针刺用补法,并用灸法,以补肾固精。
处方:肾俞　志室　命门　关元　三阴交
方义:肾俞、志室补肾以固精关;命门温肾以固封藏;关元大补元气,培元以固本,配三阴交健脾补肝益肾。

(三)湿热下注
主证:遗精频作,尿时有精液,心烦少寐,口苦而干,小便热赤不爽,舌苔黄腻,脉濡数。
治法:取任脉、足太阴经穴为主。针刺用泻法,以清热利湿,宁静精宫。
处方:中极　阴陵泉　三阴交
方义:中极为膀胱之募穴,泻之可宣通膀胱之气,使湿热由小便排出;阴陵泉、三阴交健脾利湿,清热利尿;中极、三阴交又是足三阴经交会穴,中极位于小腹,故二穴相配可固精宁宫,诸穴相配,可达清热利湿,防精外泄之效。

【其它疗法】
1　耳针
取穴:外生殖器　内分泌　神门　心　肾
方法:每次取2～3穴,轻刺激,留针15～30min,亦可用耳穴压豆。

2　穴位注射
取穴:关元　中极　志室
方法:用维生素B_1或当归注射液,每穴注入0.2～0.5ml,当进针后针感向前阴传导时将药液缓缓推入。

二十三、失眠　(附:健忘)

【概说】
失眠是以经常不能获得正常睡眠为特征的一种病证,又称"不寐",其证情不一,有初就寝即难以入睡;有的睡而易醒,醒后不能再睡;亦有时睡时醒,睡的不实,甚至整夜不能入睡者。
失眠病人,常兼有头晕,头痛,心悸,健忘以及精神萎靡等症。

【病因病机】
(一)心脾两虚:思虑劳倦,伤及心脾,心伤血亏,血不舍神;脾伤则无以化生气血,血不养心,致心神不安,导致失眠,正如张景岳所说:"劳倦思虑太过者,必致血液耗亡,神魂无主,所以不眠。"

（二）心肾不交：禀赋不足，房劳过度，或久病之人，肾阴暗耗，不能上济于心；五志过极，心火内炽，不能下交于肾，致使心火独亢伤神而不寐。

（三）肝火上扰：肝郁气结，久而化火，肝火上炎，扰动心神而致失眠。

（四）胃气不和：饮食自倍，脾胃乃伤，宿食停滞，升降失常，导致失眠，即《内经》所谓："胃不和则卧不安"。

【辨证治疗】

（一）心脾两虚

主证：难于入睡，多梦易醒，心悸健忘，体倦神疲，饮食无味，面色少华，舌淡苔薄，脉细弱。

（二）心肾不交

主证：心烦不眠，头晕耳鸣，口干津少，五心烦热，舌质红，脉细数，或兼见梦遗，健忘，心悸，腰痠等症。

（三）肝火上扰

主证：失眠，性情急躁，多梦，头痛口苦，胁胀，脉弦。

（四）胃气不和

主证：失眠而胃脘胀痛堵闷，不思饮食，大便不爽，苔腻脉滑。

治法：取手少阴和足三阴经穴为主。针刺虚证用补法，实证用泻法，以宁心安神。针治时间以下午或晚间睡前为佳。

处方：神门　四神聪　三阴交　安眠

随证配穴：心脾两虚：心俞、脾俞；心肾不交：心俞、太溪、照海；肝火上扰：行间；胃气不和：中脘、足三里。

方义：神门养心，四神聪镇静，安眠安神，三阴交健脾补肝益肾，四穴共奏宁心安神之效；心俞、脾俞补益心脾，以益气养血；太溪、照海滋肾养阴，以交通心肾；行间泻肝火以安神；中脘、足三里消食滞，健脾和胃安神。

【其它疗法】

1. 耳针

取穴：神门　心　肝　脾　皮质下

方法：每次取2~3穴，轻刺激留针20min。

2. 皮肤针

取穴：取头、背部的督脉、膀胱经线。

方法：轻轻叩刺，由上而下，腰骶部稍重，均以皮肤红润为度，每日或隔日一次，10次为1疗程。

3. 穴位注射

取穴：心俞　肝俞　脾俞　肾俞　足三里　三阴交　神门

方法：每次取2~3穴，药用维生素B_1和维生素B_{12}混合液，每穴注入0.1~0.5ml，每日或隔日一次，10次为一疗程。

附：健忘

【概说】

健忘指精气衰，记忆减弱，遇事善忘的病证。本病多由肾精虚衰，心脾不足引起。

【病因病机】

肾主藏精,生髓。脑为髓海,为"元神之府",房事不节,精亏髓减,则脑失所养,髓海不足则令人健忘。脾主思而藏意,心主神志,劳伤心脾则意不守舍,血不舍神,则遇事善忘,年高肾衰,亦多患此症。

【辨证治疗】

治法:以养心血补脾肾为主。针用补法。

取穴:四神聪 心俞 脾俞 肾俞 足三里 照海 悬钟

方义:四神聪为治健忘之效穴,功可补脑益智;心俞、脾俞以养心血;足三里以滋后天气血之源;悬钟髓会,配肾俞、照海补益肾精,以生髓充脑。

二十四、惊悸、怔忡

【概说】

惊悸、怔忡是指病人自觉心悸不宁,惊恐不安,不能自主的一类病证。

惊悸较轻,多受惊而发,怔忡较重,与惊吓无关,每由内伤日久而成,稍劳即发,病较深重;惊悸日久不愈,亦可发为怔忡。某些神经官能症,植物神经紊乱,以及各种心脏病出现的心律失常,均可出现惊悸、怔忡。

【病因病机】

(一)体虚惊吓:平素胆怯之人,突受惊吓,如耳闻巨响,目见异物,或遇险临危,以致心悸神摇,不能自主,乃成本病。《素问·举痛论》"惊则心无所倚,神无所归,虑无所定,故气乱矣。"

(二)气血两亏:久病体虚,或失血过多,或思虑过度,劳伤心脾,化源不足,致气虚血少,不能上奉于心,而心悸不宁。

(三)阴虚火旺:房劳过度,肾阴暗耗,水不济火,心肾不交而心悸怔忡。

(四)水气凌心:脾肾阳虚,心阳不振致水气凌心而发生心悸怔忡。

【辨证治疗】

(一)体虚惊吓

主证:心悸不宁,善惊易恐,烦躁不宁,多梦易醒,舌苔薄白,脉略数。

(二)气血两亏

主证:心悸不宁,面色无华,头晕目眩,气短乏力,舌质淡,有齿痕,脉细数或结代。

(三)阴虚火旺

主证:心悸不宁,头晕耳鸣,心烦少寐,舌质红少苔,脉细数。

(四)水气凌心

主证:心悸不宁,咳吐痰涎,胸脘痞满,神疲乏力,形寒肢冷,舌苔白,脉弦滑。脾肾阳虚者则见小便短少,渴不欲饮,舌苔白滑,脉弦滑等。

治法:取心俞、募穴及手少阴、厥阴经穴为主。体虚惊吓宜宁心安神,针用补法;气血两亏宜补益气血,针用补法;阴虚火旺宜滋肾养阴,交通心肾,针用补法;水饮内停宜温阳化水,针灸并用。

处方:内关 神门 心俞 巨阙

随证配穴:体虚惊悸:通里、足三里、丘墟;气血双亏:足三里、三阴交、脾俞;阴虚火旺:少府、照海;水气凌心:水分、关元、阴陵泉。

方义：惊悸、怔忡，病位在心，故总以宁心安神为主，内关为心包经络穴，通于阴维脉，对心脏有较好的调理作用，为治心悸心痛之主穴；神门为心经之原穴，心俞、巨阙为心之俞募穴，三穴共用以调理心脏之气血，宁心安神；通里为心经之络穴，丘墟为胆经原穴，足三里补益后天，三穴合用以宁心益胆，强壮体质；三阴交、脾俞以增强气血生化之源；少府为心经之荥穴以清心火，照海滋肾水以济心火，二穴合用以滋阴降火，交通心肾；水分利水，关元温脾肾强元阳，阴陵泉利水湿，三穴合用可振奋心阳，健脾化饮。

【其它疗法】

1. 耳针

取穴：心　交感　皮质下

方法：轻刺激，留针20min，留针期间捻转2～3次，每天1次，10次为一个疗程。

2. 穴位注射

取穴：心俞　脾俞　肝俞　肾俞　内关　神门　足三里　三阴交

方法：药用当归注射液或复方丹参注射液或维生素B_{12}，每次选2～3穴，每穴注射0.5～1ml，隔日注射1次。

二十五、癫狂

【概说】

癫狂是精神失常的疾病，患者以青、壮年较多。癫病表现为沉默痴呆，语无伦次，静而多喜；狂病则为喧闹不宁，狂躁打骂，动而多怒。《难经·二十难》："重阴则癫"，"重阳则狂"。王冰又有"多喜为癫""多怒为狂"的论述。

癫狂的发病原因，概以七情为要，其病机则为痰浊为患，此外，亦与遗传有一定关系。癫狂病虽见证不同，但二者亦有联系，癫病日久，痰郁化火，可转为狂病；狂病日久，郁火渐得宣泄，痰气留滞，亦能出现癫病，故常以癫狂并称。本病相当于现代医学之精神分裂症，狂躁型或抑郁型精神病，更年期精神病等。

【病因病机】

（一）癫病：思虑太过，情志抑郁，伤及肝脾，以致肝失条达，脾失健运，津液水湿凝滞为痰，上扰清窍，发为癫病。

（二）狂病：多由所求不遂，忿怒伤肝，肝失疏泄，郁而化火，炼液为痰，痰火上扰，蒙闭心窍，而致神志错乱，发为狂病。

【辨证治疗】

（一）癫病

主证：发病缓慢，先有精神苦闷，继则神志呆痴，甚则自言自语，喜笑不止；或终日不语，喜静多卧，不知饮食，不知秽洁，舌苔薄腻，脉象弦滑。

治法：取足太阳、任脉、手厥阴经穴为主。针刺用平补平泻法，以疏肝宁神，健脾化痰。

处方：

1. 心俞　肝俞　脾俞　神门　丰隆

2. 神门　膻中　大陵　丰隆

方义：本证由痰气郁结，病及心、肝、脾三脏，故取心俞开心窍宁神志；肝俞疏肝郁；脾俞健脾气以化痰浊；神门养心以治心性之痴呆；丰隆化痰以宁心神；膻中、大陵理气宽胸。

（二）狂病

主证：始则性情急躁，头痛失眠，面红，怒视，继则妄言责骂，不分亲疏，或毁物打人，力逾寻常，虽数日不食，仍精神不倦，苔黄腻，脉弦滑数。

治法：取督脉、手厥阴、足阳明经穴为主。针用泻法，以宁心安神，清热化痰。

处方：大椎　水沟　风府　内关　丰隆

随证配穴：热盛狂躁：十二井穴点刺出血以泻热。

方义：大椎泻热镇静；水沟醒脑开窍；脑为元神之府，督脉由风府穴入脑，故风府可宁神镇静；内关配丰隆清心化痰。

【其它疗法】

1. 头针

取穴：胸腔区　足运感区

方法：沿皮刺入，深达骨膜，连续捻针2min，每日1次。

2. 耳针

取穴：神门心肝脾皮质下。

方法：每次选3～4穴，癫病用轻刺激，狂病用重刺激，留针30min，每5min捻针1次。

二十六、痫证

【概说】

痫证是一种发作性神志失常的疾病，俗称羊痫风。发作时，突然仆倒，不省人事，口吐涎沫，两目上视，四肢抽搐，或发时先有鸣声，移时苏醒，醒后如常人。

痫证虽具有典型证候，但病情各异，发作持续时间有长有短，短者数秒钟至数分钟；长者数小时。发作间隔有久暂，有每日数发，有数日一发。发作时间不同，有昼发者，有夜发者，发病之前，多有头晕，胸闷，神疲等先兆。

本证一般多属实证，但反复发作可致正虚。痫证相当于现代医学的癫痫病，包括癫痫病的大发作，小发作，精神运动性发作，局限性发作等各种类型。继发性癫痫，应积极治疗其原发病。

【病因病机】

（一）大惊卒恐，惊则气乱，恐则气下，惊恐伤肾，气机逆乱，肝肾受损，阴不敛阳，化热生风而致本病。

（二）肝郁不舒，损及脾胃，湿聚成痰，痰气郁结，上蒙清窍而发病。

（三）先天遗传，多发生于儿童时期。

【辨证治疗】

（一）实证

主证：突然昏仆倒地，神志不清，牙关紧闭，面色苍白，两目上视，手足抽搐，口吐涎沫，并发出类似猪羊的叫声，甚至二便失禁，不久，渐渐苏醒，症状消失，除感疲乏无力外，饮食起居如常，舌苔白腻，脉多弦滑。

治法：取督脉、任脉、肝经穴为主。针刺用泻法。以化痰开窍，平肝熄风。

处方：

1. 水沟　鸠尾　间使　太冲　丰隆

2. 大椎　中脘　丰隆

方义：水沟、大椎醒脑开窍；鸠尾、中脘、丰隆健脾清心化痰；间使、太冲理气解郁，平肝熄风，诸穴共奏化痰开窍平肝熄风之效。

（二）虚证

主证：痫证日久，抽搐程度日渐减弱，精神萎靡，神疲乏力，头晕失眠，面色无华，食少痰多，腰膝酸软，舌淡少苔，脉细无力。

治法：取心、脾、肾经穴为主。针刺用平补平泻法，以养心安神，健脾益肾。

处方：心俞　神门　百会　三阴交　腰奇

随证配穴：白天发作：申脉；夜间发作：照海；痰浊重者：中脘、丰隆；气血大亏者：足三里、关元。

方义：虚性痫证，乃正气不足，气血双亏，痰湿凝聚所致，心俞、神门养心以安神；百会升提清脑；三阴交补肝益肾，健脾化痰；腰奇为治痫证的经验效穴；白天发作阳不足，针申脉以温阳，夜间发作阴不足，针照海以养阴，中脘、丰隆健脾化痰；关元、足三里大补气血。

【其它疗法】

1. 耳针

取穴：神门　皮质下　心　枕　缘中　胃

方法：强刺激，每次选2～3穴，留针30min，间歇捻针。隔日一次，10次为1个疗程。

2. 穴位注射

取穴：大椎　足三里

方法：药用维生素B_1或维生素B_{12}或5%当归注射液，每穴注入0.5min。

3. 挑治

取穴：取长强穴上5分、1寸、1.5寸处，共三穴。

方法：挑断皮下肌纤维，每周1次，3次为1疗程。

二十七、眩晕

【概说】

眩是眼花，晕是头晕，二者常同时并见，故统称为"眩晕"，轻者闭目片刻即止，重者如坐车船，旋转不定，不能站立，或伴有恶心，呕吐，汗出，甚则昏倒等症状。

本证可见于高血压、动脉硬化、贫血、神经官能症、耳源性眩晕等。

【病因病机】

（一）肝阳上亢：肝为风木之脏，性主疏泄，主升主动，如忧思恼怒太过，每使肝阴暗耗，肝阳上亢，干扰清窍而发眩晕；肾为先天之本，主藏精生髓，若先天不足，肾精亏虚，或房劳过度或年老体衰或久病伤肾，均可导致肾精不足，不能生髓，脑为髓海，髓海不足发生眩晕。

（二）气血两亏：病后体虚，气血两亏，或心虚伤脾，气血生化不足，不能上荣于脑，发为眩晕。

（三）痰湿中阻：肥胖之人，痰盛湿重，或饮食伤胃，劳倦伤脾，致使腐熟运化失司，聚湿生痰，痰湿中阻，清阳不升，浊阴不降，引起眩晕。

【辨证治疗】

（一）肝阳上亢

主证：眩晕每因恼怒或情绪激动加剧，急躁易怒，面红目赤，口苦，耳鸣，少寐多梦，舌质红，苔黄,脉弦数。

治法:取足厥阴、少阳、少阴经穴为主。毫针刺,补泻兼施,以平肝滋阴潜阳。

处方:风池　行间　太冲　太溪　三阴交

方义:风池熄风以平上亢之肝阳,清头明目;行间肝之荥穴,以泻肝火去目赤口苦;太冲平肝,太溪滋肾,三阴交补肝益肾,三穴共收平肝滋阴潜阳之效。

(二) 气血两亏

主证:眩晕而乏力懒言,面色㿠白,唇甲不华,心悸少寐,舌质淡,脉细弱,甚则眩晕昏倒,劳累即发。

治法:取督脉、任脉、脾胃经穴为主。针刺用补法,兼用灸法,以补益气血。

处方:百会　关元　足三里　丰隆　三阴交

方义:百会位于巅顶,灸百会可升提气血,营脑止晕,灸关元大补元气,三阴交、足三里、丰隆健脾胃以益气血生化之源。

(三) 痰湿中阻

主证:眩晕而兼见头重如裹,胸闷恶心,痰多身重多寐,舌苔白腻,脉象濡滑。

治法:取任脉、手足阳明、足太阴经穴为主。针刺用平补平泻法,以除湿化痰。

处方:中脘　曲池　丰隆　三阴交

随证配穴:胸闷恶心加内关。

方义:脾为生痰之源,中脘为胃之募穴,针之可健脾胃化痰止晕;曲池合穴,可将上逆之湿痰下引以清头明目;丰隆胃之络穴,功可健脾益胃,为化痰要穴,配三阴交共收健脾和胃,除湿化痰之效;内关为心包络穴,功可理气宽胸,和胃止呕。

【其它疗法】

1. 头针

取穴:晕听区

方法:常规消毒后,用 30 号 1.5 寸针刺入骨膜,快速捻转 2min,休息 5min,再捻转 2min,如此操作,30min,每日 1 次,10 次为一疗程。

2. 耳针

取穴:下屏尖　下脚端　心　神门

方法:每日针 1 次,10 次为 1 疗程,休息 1 周后,再行一个疗程。

3. 皮肤针

取穴:百会　太阳　印堂　华佗夹脊

方法:每天 1~2 次,中等刺激,5~10 次为一疗程。

二十八、郁证

【概述】

郁证是指由于情志不舒,气机郁滞所引起的一类病证。主要症状为情志异常,如无故喜笑、悲泣、歌唱、呻吟或痴呆、沉默;其次如突然失语、失明、胸闷、气逆、吞咽困难,甚至突然晕厥;或出现肢体麻木疼痛、瘫痪、振颤抖动等。患者以青壮年和妇女较多。文献记述的"奔豚气"、"梅核气"、"脏躁"等均属本证范畴。类似现代医学的癔病、更年期综合症。

【病因病机】

郁证的成因，总不离七情所伤，从而导致五脏气机不和。《灵枢·口问》指出："悲哀愁忧则心动，心动则五脏六腑皆摇"。就是此意。如郁怒、思虑、悲哀、忧愁之所伤，导致肝失疏泄，脾失运化，心神失常，脏腑阴阳气血失调而成郁证。

【辨证治疗】

（一）肝气郁结

主证：精神抑郁，情绪不宁，胸胁胀痛，脘闷嗳气，腹胀纳呆，大便不畅，妇女月经不调，舌苔薄腻，脉弦。

（二）气郁化火

主证：急躁易怒，头痛目赤耳鸣，大便秘结，舌红苔黄，脉弦数。

（三）痰气郁结（又称梅核气）

主证：咽中自觉有物，咳之不出，咽之不下，胸中窒闷，舌苔薄腻，脉弦滑。

（四）阴血不足（又称脏躁）

主证：无故悲伤，喜怒无常，多疑，善惊，心悸，烦躁，睡眠不安；或有突发胸闷，呃逆，暴喑，抽搐等症；严重者可昏迷，僵仆，苔薄白，脉弦细。

治法：取手、足厥阴、足太阴经穴为主。针刺平补平泻，或针刺补法，并灸。

处方：太冲　内关　三阴交

随证配穴：肝气郁结：膻中、中脘、足三里；气郁化火：行间、支沟、侠溪；痰气郁结：天突、膻中、丰隆；阴血不足：神门、足三里。

方义：郁证之病，位在心、肝、脾，故取肝经原穴太冲以疏肝解郁；太冲五行属土，故又有和胃健脾化痰之效；内关为心包经络穴，脉络三焦，故可宽胸理气，调畅气机；三阴交健脾和胃，调肝益肾。诸穴相配，共奏疏肝解郁，健脾化痰，宁心安神之效。膻中气会，理气宽中，中脘、足三里、和胃降逆，三穴增强疏肝理气作用；行间泻肝火，侠溪泻胆火，支沟泻三焦火，三穴泻火以增强疏肝解郁作用；天突降气化痰，丰隆健脾和胃化痰，膻中理气宽中，三穴合用，增强化痰散结作用；神门镇静安神，足三里补益气血，二穴合用，增强安神补血的作用。

【其它疗法】

1. 耳针

取穴：心　皮质下

方法：轻刺激，留针 20min。

2. 电针

取穴：发作时取水沟、合谷、内关、神门、足三里、太冲；不发作期取内关、神门、足三里、三阴交；癔病性瘫痪加曲池、阳陵泉。

方法：选用疏密波或连续波，发作时用强刺激，每次 5～10min，不发作期用弱刺激或中度刺激，以病人能耐受为度，每次 10～20min，每日或隔日一次，10 次为一疗程。

3. 皮肤针

取穴：颈项部、背部督脉和膀胱经。

方法：轻度叩刺，以皮肤红润为度，每日或隔日一次，10 次为一疗程。

4. 穴位注射

取穴：心俞　肝俞　脾俞　间使　足三里

方法：用维生素 B_1 和维生素 B_{12} 混合液，每穴注入 0.1～0.5ml，隔日治疗一次。

二十九、肥胖症

【概说】

正常成人标准体重(公斤)＝身高(厘米)－100。肥胖症是指人体内脂肪贮存过多,超过正常体重15～20%即为肥胖。肥胖如兼见颈、小腹和臀部脂肪明显积聚,可出现一定的代谢失调现象,如容易疲劳,乏力,出汗或兼见各种神经官能症如头痛、心悸、腹胀等,则为肥胖症。现代医学揭示肥胖与脑血管疾病、心血管疾病、高血压、动脉硬化、糖尿病等有密切关系,肥胖可以加速人的衰老,导致各种疾病的发生。本病包括单纯性肥胖症和继发性肥胖症。

【病因病机】

(一) 过食厚味,致油脂堆积,影响脾之运化,痰湿内停成病。

(二) 肺失肃降,肾失温煦,痰湿内停致病。

【辨证治疗】

(一) 脾失健运

主证:纳差,体虚,大便溏薄,肌肉松驰,舌体胖,脉弱濡缓。

(二) 湿热内蕴

主证:饮食量多,便秘,口渴,口臭,肌肉结实而胖,舌红苔腻,脉滑数。

(三) 冲任失调

主证:腹部、臀部胖甚,腰痠腿软,月经不调,量少,舌胖淡,脉沉细。

治法:取手足阳明、足太阴经穴为主。针刺用平补平泻法,以健胃脾,化痰湿,通肠导滞。

处方:曲池　足三里　三阴交　天枢　梁丘　公孙

方义,肥胖多由痰湿内停所致,病位在脾胃、大肠。方中公孙、三阴交健脾和胃,以促运化,祛痰湿;足三里、梁丘健胃,以助消化;曲池、天枢通肠导滞,使痰湿由大肠而泄。诸穴协同,共奏健脾胃,化痰湿,通肠导滞之效,痰湿积滞排除,则人体负担减轻,体重下降而达减肥目的。

【其它疗法】

1. 耳针

(1) 取穴:内分泌　卵巢　脑点　饥点　神门　脾　胃　交感

方法:针刺泻法,强刺激,不留针或留针20min左右,每次取6穴,两耳交替用或同时用,每日一次,10次为一疗程。

(2) 取穴:胃　肺　饥点

方法:任选一穴埋针,于饥饿感和食前自行按压。

(3) 取穴

内分泌紊乱:内分泌、皮质下、缘中;食欲过盛:饥点、渴点、脾、胃;嗜睡:丘脑、神门。

方法:每次取4～6穴,5次为一疗程,1疗程后休息1周,再进行第二疗程。

三十、头　痛

【概说】

头痛是临床上常见的一种自觉症状,可见于多种急、慢性疾病中。本节仅讨论内科范围内以头痛为主要症状的一般辨证治疗规律。

头痛的发生,常见于高血压,颅内肿瘤,神经机能性头痛,偏头痛,五官科疾患,感染性发热性疾病等。

【病因病机】

头居人体最高部位，脏腑之气血皆上注于头，手、足三阳经脉和主一身之阳的督脉亦均上至于头部，所以说"头为诸阳之会。"

（一）外感诸邪，内伤诸疾都能直接或间接地引起头部气血失和，经络阻滞而导致头痛，如六淫之邪外袭，上犯巅顶，阻抑清阳。

（二）肝失条达，郁久化热，上扰清空；肝肾阴虚，肝阳上亢。

（三）禀赋虚弱，气血素亏，脑失所养等均能导致头痛。

【辨证治疗】

（一）风邪袭络

主证：头痛时作，遇风则发，痛连项背，痛势剧烈，如锥如刺，痛有定处，甚则头皮肿起，脉弦，舌苔薄白。本病亦名头风。

（二）肝阳上亢

主证：头痛目眩，尤以头之两侧为重，烦躁易怒，心烦失眠，面赤口苦，脉弦，舌质红苔黄。

（三）气血不足

主证：痛势绵绵，头晕目眩，神疲乏力，面色无华，喜暖畏冷，操劳或用脑过度则加重，脉细弱，舌质淡，苔薄白。

治法：头痛一症，虽有风邪袭络，肝阳上亢，气血不足等各种原因引起，而针灸临床上则以分经辨证为主，在分经的基础上，采取循经取穴加局部取穴。

处方：百会　风池　太阳

随证配穴：前额痛（阳明头痛）：阳白、印堂、攒竹、合谷、内庭；侧头痛（少阳头痛）：头维透率谷、外关、足临泣；后头痛（太阳头痛）：天柱、大椎、后溪、金门；头顶痛（厥阴头痛）：四神聪、太冲、内关、涌泉；感受外邪者加：合谷、列缺；肝阳上亢者加：太冲、三阴交；气血虚者加：气海、足三里、脾俞。

方义：本方系按部分经，即病部近取与循经远取相配，旨在疏通经络之气，含通则不痛之意；足厥阴经脉会于巅，足少阳胆经布于头之两侧，取两经之病部风池、率谷、头维等与循经远取之太冲、足临泣等穴，以平熄亢逆之风阳；取脾俞、足三里、合谷、三阴交能运化水谷，生精化血，以资生化之源，使髓海得以充养而痛自止。

【其他疗法】

1. 皮肤针

皮肤针重叩太阳、印堂及头痛处出血，加拔火罐。本法适用于风邪袭络，肝阳上亢引起之头痛。

2. 耳针

选穴：枕　额　脑　神门

方法：每次取2～3穴，留针20～30min，间隔5分钟行针一次，或埋针3～7天。顽固性头痛可在耳背静脉放血。

【附注】

针灸治疗头痛有较好的疗效，由于引起头痛的病因较复杂。如治疗多次无效，或头痛持续而又逐步加重者，须查明原因，防止贻误病情。

三十一、面痛

【概说】

面部一定部位出现阵发性、暂短性剧烈疼痛称为面痛。本病多发生于面部一侧的额部、上颌部或下颌部。疼痛常突然发作,呈闪电样、刀割样、难以忍受。本病常反复发作,表现为慢性疾病。发病年龄多在中年以后,女性患者较多。

本病常见于现代医学的三叉神经痛。

【病因病机】

(一)外感风寒:感受风寒之邪,客于面部经络,致使经络拘急收引,气血运行受阻,而卒然疼痛。

(二)肝胃郁火:肝气郁结,郁而化火,饮食不节,食滞生热,肝胃之火上冲于面,可导致面痛。

(三)阴虚火旺:素体阴虚,房劳伤精,可使阴虚火旺,亦可导致本病。

此外,牙病、口腔病、耳鼻病患、神志病等都能诱发本病。

【辨证治疗】

(一)感受风寒

主证:疼痛突然发作,呈阵发性闪电样剧痛,其痛如刀割、针刺、火灼,病人难以忍受,每次发作持续时间短暂,数秒或1～2分钟,一天可以发作多次。常因触及面部的某一点而诱发。常伴有面部肌肉抽搐、流泪、流涕及流涎等症,或有外感症状,脉弦紧。

(二)肝胃郁火

主证:除上述典型疼痛症状外,兼有烦躁,易怒,口渴,便秘,苔黄而干,脉多弦数。

(三)阴虚火旺

主证:痛势较缓并兼有形质消瘦,颧红,腰痠,神倦,每遇劳累则面痛发作加剧,脉细数,舌红少苔。

治法:以分部近取与循经远取相结合。毫针刺用泻法,持续捻针。

处方:

眶上痛:阳白　鱼腰　攒竹　太阳　合谷

上颌痛:四白　颧髎　迎香　合谷

下颌痛:下关　颊车　大迎夹　承浆　合谷

随证配穴:感受风寒加风池;肝胃郁火加太冲、内庭;阴虚火旺加照海、三阴交。

方义:上方局部腧穴具有疏通患部经气,泻实止痛的作用;合谷、内庭泻阳明胃热;外关、太冲泻肝胆之热;风池疏风止痛;照海、三阴交益阴降火。

【其他疗法】

1. 耳针

选穴:面颊　上颌　下颌　神门

方法:每次取2～3穴,留针20～30min,每隔5min捻转一次,或埋针。

2. 穴位注射

方法:用维生素B_{12}或B_1注射液或1%普鲁卡因注射液注射压痛点,每穴0.5～1ml。每隔2～3天注射一次。

【附注】

针刺治疗三叉神经痛止痛效果较好。对继发性三叉神经痛或三叉神经麻痹须查明原因,采取适当措施。

三十二、胁 痛

【概说】

胁痛是指一侧或两侧胁肋疼痛而言,是病人的一个自觉症状。因肝居胁下,胆附于肝,肝胆之脉又布胁肋,说明胁痛之形成,与肝胆疾患甚为密切。

本病常见于肝脏、胆囊、胸膜等急、慢性疾患、胸胁外伤以及肋间神经痛等。

【病因病机】

(一)肝郁气滞:肝居于胁部,其脉分布两胁,若情志郁结,肝气失于条达,络脉受阻,经气运行不畅,可发为胁痛。

(二)精血亏损:因精血亏损,血少不能濡养肝络。

(三)外伤:跌仆闪挫,络脉停瘀等,均能导致胁痛。

【辨证治疗】

(一)肝郁气滞

主证:胁痛多见于一侧,或两侧皆痛,而以胀痛为主,每因情志变动而增减,痛无定处,胸闷不舒,善太息,饮食不振,口苦,苔薄白,脉弦。

(二)气滞血瘀

主证:胁痛如刺,痛有定处,痛处拒按,入夜痛甚,舌质紫暗,脉沉涩。

(三)肝阴不足

主证:胁肋隐痛,其痛绵绵不止,头晕目眩,口干心烦,舌质红少苔,脉虚弱或细数。

治法:取足厥阴、少阳经穴为主,配以局部及背俞穴。毫针刺,实证用泻法,虚证用补法,或平补平泻。

处方:支沟　阳陵泉　期门　太冲

随证配穴:气滞血瘀者加膈俞、三阴交;肝阴不足者加肝俞、肾俞、足三里、三阴交。

方义:取肝募期门,原穴太冲,配少阳经支沟、阳陵泉,以疏肝胆之经气,使气机通畅,奏理气止痛之功;血会膈俞配三阴交以活血化瘀;肝俞、肾俞配期门、太冲可益精养血,调肝止痛;足三里配三阴交,扶助脾胃以资生化之源。

【其他疗法】

1. 皮肤针

用皮肤针叩打胁肋痛处,加拔火罐。适用于劳伤胁痛,有止痛化瘀作用。

2. 耳针

取穴:胸　神门　肝

方法:取患侧 2～3 穴,留针 20～30min,痛时针刺。

【附注】

1. 针刺治疗胁痛,同时须进行有关检查,必要时采取病因治疗。

2、肋间神经痛,可根据疼痛部位,选取相应节段的华佗夹脊穴,有较好的止痛效果。

三十三、腰 痛

【概说】

腰痛，又称"腰脊痛"，疼痛的部位或在脊中，或在一侧，或两侧俱痛，是临床上常见证候之一。腰为肾之府，腰脊内属于肾，外络诸经，可见腰痛与肾之关系甚密。本证较常见于腰部软组织损伤、肌肉风湿以及脊柱和内脏病变等。

本篇主要讨论寒湿腰痛、腰肌劳损以及肾虚腰痛。

【病因病机】

(一)寒湿腰痛：多由感受风寒，或坐卧湿地，或涉水冒雨或汗出当风，风寒湿之邪客于经络，经络之气阻滞而发病。

(二)腰肌劳损：用力过度或外伤闪挫，使经脉气血受损，引起气滞血瘀而导致腰痛。

(三)肾虚腰痛：房劳过度，精气耗损，可以导致肾虚腰痛。

【辨证治疗】

(一)寒湿腰痛

主证：腰痛发于感受寒湿之邪以后，腰背冷痛重着，转侧不利，或拘急强直不能俯仰，或痛连臀部下肢，每遇阴雨天则加重，静卧休息疼痛不减，舌苔白腻，脉沉弱或沉迟。

(二)劳损腰痛

主证：有腰部扭伤史，腰脊强痛，一般痛处固定不移，轻则俯仰不便，重则不能转侧，痛处拒按，舌质淡红或紫暗，脉弦或涩。

(三)肾虚腰痛

腰痛痠软，隐隐作痛，膝软无力，日久不愈，精神倦怠，反复发作，遇劳则甚，卧息可减。偏于阳虚者，手足不温，少腹拘急，腰部冷感；偏于阴虚者伴五心烦热，心烦，失眠，口燥咽干，舌质淡，脉沉迟，或舌质红，脉细数。

治法：取足太阳、督脉经穴为主。根据证侯虚实，酌用毫针补泻，或平补平泻，或针灸并用。

处方：肾俞　腰阳关　夹脊　委中

随证配穴：寒湿：大肠俞、关元俞；肾阳虚：命门、腰眼；肾阴虚：志室、太溪；劳伤：水沟、腰痛点、阿是穴。

方义：腰为肾之府，取肾俞以益肾气，灸之能除寒去湿；腰阳关是局部取穴，委中是四总穴之一，是治疗腰背痛的远道取穴；取大肠俞、关元俞以祛风散寒，通经止痛；命门、腰眼针灸并用，可补肾阳，益肾精；志室、太溪可补益肾阴；督脉行于脊里，取水沟是循经远道取穴法，可治疗腰脊强痛；腰痛点是治疗扭伤所致腰痛的有效奇穴。

【其他疗法】

1. 刺络拔罐：选择压痛部和委中，用皮肤针重叩出血，加拔火罐。本法适用于寒湿腰痛和慢性腰肌劳损。

2. 穴位注射：用10%葡萄糖注射液5~10ml加维生素B_1注射液100mg，或用复方当归注射液，注入压痛点肌层。隔日一次，10次为一疗程。本法适用于慢性腰肌劳损。

【附注】

针灸治疗各种类型的腰痛，均有较好的效果。如因脊椎结核，肿瘤等引起的腰痛，不宜在病灶局部针刺，并须给予病因治疗。

三十四、痹 证

【概说】

痹,有闭阻不通之意。凡外邪侵入肢体的经络、肌肉、关节,气血运行不畅,引起疼痛、肿大、重胀或麻木等证,甚至影响肢体运动者,总称痹证。

本证可包括风湿热、风湿性关节炎、类风湿关节炎、肌纤维组织炎、痛风、神经痛等病。

【病因病机】

痹证的成因,多由卫气不固,腠理空疏,或劳累之后,汗出当风,涉水冒寒,久卧湿地等,以致风寒湿邪乘虚而入,经络痹阻,发为风寒湿痹。《素问·痹论》说:"风寒湿三气杂至,合而为痹也"。由于感受风寒湿三气各有偏胜,故以风气胜者为行痹,寒气胜者为痛痹,湿气胜者为着痹。如素有蓄热,复感风寒湿邪,寒从热化,则为风湿热痹。

【辨证治疗】

(一) 行痹

主证:肢体关节酸痛,游走不定,上下左右走窜疼痛,以腕、肘、膝、踝等处为甚,关节运动不利,或见恶寒发热,舌苔薄腻,脉多浮紧或浮缓。

(二) 痛痹

主证:遍身或局部关节疼痛剧烈,痛有定处,得热则减,遇寒则甚,局部不红不热,舌苔薄白,脉浮紧。

(三) 着痹

主证:肌肤麻木不仁,肢体关节痠痛,沉重,痛有定处,遇阴雨天则加重,苔白腻,脉濡缓。

(四) 热痹

主证:关节疼痛,痛不可触,痛处灼热红肿,活动受限,可涉及一个或多个关节,兼有发热,口渴,苔黄,脉滑数。

治法:以局部取穴,循经取穴和按病证取穴为主,辅以阿是穴。行痹、热痹用毫针刺,泻法浅刺,亦可用皮肤针叩刺;痛痹深刺留针,多灸,或温针灸;着痹针灸并施,并配以拔火罐法。

处方:

肩部:肩髃　肩髎　臑俞

肘臂:曲池　合谷　天井　尺泽　外关

腕部:阳池　外关　阳溪　腕骨

背脊:水沟　身柱　腰阳关

髀部:环跳　居髎　悬钟

股部:秩边　承扶　阳陵泉

膝部:犊鼻　梁丘　阳陵泉　膝阳关

踝部:申脉　照海　昆仑　丘墟

随证配穴:行痹加膈俞、血海、三阴交;痛痹加肾俞、关元;着痹加足三里、商丘、阴陵泉;热痹加大椎、曲池。

方义:上述处方,针对痹证的性质制定。如行痹为风胜,取膈俞、血海、三阴交,有活血、养血作用,含血行风自灭之意;着痹取足三里、阴陵泉、商丘,是因水湿仃留,必先由中土不运,运脾为治湿之本,取之以健运脾胃而化湿;痛痹久延,可致阳气衰惫,取关元、肾俞以益火之原,振奋阳气而驱散寒邪;大椎、曲池清热解表以治热痹。分部处方,主要根据病所的经络循行部位选穴,旨在疏通经络气血的阻滞,使营卫调和则风寒湿邪无所依附而痹痛遂解。并视病痛部位和邪之深浅,决定进针深度,随其证情变化,运用各种不同的治疗和操作方法。

【其他疗法】

1. 刺络拔罐

用皮肤针重叩背脊两侧或关节局部,使叩处出血少许,并加拔火罐。本法适用于热痹关节肿痛。

2. 穴位注射

采用当归、防风、威灵仙等注射液,注射于肩、肘、髋、膝部穴位,每穴0.5～1ml。注意勿注入关节腔,每隔1～3日注射一次,10次为一疗程。每次取穴不宜过多,如为多发性关节病变,可选取重点部位注射,以后轮换进行。

【附注】

1. 针灸治疗痹证有较好效果,但类风湿性关节炎病情缠绵,非一日可获效。
2. 本证还须与骨结核、骨肿瘤鉴别,以免延误病机。

三十五、面 瘫

【概说】

面瘫,即面神经麻痹。中医学称为"口眼㖞斜"。春、秋两季发病较高。可发生于任何年龄,而多数患者为20～40岁,男性略多。

临床分为周围性与中枢性两类,两者在发病原因和见症方面有很大区别,前者多由面神经炎所引起,后者可因脑血管病或脑肿瘤等引起,本篇仅叙述周围性面瘫。

【病因病机】

本病致病原因,多由脉络空虚,风寒之邪乘虚侵袭阳明、少阳脉络,以致经气阻滞,经筋失养,筋肌纵缓不收而发病。

【辨证治疗】

临床发病突然,一侧面部板滞、麻木,继之面部表情肌瘫痪,而出现额纹消失,眼闭合不紧露睛流泪,鼻唇沟变浅,口角歪向健侧,食物常嵌在齿颊间,患侧不能作蹙额、皱眉、示齿、鼓腮等动作,部分病人初起时有耳后、耳下及面部疼痛,还可出现患侧舌前2/3味觉减退或消失,听觉过敏等症。病程延久,可因瘫痪肌挛缩,口角歪向病侧,称"倒错"现象。

治法:取手、足阳明经穴为主,辅以少阳经穴。面部穴位可采取透刺。

处方:阳白 四白 攒竹 下关 颧髎 巨髎 地仓透颊车 合谷 足三里

随证配穴:鼻唇沟平坦加迎香;人中沟平坦加人中;颏唇沟歪斜加承浆;乳突部疼痛:加风池、翳风、外关。

方义:合谷、足三里以疏通阳明经气,能祛除头面之风邪;翳风、风池、外关能祛除少阳之风邪止痛;阳白、四白、攒竹、下关、颧髎、巨髎、地仓、颊车均为局部取穴,以疏通患部之经气。

【其他疗法】

1. 皮肤针

用皮肤针叩刺阳白、太阳、四白、牵正等穴,用小火罐吸拔5～10min,隔日一次。本法适用于发病初期,或面部有板滞感觉等面瘫后遗症。

2. 穴位注射

用维生素 B_1 100mg 或 B_{12} 100ug 注射液注射翳风、牵正等穴，每穴 0.5～1ml，每日或隔日一次。以上穴位可交替使用。

3、穴位贴敷

将马钱子锉成粉，约 1～2min，撒于膏药或胶布上，贴在患侧的下关穴，隔 2～3 日更换一次，一般须更换 4～5 次。

【附注】

1. 面神经麻痹有周围性和中枢性二种，应注意鉴别。
2. 本病初起时针刺不宜过强。
3. 治疗期间避免风吹受寒，面部可作按摩和热敷。
4. 防止眼部感染，可用眼罩和眼药水点眼，每日 2～3 次。

三十六、痿　证

【概说】

痿证，是指肢体痿弱无力，不能随意活动，或伴有肌肉萎缩的一类病证，其证以下肢痿弱较多见，故又称"痿躄"。

本证常见于多发性神经炎，小儿麻痹后遗症，早期急性脊髓炎，重症肌无力，癔病性瘫痪及周围性瘫痪等。

【病因病机】

（一）肺热津伤：外受风热，侵袭于肺，耗伤肺之津液，以致筋脉失去濡润。

（二）湿热侵淫：由湿热之邪蕴蒸阳明，阳明受病则宗筋弛缓，不能束筋骨利关节。

（三）肝肾阴亏：因病久体虚，房劳过度，肝肾精气亏损。

（四）外伤瘀阻：筋脉失于荣养，均能引起本证。

【辨证治疗】

（一）肺热津伤

主证：两足痿软不用，兼有发热，咳嗽，心烦，口渴，小便短赤，舌红苔黄，脉细数或滑数。

（二）湿热侵淫

主证：两足痿软或微肿，押之微热，身重，胸脘痞满，小便赤涩热痛，舌苔黄腻，脉濡数。

（三）肝肾阴亏

主证：下肢痿弱不用，兼有腰背痠软，遗精早泄，带下，头晕，目眩，舌红，脉细数。

（四）外伤瘀阻

主证：有外伤病史，肢体麻木，痿废不用，或有大小便失禁。脉缓或涩，舌苔薄白，舌质淡红或紫暗。

治法：以取阳明经穴为主。上肢多取手阳明；下肢多取足阳明；属于肺热及湿热者，单针不灸，用泻法，或兼用皮肤针叩刺；肝肾阴亏者，针用补法。

处方：

上肢：肩髃　曲池　合谷　外关

下肢：髀关　环跳　血海　梁丘　足三里　阳陵泉　解溪　悬钟

随证配穴：肺热：尺泽、肺俞；湿热：脾俞、阴陵泉；肝肾阴虚：肝俞、肾俞；外伤：相应节段华

佗夹脊穴;小便失禁:中极、三阴交;大便失禁:大肠俞、次髎

方义:本方以阳明经穴为主,是根据《素问·痿论》所说:"治痿独取阳明"之意。取筋会阳陵泉,髓会悬钟以增强濡养筋骨的作用;取肺俞、尺泽以清泻肺热;取脾俞、阴陵泉以清利湿热;取肝俞、肾俞以补肝肾之阴;取华佗夹脊穴以通调督脉之气;中极、三阴交调肾与膀胱之气;大肠俞、次髎调理大肠功能。

【其他疗法】

1. 皮肤针

用皮肤针叩刺上述阳明经穴。上肢加夹脊(3～5椎);下肢加夹脊(13～21椎)。病变部位腧穴须反复叩刺。

2. 穴位注射

取穴:肩髃　曲池　手三里　外关　髀关　足三里　阳陵泉　绝骨

方法:采用维生素$B_1$100mg,$B_6$50mg,B_{12}100ug等注射液注射于上列穴位,每次2～4穴,每穴注入0.5～1ml,隔日一次,10次为一疗程。

【附注】

1. 痿证疗程较长,需要患者配合,耐心治疗。针刺对某些患者可有不同程度的效果。
2. 为明确其病灶所在和发病原因等,应进行必要的检查。
3. 在针刺治疗的同时,还可以配合药物、推拿和理疗等方法,以提高疗效。
4. 在医生指导下,进行适量的针对性的功能锻炼,具有重要的意义。

第二节　妇儿科病证

一、月经不调

【概说】

月经不调,是指月经周期、经量、经色、经质等发生改变,并伴有其他症状而言。常见的有经行先期、经行后期、经行先后不定期等。常见于垂体前叶或卵巢功能异常而致的月经紊乱等病。

【病因病机】

(一)经行先期:多由忧思气结,久郁化火,或热蕴胞宫,以致血热妄行而经期超前。

(二)经行后期:每因寒邪留滞胞宫,或阳虚血衰,影响冲任,经血不能应期来潮。

(三)经行不定期:生育过多,房事劳倦,或长期患有失血疾病,或脾胃素弱等,损伤肝肾,以致冲任失职,则可导致经行错乱而无定期。

【辨证治疗】

(一)经行先期

1、血热

主证:月经先期,量多,色紫红,质粘稠,心胸烦闷,小便短赤,舌红苔黄,脉数有力。

2、气虚

主证:月经超前,量多,色淡,质清稀,精神疲倦,心悸气短,自觉小腹空坠,舌淡苔薄,脉弱无力。

(二)经行后期

1、血虚

主证：经行后期，血少色淡，小腹空痛，身体瘦弱，面色萎黄，皮肤不润，头晕眼花，或心悸少寐，舌淡红，少苔，脉虚细。

2、血寒

主证：经期延后，色黯而量少，小腹绞痛，得热稍减，肢冷畏寒，苔薄白，脉沉迟。

3、气滞

主证：经期后延，色黯量少，小腹胀满而痛，精神抑郁，胸痞不舒，噫气稍减，胁肋乳房作胀，舌苔薄白，脉弦。

(三) 经行先后无定期

1、肝郁

主证：经期先后不定，经量或多或少，色紫红，质粘稠，经行不畅，胸胁乳房作胀，少腹胀痛，抑郁不乐，时欲叹息，苔薄白，脉弦。

2、肾虚

主证：经期先后不定，经血量少，色淡质稀，头晕耳鸣，腰膝痠软，夜尿较多，大便不实，舌淡苔薄，脉沉弱。

治法：取任脉、足太阴经穴为主。经早只针不灸，用平补平泻法；经迟、经乱，针灸并用。

处方：气海　三阴交

随证配穴：经早：太冲、太溪；经迟：血海、归来；经乱：肾俞、交信、脾俞、足三里。

方义：本方配穴主要作用是通调冲任，理气活血，任主胞胎，任脉之气畅旺，则月事调和；气海为任脉经穴，可调一身元气，以气为血帅，气充则能统血；脾胃为生血之本，脾旺则血有所统，故取三阴交穴；血热经早，加太冲清肝热，太溪益肾水而调经；经迟因血瘀者，泻血海、归来、气海等穴，以行气活血，血虚者用补法并灸，能温经养血；经乱为先天肾气和后天气血均虚，故配肾俞、交信以培本固元，脾俞、足三里扶助中焦而资气血生化之源。

【其他疗法】

耳针

取穴：屏间　卵巢　子宫　肾　肝

方法：每次取 2～4 穴，中、强刺激，留针 15～20min。也可用耳穴埋针。

【附注】

1. 注意经期卫生，忌食生冷或刺激性食物，减轻体力劳动。
2. 本病一般多在经前 3～5 天开始针治，连续 3～5 次，至下次月经来潮前再针。

二、痛　经

【概说】

妇女每逢经期或行经前后，少腹部疼痛，甚至剧痛难忍者，称为痛经。多见于青年妇女。可见于子宫发育不良，过度前倾和后倾，子宫颈管狭窄，子宫内膜异位，盆腔炎等疾病。

【病因病机】

本病可分为虚实两类。其发病原因，实证多由行经期受寒饮冷，以致血因寒而凝滞，瘀血停滞胞中，经行受阻，不通则痛；或因情志郁结，气滞经行不畅而成。虚证每因体质素弱，或大病、久病之后，气血不足，渐至血海空虚，胞脉失养所致。

【辨证治疗】

(一) 实证

主证：多在经前即开始小腹疼痛。如小腹胀痛，经行不畅，量少，色紫暗有块，血块排出后腹痛减轻，胸胁乳房作胀，舌边尖紫，或舌边有瘀点，脉沉弦者，为气滞血瘀证；如少腹冷痛，痛连腰脊，得热则缓，经行量少，色黯有块，苔白腻，脉沉紧者，为寒湿凝滞证。

治法：取任脉、足太阴经穴为主。针用泻法，寒证针灸并用。

处方：中极　次髎　合谷　血海　地机　太冲

方义：中极是任脉经穴，可通调冲任脉气；地机是脾经郄穴，与血海相配可活血通经；太冲是肝经原穴，可疏肝解郁，配合谷可调气行血，通经止痛；次髎是治疗痛经的经验效穴。

(二) 虚证

主证：多在经行末期或经净之后小腹疼痛，痛势绵绵，喜暖喜按，经色淡而量少，质清稀，甚者见形寒怕冷，面色苍白，心悸，头晕等证，脉细无力。

治法：取任脉、背俞穴为主。毫针刺用补法，并灸。

处方：关元　脾俞　肾俞　足三里　三阴交

方义：关元是任脉与足三阴交会穴，配以肾俞，灸之可暖下焦，益精血，以温养冲任；脾俞与足三里、三阴交相配可补脾胃而益气血。气血充足，胞脉得养，冲任调和，则痛经自止。

【其他疗法】

1. 穴位注射

方法：用1%普鲁卡因注射液1ml注射于上髎、次髎穴的皮下，每天一次。

2. 耳针

取穴：子宫　卵巢　屏间　肾

方法：每次取2～4穴，中，强刺激，留针15～20min。也可用耳穴埋针。

【附注】

1、注意经期卫生，避免精神刺激，防止受凉和过食生冷。

2、痛经原因很多，必要时作妇科检查，以明确诊断。

三、经　闭

【概说】

凡发育正常的女子，年龄在14岁左右月经便按时来潮，如超过18周岁而尚未来潮，或已形成月经周期，复停止三个月以上(妊娠和哺乳期除外)，均可称为经闭。常见于神经、精神等因素所致之经闭和卵巢、内分泌功能障碍所致的经闭。

【病因病机】

本病分为虚实两类。根据发病原因、症状、脉象等，分为血枯经闭和血滞经闭。

(一) 血枯经闭：由于多产，思虑过度，素体亏虚，久病体弱等原因致使脾胃生化功能减弱，阴血亏耗过甚，因而血源枯竭，乃致血枯经闭。

(二) 血滞经闭：受寒饮冷，邪气客于胞宫，或情志抑郁气机不畅，瘀血凝结，经脉阻滞，成为血滞经闭。

【辨证治疗】

(一) 血枯经闭

主证：经期延后，经量逐渐减少以至闭止，日久则面色萎黄，精神不振，头晕目眩，食少，便溏,皮肤干燥,舌淡苔白,脉缓弱者为气血虚弱;如见头晕耳鸣,腰膝痠软,口干咽燥,五心烦热,潮热盗汗,舌淡苔少,脉弦细,为精血不足。

治法:取任脉经穴及背俞穴为主。毫针刺用补法,并灸。

处方:关元　肝俞　脾俞　肾俞　足三里　三阴交

方义:脾为后天之本,主消化水谷,化精微而为气血,血源充足,则经血自行,故取脾俞、足三里、三阴交以健脾胃;肾为先天之本,肾气旺则精血自充,故取肾俞、关元以补肾气;肝藏血,故取肝俞以补养肝血。脾能统血,肝能藏血,肾能藏精,冲任得养,则经闭可通。

(二)血滞经闭

主证:月经数月不行,少腹胀痛,拒按,或少腹有痞块,胸胁胀满,舌边紫黯,或有瘀点,脉沉紧。

治法:任脉、足太阴、足厥阴经穴为主。毫针刺用泻法。

处方:中极　归来　血海　太冲　合谷　三阴交

方义:中极是任脉与足三阴经交会穴,能调理冲任而疏导下焦;归来为局部取穴,能疏通胞宫血滞;血海为足太阴经穴,太冲为足厥阴经穴,二穴能疏通肝气,行瘀化滞;合谷、三阴交调理气血,可使气血下行而达通经的目的。

【其他疗法】

1、耳针

取穴:子宫　内分泌　肝　脾　肾　神门　皮质下　卵巢

方法:每次取2～3穴,中等刺激,隔日一次,10次为一个疗程,也可用耳穴埋针。

2、皮肤针

用皮肤针轻度或中度叩刺督脉、膀胱经腰骶部,隔日一次,10次为一个疗程。

【附注】

1、经闭首先应与早期妊娠鉴别。

2、针刺同时必须进行有关检查,以明确发病原因,采取相应的治疗措施。

四、崩　漏

【概说】

妇女非周期性子宫出血,称为崩漏。凡发病急骤,暴下如注,大量出血为崩;发病势缓,经血量少,淋漓不净为漏。崩和漏可互相转化,血崩经急救止血处理,有时可转变为漏下;漏下历时较久,也可转变为血崩。青春期和更年期妇女较为多见。

【病因病机】

本病发生的原因,多由冲任损伤,肝脾失调所致。

(一)肾虚不固:肾主闭藏,房劳过度则伤肾,损及冲任,不能固摄血脉,以致经血非时而下。

(二)肝郁化火:如情志不舒,肝失条达,气血壅滞,郁结化热,藏血失职,以致邪热迫血妄行。

(三)脾气虚弱:如饮食失节,或思虑太过伤脾,脾虚不能统血,轻则漏下不止,重则崩注不止。崩漏分虚实两类。

【辨证治疗】

(一) 实热
主证:阴道骤然大量下血,或淋漓日久,血色深红,烦躁不寐,头晕,舌质红苔黄,脉数。
(二) 气虚
主证:骤然血崩,下血甚多,或淋漓不绝,色淡红,质清稀,身体倦怠,气短懒言,不思饮食,舌质淡,脉细弱。
治法:取任脉、足太阴经穴为主。实热证毫针刺,泻法,不灸;虚寒证毫针刺,补法,多灸。
处方:关元　三阴交　隐白
随证配穴:实热者加血海、水泉;阴虚加内关、太溪;气虚加脾俞、足三里;虚脱加灸百会、气海。
方义:本方主要作用以调补冲任之气为主,并佐以清热化瘀;关元为足三阴、冲任之会,可以调补冲、任脉之气,以加强固摄,制约经血妄行;三阴交为足三阴经之交会穴,有补脾统血作用,为治疗妇科病之要穴;隐白为脾经之井穴,治崩漏常用,偏热加血海、水泉可泄血中之热,以止血热之妄行;气虚加足三里、脾俞以培补中气,使气充而能摄血;阴虚加内关、太溪调养心肾而退虚热;灸百会、气海以振元气,而收回阳固脱之功。

【其他疗法】
1、耳针
取穴:皮质下　内分泌　子宫　卵巢　肾上腺
方法:找寻敏感点。留针1～2h,可间歇行针。
2、穴位注射
选取生殖区左右,两侧同时捻转,约3～5min,间歇5min左右,再捻第二遍,共捻三遍。

【附注】
1、绝经期妇女,如反复多次出血,需作妇科检查,应警惕肿瘤。
2、大量出血时,出现虚脱,应及时采取抢救措施。

五、带　下

【概说】
带下,是指妇女阴道分泌物增多,连绵不断而言。临床以带下白色较为多见,所以通常称为白带。
本证常见于阴道炎、宫颈炎、盆腔炎和子宫颈癌等疾患中。

【病因病机】
带下的病因,多由任脉不固,带脉失约、以致水湿浊液下注而成。
(一) 脾虚:饮食劳倦、损伤脾胃,运化失职,聚湿下行,发为带下。其中黄带多为脾经湿热,白带多属虚寒。
(二) 脾肾阳虚:肾阳不足,脾肾阳虚,水湿下注,而成白带。

【辨证治疗】
(一) 脾虚
主证:带下量多,色白或淡黄,质粘稠,无臭,如涕如唾,连绵不断,面色萎黄或㿠白,精神疲倦,纳少便溏,下肢浮肿,舌淡苔白腻,脉缓弱。
(二) 湿热

主证：带下色黄量多，质粘稠，其气秽臭，阴中瘙痒，大便干结，小便短赤，脉濡数，舌苔黄腻；或带下色黄兼赤，口苦咽干，烦热，心悸失眠，急躁易怒，舌苔黄，脉弦数。

（三）肾虚

主证：带下量多，质清而稀，淋漓不断，腰痠如折，小腹发冷，小便频数清长，大便溏薄，舌淡苔薄白，脉沉。

治法：取任脉、足太阴、足少阴经穴为主。湿热，毫针泻法，不灸；脾虚、肾虚，用毫针刺，平补平泻，多灸。

处方：带脉　中极　次髎　气海　三阴交　太冲

随证配穴：湿热加行间、阴陵泉；脾虚加关元、足三里；肾虚加肾俞、关元、复溜、大赫；阴部瘙痒加蠡沟；带下赤色加血海；热重者加曲池。

方义：中极为任脉经穴，膀胱募穴，泻之可清利下焦湿热；带脉穴为带脉与足少阳的交会穴，能固摄带脉，主治带下；次髎为近取穴，可清热利湿，功可止带；三阴交、太冲既能健脾利湿，又能清泻肝火；阴陵泉、足三里穴相配，有健脾利湿之效；肾俞、关元、大赫、复溜四穴，为邻近与远端取穴相结合，有助阳补肾的作用，使肾能闭藏，任固带约，可止带下；蠡沟可清肝经湿热，血海清泻血热；热重配曲池以清热，可相得益彰，提高疗效。

【其他疗法】

1、耳针

取穴：子宫　卵巢　内分泌　膀胱　肾

方法：每次3～5穴，留针15～20min。

2、艾条灸

取穴：命门　神阙　中极　隐白　三阴交

方法：艾条熏灸，每穴5min，隔日一次，10～15次为一个疗程。本法适用于虚寒带下。

【附注】

1、针灸治疗白带有一定疗效，如发现黄、赤带须作妇科检查。

2、注意卫生，保持外阴部清洁。

六、阴　挺

【概说】

阴挺，即子宫脱垂。正常子宫位置在盆腔中央，呈前倾前曲位，子宫底平耻骨联合，子宫颈平坐骨棘。凡子宫位置沿阴道下移，低于坐骨棘水平以下，甚至脱出阴道口外者，称为阴挺。

【病因病机】

发病原因，主要由于素体虚弱，产后气血未复，过早地参加体力劳动，或因多产伤气，以致气虚下陷，胞络松弛，不能收摄胞宫所致。

【辨证治疗】

（一）气虚

主证：阴道中有物下坠，或下坠于阴道口，或阴道口外，甚者坠出数寸，状如鹅卵，其色淡红，自觉小腹下坠，精神疲惫，心悸气短，小便频数，白带较多，舌质淡，苔薄，脉虚弱。

（二）肾虚

主证：阴中有物脱出阴道口外，腰腿痠软，小腹下坠，或阴道干涩，小便频数，头晕耳鸣，舌淡红,脉沉弱。

治法:取任脉、督脉经穴为主。毫针刺,补法并灸。

处方:百会 关元 气海 子宫 中脘

随证配穴:气虚者加足三里、三阴交;肾虚者配大赫、照海。

方义:本方以升举阳气,固摄胞宫为目的。百会为督脉经穴,位于巅顶,取百会乃"下病高取"、"陷者举之"之意;气海、关元有益气固摄之功;子宫为经外奇穴,是治疗阴挺有效穴位;中脘补益中气,气虚者配足三里、三阴交,可健脾益气,并补中气;肾虚者配大赫、照海,以补益肾气,固摄胞宫。

【其他疗法】

1、穴位注射

取穴:脾俞 肝俞 提托穴 维胞

方法:用5%当归注射液,每穴0.5～1.0ml,隔日一次,两侧交替取穴,进针0.8～1寸,注入药液,10次为一疗程。

2、电针

取穴:子宫 足三里

方法:足三里用补法,子宫穴用二寸毫针向子宫方向斜刺,以病人感到子宫上抽,腰部和阴部酸胀为度,通电15～20min。

3、头针

选取两侧生殖区、足运感区,间歇捻针,留针15～20min。

【附注】

1、针灸治疗不同程度的子宫脱垂均有效果。

2、体质虚弱或有继发感染者可配合药物治疗。

3、治疗期间不宜参加重体力劳动,并嘱患者作提肛肌运动锻炼。

七、妊娠恶阻

【概说】

妊娠恶阻是指妇女妊娠二、三月,出现恶心,呕吐,头晕,厌食或食入即吐的一种病证,是孕妇早期最常见的疾患。严重的恶阻可使孕妇迅速消瘦,或诱发其它疾病。

产生恶阻的原因,多由于平时胃气虚弱,受孕后胎气上逆犯胃,致胃气不降,发生恶阻。

【病因病机】

(一)脾胃虚弱:胃气素虚,受孕之初,月经停闭,血海不泻,冲脉之气较盛,其气上逆犯胃,胃气不得下降,反随冲气上逆而发为恶阻。

(二)肝胃不和:孕后阴血聚以养胎,肝血虚少,致肝阳偏盛,木旺克土,上逆犯胃,胃气不降,反而上逆,发为恶阻。

【辨证治疗】

(一)脾胃虚弱

主证:孕后二、三个月,恶心,呕吐,或食入即吐,或呕吐清涎,脘腹胀满,神疲思睡,舌淡苔白,脉滑而无力。

(二)肝胃不和

主证：妊娠初期，呕吐苦水或酸水，脘闷胁痛，嗳气叹息，精神抑郁，头晕目胀，舌苔微黄，脉弦滑。

治法：取足阳明、任脉、手厥阴经穴为主。针刺平补平泻法，以健脾和胃，疏肝解郁，降逆止呕。

处方：中脘　内关　足三里

随证配穴：脾胃虚弱加公孙；肝胃不和加膻中、太冲。

方义：中脘穴为腑会，胃之募穴，六腑皆禀气于胃，中脘又是任脉，手太阳，手少阳、足阳明四脉之会，故中脘可和胃降逆，疏调三焦气机，足三里为胃经合穴，功可降逆气，又为全身强壮要穴，可补益气血，为气血不足之主穴，与中脘相配，起到健脾和胃，补益气血，降逆止呕作用；内关为手厥阴经络穴，功可理气宽胸，和胃降逆、止呕，与中脘相配更增强疏调三焦气机之效；脾胃虚弱加公孙穴，因公孙为脾经络穴，功可健脾和胃；公孙又为八脉交会穴，通冲脉，冲脉起于胞宫，冲脉又为血海，十二经之海，故公孙穴可以补气降冲逆，而止呕吐；肝胃不和加膻中者，因膻中为心包之募穴，又为八会穴之气会，故膻中穴可理气活血，通调三焦气机，以治胁胀痛，叹息嗳气，精神抑郁之症；太冲为肝经原穴，功可平肝降逆气，疏肝、降逆和胃止呕。

【附注】

1、妊娠早期，胞胎本固，针治时，取穴不宜过多，手法不宜过重，以免影响胎气。

2、病者宜保持安静，卧床休息，切忌恣食生冷，或油腻之品，宜少食多餐，调养胃气。

八、胎位不正

【概说】

胎位不正是指妊娠30周后，胎儿在子宫体内的位置不正，多见于经产妇或腹壁松弛的孕妇。产妇本身多无自觉症状，经产科检查后才明确诊断，常见的有臀位、横位等。

【病因病机】

胞脉系于肾，若素体肾虚，或房劳过度，或多产伤肾，精血亏损，复加受孕之后，精血聚而养胎，如精血不能通过胞脉濡养胞宫，因此胎位难以维持常态。

【辨证治疗】

产妇一般无自觉症状，需经产科检查后才能明确诊断。

取穴：双侧至阴穴。

方法：治疗时患者松解腰带，坐在靠背椅上或仰卧在床上，以艾条灸两侧至阴穴15～20min，每日1～2次，至胎位转正为止。据报道，成功率达80%以上，经产妇较初产妇效果更好，以妊娠七个月者成功率最高，八个月以上者较差，也有采用针刺，但多数用灸法。

【附注】

胎位不正原因很多，须详细检查，如因骨盆狭窄，子宫畸形等引起，应作其他处理。

九、滞产

【概说】

产妇临产后总产程超过24小时者称为滞产。古人称为"难产"或"产难"。

【病因病机】

多由初产妇精神紧张，或临盆过早，致胞浆早破，下血过多。或因体弱气血不足，胞宫收缩无力等引起。

【辨证治疗】

(一) 气血虚弱

主证:产时少腹阵痛微弱,坠胀不甚,或下血量多色淡,久产不下,面色苍白,精神倦怠,心悸气短,舌淡,脉虚弱。

(二) 气滞血瘀

主证:腰腹剧痛,下血量少,色黯色,久产不下,面色青黯,精神抑郁,胸脘胀满,时欲呕恶,舌质黯红,脉沉实。

治法:取足太阴、手阳明经穴为主。毫针刺,虚者用补法,实者用泻法。

处方:合谷　三阴交　至阴　独阴

随证配穴:气血虚弱者配足三里、复溜;气滞血瘀者配太冲、肩井。

方义:合谷为手阳明经原穴,可行气理气,活血化瘀,三阴交为足三阴之会,既可行气治瘀,又可益气养血;再配膀胱经井穴至阴,奇穴独阴,以增强催产之力。气血虚弱者配足三里,强壮脾胃,生化气血,复溜补肾,以助产力;气滞血瘀者配太冲行气活血,肩井理气催产。

【其他疗法】

耳针

取穴:子宫　皮质下　内分泌　肾　膀胱

刺法:中等刺激,每隔3～5分钟捻转一次。

【附注】

针灸对子宫收缩无力的滞产,具有催产作用。如因子宫畸形,骨盆狭窄等引起的滞产,应作其他处理。

十、乳　少(附回乳)

【概说】

产妇分娩后2～3天开始分泌乳汁。如果乳汁分泌不足,有的甚至全无乳汁者,称为乳少,或乳汁不行。

【病因病机】

(一) 气血虚弱:乳汁为气血所化,如果产妇体质虚弱,脾胃运化功能减退,或临产失血过多,以致气血不足,不能生化乳汁。

(二) 肝郁气滞:亦有因情志失调,如忧虑紧张,以致气机失畅,经脉运行受阻而乳汁不行者。

【辨证治疗】

(一) 气血虚弱

主证:产后乳汁分泌不足,甚至点滴不下,或哺乳期中日见减少,乳房无胀痛感,面色苍白,皮肤干燥,心悸,神疲,食少,便溏,舌淡苔少,脉虚细。

(二) 肝郁气滞

主证:产后乳汁不行,乳房胀满而痛,精神抑郁,胸闷胁痛,胃脘胀满,食欲减退,舌淡红,脉弦。

治法:取足阳明经穴为主。气血虚弱者,毫针刺用补法并灸;肝郁气滞者,毫针刺用泻法,或平补平泻。

处方：乳根　膻中　少泽

随证配穴：气血虚弱者加脾俞、足三里、三阴交；肝郁气滞者加期门、内关、太冲。

方义：乳房为足阳明经所过，乳根属胃经穴，又在乳部，取之可疏通阳明经气而催乳；气会膻中，可理气通乳；少泽为通乳经验效穴；脾俞、足三里、三阴交有调补脾胃，生血化乳的功能；期门、太冲可疏肝解郁，配内关以宽胸理气而通乳。

【其他疗法】

耳针

取穴：乳腺　内分泌　胸　肾上腺

方法：找敏感点，捻针数分钟，或埋针1～7天。

【附注】

乳少，在治疗同时宜补充营养，多吃汤类。

附：回乳

若产后不欲哺乳者，可用针灸回乳。

取穴：足临泣　光明。

方法：针后加灸，每穴艾灸10min，每天1次，连续针灸3～5次。

十一、急惊风

【概说】

急惊风类似今之惊厥，为儿科常见急症之一。临床以神昏、四肢抽搐、口噤、角弓反张等为主症。因其发病迅速，症情急暴，故称为急惊风。多见于三周岁以下小儿。

本证常见于小儿高热、脑膜炎、脑炎、血钙过低、脑发育不全、癫痫等疾病。

【病因病机】

（一）外感时邪：小儿形气未充，质属纯阳，如外感时邪，易致阳气不得宣泄，实热内郁，引起肝风。

（二）痰火积滞：因乳食不节，脾胃受损，以致水精布散失常，水液凝滞成痰，痰浊内蕴，生热化风而成。

（三）暴受惊恐：亦有暴受惊恐，而突发惊厥抽风者。

【辨证治疗】

主证：本病初起壮热面赤，摇头弄舌，咬牙龂齿，睡中惊悸，手足乱动，烦躁不宁，继即神志昏迷，两目直视，牙关紧闭，四肢抽搐、颤动，或阵发，或持续不已。呼吸迫促，便秘溲赤，脉浮数或弦滑，指纹青紫相兼。

治法：取督脉和手阳明经穴为主，辅以足厥阴经穴。毫针浅刺，疾出不留，用泻法；或三棱针点刺出血。

处方：水沟　印堂　十宣　合谷　太冲

随证配穴：壮热加大椎、曲池；痰多加列缺、丰隆；口噤加颊车、合谷。

方义：本方旨在熄风镇惊。水沟、印堂位居督脉，两穴有开窍醒脑镇惊作用；刺十宣出血能泄诸经邪热；合谷、太冲二穴合用，谓之开四关，能治小儿惊厥；热甚者配大椎、曲池，共泻阳热之亢盛；取肺、胃络穴列缺、丰隆，具有宣肺化痰之功；口噤者配合谷、颊车以松缓口颊。

【其他疗法】
耳针
取穴:交感　神门　皮质下　脑点　心
方法:重证强刺激,可留针 1h。
【附注】
针刺对惊厥的缓解有较好效果,但必须查明发生惊厥的原因,采取针对病因治疗的措施。

十二、慢惊风
【概说】
慢惊风又称"慢脾风",以抽风、形瘦、腹泻等为主要证候。多见于三周岁以下小儿,久病中虚或大病之后,证情每多严重。
【病因病机】
慢惊风多见于大吐大泻之后,或脾胃虚弱,化源不足;或过服寒凉攻伐药物,脾胃受戕,中阳衰竭;或热病伤阴,肾阴不足,肝血亏损,木失濡养,虚风内动,亦有因急惊风失治迁延所致。
【辨证治疗】
主证:面黄肌瘦,形神疲惫,四肢倦怠或厥冷,呼吸微弱,囟门低陷,昏睡露睛,时有抽搐,因于脾阳虚弱者可见大便溏薄,色青带绿,足跗和面部浮肿,脉象沉迟无力,舌质淡白;因于肝肾阴亏者,还可见神倦虚烦,面色潮红,舌光少苔或无苔,脉沉细而数。
治法:取任脉、足阳明及背俞穴为主。毫针刺用补法并灸。
处方:中脘　章门　气海　天枢　足三里　太冲　脾俞　胃俞　肝俞　肾俞
方义:取腑会中脘及足阳明合穴足三里,培补脾胃,以扶后天之本;取脾之募穴章门,以温补脾阳;气海培元以助健运;天枢为大肠之募穴,灸之能温调脾胃虚寒,助运化而治便溏;太冲为肝之原穴能养血熄风;脾、胃、肝、肾俞能健脾益肾,平肝熄风。综合本方具有温补脾胃,培元熄风之效。
【其他疗法】
皮肤针
主穴:大椎　身柱　气海　足三里　胃俞　脾俞　胸$_5$～腰$_2$夹脊
备穴:关元　百会　章门　天枢
【附注】
慢惊风类似慢性脑脊髓膜炎,针灸对本病仅能改善症状。应配合中西药物同时治疗。

十三、小儿腹泻
【概说】
小儿腹泻,是以大便次数增多,便下稀薄,或水样便为特征的一种病证。本病为儿科常见疾病,四季皆可发生,夏秋两季多见。
【病因病机】
小儿脾胃薄弱,饮食不节或不洁,调护失宜,均可使脾胃受损,运化失职,不能腐熟水谷,水谷不分,并走大肠,则成腹泻。故内伤饮食是形成腹泻一个重要因素。小儿脏腑娇嫩,若不慎感受外邪,困扰脾胃,亦可使脾胃的运化失常而生本病。

【辨证治疗】
主证:腹胀肠鸣,时时作痛,痛即欲泻,泻后痛缓;一日可泻多次,泻物酸腐臭秽,或完谷不化,频作嗳气,不思饮食,舌苔腻,脉滑而实者,属伤食腹泻;如泻下稀薄,色黄而臭,腹部疼痛,身热口渴,肛门灼热,小便短赤,舌苔黄腻,脉滑数者为湿热泻。

治法:取足阳明经穴为主。刺法不留针。

处方:天枢　上巨虚　四缝

随证配穴:伤食者加建里、气海;湿热泻加曲池、合谷、阴陵泉。

方义:天枢属足阳明胃经,又为大肠募穴,上巨虚为大肠腑下合穴,二穴同用可调肠腑而止泻;四缝能消食导滞,健运止泻;建里、气海具有消食滞,除胀满,健脾胃的作用;曲池、合谷可以清热,配阴陵泉以利湿止泻。

【附注】
1、泄泻严重者,易导致阴阳俱伤,气脱阴竭的重证,应予以注意。
2、治疗时应控制饮食,或给少量容易消化的食物。

十四、小儿疳积

【概说】
疳疾亦称疳积,是以形体干枯羸瘦,头发稀疏,腹部胀大,青筋暴露,饮食异常,精神疲惫为特征的一种儿科病证。

本病可见于小儿喂养不足,饮食失调,以及慢性腹泻,肠寄生虫病,结核病等。

【病因病机】
多由饮食不节,断乳过早,喂养不当,病后失调,药物攻伐太过,以及虫积等因素,使脾胃功能受损,津液耗伤,不能消磨水谷,久之积滞生热,迁延成为疳症。

【辨证治疗】
主证:发病缓慢,初起身有微热,或午后潮热,口干腹胀,便泻秽臭,尿如米泔,烦躁啼哭,不思饮食;继则积滞内停,腹大脐突,面色萎黄,形体消瘦,肌肤甲错,毛发稀疏,舌苔浊腻或光剥,脉象虚弱者属脾胃虚损证。如症见饮食异常或饥饱无度,或嗜食异物者,多属虫积。

治法:取足太阴、阳明经穴为主。毫针浅刺不留针。

处方:下脘　足三里　太白　四缝

随证配穴:虫积配百虫窠;潮热加大椎。亦可点刺脾俞、胃俞、肝俞。

方义:疳积的病机,不外乎脾胃运化失常所致。脾胃为后天之本,下脘处于胃之下口,故可消积化滞;足三里为胃之下合穴,可扶土以补中气;太白为脾经原穴,可健脾而化积消滞;四缝,是治疗疳疾有效奇穴;百虫窠是治虫积的有效穴位。点刺脾、胃、肝俞可以振奋脾胃之气,恢复其健运动能。

【附注】
1、疳疾患儿饮食须定时定量,不宜过饥过饱或过食香甜油腻。
2、婴儿断乳时,应给予适量营养食物。
3、凡因寄生虫病或结核病引起的,须治疗原发病。

十五、小儿瘫痪

【概说】

小儿瘫痪属于"痿证"范围。本篇所述为"小儿麻痹后遗证"。

【病因病机】

本病主要由于感受风、湿、热邪,时疫邪毒,从口鼻侵犯脾胃,蕴积成热,内窜经络,致经络壅阻,气血失调,筋脉肌肉失养,则出现肢体痿软瘫痪。病久精血亏损,病及肝肾,筋骨肌肉枯萎,故病变后期出现筋软骨萎、肌肉萎缩、弛缓不收及骨骼畸形等症。

【辨证治疗】

主证:本病主症瘫痪,表现肢体瘫痪呈弛缓性,以下肢为多见,或现单瘫、半身瘫痪。亦有腹肌、肋间肌、膈肌瘫痪者,病情比较严重。若病久不愈,则患者肌肉逐渐萎缩,躯干各部发生畸形,形成顽固性瘫痪。

治法:以手足阳明经穴为主。辅以病部取穴。根据病情采用泻法或补法。

处方:

上肢瘫痪:肩髃　曲池　外关　合谷　大椎　天柱

下肢瘫痪:环跳　髀关　足三里　阳陵泉　悬钟　昆仑　三阴交　解溪　腰$_{1-5}$夹脊穴

腹肌瘫痪:梁门　天枢　带脉　关元

随证配穴:膝反屈加承扶、委中、承山;足内翻加风市、申脉;足外翻加太溪、照海;腕下垂加阳池、中泉。

方义:本方根据《素问·痿论》"治痿独取阳明"之意,故以取手足阳明经穴为主,方中用筋会阳陵泉,髓会绝骨以增强濡养筋骨的作用。其它腧穴均为局部近取,用以疏通经气。夹脊穴为经外奇穴,有调节脏腑,疏通经络的作用,亦属近部取穴的范畴。

【其他疗法】

1、皮肤针

取穴可参照以上配方,方法每日或隔日一次,10~15次为一个疗程。

2、穴位埋线

取穴参照以上配方。

【附注】

本病近年来采用口服脊髓灰质炎减毒活疫苗进行预防,发病已明显减少。后遗症应及时治疗,并配合功能锻炼,关节严重畸形者,可做患肢矫形手术。

十六、痄腮

【概述】

痄腮,又名"蛤蟆瘟",是以发病急,耳下腮部肿胀疼痛为特征的一种急性传染性疾病。现代医学称"流行性腮腺炎"。

本病主要是由于风热疫毒所引起。风热疫毒从口鼻而入,客于少阳,郁而不散,气血壅滞,结于腮颊所致。

【辨证治疗】

主证:轻症,仅觉耳下腮部疼痛,继而肿胀,如无其他见症,可在数日后逐渐消退。较重的,初起有恶寒、发热、头痛、呕吐等症,并渐见腮部焮热红肿,咀嚼困难,病发一侧或两侧。严重的,则见高热烦渴,并发睾丸肿大,舌苔黄腻,脉浮数或滑数。

治法:取手少阳、阳明经穴为主。毫针浅刺泻法。

处方:翳风　颊车　外关　曲池　合谷

随证配穴:恶寒发热加列缺;高热加大椎、十二井穴;睾丸肿痛加太冲、曲泉。

方义:本病患部属于少阳经,翳风为手足少阳之会穴,能宣散局部气血之壅滞;手阳明经上循面颊,故取颊车、曲池、合谷以疏泄邪热而解毒;远取外关以利少阳气机,可奏清热消肿之功;列缺散风解毒;大椎、十二井清热;太冲、曲泉以疏解厥阴之经气。

【其他疗法】

灯火灸

方法:先将病侧角孙穴处头发剪短,用灯心草蘸香油点燃,迅速触点穴位,闻及"叭"的响声,立即提起,灸治1~2次即可,若肿热不退,次日再灸一次。

【附注】

1、针灸治疗腮腺炎效果良好。如有严重合并症,应配合其他疗法。

2、患者自起病至腮肿完全消退时,须进行隔离。

3、流行季节针刺颊车、合谷,每日二次,可作为预防。

第三节　外科病证

一、风　疹

【概说】

风疹,即荨麻疹。又有"瘾疹"、"风疹块"等名称,是一种常见的皮肤病。其特征是皮肤上出现鲜红色或苍白色的瘙痒性风团。急性期短期发作后可痊愈。

【病因病机】

(一)风邪侵袭:本病多因腠理不固,为风邪侵袭,遏于肌肤而成。

(二)胃肠积热:因胃肠积热,内不得泄,外不能达,郁于肌肤而发。

(三)肠内寄生虫:因体质因素,过食鱼虾或患肠道寄生虫病而诱发者。

【辨证治疗】

主证:本病可发生于身体任何部位,以肱股内侧较多,发病迅速,突然在皮肤上出现大小不等形状不一的皮疹,多成块成片;有的呈丘疹样,此起彼伏,疏密不一,并伴有皮肤异常瘙痒,并常因气候冷热而减轻或加剧。本病皮疹的发生与消失都很迅速,不留任何痕迹。如同时发于咽喉可见呼吸困难;发于胃肠兼有恶心、呕吐、腹痛、腹泻等症状。

治法:取手阳明、足太阴经穴为主。毫针刺用泻法。

处方:曲池　合谷　血海　膈俞　委中　天井

随证配穴:呼吸困难加天突;恶心、呕吐者加内关;腹痛腹泻加天枢。

方义:本病为风邪遏于肌表,曲池、合谷同属阳明,取之可疏通肌表,清泄阳明;血海主血分病,配合谷、曲池用泻法可疏风邪,清血热;委中为血郄,膈俞为血之会穴,凡热毒瘾疹,蕴于血分等尤为相宜;天井为三焦之合穴,取之以利三焦之通调而宣郁热。

【其他疗法】

耳针

取穴：神门　肺　枕　内分泌　肾上腺

方法：捻转并留针15～30min。或在耳后划刺，或耳后静脉放血，每日一次。

【附注】

针灸治疗风疹效果良好。慢性者，尽可能查明其原因，进行病因治疗。皮肤瘙痒症亦可参照上方治疗。

二、痤　疮

【概论】

本病是指面部生粟疹脓疱，破时出白粉汁为特征的面部皮肤病。本病又称"酒刺"、"痤"、"肺风粉刺"，多见于青年男女，好发于颊面，偶可累及胸背，其发病多与血热有关。

【病因病机】

（一）过食肥甘厚味，脾胃湿热内蕴，上蒸于面，发为痤疮。

（二）肺经蕴热，外受风邪，风热上蒸于面，而发痤疮。

（三）体热冷渍，血热蕴结头面，发为痤疮。

【辨证治疗】

主证：初起患处有针尖至粟米大小黑头粉刺，挤压时可出线状膏脂，渐至顶部生脓疱，硬结，微疼，消退后结疤。

治法：取手太阴、足太阳经穴为主。毫针刺用泻法，以清热解毒。

处方：鱼际　中府　肺俞　合谷

方义：肺主皮毛，鱼际为肺经荥水穴，中府为肺之募穴，二穴相配以清肺热；肺俞宣肺，开发腠理；合谷理气，解表清热，四穴共奏清肺泄火解毒之效。

【其它针法】

1、电针

取穴：曲池　合谷　大椎　肺俞　足三里　三阴交

方法：针刺得气后，通电，每次通电2～3穴，留针20min，日1次，20次为一疗程。

2、耳针

取穴：肺　神门　交感　内分泌　皮质下

方法：耳穴常规消毒，将中药王不留行籽压于穴上，胶布固定，嘱患者每天按压3～5次，每次3min，以微痛为度。两耳轮换贴，5次为一疗程。

3、火针

取穴：膈俞　肺俞　大椎

操作：将针烧红、迅速刺入穴位、深2～3分，10次一疗程，隔日一次。

4、自血穴位注射

取穴：足三里单侧或双侧。

方法：先抽好自血约4ml左右，迅速注入足三里穴，每穴2ml，每周一次，5次一疗程。

三、丹　毒

【概说】

丹毒是一种急性传染性皮肤病,发病时皮肤突然变赤,状如涂丹,因此名为丹毒。因其发病部位不同而有多种名称,如发于头面的称"抱头火丹",游走全身的称"赤游丹",生腿足的名为"流火"。

【病因病机】

本病多由脾胃湿热蕴积,或风邪热毒外袭,以致血分生热,郁于肌肤;或因皮肤破损,毒邪侵入所致。发于头面者,多偏于风热;发于下肢者,多偏于湿热。

【辨证治疗】

主证:发病急速,患处皮肤鲜红灼热疼痛,状如云片,边缘清楚,很快向四周蔓延。中间由鲜红转为暗红,经数天后脱屑而愈。如兼见发热恶寒,头痛,苔薄黄,舌质红,脉浮数者为风热证;兼见发热心烦,口渴胸闷,胃纳不香,便秘溲赤,舌苔黄腻,脉濡数者为湿热证;如见壮热呕吐,神昏谵语,时有痉厥,为邪毒内攻之证。

治法:取手足阳明、足太阳经穴为主。毫针刺用泻法,或局部点刺出血。

处方:曲池 合谷 曲泽 委中 血海 阿是穴

随证配穴:风热加风池;湿热加足三里、阴陵泉;身热加大椎;邪毒内攻加十二井穴、劳宫;便秘加支沟。

方义:曲池、合谷可疏散阳明风热;泻血海、委中、曲泽、阿是穴点刺出血,可清血分之热;足三里、阴陵泉可清利湿热;刺十二井出血和泻劳宫有泻热启闭,清心开窍的作用;泻大椎、风池有退热解表之功;取支沟有清热通便之效。

【其他疗法】

刺络拔罐

方法:在红肿部用三棱针散刺或用皮肤针叩刺,放出血液,必要时,在针刺后加拔火罐。每日1～2次。

【附注】

针刺治疗本病应注意消毒,防止感染。如因混合感染而形成溃疡,或出现败血症及脓毒血症时,必须考虑中西医综合治疗。

四、蛇 丹

【概说】

本病为在皮肤上出现簇集成群,累累如串珠的疱疹,疼痛剧烈的皮肤病。因此它每多缠腰而发,故又名缠腰火丹。亦有发生于胸部及面部者。多发生于春、秋两季。

本病相当于现代医学之带状疱疹。

【病因病机】

本病多由肝经郁火和脾胃湿热内蕴,又复感受火热时邪,以致引动肝火,湿热蕴蒸,浸淫皮肤、脉络而发为疱疹。

【辨证治疗】

主证:初起患部有束带状刺痛,局部皮肤潮红,伴有轻度发热,乏力,食欲不振等全身症状。皮疹呈簇集状水泡,水疱如绿豆或黄豆大小,中间夹以血疱或脓疱,排列如带状。皮疹多数发生在单侧,常见于肋间,次为头面部。疱疹在2～3周后,渐见干燥结痂,最后痂退而愈。愈后一般不留瘢痕。少数患者有时疼痛可延续较长时间。

治法:循经取穴为主,辅以局部取穴。毫针刺用泻法。
处方:曲池　合谷　血海　委中　阳陵泉　太冲
方法:先辨清疱疹的头尾,先在距头尾5分处用三棱针点刺4～5针,疱疹两侧酌情点刺数针,微出血为宜。然后再针上组穴。日针治一次。留针20～30min

方义:三棱针局部围刺,点刺出血,可清泻邪毒;曲池、合谷疏风解热;血海、委中清血中之热;阳陵泉、太冲可清肝胆湿热。

【其他疗法】
耳针
取穴:相应敏感点　肺　肝　下屏尖　屏间
方法:取2～3个穴,捻转强刺激,留针20～30min。

【附注】
针刺带状疱疹镇痛效果明显。少数病例合并化脓感染者须外科处理。

五、疔　疮

【概说】
疔疮是常见的外科急症,好发于面部和指端。因其初起形小根深,底脚坚硬如钉,故名疔疮。又因发病部位和形状各异,又有不同的名称,如生于人中部的称"人中疔",生于指头上的称"蛇头疔",疔疮上有一条红丝蔓延直上的称"红丝疔"。

【病因病机】
本病多由恣食辛辣,膏梁厚味等,以致脏腑积热,毒由内发;或因肌肤不洁,邪毒外侵,气血阻滞,发于腠理而成。若毒邪盛则流窜经络,内攻脏腑而成危候。

【辨证治疗】
主证:本病初起状如粟粒,色或黄或紫,或起水疱、脓疱,根结坚硬如钉,自觉麻痒而疼痛轻微,继则红肿灼热,疼痛增剧,多有寒热。如见壮热烦躁,眩晕呕吐,神识昏愦,舌质红,舌苔黄,脉数者,为疔毒内攻之象,称为"疔疮走黄"。如发生于四肢,患处有红丝上窜的,名为"红丝疔。"

治法:取督脉、手阳明经穴为主。毫针刺用泻法,或三棱针点刺出血。
处方:身柱　灵台　合谷　委中
随证配穴:根据患部所属经脉选穴。如生于面部的配商阳、曲池;生于食指端的加曲池、迎香;生于颞部的加阳陵泉、足窍阴;生于足小趾、次趾的加阳陵泉、听会;如系红丝疔,可沿红丝的止点,依次点刺到起点,以泄其恶血。

方义:督脉统率诸阳,泻身柱、灵台以疏泄阳邪火毒,二穴又为治疔疮的经验穴。合谷为手阳明经之原穴,阳明多气多血,泻之以泄阳明火毒,面唇疔疮尤为适宜。委中为足太阳之合穴,刺血以清泄血热。随证配穴是根据"经脉所通,主治所及"的原理进行取穴治疗的。

【其他疗法】
挑治
方法:在背部脊柱两旁,寻取丘疹样突起处,用粗针挑治,每日一次。

【附注】
1、疔疮初起,切忌挤压、挑治。患部不宜针刺和拔罐。红肿发硬时忌手术切开,以免引起感染扩散。

2、疔疮走黄,症情凶险,须及时抢救。疔疮如已成脓,应转外科处理。
3、治疗时忌食鱼腥、虾、蟹等发物。

六、乳　痈

【概说】

乳痈是乳房急性化脓性疾病。多发于产后哺乳期,发生于怀孕期者较为少见。

本病相当于现代医学之急性乳腺炎。

【病因病机】

(一)肝郁气结:忧思恼怒,肝气郁结。

(二)胃经积热:多食厚味,胃经积热。

(三)乳头破裂:因乳头皮肤破裂,外邪火毒侵入乳房,致使脉络阻塞,排乳不畅,火毒与积乳互凝,而结肿成痈。

【辨证治疗】

主证:乳房红肿疼痛,多发生于产后。初起乳房结块,肿胀疼痛,排乳困难,寒热头痛,恶心烦渴,此时痈脓尚未形成;若乳部肿块增大,焮红疼痛,时有跳痛者,为化脓征象。

治法:取足厥阴、少阳、阳明经穴为主。毫针刺用泻法。

处方:肩井　膻中　乳根　少泽　足三里　太冲

随证配穴:寒热加合谷、外关;乳房胀痛加足临泣。

方义:乳痈乃胃热肝郁所致,故取太冲以舒肝解郁,取足三里、乳根以降胃火,消阳明之结滞;膻中可疏调气机,解郁通乳;肩井能疏理胸胁之气,是治疗乳痈有效穴位;少泽为治疗乳痈经验效穴;合谷能治阳明之热,外关通于阳维,主治寒热;足临泣可宣散气血,疏通乳汁之凝滞,以治疗乳房胀痛。

【其他疗法】

1、灸法:初起时用葱白或大蒜捣烂,敷患处,用艾条薰灸10～20min,每天1～2次。本方适应于乳痈尚未成脓。

2、拔罐法:选用适当大小玻璃火罐在溃破处吸拔脓液。本法适应于痈脓形成阶段。

七、肠　痈

【概说】

肠痈是肠内发生痈肿的急性腹部外科疾患。古代文献根据疼痛部位分为大肠痈和小肠痈。凡痛在天枢附近者称为"大肠痈",病在关元附近者,称为"小肠痈"。又因本病有右足不能伸直的症状,故又有"缩脚肠痈"之称。

本病相当于现代医学之急性阑尾炎。

【病因病机】

本病多由饮食不节,宿食停滞,恣食生冷,寒湿失调,或饱食之后急促奔走,肠腑传导功能失常,湿热蕴结于肠内,气机壅塞,气血瘀阻而致。热瘀互结,可使血败肉腐而成痈脓。

【辨证治疗】

主证:初起脘部或绕脐疼痛,旋即转移至右下腹,以手按之其痛加剧,痛处固定不移,右腿屈而难伸,并有发热恶寒,恶心呕吐,便秘,尿黄,舌苔薄腻而黄,脉数有力等证。若痛势剧烈,腹皮拘急,拒按,局部可触及肿块,壮热自汗,脉象洪数等,则属重证。

治法:取手足阳明经穴为主。毫针刺用泻法,留针20~40min,一般每日针1~2次,重证可每隔4h针刺一次。

处方:天枢 阑尾穴 曲池 上巨虚

随证配穴:发热加大椎、合谷;呕吐加内关、中脘。

方义:阑尾穴是治疗肠痈的经验效穴,上巨虚为大肠的下合穴,配大肠募穴天枢,以通调肠中积滞,化湿除热,行气止痛;曲池是大肠经合穴,可通导肠腑,兼泻积热。配大椎、曲池加强退热作用;配中脘、内关以和胃止呕。

【其他疗法】

1、穴位注射

取穴:阑尾穴、腰部压痛点。

方法:用10%葡萄糖注射液5ml,注射深度0.5~0.8寸,每日一次。

2、耳针

取穴:阑尾 下脚端 大肠 神门

方法:间歇捻转,留针2~3h。

【附注】

1、针灸治疗单纯性阑尾炎效果较好。若症状严重,有阑尾穿孔或坏死倾向者,须及时进行外科处理。

2、慢性阑尾炎可参照以上用穴。每日或隔日一次。局部并可采用艾条点灸或隔姜灸。

八、瘿 病

【概说】

瘿病是以颈部肿大,或明显粗大为主要症状的疾患,俗称"大脖子"病。其特点是:颈部漫肿或结块,皮色不变,不痛,缠绵难消,且不溃破。

本病包括单纯性甲状腺肿大、甲状腺机能亢进。

【病因病机】

本病多由恼怒忧思,情志抑郁,以致气结不化,津液凝聚成痰,气滞久则血瘀,气、痰、瘀三者互凝于颈部而成;或因水土不宜所致。

【辨证治疗】

主证:颈部呈弥漫性肿大,肿势逐渐增加,边缘不清,皮色如常,不痛。部分患者肿胀过大而下垂,往往遇喜则减,遇怒则长,肿胀严重者,可有呼吸困难,声音嘶哑等证。有的兼见胸闷、心悸气促,手指颤动,急躁易怒,容易汗出,眼球突出,脉弦滑而数。

治法:取手少阳、阳明经穴为主。毫针刺用泻法。

处方:臑会 天鼎 天突 天容 合谷 足三里

随证配穴:肝郁气滞加膻中、太冲;心悸加内关、神门;眼球外突加丝竹空、攒竹、睛明、风池;烦躁易怒,汗出加复溜、三阴交。

方义:臑会穴为手少阳、阳维脉之会穴,针之能宣通三焦之经气,以疏导经脉之壅滞;阳明经循行于颈部,取合谷、足三里以疏理阳明之经气,消气血痰浊之凝聚;天突、天容、天鼎三穴均分布在颈部,属近部取穴,以疏通气血,共奏行气化瘀,祛痰散结之效;膻中为气会、太冲为肝经原穴,二穴可疏肝理气;神门、内关可养心安神治心悸;丝竹空、攒竹、睛明为局部取穴,风池通于目,四穴合用,可通调眼部气血,抑其向外突出;复溜、三阴交可补阴抑阳,可治疗烦躁易怒,多汗。

【其他疗法】
耳针
取穴:神门　皮质下　内分泌　相应部位
方法:每次取2～3穴,每日一次。用于单纯性甲状腺肿。甲状腺机能亢进者,酌加心、脾、脑点、神门。

【附注】
1、在瘿肿周围针刺,中心部直刺一针,对消除肿块有较好效果。
2、针刺治疗单纯性甲状腺肿,同时给予碘剂内服,可增强疗效;甲状腺显著增大,出现压迫症状者,可考虑手术;甲状腺机能亢进,如出现高热,呕吐,谵妄,脉细数等症状,为甲状腺危象,应迅速进行抢救。

九、扭　伤(附:落枕)

【概说】
扭挫伤是指四肢关节或躯体部软组织损伤,如皮肤、肌肉、肌腱、韧带、筋脉等,而无骨折、脱臼、皮肤破损,俗称"伤筋"。
临床主要表现为受伤部肿胀疼痛。

【病因病机】
由于持重不当或运动失度,不慎跌仆、闪挫、牵拉以及过度扭转等原因,引起筋脉关节损伤,使局部气血瘀滞,经脉闭阻而成。

【辨证治疗】
主证:扭伤局部因瘀阻而肿胀疼痛,伤处肌肤出现红肿青紫。新伤局部有微肿,按压疼痛,表示伤势较轻;如红肿高大,关节屈伸不利,表示伤势重。陈伤一般肿胀不明显,常以风寒湿邪侵袭而反复发作。损伤部位常发生于肩、肘、腕、腰、髋、膝、踝等处。
治法:以受伤局部取穴为主。毫针刺用泻法。陈伤留针加灸,或用温针。
处方:
肩部:肩髃　肩髎　肩贞
肘部:曲池　小海　天井
腕部:阳池　阳溪　阳谷
腰部:肾俞　腰阳关　委中
髋部:环跳　秩边　承扶
膝部:膝眼　梁丘　膝阳关
踝部:解溪　昆仑　丘墟
颈部:天柱　风池　大杼　后溪
方义:扭伤取穴,一般是根据损伤部近取的原则,以达到行气血通经络的目的,使受伤组织功能恢复正常。伤势较重的,可应用循经近刺和远刺相结合的方法。

【其他疗法】

1、刺络拔罐

方法：皮肤针重叩压痛部至微出血，加拔火罐。适用于新伤局部血肿明显，陈伤瘀血久留，寒邪袭络等病证。

2、穴位注射

方法：用10％葡萄糖液10ml或加入维生素B_1注射液100mg，注入压痛肌束，如原有放射痛者针感要与其疼痛部相一致，每日或隔日一次。本法适用于急性腰扭伤。

3、耳针

取穴：相应敏感点　皮质下　神门　肾上腺

方法：中、强刺激，留针10～30min。每天或隔天一次。适用于各部急性扭伤，有明显止痛效果。

【附注】

1、针刺治疗扭伤有一定疗效。对骨折、脱臼以及韧带断裂等须注意排除。

2、必要时可配合推拿、药物治疗。

附：落枕

落枕，又称颈部伤筋。是由睡眠时姿势不当，或风寒侵袭项背，局部经气不调所致。

主证：多在早晨起床后，一侧项背发生牵拉痛，甚至向同侧肩部及上臂扩散，颈项活动受限制。

治法：取督脉、手足太阳经穴为主。毫针刺泻法，针后可灸。

处方：大椎　天柱　肩外俞　绝骨　后溪

随证配穴：不能前后俯仰加昆仑、列缺；不能左右回顾加支正。并可在患部附近拔火罐。此外可以单用落枕穴治疗。

【附注】

1、针刺治疗落枕效果较好，针后可配合推拿及热敷。

2、睡眠枕头高低须适度，避免受冷，以防止复发。

第四节　五官科病证

一、耳鸣、耳聋

【概说】

耳鸣、耳聋，都是听觉异常疾患的症状，可因多种疾病引起。耳鸣以自觉耳内鸣响为主症，耳聋以听力减退或听觉丧失为主症。因两者在病因及治疗方面，大致相同，故合并介绍。

【病因病机】

(一)肝胆火盛：因暴怒，惊恐，肝胆之火上逆，以至少阳经气闭阻。

(二)外感风邪：外感风邪侵袭，壅遏清窍。

(三)肾精亏虚：肾虚气弱，精气不能上达于耳而成。本病可分为虚实二类。

【辨证治疗】

(一)实证

主证：暴病耳鸣，或耳中觉胀，鸣声不断，按之不减；如系肝胆风火上逆，可见头胀，面赤，咽干，烦躁易怒，脉弦；如因外感风邪，多见头痛，畏寒，发热，脉浮数等证。

(二) 虚证

主证：久病耳聋，耳中如蝉鸣，时作时止，劳累则加剧，按之鸣声减弱。兼见头晕、腰膝痠软乏力、遗精、带下，脉虚细等证。

治法：取手、足少阳经穴为主。毫针刺，实证用泻法；虚证用补法，并可用小艾炷灸患处腧穴。

处方：翳风 听会 侠溪 中渚

随证配穴：肝胆火盛加太冲、足临泣；外感风邪加外关、合谷；肾虚加肾俞、命门、关元、太溪。

方义：手、足少阳经脉均绕行于耳之前后，故取手少阳之中渚、翳风，足少阳之听会、侠溪，四穴参合，疏导少阳经气，为治疗本病之主方。肝胆火盛者，配取肝经穴太冲，胆经穴足临泣，以清泻肝胆之火，取"病在上，取之下"和"盛则泻之"之意；配外关、合谷以疏解风邪；配肾俞、命门、关元以调补肾之元气，使精气上输耳窍，奏止鸣复聪之效。

【其他疗法】

1. 穴位注射

取穴：听宫 翳风 肾俞 完骨

方法：采用654—2注射液，每次两侧各选一穴，每穴注射5ml；或用维生素B_{12}100ug注射液，每穴0.2～0.5ml。进针0.5～1寸。

2. 头针

选取两侧晕听区，间歇运针，留针20min。每日或隔日一次。适用于神经性耳鸣，听力下降。

【附注】

耳聋、耳鸣的发生，其原因很多，针灸对神经性耳鸣、耳聋效果较好。

二、目赤肿痛

【概说】

目赤肿痛，为多种眼疾患中的一个急性症状，以目赤、睑肿、疼痛为主症。俗称"红眼"或"火眼"。古代文献根据发病原因、症状急重和流行性，有称"风热眼"、"暴风客热"、"天行赤眼"等。本证常见于急性结膜炎、假膜性结膜炎以及流行性角结膜炎等。

【病因病机】

(一)外感时邪：外感风热时邪，致经气阻滞，郁而不宣。

(二)肝胆火盛：因肝胆火盛，循经上扰，以致经脉闭阻，血壅气滞而成。

【辨证治疗】

主证：目赤肿痛，畏光流泪，眵多而且难开。如兼有头痛，发热，脉浮数等为风热；如兼有口苦，烦热，便秘，脉弦滑者属肝胆火盛。

治法：取手阳明、足厥阴肝经穴为主。毫针刺用泻法。

处方：睛明 风池 太阳 合谷 行间

随证配穴：风热加外关；肝胆火旺加太冲。

方义：肝开窍于目，太阳、少阳、阳明经脉均循行于目部，故取风池、合谷调节阳明、少阳经气以疏风清热；睛明为太阳、阳明经会穴，能宣泄患部之郁热；行间为肝经荥穴，能引导厥阴经气下行，以泻肝热；太阳邻近患部，点刺出血，可以泄热消肿。外关可宣散风热，清利头目；肝经原穴太冲,以清泻肝胆之火。

【其他疗法】

1. 耳针

取穴:眼　目₁　目₂　肝

方法:留针20min,间歇运针。亦可在耳尖或耳后静脉点刺出血。

2. 挑治

可在肩胛间按压过敏点,或大椎穴两旁0.5寸处选点挑治,本法适用于急性结膜炎。

【附注】

针刺眼眶内穴位时,针具应严格消毒,进出针须缓慢,轻捻转不宜提插,以防止感染或出血。

三、鼻渊

【概说】

鼻渊是指鼻流腥臭浊涕,鼻塞,嗅觉减退为主症的一种疾病。因流涕不止,如泉如渊,故名鼻渊;又名"脑渗","脑漏"。多见于慢性鼻炎及慢性副鼻窦炎等病。

【病因病机】

本病多由外感风寒之邪,侵袭肺脏,蕴久化热,上扰鼻窍;或感受风热之邪,肺气失宣,邪气上扰,壅于鼻窍;或外邪已解,尚有余热,拘于鼻窍而成鼻渊。

【辨证治疗】

主证:鼻流腥臭浊涕,色黄,鼻塞,嗅觉减退。经久不愈,反复举发者,则兼见头昏、鼻额胀痛,记忆减退,舌红,苔黄腻,脉数等。

治法:取手太阴、阳明经穴为主。毫针刺用泻法,以清热宣肺,通窍止涕。

处方:尺泽　列缺　合谷　迎香　风池　足三里

方义:尺泽为肺经合水穴,功可泄肺清热;列缺为肺经络穴,与大肠经相表里,大肠经上挟鼻孔,列缺配迎香通鼻窍,泻热止涕;合谷、风池,宣肺解表;足三里为胃经合穴,胃起于鼻,足三里既可健脾胃,补气血,又可化痰浊,降逆气,为治慢性鼻病之效穴。

【其他疗法】

耳针

取穴:内鼻　下屏尖　肺　额

方法:轻刺激,留针20min。

四、鼻衄

【概说】

鼻衄,即鼻出血。血不循常道,上溢鼻窍,破脉由鼻而出,谓之鼻衄。多见于外伤、鼻部疾患和一些急性、热性病以及高血压,肝硬化,血液病,及妇女倒经等疾病。

【病因病机】

引起鼻衄的原因是血热灼伤络脉,肺气通于鼻,足阳明胃脉起于鼻,手阳明大肠脉止于鼻,如肺蕴风热,或阳明火邪上迫肺窍,或阴虚火旺,虚火上炎,迫于肺窍,均能热伤血络,而发生鼻衄。

【辨证治疗】

(一)肺胃热盛

主证:鼻衄,伴有发热,咳嗽,舌红,脉浮数;或伴有口渴引饮,口臭便秘,舌红,苔黄,脉洪数。

(二)阴虚火旺

主证:鼻衄,颧红,口干,五心烦热,盗汗,午后潮热,舌红,脉细数。

治法:取手阳明、督脉经穴为主。肺胃热盛者,用泻法,以清热止血;阴虚火旺者,针用平补平泻,以滋阴降火。

处方:迎香 合谷 上星

随证配穴:肺热:孔最;胃热:内庭;阴虚火旺:照海。

方义:手阳明之脉,上挟鼻孔,取迎香、合谷清鼻热,以止衄;上星为督脉穴,督脉总督诸阳,泻上星以泻阳热;孔最为肺之郄穴,功善止血;内庭为胃之荥水穴,功善清胃热;照海滋阴以降虚火,诸穴共奏清热止衄之功。

五、牙 痛

【概说】

牙痛为口腔常见病,依病因不同有风火牙痛、胃火牙痛、虚火牙痛和龋齿牙痛等不同类型。多见于急、慢性牙髓炎、龋齿、冠周炎等病。

【病因病机】

牙痛多因火热或牙质损坏而发病。手、足阳明经分别入上、下齿,如阳明腑热,随经上扰则可导致牙痛;或风邪袭外,内郁阳明,胃火循经上炎;或肾阴亏损,虚火上炎;或多食甘酸,口齿不洁,垢秽蚀齿,均可导致牙痛。

【辨证治疗】

(一)胃火牙痛

主证:牙痛甚剧,兼有口臭口渴,便秘,舌苔黄,脉洪数等。

(二)风火牙痛

主证:牙痛龈肿,兼恶寒发热,脉浮数等。

(三)肾虚牙痛

主证:牙痛隐隐,时作时止,牙齿浮动,舌红体瘦,脉细数。

治法:取手足阳明经穴为主。针用泻法,以清热泻火止痛;风火牙痛加手少阳经穴。针刺用泻法,以祛风泻火;肾虚牙痛加足少阴经穴,针刺用平补平泻法,以滋阴降火。

处方:合谷 内庭 下关 颊车

随证配穴:风火牙痛:翳风,液门;肾虚牙痛:太溪。

方义:手阳明经入下齿,足阳明经入上齿,故取合谷、颊车二穴,远近相配,以清阳明之火,治上下齿疼痛;内庭为胃经荥水穴,善清胃火,与局部之颊车相配治疗下牙痛。液门为三焦经之荥水穴,与翳风穴远近相配可祛风泻火以止风火牙痛;太溪为肾之原穴,可滋肾阴以降虚火,用于肾虚牙痛。

【其他疗法】

耳针

取穴：神门　皮质下　牙痛点
方法：强刺激，留针20～30min。

六、咽喉肿痛

【概说】

咽喉肿痛是以咽喉红肿疼痛为主证的一种病症。祖国医学中的"喉痹"、"乳蛾"、"喉痛"多指此病。风热、痰火及阴虚为三大致病因素，临床上常依症状表现而分为虚实两类。多见于急性扁桃体炎、急性咽炎、单纯性喉炎、以及扁桃体周围脓肿等。

【病因病机】

(一) 外感风热邪毒，熏灼肺系，郁于咽喉。

(二) 过食辛辣煎炒，引动胃火上蒸，消烁津液，痰火蕴结于咽喉。

(三) 肾阴亏耗，虚火上炎，阴液不能止润咽喉。

【辨证治疗】

(一) 实热

主证：起病急骤，咽喉肿痛，并恶寒发热，头痛，口渴，便秘，舌红，苔薄黄，脉浮数。

治法：取手太阴、足阳明经穴为主。针刺用泻法，以疏风清热。

处方：少商　合谷　内庭　天容

方义：少商点刺出血，可清泄肺热而止咽痛；合谷解表邪以清阳明之郁热；内庭为胃经荥穴，功能清泄胃火；天容位邻咽喉，针之可通利咽喉而止疼痛。

(二) 阴虚

主证：咽痛不甚，起病缓慢，咽干，瘖哑咽部稍红，说话多时则咽喉疼痛，或吞咽时微觉痛楚，手足心热，咽干以夜间尤甚。舌红无苔，脉细数。

治法：取足少阴、手太阴经穴为主。针刺补泻兼施，以滋阴清热止痛。

处方：照海　列缺　廉泉　扶突。

方义：照海、列缺为八脉交会穴，能通利咽喉，引虚火下泻，列缺清肺火，照海滋肾阴，二穴相配泻火增液，故为治咽喉干痛之主穴；廉泉位近咽喉，功可增液润喉；扶突通利咽喉以止疼痛。

【其它针法】

耳针

取穴：咽喉　扁桃体　轮1～6

方法：中强刺激，捻转2～3min，留针1h，每天1次。

七、青盲

【概说】

青盲，是指视力逐渐减退的一种慢性眼病。初起自觉视物昏渺，蒙昧不清者，称"视瞻昏渺"。日久失治，不辨人物，不分明暗者，即为青盲。多由肝肾阴亏，气血两虚，肝郁气滞引起。多见于视神经萎缩等病。

【病因病机】

(一) 肝肾不足，精血耗损，精气不能上荣，目失涵养。

(二)饮食不节,劳伤过度,脾气受损,精微不化,不能运精于目。
(三)七情郁结,肝失疏泄,气滞血瘀,精气不能上荣于目。

【辨证治疗】

(一)肝肾阴亏

主证:视物不清,眼内干涩,头晕耳鸣,遗精、腰痠,脉象细弱,舌红少苔。

(二)气血两虚

主证:视物不清,神疲乏力,懒言声低,纳少便溏,脉细弱,舌质淡,苔薄白。

(三)肝气郁结

主证:视物不清,两胁胀痛,头晕目眩,口苦咽干,脉弦。

治法:取足少阳、太阳经穴为主。肝肾阴虚,气血两虚,针用补法以补益肝肾,濡养气血;肝气郁结,针用平补平泻法,以疏肝解郁。

处方:风池 睛明 球后 光明

随证配穴:肝肾阴虚:太冲、太溪、肝俞、肾俞。气血两虚:足三里、三阴交。肝气郁结:期门、太冲、内关。

方义:足少阳、太阳两经均通于眼部,故取风池、光明、睛明,疏通眼部经气以明目;球后为经外奇穴,是治疗本病的有效穴位;肝俞、肾俞、太溪、太冲,以补益肝肾;足三里,三阴交以补益气血;期门、太冲、内关以疏肝解郁。

【其它疗法】

耳针

取穴:眼 肝 肾 脾 心 目$_1$ 目$_2$

方法:每次针3～4穴,中等刺激,留针20～30min,10次为一疗程。

八、近 视

【概说】

近视是指视近物正常,视远物则模糊不清的一种疾病。古称"能近怯远症"。先天禀赋不足,肝肾亏损及不良的用眼习惯是近视发病的主要原因。多见于近视眼、弱视、散光等病。

【病因病机】

(一)用眼过度:肝藏血,开窍于目,目得血而能视。如看电视过久,或在暗处,或在强光下,或卧床,或在车上摇动处看书过久,久视则伤血,肝血不能上荣于目则发为近视。

(二)肝肾不足:各种原因造成肝肾亏损,阴精不足,肾精不能上注于目,发为近视。

(三)亦有饮食不节,偏食一物,脾胃受损,气血化源不足,目失所养而成近视者。

【辨证治疗】

(一)久视伤血

主证:视力逐渐减弱,视物初时尚可,时间稍长即模糊不清,眼痠胀不适,休息后可稍有改善者,舌正脉平。

(二)肝肾不足

主证:视力逐渐减弱,眼睛干涩,头晕失眠,记忆力减退,或伴腰膝痠软者,舌红,脉细。

(三)脾胃虚弱

主证:近视,偏食一物,寒食不断,面色萎黄,或有虫斑,精神不振,记忆减退,舌淡脉弱,乃气血不足之象。

治法:取足太阳、少阳经穴为主。针用补法,以补肝益肾,益气明目。

处方:风池 光明 睛明 承泣 透眼 内角 肝俞 肾俞 合谷

方义:肝藏血,目得血而能视,肝胆相表里,取风池、光明、肝俞、肾俞以补肝益肾,使肝血肾精上荣于目;睛明为足太阳、阳明、手太阳、阴跷阳跷五脉之会;承泣为阳跷、任脉、足阳明之会,合谷为大肠原穴,阳明经多气多血,故三穴合用可以益气血以明目。

【其它疗法】

1. 耳针

取穴:眼 肝 肾 脾 目$_1$ 目$_2$

方法:毫针刺,每次 2～3 穴,每次留针 30～60min,间歇运针,或用揿针埋藏,或王不留行贴压,每 3～5 日更换 1 次,双耳交替,嘱患者每日自行按压数次。10 次为 1 疗程。

2. 皮肤针

取穴:眼区周围

方法:用皮肤针沿眼周围由内向外转圈轻叩 3～5 次,每日 1 次,10 次为 1 疗程。

亏血亦虚之象。

治则：滋阴养血，少阳经交会主，针用补法，以养肝益精，益气明目。

处方：以足少阳胆经、肝俞、胆俞、肾俞、脾俞、合谷。

方义：肝藏血，目得血而能视，肝俞补血能柔肝，取风池、肝俞、脾俞、肾俞、胆俞以补益肝肾，精上荣于目，睛明为足太阳、阳跃脉与手太阳、阴跃脉的五脉交会，养血为明目，主穴，足阳明之合谷及太阴脾经之三阴交，用间接灸之也。取二、三穴用以养气血以明目。

【其它疗法】

1. 耳针

取穴：眼、肝、肾、目1、目2。

方法：毫针浅刺，每次 2～3 穴，留针留针 30～60min，间歇运针；亦用耳针埋藏，每隔不留针5～7日更换 1 次，双耳交替，隔耳贴穴的特按摩数次，10次为 1 疗程。

2. 皮肤针

取穴：睛周围区。

方法：轻度刺激眼眶周围由内向外移环推叩 3～5 次，每日 1 次，10次为 1 疗程。